AF520841

Comprehensive Textbook of
Cosmetic Dermatology, Laser and Energy-based Therapies

Comprehensive Textbook of
Cosmetic Dermatology, Laser and Energy-based Therapies

Editors

Zeina Tannous MD
Professor and Chair
Department of Dermatology
Lebanese American University School of Medicine
Lebanon
Affiliate Faculty
Wellman Center for Photomedicine
Massachusetts General Hospital
Harvard Medical School
Boston, Massachusetts, USA

Molly Wanner MD MBA
Assistant Professor
Department of Dermatology
Harvard Medical School
Massachusetts General Hospital
Boston, Massachusetts, USA

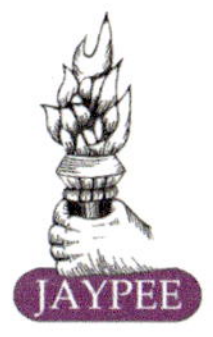

JAYPEE BROTHERS MEDICAL PUBLISHERS
The Health Sciences Publisher
New Delhi | London

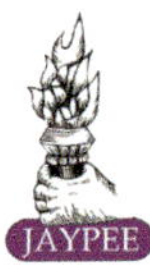

Jaypee Brothers Medical Publishers (P) Ltd

Headquarters
EMCA House
23/23-B, Ansari Road, Daryaganj
New Delhi 110 002, India
Landline: +91-11-23272143, +91-11-23272703
+91-11-23282021, +91-11-23245672
E-mail: jaypee@jaypeebrothers.com

Corporate Office
Jaypee Brothers Medical Publishers (P) Ltd.
4838/24, Ansari Road, Daryaganj
New Delhi 110 002, India
Phone: +91-11-43574357
Fax: +91-11-43574314
E-mail: jaypee@jaypeebrothers.com

Overseas Office
JP Medical Ltd.
83, Victoria Street, London
SW1H 0HW (UK)
Phone: +44-20 3170 8910
E-mail: info@jpmedpub.com

EU GPSR Authorised Representative
Logos Europe, 9 rue Nicolas Poussin
17000, La Rochelle, France
Phone: +33 (0) 6 67 93 73 78
E-mail: Contact@logoseurope.eu

Website: www.jaypeebrothers.com
Website: www.jaypeedigital.com

Inquiries for bulk sales may be solicited at: jaypee@jaypeebrothers.com

Comprehensive Textbook of Cosmetic Dermatology, Laser and Energy-based Therapies / Zeina Tannous, Molly Wanner

First Edition: **2022**

Reprint: 2026

ISBN: 978-93-5270-167-4

Printed at: Replika Press Pvt. Ltd.

DEDICATIONS

This book is dedicated to my late parents,
Salem and Jeannette Tannous,
for loving me unconditionally and
raising me to believe that everything is possible.
Forever they remain in my soul.

Zeina Tannous, MD

This book is dedicated to my parents
for their unwavering support and
to my husband and children,
Maya and Camila,
for their love and encouragement.

Molly Wanner, MD MBA

CONTRIBUTORS

Editors

Zeina Tannous MD
Professor and Chair
Department of Dermatology
Lebanese American University School of Medicine
Lebanon
Affiliate Faculty
Wellman Center for Photomedicine
Massachusetts General Hospital
Harvard Medical School
Boston, MA, USA

Molly Wanner MD MBA
Assistant Professor
Department of Dermatology
Harvard Medical School
Massachusetts General Hospital
Boston, MA, USA

Contributing Authors

Ali Rajabi-Estarabadi MD
Resident
Department of Dermatology
Broward Health, Fort
Lauderdale, Fl, USA

Arielle NB Kauvar MD
Clinical Professor of
Dermatology
New York University Medical
Center Director, New York
Cosmetic, Skin & Laser Surgery
Center, New York, USA

Caiwei Zheng BS
Medical Student
University of Miami Miller
School of Medicine
Miami, Fl, USA

Cameron Rokhsar MD
Associate Clinical Professor
The Mount Sinai Hospital
New York
Founder and Medical Director
New York Cosmetic, Skin &
Laser Surgery Center
New York, USA

Catherine DiGiorgio MS MD
Dermatologist
Boston Center for Facial
Rejuvenation
Boston, MA, USA

Christine Caroline Dierickx MD
Director, Skinperium Laser and
Cosmetic Dermatology Clinic,
Luxembourg, Luxembourg

Christine Chen BS
Medical Student
Lewis Katz School of Medicine
at Temple University
Philadelphia, PA, USA

David M Ozog MD
Chairman and Clarence S.
Livingood Chair, Department
of Dermatology, Henry Ford
Hospital, Detroit, MI, USA

Elizabeth L Tanzi MD
Associate Clinical Professor
Department of Dermatology
George Washington School of
Medicine, Washington DC
Director, Capital Laser & Skin
Care, Chevy Chase, MD, USA

Emily O McLean MD
Dermatologist
Novant Health Dermatology – SouthPark
Charlotte, NC, USA

Emmy Graber MD MBA
President and Founder
The Dermatology Institute of Boston
Boston, MA, USA

Frank Beerwerth PhD
Scientist, Procter & Gamble Company, Kronberg
DE, Germany

Gary D Monheit MD
Clinical Professor
Department of Ophthalmology and Dermatology
University of Alabama
Physician
Total Skin and Beauty Dermatology Center
Birmingham, Alabama, USA

Girish C Mohan MD
Director of Laser and Cosmetic Dermatology
Hartford Hospital
Farmington, CT, USA

Hana Jeon MD
Mohs Surgery, Laser and Cosmetic Specialist
Lumos Dermatology®
New York, USA

Hao Feng MD MHS
Assistant Professor
Department of Dermatology
University of Connecticut Health Center
Farmington, CT, USA

Henry HL Chan MBBS MD PhD
Honorary Clinical Professor
Division of Dermatology
Department of Medicine
The University of Hong Kong
Hong Kong SRA, China
Visiting Scientist
Wellman Center for Photomedicine, Massachusetts General Hospital
Boston, MA, USA

H Ray Jalian MD
Dermatologist
Rebecca Fitzgerald, MD Inc
Los Angeles, CA, USA

James Alastair Carruthers MBBS MSC FRCPC
Clinical Professor Emeritus
Department of Ophthalmology
University of British Columbia
Vancouver, BC, Canada

Jean Diana Carruthers MD FRCSC FRC (Ophth)
Clinical Professor
Department of Ophthalmology
University of British Columbia
Vancouver, Canada

Jeffrey S Dover MD FRCPC
Co-founder
SkinCare Physicians, Chestnut Hill, MA, USA
Associate Clinical Professor
Department of Dermatology
Yale University School of Medicine
New Haven, CT, USA
Adjunct Associate Professor
Department of Dermatology
Brown Medical School
Providence, RI, USA

Jennifer Lynn Goodrich LCDR MC USN
Service Chief
Department of Otolaryngology
Walter Reed National Military Medical Center
Bethesda, Maryland, USA

J Frank Nash PhD
Senior Director – Research Fellow
Procter & Gamble Company
Cincinnati, OH, USA

Jill Katherine Cotseones DO
Dermatologist, Northwestern Medicine Regional Medical Group Dermatology
Geneva, IL, USA

John P Tsatalis BS
Medical Student
University of Miami Miller School of Medicine
Miami, Fl, USA

J Stuart Nelson MD PhD
Distinguished Professor
Department of Surgery and Biomedical Engineering
University of California
Irvine, CA, USA

Kachiu C Lee MD MPH
Assistant Professor of Dermatology
Temple University
Cosmetic Dermatologist and Laser Specialist
Main Line Center for Laser Surgery, Ardmore, PA, USA

Kelly Stankiewicz MD
Founder and Owner
The Dermatology House
Park City, UT, USA

Keyvan Nouri MD, MBA
Professor, Director of Mohs/ Laser/Dermatologic Surgery
Doctor Philip Frost Department of Dermatology and Cutaneous Surgery University of Miami Miller School of Medicine, Miami, Fl, USA

Lauren Meshkov Bonati MD
Associate Dermatologist
Mountain Dermatology Specialists
Edward Village, Blvd, CO, USA

Lindsay Rachel Sklar MD
Dermatologist
West Bloomfield Dermatology and Mohs Surgery, West Bloomfield Township
MI, USA

Macrene Renee Alexiades MD PhD FAAD
Associate Clinical Professor
Department of Dermatology
Yale University Scholl of Medicine
Director and Founder
Dermatology & Laser Surgery Center of New York
NY, USA

Marc R Avram MD
Clinical Professor
Department of Dermatology
Weill-Cornell Medical Center
New York, USA

Mathew M Avram MD JD
Associate Professor of Dermatology
Harvard Medical School
Director, MGH Dermatology Laser and Cosmetic Center
Massachusetts General Hospital, Boston, MA, USA

Meera Kohli BA
Medical Student
Sidney Kimmel Medical College of Jefferson University
Philadelphia, PA, USA

Molly Wanner MD MBA
Assistant Professor
Department of Dermatology
Harvard Medical School
Massachusetts General Hospital
Boston, MA, USA

Mona Sadeghpour MD
Co-Founder, SkinMed Institute
Lone Tree, Colorado, USA

Murad Alam MD
Professor and Vice-Chair
Department of Dermatology
Northwestern University
Chicago, IL, USA

Neil Sadick MD
Clinical Professor
Department of Dermatology
Weill Medical College of Cornell University
New York, USA
Faculty
Department of Dermatology
University of Minnesota
Minneapolis, USA

Oge C Onwudiwe MD
Researcher
Wellman Center for Photomedicine/Massachusetts General Hospital
Boston, MA, USA

Omar A Ibrahimi MD, PhD
Founder and Medical Director
Connecticut Skin Institute
Stamford, CT, USA

Omer Ibrahim MD
Adjunct Professor
Cleveland Clinic Foundation
Department of Dermatology
Cleveland, OH, USA
Associate
Chicago Cosmetic Surgery and Dermatology
Chicago, IL, USA

Roy G Geronemus MD
Director
Laser & Skin Surgery Center of New York
Clinical Professor
Department of Dermatology
New York University Medical Center
New York, USA

Saami Khalifian MD
Clinical Instructor
Department of Dermatology
David Geffen School of Medicine, UCLA
Santa Monica, CA, USA

Samantha L Schneider MD
Dermatologist and Mohs Surgeon
Skin Cancer and Dermatology Institute
Carson City, Nevada, USA

Sandy S Tsao MD
Assistant Professor
Harvard Medical School
Co-Director, Ethnic Skin of Color Program
Department of Dermatology
Massachusetts General Hospital
Boston, MA, USA

Shivani Sharma BA
Medical Student
UT Southwestern School of Medicine, Dallas, TX, USA

Suzanne Linsmeier Kilmer MD
Founder
Laser & Skin Surgery Center of Northern California
Sacramento, CA, USA

Thomas E Rohrer MD
Dermatological Surgeon, SkinCare Physicians, Chestnut Hill, MA, USA

Wai Man Mandy Chan MBBS MRCP FAMS
Clinical Assistant Professor
Department of Medicine
The University of Hong Kong
Hong Kong, China

Yakir Levin MD PhD
Instructor, Harvard Medical School, Department of Dermatology and Wellman Center for Photomedicine
Massachusetts General Hospital, Boston, MA, USA

Zeina Tannous MD
Professor and Chair
Department of Dermatology
Lebanese American University School of Medicine, Lebanon
Affiliate Faculty
Wellman Center for Photomedicine
Massachusetts General Hospital
Harvard Medical School
Boston, MA, USA

Zoe Diana Draelos MD
Clinical and Research Dermatologist, Dermatology Consulting Services, High Point, North Carolina, USA

PREFACE

Minimally invasive cosmetic procedures have become extremely popular, and the use of lasers and energy-based devices to treat cosmetic and medical conditions has dramatically increased in the past 20 years. The cutting-edge research in the fields of Dermatology and Plastic Surgery has led to rapid advancement of lasers and energy-based devices that have become more targeted and effective. While anyone can turn on a laser or an energy-based device, using this precise surgical tool to obtain the best results requires more than a key.

This book provides a comprehensive approach to lasers and energy-based devices. It is divided into multiple sections that cover (1) Basics, (2) Vascular, (3) Hair, (4) Pigmentary disorders and tattoos, (5) Rejuvenation, scar remodeling, and body contouring, (6) Soft-tissue fillers and neuromodulators, and (7) Medical applications. Each chapter pulls key pieces of information into tables, making it simple for the reader to access crucial teaching points. Not only does the book explain the science of energy-based devices, but it also provides a practical approach. There is a special emphasis on practical tools and techniques for everyday practice.

The authors of "*Comprehensive Textbook of Cosmetic, Laser, and Energy-based Therapies*" have vast experience and have distilled their knowledge to the essential components. They have meticulously outlined strategies to help avoid pitfalls that can lead to complications. Fundamentally, the goal of this book is to help the healthcare provider to execute at the highest level.

Zeina Tannous
Molly Wanner

ACKNOWLEDGMENTS

We would like to thank the authors of this book for sharing their combined decades of experience. We would like to acknowledge the professional staff at Jaypee Brothers Medical Publishers (P) Ltd, for the excellent job they have done in the production of this book. We would like to also thank the patients who shared their photos in support of teaching. Lastly, we would like to give special thanks to R Rox Anderson and Bill Farinelli for teaching us about lasers, and to Beverly Dammin for supporting us at every step of the way.

CONTENTS

SECTION 1: BASICS

SECTION 2: VASCULAR

SECTION 3: HAIR

SECTION 7: MEDICAL APPLICATIONS

1 SECTION

BASICS

1

CHAPTER

Analysis of the Aging Face

Emily O McLean, Emmy Graber

BACKGROUND

With credit to Jane Austen, it is a truth universally acknowledged, that an adult, in possession of a face, must be in want of a pleasing appearance. The drive to optimize one's attractiveness is not a superficial desire. In fact, numerous studies have found positive associations between physical attractiveness and economic mobility, successful personal relationships and professional achievement.[1] Interestingly, groups of people do generally agree on who is and who is not attractive regardless of cultural background. Features common to beautiful faces are established as the fundamental tenets of facial beauty: A youthful appearance, symmetry, sexual dimorphism, and averageness (prototypicality).[2] The cosmetic dermatologist must be aware of these fundamental tenets in order to best analyze the aging face.

Youthfulness is characterized by clarity, even pigmentation, and smooth shadowless contours that together create a harmonious face. Symmetry—two halves appearing similar to each other—is also a common feature of faces rated as beautiful. Both youthfulness and symmetry serve as outward, subconscious markers of health, and vigor. Averageness refers to how similar a face is to the majority. For example, composite photographs combining many faces into one image are typically thought to be more beautiful than an image representing just one or a few faces. It makes sense, from an evolutionary perspective, that humans are preconditioned to find these features attractive as the survival of the species depends on mating with healthy partners with genetic diversity.[1]

As classically beautiful faces are typically readily identifiable as either feminine or masculine, a quality known as sexual dimorphism, practitioners of aesthetic medicine must consider the facial traits that are traditionally associated with gender. Female faces have prominent or high cheekbones, relative hairlessness, and smooth skin relative to men. Additionally, the brows are thinner and higher, and the jaw shorter and more narrow in female as compared to male faces. These differences are important to understand so as to avoid inadvertently feminizing a male face or masculinizing a female face.[2] On the other hand, a skilled physician may intentionally exploit these features in certain situations. For example, a transgender woman may desire a more feminine-appearing face and therefore may benefit from filler placement to enhance the malar cheeks.

It is imperative for the astute clinician to be sensitive to the fact that there are differences in the process of aging between ethnicities and genders. As compared to Caucasian skin, the color of the skin has a higher concentration of epidermal melanin and a thicker dermis leading to differences in the photoaging process. Darker skin is more prone to dyspigmentation with both hypopigmentation and hyperpigmentation, but less likely to develop deep rhytids.[3] Furthermore, the risk for complications with cosmetic procedures varies based on skin color with darker skinned patients at higher risk for hypertrophic or keloidal scarring and post-inflammatory hyperpigmentation.

THE AGING PROCESS

Knowledge of the intrinsic and extrinsic aging processes allows for thorough understanding of how changes impact appearance over time. Intrinsic aging refers to chronologic changes that occur in heritable patterns based on the underlying molecular biology of the skin and subcutaneous structures. The intrinsic aging process is not modifiable and leads to subtle changes in the skin including fine wrinkling, the development of benign neoplasms such as cherry angiomas, and varying degrees of skin laxity and fat redistribution.

In contrast, extrinsic aging refers to effects on the skin and subcutaneous structures that result from environmental factors such as sun exposure, smoking, diet, sleep habits, and exercise. The most well understood contributor to extrinsic aging is chronic ultraviolet radiation that causes tissue injury leading to surface changes including erythema, irregular pigmentation, telangiectasias, and rough skin texture. Photodamage also serves to accelerate the changes of intrinsic aging resulting in more pronounced wrinkling and lipoatrophy. Tobacco smoking has also been proven to cause premature skin aging, likely mediated by similar pathophysiologic pathways as photoaging.[4] Photos of twins, one of who had an extensive smoking history, demonstrate the effects that tobacco smoking has on aging (**Fig. 1**).[5]

The link between other extrinsic factors and aging are less well studied, though are of great interests to researchers. The relationship between facial aging and exercise is complex and remains to be fully elucidated, but there have been publications demonstrating a link between endurance exercise and the attenuation of age-related changes in the skin. In one study, subjects who exercised regularly had thinner strata cornea and thicker dermises than controls who did not exercise regularly than would be expected based on their age.[6] Of course, the benefits of exercise on skin aging may be outweighed by sun exposure during outdoor activity if the skin is not protected adequately with sunscreen and clothing. Additionally, poor dietary choices such as eating a diet high in simple sugars or fried foods may accelerate aging by promoting the accumulation of pro-inflammatory advanced glycation end products in the skin.[7,8] Air pollutants such as particulate matter and volatile organic compounds that arise from motor vehicles or industrial facilities have also been shown to be detrimental to the skin, especially in the development of dyspigmentation.[9,10]

A summary of the changes in the upper face, lower face, and epidermis as the skin ages is presented in **Figure 2**.

INITIAL APPROACH

During an initial cosmetic consultation visit, the primary goal of the clinician should be to ascertain the patient's primary aesthetic concern(s), his or her treatment goal, and the underlying motivation for seeking treatment.

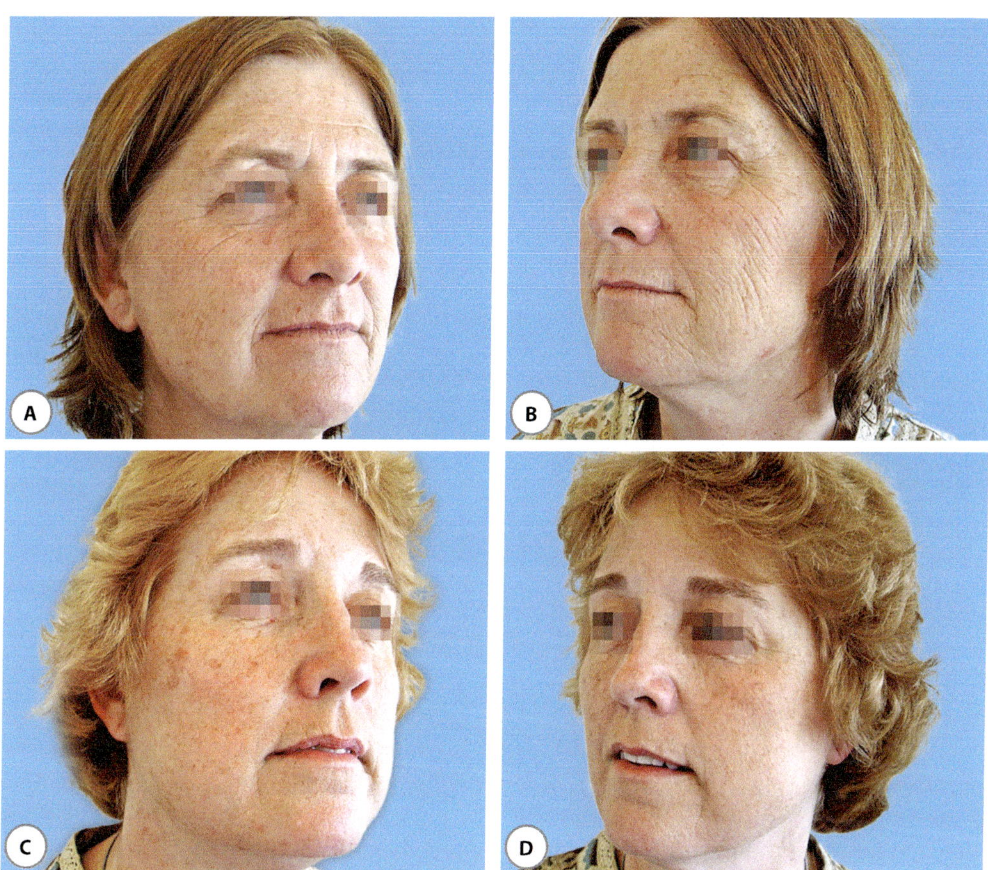

FIGS. 1A TO D: Top: Twin 1 (smoker), right (A) and left (B) profiles. Bottom: Twin 2 (non-smoker), right (C) and left (D) profiles. Note the extensive deep wrinkling, widespread lentigines, scattered hypopigmentation, and moderate skin laxity of twin 1 versus twin 2's mild fine wrinkling, few scattered lentigines, mild-density hypopigmentation, and mild skin laxity.[5]

Assessing the patient's expectations of treatment outcome is essential to a successful therapeutic patient-physician alliance.

A well-trained dermatologist with a honed eye should perform a complete physical exam of the face paying particular attention to skin texture, wrinkles, pigment irregularities, vascular abnormalities such as telangiectasias, distribution and fullness of subcutaneous fat, and the presence of lax or redundant skin. As part of the physical exam, it is important to have the patient speak and animate in order to analyze wrinkles both at rest and with muscle contraction. It may be helpful to ask the patient to highlight his or her areas of concern with a mirror as part of the examination.

The four R's—*r*elax, *r*efill, *r*edrape, and *r*esurface—provide a useful framework for developing a comprehensive, multimodal treatment plan to address the patient's aesthetic concerns. The thoughtful clinician can utilize this framework to *relax* the muscles, *refill* lost volume, and *redrape* and *resurface* the skin.[11]

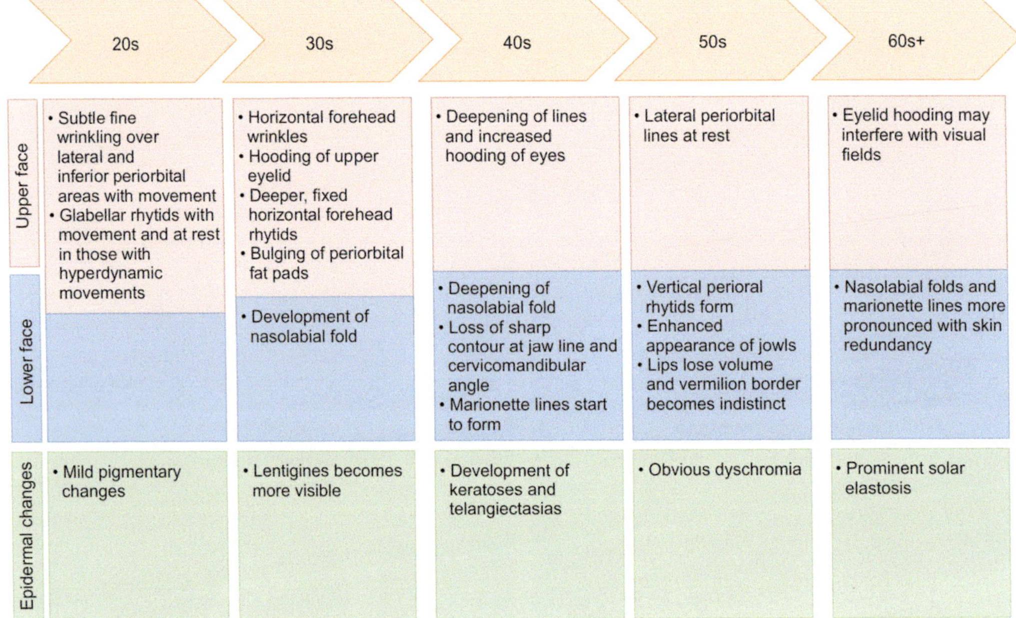

FIG. 2: Timeline.

Relaxation refers to muscle-related rhytids that are most readily addressed via the use of injected neuromodulatory agents such as botulinum toxin. Treatment of fine lines of the upper face such as horizontal forehead lines and crow's feet—a common complaint especially in patients who tend to squint—is often the first cosmetic intervention a patient will undertake and is appropriate for patients even in their twenties. Neuromodulators may also be used in older patients for *relaxing* static rhytids of the glabella and forehead. In the lower face, people with strong orbicularis oris muscles such as smokers or people who habitually purse their lips benefit from botulinum toxin injection. Additionally, skillfully placed neuromodulator to *relax* the depressor anguli oris muscle can improve the appearance of prominent frown lines. Neuromodulators injected in the mentalis muscle can also be used to *relax* a dimpled chin.

Refilling refers to the use of soft tissue fillers to address fat atrophy and volume loss which begin to contribute to the overall aged appearance of the face as early as the late twenties or early thirties. Usually, the first areas of the face to show signs of volume loss are the tear troughs and nasolabial folds. Overtime, the fat pads in the buccal and malar cheeks, temples, and chin begin to waste away creating a flat or hollow contour. A common request for patients in their thirties and early forties is to *refill* the tear trough area of the lower eye lid with hyaluronic acid fillers which improve the contour and minimize the dark shadows and creases that contribute to a tired and aged appearance. Midface augmentation to *refill* for the malar cheeks is also a relatively common way to not only improve the contour of the cheek, but also to lift the jowls.

Redraping allows the cosmetic dermatologist to address the skin sagging and laxity that tend to become bothersome in the late forties to fifties and beyond. For these patients, it is especially important to carefully consider the risks and benefits of any minimally invasive procedure, as nonsurgical interventions are less likely to yield the desired results in cases of severe laxity. Non-surgical tightening procedures such as radiofrequency skin tightening or thread lifts work optimally for patients with mild-to-moderate laxity. Neuromodulators may also be employed to address laxity of the upper eyelid with specific injection techniques. However, patients with severe laxity often require surgical interventions such as blepharoplasty or facelifts to *redrape* the skin.

Resurfacing techniques are akin to polishing and aim to improve the texture and color of the skin. Telangiectasias, lentigines, acneiform lesions, atrophic scars, pore size, and static fine lines that persist at rest despite botulinum toxin are all appropriate targets for *resurfacing*. A multitude of treatment options exist to address these complaints including ablative and nonablative lasers, percutaneous collagen induction therapy or microneedling, chemical peels, microdermabrasion, and cosmeceuticals. The treatment of choice depends not only on the cosmetic concern, but also on the patient's willingness to tolerate postprocedure down time, availability for repeat procedures, and budget.

In conjunction with any procedures, the importance of vigilant photoprotection, smoking avoidance, and the importance of a healthy diet and exercise should be emphasized to all patients as means to potentially slow the extrinsic aging process.

COMMON PITFALLS

Knowing when to advise against a treatment for a patient is a critical skill in analyzing the face. The skilled cosmetic dermatologist must be able to navigate situations when it would be in the patient's best interest to decline or to perform a procedure. Sometimes, this takes analysis of not just the face, but also the psyche. For example, a patient who suffers from body dysmorphic disorder (BDD) will likely remain unsatisfied with his or her appearance despite many procedures due to distorted perception, which increases the risk of adverse outcomes with little chance of satisfying the patient.

Body dysmorphic disorder is a psychiatric disease recognized by the diagnostic and statistical manual of mental disorders, fifth edition (DSM-5) that is characterized by a preoccupation with a perceived flaw in physical appearance that is either slight or nonobservable that causes significant distress and impairs functioning in either occupational or social situations.[12] Though the prevalence of BDD in the general population is 2.4%, one survey found that up to 14% of cosmetic dermatology patients have BDD.[12,13] Diagnosing BDD poses an important challenge to cosmetic dermatologists as patients often have poor insight into their condition, may not readily disclose their pervasive thoughts and compulsions, and are not usually overtly psychotic. A history of seeing several physicians for the same problem, requesting additional treatments on an area that has previously been treated, and dissatisfaction with prior procedures are all clues to the diagnosis. Rarely are nonpsychiatric treatments such as aesthetic dermatologic procedures effective in minimizing the distress of BDD. While it is appropriate and ethical to refuse to perform a procedure on a patient suffering with BDD, it is important not to dismiss the patient's concerns and consider a referral to a mental health care provider.

More commonly, the cosmetic dermatologist will be confronted with a patient with a single, localized complaint who requests a specific treatment modality based on his or her exposure to media reports, the patient's own research, or anecdotal reports from friends or family. In these situations, it is important to identify the patient's goal and guide him or her to the most optimal treatment option if the requested treatment would not achieve the patient's goals or presents an unfavorable risk-benefit ratio. The preferred treatment approach may involve a single treatment of another part of the face, a different modality, or a multimodal treatment plan. One example would be a patient requesting microneedling to address telangiectasias. As microneedling would not improve the appearance of telangiectasias, the patient should be guided instead to an indicated modality such as laser.

CONCLUSION

Analyzing the aging face is a complex task that requires the ability to be not only an adept dermatologic surgeon, but also to be a visionary, artist, and psychiatrist. An understanding of the aging process, the anatomy of the face, and the goals of the patient will allow for the tailoring of an appropriate treatment plan which may include a single treatment or a complex plan consisting of multiple modalities performed overtime.

REFERENCES

1. Little AC, Jones BC, DeBruine LM. Facial attractiveness: Evolutionary based research. Philos Trans R Soc Lond B Biol Sci. 2011;366(1571):1638-59.
2. Bashour M. History and Current Concepts in the Analysis of Facial Attractiveness. Plast Reconstr Surg. 2006;118(3):741-56.
3. Vashi NA, Maymone MBDC, Kundu RV. Aging differences in ethnic skin. J Clin Aesthet Dermatol. 2016;9(1):31-8.
4. Morita A. Tobacco smoke causes premature skin aging. J Dermatol Sci. 2007;48(3):169-75.
5. Doshi DN, Hanneman KK, Cooper KD. Smoking and skin aging in identical twins. Arch Dermatol. 2007;143(12):1543-6.
6. Crane JD, MacNeil LG, Lally JS, Ford RJ, Bujak AL, Brar IK, et al. Exercise-stimulated interleukin-15 is controlled by AMPK and regulates skin metabolism and aging. Aging Cell. 2015;14(4):625-34.
7. Gkogkolou P, Böhm M. Advanced glycation end products: Key players in skin aging? Dermatoendocrinol. 2012;4(3):259-70.
8. Danby FW. Nutrition and aging skin: Sugar and glycation. Clin Dermatol. 2010;28(4):409-11.
9. Krutmann J, Liu W, Li L, Pan X, Crawford M, Sore G, et al. Pollution and skin: From epidemiological and mechanistic studies to clinical implications. J Dermatol Sci. 2014;76(3):163-8.
10. Vierkötter A, Schikowski T, Ranft U, Sugiri D, Matsui M, Krämer U, et al. Airborne Particle Exposure and Extrinsic Skin Aging. J Invest Dermatol. 2010;130(12):2719-26.
11. Kaminer MS, Bogle MA, Arndt KA, Dover JS. Evaluation of the Aging Face. In: Atlas of Cosmetic Surgery; 2nd ed. WB Saunders, Philadelphia. Elsevier. 2009:37-44.
12. Kuhn H, Mennella C, Magid M, Stamu-O'Brien C, Kroumpouzos G. Psychocutaneous disease: Clinical perspectives. J Am Acad Dermatol. 2017;76(5):779-91.
13. Conrado LA, Hounie AG, Diniz JB, Fossaluza V, Torres AR, Miguel EC, et al. Body dysmorphic disorder among dermatologic patients: Prevalence and clinical features. J Am Acad Dermatol. 2010;63(2):235-43.

2

CHAPTER

Principles of Laser, Light, and Tissue Interactions

Omer Ibrahim, Jeffrey S Dover

INTRODUCTION

Light is released, transferred, and absorbed in specific amounts of energy called quanta.[1] In dermatology, quanta of light have been harnessed and used in lasers and other light-based devices as integral sources of therapeutic energy in the treatment of many ailments, from photoaging to cutaneous neoplasia. Laser is an acronym for *light amplification by the stimulated emission of radiation*. In his "The Quantum Theory of Radiation," Einstein described the transfer of energy from light to atoms, ultimately leading to the emission of electromagnetic radiation. Most atoms exist in a ground-energy state, and upon absorbing light energy are converted to higher energy levels. Upon their return to their ground state, they release energy as photons or electromagnetic waves. When a photon of a specific wavelength collides with an excited atom, two photons are released concurrently with equal frequencies, a phenomenon known as "stimulated emission".[2,3] The first laser was created in 1960 by using an energy source to energize solid ruby crystals.[4] Since this crucial discovery, lasers and light-based devices have evolved rapidly, and their applications have spanned almost every field in modern medicine.

LASER FUNDAMENTALS

Light and other forms of electromagnetic radiation are composed of photons (particles or quanta of light) that travel in a vacuum at a constant velocity, also referred to as the speed of light ($c = 2.998 \times 10^8$ m/s).[5] The speed of light, c, is correlated to wavelength λ and frequency ν, by which: $c = \lambda\nu$. The energy of a photon is therefore proportional to its frequency, such that the energy of radiation increases with increasing frequency (and decreasing wavelength). Visible light, the only wavelengths visible to the human eye, ranges from 390 nm (violet) to 700 nm (red), and represents a relatively small portion of the electromagnetic spectrum.[5] Most lasers used in dermatology employ wavelengths within the visible light range and the near infrared spectrum.

Natural sunlight and spontaneously emitted light such as that from a light bulb are formed as a result of excited atoms that emit photons at different times, in any direction and usually with different wavelengths. This results in electromagnetic radiation that is broadband (multiple wavelengths), incoherent, and divergent. In contrast, lasers are fundamentally different (**Table 1**). A laser device creates energy in the form of a monochromatic,

TABLE 1: Comparison of three types of light sources.

	Lasers	Intense pulsed light	Ambient light
Properties	Monochromatic, coherent, collimated	Broadband, incoherent, divergent	Broadband, incoherent, divergent
Energy source	Flashlamp, electrical current, or another laser	Flashlamp	Pre-existing source (e.g., sunlight, lamp, flashlight, etc.)
Wavelengths	193–10,600 nm (monochromatic)	420–1,200 nm (broadband, but with filter capability to narrow wavelength band)	Depends on light source
Output	Continuous or pulsed	Pulsed	N/A
Pulse duration	Milliseconds to picoseconds	Milliseconds	N/A

coherent, and collimated beam of light that interacts with its target tissue. All laser devices contain an energy source and an optical resonator (**Fig. 1**). The function of the energy source is to excite atoms and electrons to an elevated energy state; the energy source can be in the form of an electrical current, flashlamp, or even another laser.[6] The resonator is comprised of a medium (solid, liquid, liquid crystal, or gas) that determines the resultant wavelength and properties of the laser. The medium is enclosed within a tube that contains two parallel mirrors. One of the mirrors is completely opaque and the other is partially transmissible. The laser's energy source pushes the electrons in the medium to an excited state, a process referred to as "pumping." After pumping, the excited atoms or molecules return from the excited to the ground state and in doing so release photons with a specific wavelength. The combination of multiple atoms and molecules undergoing this transition with resultant emissions of wavelengths of identical frequencies allows another process to occur: The stimulated emission of photons, as described by Albert Einstein.[2] When a photon of a certain wavelength collides with an electron in an excited state, a second photon of the same wavelength is emitted (**Fig. 2**). Therefore, one photon stimulates the next atom or molecule to emit a photon. The resulting two photons stimulate another two atoms or molecules, resulting in the release of four photons and so on (**Fig. 2**). The photons oscillate back and forth between the parallel mirrors, colliding with and exciting other atoms in the process. This chain reaction increases the number of photons exponentially, while maintaining their energy. Inversion occurs when the number of excited atoms outweighs the number of atoms in the ground state. Finally, the photons that are traveling in a perfectly parallel direction exit the resonator through the partially transmissible mirror at the distal end of the resonator as a laser beam (**Fig. 1**).

The resulting laser beam exiting the resonator is monochromatic, coherent, and collimated (**Table 1**).[5] Unlike natural or incandescent light that emits light across the entire visible spectrum, the monochromatic nature of a laser describes its temporal coherence—laser light is composed of a single wavelength. This property of laser light is important therapeutically as it allows for the selective absorption of the laser by specific chromophores (light-absorbing compounds). Laser light is also coherent, in that the waves are in phase in space and time. This allows the beam to travel larger distances with minimal

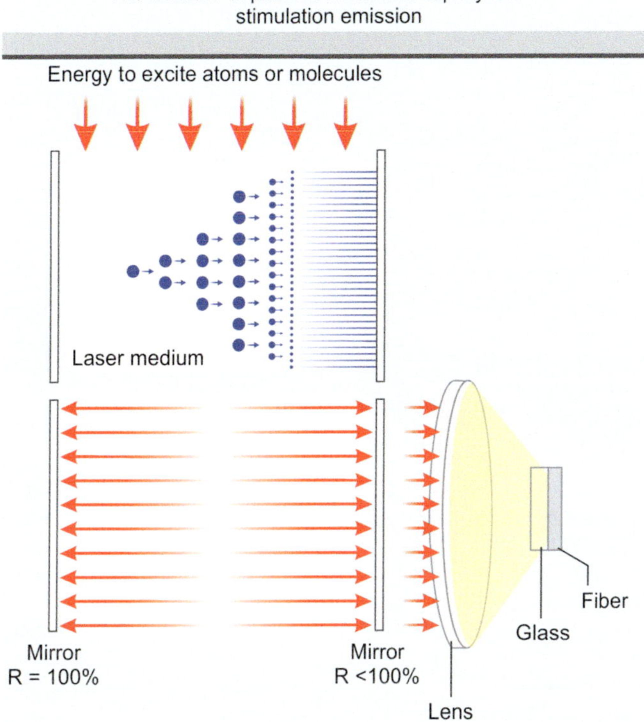

FIG. 1: A laser is composed of an energy source and an optical resonator. The energy source excites atoms and electrons to an elevated energy state. The resonator is comprised of a medium that determines the wavelength of a laser, and two parallel mirrors. Photons oscillate back and forth between the parallel mirrors. The photons that are traveling in a perfectly parallel direction exit the resonator through the partially transmissible mirror at the distal end of the resonator as a laser beam.

Source: Used with permission from Landthaler M, Bäumler W, Hohenleutner U. Chapter 239. Lasers and Flashlamps in Dermatology. In: Goldsmith LA, Katz SI, Gilchrest BA, Paller AS, Leffell DJ, Wolff K (Eds). Fitzpatrick's Dermatology in General Medicine, 8th Edition. New York, NY: McGraw-Hill. 2012.

divergence and without substantial loss of intensity. Finally, laser light is collimated, in that all the photons are parallel to each other. This allows the light to travel long distances with minimal distortion and dispersion. Collimation also allows the dense packing of energy into a relatively small volume of light.

Laser light can be continuous or shuttered, depending on the temporal behavior of the excitation of the atoms or molecules. When the energy supply to the laser medium is continuous, the emission of the laser is considered continuous-wave emission, and a continuous beam of laser light is produced with little or no variation in power output overtime. Shutters may be opened or closed to either permit or obstruct the laser beam from exiting the device.

Pulsed excitation occurs when the energy supply of the laser is limited to a certain time interval by gas discharge or flashlamp and the laser emits pulses accordingly. These laser pulse durations can vary from microseconds to milliseconds. Pulsed excitation allows for

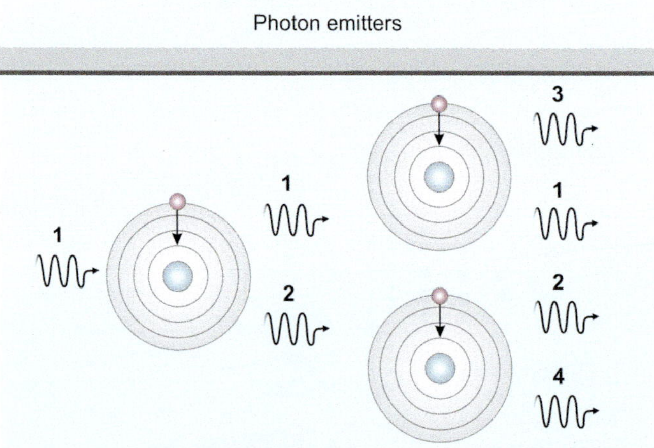

FIG. 2: The stimulated emission of radiation: When a photon (photon 1) of a certain wavelength collides with an electron in an excited state, a second photon (photon 2) of the same wavelength is emitted. Photon 1 then stimulates another excited electron, as does photon 2, both emitting photon 3 and photon 4, respectively. This chain reaction continues until a laser beam of coherent and parallel photons exits the resonator.

Source: Used with permission from Landthaler M, Bäumler W, Hohenleutner U. Chapter 239. Lasers and Flashlamps in Dermatology. In: Goldsmith LA, Katz SI, Gilchrest BA, Paller AS, Leffell DJ, Wolff K (Eds). Fitzpatrick's Dermatology in General Medicine, 8th Edition New York, NY: McGraw-Hill. 2012.

peak power outputs up to 100-fold greater than continuous wave lasers. To achieve very short pulse durations in the nanosecond or picosecond range, the resonator is additionally equipped with an optical polarizer and a non-linear crystal. The polarizer sets the linear polarization of the laser beam that passes through the crystal. However, if an appropriate electrical voltage is applied to the crystal, the polarization of the photons is changed inside the crystal and subsequently blocked by the optical polarizer. This prevents photons from running back and forth inside the resonator (oscillation), which hampers light amplification and which is equivalent to a low circuit quality of the resonator. In such a case, the stimulated emission is minimized and the pumping of the laser medium produces a maximum number of excited atoms or molecules in the laser medium. When this maximum number is achieved, the electrical voltage of the crystal is switched off within nanoseconds and the photons can easily pass the crystal, which is equivalent to a high circuit quality of the resonator. Now, the laser oscillation immediately starts and the light amplification yields a very high number of photons per time unit due to the high number of excited atoms or molecules in the laser medium. The outcome of this circuit quality switch (Q-switch) is a very intense laser pulse with pulse durations in the range of nanoseconds to picoseconds.

INTENSE PULSED LIGHT FUNDAMENTALS

Intense pulsed light (IPL) devices are not lasers; they contain a flashlamp that delivers noncoherent light ranging from approximately 420 nm to 1,200 nm. IPL devices can be modified to emit different bands of light, fluences, and pulse durations (**Table 1**).[7] The monochromatic light can be tuned using different cutoff filters and separate handpieces in order to maximize certain desired wavelengths depending on the target chromophore and the skin type of the patient. The filter cuts off emitted light, permitting only wavelengths longer than a certain threshold value to pass through. For example, a 560-nm filter allows only wavelengths longer than 560 nm to pass through. Therefore, given the vascular absorption peak of 585–595 nm, a 560-nm filter can be used to treat vascular lesions.[7]

LASER-TISSUE INTERACTIONS

When a laser light comes into contact with skin, it may undergo reflection, transmission, absorption, and scattering.[8] The fundamental action or effect of the laser depends on its absorption. Absorption describes the conversion of laser energy to heat when its photons strike the target chromophore. Reflection occurs when the laser beam strikes the skin's surface at an oblique angle and a portion of the beam bounces off the surface in a different direction. Of note, even laser beams positioned exactly perpendicular to the skin still undergo up to 5% reflectance due to the inherent reflective property of the stratum corneum; therefore, safety goggles are necessary when wielding lasers at all times.[5] Scattering of a laser beam describes the deviation of laser light once it passes through the stratum corneum into the tissue, due to contact with small molecules in the skin. Scattering occurs more readily with shorter wavelengths. The size of the scattering objects ranges from a few nanometers (small cell organelles and cell membranes) to a few microns (large cell organelles, cells, and collagen fibers) to hundreds of microns (hair follicle and sweat glands). As expected scattering increases the effective area treated by the laser due to aberrant scattered laser light, thereby increasing the effective heated area. Finally, transmission of the laser occurs when the beam is not absorbed by the target chromophore and is conducted to deeper structures. Transmission is more likely to occur with longer wavelengths and larger spot sizes.[5] Once the length of the wavelength surpasses approximately 1,100 nm, the increase in penetration depth reverses because radiation >1,100 nm is increasingly absorbed by water in skin.

For monochromatic lasers, photons of a single wavelength are absorbed by specific chromophores (targets) according to their absorption coefficient. Given the polychromatic nature of IPL radiation, photons of different wavelengths are absorbed by different chromophores, thereby necessitating the use of cut off filters.

The absorption of laser or IPL light by a chromophore can result in a several reactions: Chemical (photochemical), mechanical (photoacoustic or photodisruptive), or thermal.[5] A photochemical reaction is one in which a microscopic chemical or biological response is induced by the light energy. For example, low-level laser energy to the scalp is absorbed by the mitochondria, thereby activating the cellular respiratory chain to induce hair growth.[9] A photoacoustic or photodisruptive response describes the generation of high energy acoustic waves within the target chromophore, as exemplified by the use of nanosecond or picosecond lasers in the treatment of pigmented lesions and tattoos: High-energy photons absorbed by pigment particles generate acoustic waves within the particles leading to their break up.[10]

The photothermal response is the mechanism on which most lasers rely. This response refers to the transformation of light energy into heat when absorbed by a chromophore, causing direct damage to adjacent structures. The neodymium-doped yttrium aluminum garnet (Nd:YAG) laser (1,064 nm frequency doubled to 532 nm) and pulsed dye lasers (585–600 nm) are absorbed both by hemoglobin and melanin but they sit near peaks of absorption of oxyhemoglobin. Radiation of ruby lasers (694 nm), alexandrite lasers (755 nm), and diode lasers (around 810 nm) are less well absorbed by oxyhemoglobin and more suitable for pigmented chromophores in benign pigmented lesions and for hair removal. Radiation of the Nd:YAG laser (1,064 nm) is minimally absorbed by all skin chromophores; however, at high radiant exposures, the Nd:YAG laser can be used for pigmented or vascular lesions with either a short or long pulse. Longer wavelength lasers such as the erbium-doped yttrium aluminum garnet (Er:YAG) and carbon dioxide (CO_2) lasers are absorbed solely by water, and therefore heat up tissue for vaporization or ablation. These ablative lasers induce thermal damage to the epidermis and dermis, whereas nonablative lasers (1,440, 1,540, 1,550, 1,565, and 1,927 nm) target dermal tissue to induce bulk heating of dermal collagen and avoid damage to the epidermis. Unlike photochemical effects, photothermal reactions necessitate relatively high energy levels.[11]

At temperatures below 50°C, reversible thermal damage, local vasodilation, and inflammatory cascade activation are produced.[12] At temperatures between 50°C and 100°C, tissue and its proteins undergo irreversible coagulation or denaturation. At temperatures >100°C, tissue vaporization occurs, generating plume containing water vapor and tissue components.[12] At temperatures >100°C, and with sufficiently high energy levels, steam can be formed deep within tissue cavities, leading to explosion and mechanical damage to tissue.

By changing the intensity and pulse duration parameters, the temperature can be modulated to achieve coagulation, vaporization or explosion of a specific target in skin. In general, using higher intensities (W/cm^2) and shorter pulse durations results in higher maximum temperatures inside the target, more tissue vaporization and less surrounding coagulative necrosis. Using lower power and longer pulse widths results in less vaporization and more coagulative necrosis at the edge of the vaporized tissue.

SELECTIVE PHOTOTHERMOLYSIS

The model of selective photothermolysis was first described in the early 1980s by Anderson and Parrish, and since then, this model has revolutionized the use of lasers in the treatment of cutaneous disorders.[13] The two key concepts of this theory require that the selected wavelength of the laser must be absorbed by a specific target chromophore and the correct pulse duration (exposure time) must be used for spatial confinement of heat in the target. This was demonstrated using a 577-nm wavelength for vessels and 351-nm wavelength for pigment. By selecting a wavelength that can be absorbed by a specific chromophore with pulse duration shorter than the thermal relaxation time (TRT), the damage to the peripheral tissue is minimized. The TRT is the time needed for the irradiated tissue to cool down to half of its heated temperature.[14] The TRT is proportional to the diameter of the target. Therefore larger chromophores require longer pulse durations, and thereby demonstrate greater overall heating.

Wavelength

The main chromophores in skin on which many lasers exert their action are water, melanin, and hemoglobin. The CO_2 laser (10,600 nm) is absorbed by water in the tissue, and penetrates <0.1 mm deep.[15] The Er:YAG laser (2,940 nm) is also preferentially absorbed by water. Argon-ion lasers (488 and 514 nm), potassium titanyl phosphate (KTP) lasers (532 nm), and pulsed dye lasers (585–595 nm) may be absorbed by both hemoglobin and melanin. Ruby lasers (694 nm) are absorbed mainly by melanin pigment although a small amount of hemoglobin absorption also occurs. Alexandrite lasers (755 nm) are preferentially absorbed by melanin. As mentioned earlier, although there is no specific chromophore for the Nd:YAG laser (1,064 nm), this wavelength is absorbed to a small extent by hemoglobin and melanin and at higher fluences it can be used to treat pigmented or vascular lesions.

Pulse Duration

The pulse duration must correlate with the size of the target. Coagulation of blood vessels, including larger leg veins, requires pulse durations in the millisecond range.[16-19] With proper pulse duration selection, only the temperature in the vessel increases, coagulating the vessel. Longer pulse durations than necessary result in excessive heat flow to the adjacent dermis, which may cause unnecessary adverse reactions.

The pulse duration necessary to effectively treat pigment in hair, epidermal and dermal melanocytic lesions, and tattoos depends on the size of the target chromophore. Hair follicles are 0.02–0.2 mm in diameter and are targeted by pulses in the range of 10–50 ms.[20] Melanocytes are typically several micrometers in diameter (average 7 micrometers) and therefore require pulse widths ranging from milliseconds to nanoseconds. Melanosomes are smaller in size, with diameters ranging from 1 to 1.5 μm, and therefore can be targeted with nanosecond and picosecond pulses.[21] Tattoo pigment particles are on average 100 nm (0.1 μm) in diameter and are targeted by nanosecond and picosecond pulses.[22]

FRACTIONAL PHOTOTHERMOLYSIS

In the late 20th century, ablative lasers (CO_2 and Er:YAG) revolutionized the treatment of facial photodamage and skin laxity. By ablating aged, damaged skin, the induced heating and ensuing repair response made way for younger, tighter collagen, and skin. Although effective, fully ablative lasers carried high-risk profiles and prolonged recovery times, leading to their ultimate downfall. In addition, the nonablative lasers of the time fell short of the dramatic results that ablative ones offered. In order to fill the prominent gap between fully ablative and nonablative lasers, the concept of fractional photothermolysis emerged.[23] Fractional photothermolysis uses focused laser irradiation to create spatially distributed columns of microthermal injury within the treatment area, called microscopic treatment zones (MTZs). Each MTZ consists of a micro ablation zone (MAZ) and a surrounding area of coagulation known as the coagulation zone (CZ) (**Fig. 3A**). The depth and size of the MAZ and CZ depend on the laser and laser settings. For instance, the CZ of the Er:YAG laser is much smaller than the CO_2 laser. With proper technique and settings, there is enough energy in each column of MTZ to induce thermal heating or ablation without spread to adjacent tissue. Fractional irradiation allows relatively deeper penetration of the laser beam into the dermis, causing controlled vaporization or coagulation, transepidermal elimination of the coagulated debris, and reactive collagen remodeling. By maintaining the integrity of most of the intervening epidermis, fractional irradiation shortens healing times and decreases side effects.[15]

Fractional photothermolysis can be either ablative (CO_2 and Er:YAG) or nonablative (1,440, 1,540, 1,550, 1,565, and 1,927 nm). In ablative fractional photothermolysis, there is controlled vaporization and removal or ablation of thin columns of both epidermis and dermis. In nonablative fractional photothermolysis, the tissue is more gently heated yielding coagulated columns in the epidermis and dermis without any tissue ablation (**Fig. 3B**).[23,24] Intense heating of columns

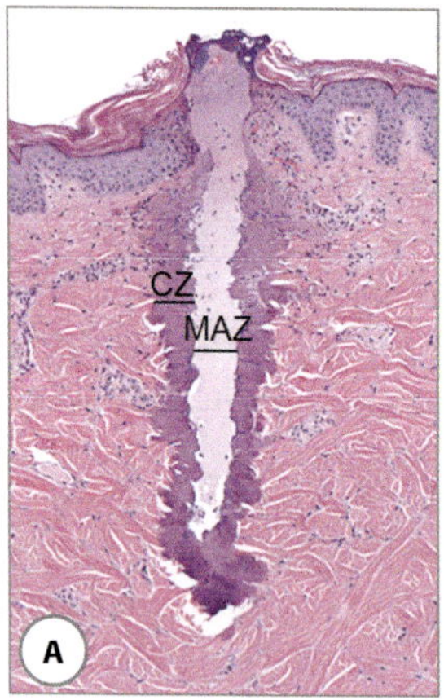

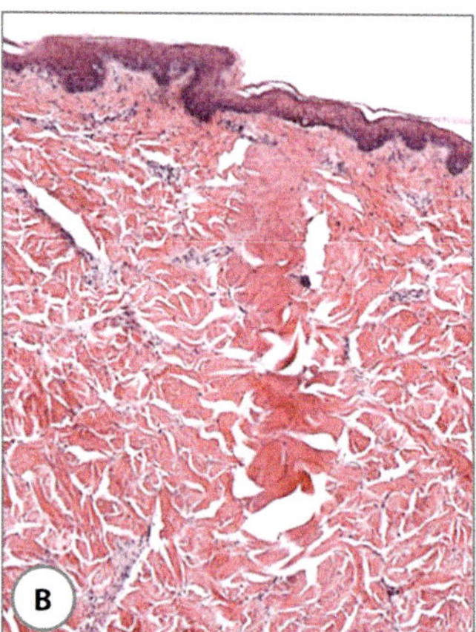

FIGS. 3A AND B: (A) Microscopic treatment zone (MTZ) of fractional ablative carbon dioxide laser, demonstrating the central ablated channel [micro ablation zone (MAZ)], and surrounding area of coagulation [coagulation zone (CZ)]. (B) microscopic treatment zone (mtz) of nonablative 1,540 nm, demonstrating coagulation within the treated dermis, and an intact overlying epidermis.

Courtesy: Dr. Emily Wenande, MD.

Source: Used with permission from Lapidoth Moshe, Adatto Maurice, Shlomit Halachmi. Treatment of actinic keratoses and photodamage with non-contact fractional 1540-nm laser quasi-ablation: An ex vivo and clinical evaluation. Lasers Med Sci. 2013;28(2):537-42.

within the dermis while leaving normal intervening skin intact can induce enough protein denaturation, release of heat shock proteins, and an inflammatory cascade that ultimately leads to collagen remodeling and synthesis. Nonablative fractionation allows for columns of thermal damage in comparison to nonfractionated, nonablated lasers that merely induce a homogenous layer of dermal heat.[23] Although, nonablative fractional lasers are much better tolerated, with fewer side effects and shorter healing time, their results may not be as impressive as ablative fractional lasers. Fractional photothermolysis has been used to treat many conditions including photoaging, acne scarring, traumatic scarring, skin laxity, and dyschromias.[24] Fractionation has also made laser-assisted topical drug delivery possible.[25-28]

CONCLUSION

Lasers and light-based devices harness the energy of light quanta in order to treat a myriad of cutaneous conditions in aesthetic and surgical dermatology. Prior to wielding these complicated and powerful devices, the clinician should have a solid knowledge base of the fundamentals and scientific basis of these devices. Herein we described the mechanism by which lasers exert their effect on their targets; we described the differences between lasers, IPL, and ambient light; and we elucidated the different types of interactions light can have with skin and tissues. Knowledge of these basic laser and light-based principles will allow the clinician to safely and effectively employ these devices in the treatment of a plethora of skin conditions.

REFERENCES

1. Dicke RH. Coherence in Spontaneous Radiation Processes. Phys Rev. 1954;93(1):99-110.
2. Einstein A. Zur Quantentheorie der Strahlung. Phys Zeitschrift. 1917;18:121-8.
3. Azadgoli B, Baker RY. Laser applications in surgery. Ann Transl Med. 2016;4(23):452.
4. Maiman TH. Stimulated optical radiation in ruby. Nature. 1960;187:493-4.
5. Franck P, Henderson PW, Rothaus KO. Basics of Lasers: History, Physics, and Clinical Applications. Clin Plast Surg. 2016;43(3):505-13.
6. De Felice E. Shedding light: laser physics and mechanism of action. Phlebology. 2010;25(1):11-28.
7. Raulin C, Greve B, Grema H. IPL technology: a review. Lasers Surg Med. 2003;32(2):78-87.
8. Dover JS, Arndt KA, Geronemus RG, Olbright SM, Noe JM, Stern RS. Illustrated cutaneous laser surgery: a practitioner's guide. Norwalk Conn: Appleton & Lange; 1990.
9. Gupta AK, Foley KA. A Critical Assessment of the Evidence for Low-Level Laser Therapy in the Treatment of Hair Loss. Dermatol Surg. 2017;43(2):188-97.
10. Ho DD, London R, Zimmerman GB, Young DA. Laser-tattoo removal--a study of the mechanism and the optimal treatment strategy via computer simulations. Lasers Surg Med. 2002;30(5):389-97.
11. Allemann IB, Kaufman J. Laser principles. Curr Probl Dermatol. 2011;42:7-23.
12. Herd RM, Dover JS, Arndt KA. Basic laser principles. Dermatol Clin. 1997;15(3):355-72.
13. Anderson RR, Parrish JA. Selective photothermolysis: precise microsurgery by selective absorption of pulsed radiation. Science. 1983;220(4596):524-7.
14. Goldman L, Wilson RG, Hornby P, Meyer RG. Radiation from a Q-switched ruby laser. Effect of repeated impacts of power output of 10 megawatts on a tattoo of man. J Invest Dermatol. 1965;44:69-71.
15. Borges J, Manela-Azulay M, Cuzzi T. Photoaging and the clinical utility of fractional laser. Clin Cosmet Investig Dermatol. 2016;9:107-14.
16. Brightman LA, Geronemus RG, Reddy KK. Laser treatment of port-wine stains. Clin Cosmet Investig Dermatol. 2015;8:27-33.
17. Morton LM, Smith KC, Dover JS, Arndt KA. Treatment of purpura with lasers and light sources. J Drugs Dermatol. 2013;12(11):1219-22.
18. Franca K, Chacon A, Ledon J, Savas J, Izakovic J, Nouri K. Lasers for cutaneous congenital vascular lesions: a comprehensive overview and update. Lasers Med Sci. 2013;28(4):1197-204.
19. Meesters AA, Pitassi LHU, Campos V, Wolkerstorfer A, Dierickx CC. Transcutaneous laser treatment of leg veins. Lasers Med Sci. 2014;29(2):481-92.
20. Zandi S, Lui H. Long-term removal of unwanted hair using light. Dermatol Clin. 2013;31(1):179-91.
21. Thong HY, Jee SH, Sun CC, Boissy RE. The patterns of melanosome distribution in keratinocytes of human skin as one determining factor of skin colour. Br J Dermatol. 2003;149(3):498-505.
22. Hogsberg T, Loeschner K, Lof D, Serup J. Tattoo inks in general usage contain nanoparticles. Br J Dermatol. 2011;165(6):1210-8.
23. Manstein D, Herron GS, Sink RK, Tanner H, Anderson RR. Fractional photothermolysis: a new concept for cutaneous remodeling using microscopic patterns of thermal injury. Lasers Surg Med. 2004;34(5):426-38.
24. Saedi N, Jalian HR, Petelin A, Zachary C. Fractionation: past, present, future. Semin Cutan Med Surg. 2012;31(2):105-9.
25. Waibel JS, Wulkan AJ, Shumaker PR. Treatment of hypertrophic scars using laser and laser assisted corticosteroid delivery. Lasers Surg Med. 2013;45(3):135-40.
26. Rkein A, Ozog D, Waibel JS. Treatment of atrophic scars with fractionated CO2 laser facilitating delivery of topically applied poly-L-lactic acid. Dermatol Surg. 2014;40(6):624-31.
27. Waibel JS, Mi QS, Ozog D, Qu L, Zhou L, Rudnick A, et al. Laser-assisted delivery of vitamin C, vitamin E, and ferulic acid formula serum decreases fractional laser postoperative recovery by increased beta fibroblast growth factor expression. Lasers Surg Med. 2016;48(3):238-44.
28. Haak CS, Hannibal J, Paasch U, Anderson RR, Haedersdal M. Laser-induced thermal coagulation enhances skin uptake of topically applied compounds. Lasers Surg Med. 2017;49(6):582-91.

3

CHAPTER

Laser, Light and Energy-based Devices

Murad Alam

INTRODUCTION

Light, laser and energy devices have revolutionized dermatology, as well as many other medical specialties. Selective modalities for targeting specific skin complaints have been created, refined, and widely adopted over the past five decades. Collectively, these have enabled more effective treatment of previously resistant conditions with concomitant mitigation of adverse events.

Much of the credit belongs to the visionary scientists who have made such advances possible. Therapies have been rationally and systematically developed from first principles in order to maximize effectiveness while minimizing collateral tissue injury. The review below considers the mechanisms of action and practical applications of some of these technologies.

NONABLATIVE LASERS

Traditional nonablative lasers are those that neither vaporize skin nor physically breach the epidermis (see traditional ablative, and fractional nonablative lasers, later).[1,2] Some of these target chromophores such as pigment or hemoglobin, and may also be further discussed later with regard to these indications.

Traditional nonablative lasers also have a secondary effect of inducing collagen remodeling.[3,4] First documented with the pulsed-dye laser, this has now been substantiated with virtually every type of nonablative laser and energy device. Histology after treatment shows growth in collagen bundles and the thickness of the collagen layer. Some have suggested that this may be analogous to a deep scar, but regardless of the nosology or provenance of this effect, it often improves the physical appearance of the skin.

TRADITIONAL ABLATIVE LASER

Ablative lasers are useful for reducing fine and coarse wrinkles, and epidermal color and texture abnormalities, as well as tightening atrophic skin.[1,2,5] Both carbon dioxide (CO_2) and erbium (typically, Er:YAG) lasers vaporize skin by targeting water within and around cells. Carbon dioxide lasers emit a wavelength of 10,600 nm, and Er:YAG lasers, of 2,940 nm. Continuous wave carbon dioxide lasers can induce a broad area of thermal necrosis, but pulsed devices with pulse duration of under 1 ms, which have been available since the late 1990s, are more selective. After several passes, pulsed CO_2 lasers may vaporize a layer of

100 μm while producing an underlying zone of thermal necrosis, or residual thermal damage (RTD) of 100–200 μm. The collateral thermal injury associated with CO_2 lasers can slow healing, generate erythema lasting weeks to months, and rarely, result in hypopigmentation verging on depigmentation, and even scarring. However, this same coagulative thermal effect is responsible for immediate and delayed tissue contraction, a desirable outcome in most cases. Immediate tissue contraction occurs at the time of laser application, as tissue coagulates and deforms. Intense neutrophil-rich inflammation then develops high in the dermis, just below the level of the ablative zone, with this developing into fibrosing granulation tissue, and resolving with elastophagocytosis, fibrosis, and additional contraction in weeks to months.

Er:YAG lasers vaporize tissue more efficiently, as their wavelength closely corresponds with a wavelength at which water absorbs energy. This reduces the incidence of necrotic tissue injury, delayed erythema, hypopigmentation, and scar, but also means that tissue contraction occurs to a much lesser extent. If many multiple passes of Er:YAG are performed to create a much deeper injury, risks of hypopigmentation and scar increase, but even so, the same degree of tightening seen with equivalent depth ablation with CO_2 is not seen.

Carbon dioxide and Er:YAG lasers can be used in combination. The CO_2 laser may be used first, to ablative and tighten tissue, and the Er:YAG laser may then be used to vaporize and remove the residual layer of thermal necrosis, hence speeding healing. Modified erbium lasers include a coagulative setting to achieve this same effect.

Regardless of the approach used, one limitation of fully ablative pulsed lasers is the relatively protracted downtime after treatment. For full-field carbon dioxide ablation of the face, 2 weeks away from work and social events is likely required, and even with Er:YAG resurfacing, a period of 1 week is to be expected. Moreover, the character of postoperative downtime after full-field ablation is severe, with extensive desquamation, serous crust, and an inability to apply makeup for days to weeks.

FRACTIONAL NONABLATIVE LASERS

Fractional photothermolysis, a process invented by Manstein and Anderson, is a modified method of skin resurfacing designed to reduce the risk of complications and delayed healing associated with full-field resurfacing while providing greater effectiveness than fully nonablative treatments.[1,2,6,7] In fractional photothermolysis, water-absorbing wavelengths are used to create a gridline pattern of microscopic, vertically oriented columns of coagulated skin. These are called microthermal zones (MTZs), these areas can be 100–200 μm in diameter and up to 1,600 μm deep. The spacing on the skin surface between these columns, as well as the depth of the columns, can be changed using appropriate laser settings.

Unlike full-field resurfacing, fractional resurfacing does not result in tissue damage to the entire treated skin surface. Spared areas between the MTZs enable rapid healing, while also preserving the structural integrity of the skin, which does not fully desquamate.

The first fractional nonablative device was the 1,550 nm erbium doped laser, and similar other devices such as the 1,540 nm Er:glass and the 1,440 nm device soon followed. In each case, posttreatment erythema and edema persist for several days, followed by several days of transepidermal elimination of the necrotic tissue columns as microcrusts. Wound care is relatively simple, with bland emolliation for the first several days, and make-up can be applied soon thereafter. Other benefits of this approach include the sufficiency of preoperative topical anesthetic for pain management, and the safety of use in darker skinned patients. Dyschromia, scars, striae, and fine textural abnormalities may be improved by fractional nonablative lasers, often after multiple treatments spaced many weeks to a month or more apart. Wrinkles and laxity are less responsive.

FRACTIONAL ABLATIVE LASER

The fractional ablative laser, specifically the index carbon dioxide device, has been available since 2007.[1,2,7,8] The underlying premise and mechanism is the same as that of fractional nonablative lasers, but the degree of injury is ablative rather than nonablative. Downtime after ablative fractional lasers may be several days longer, as much as a week on average. Effectiveness is greater than with nonablative fractional devices, particularly for textural abnormalities such as acne scarring. Fewer treatments may also be required than with fractional nonablative lasers to achieve the same effect. Fractional ablative devices are less safe for those with ethnic skin, in whom there is a risk of pigmentary abnormality. While lower than with full-field ablative resurfacing, the risk of scar and hypopigmentation in lighter skinned patients is also a concern, particularly when a relatively greater surface area is treated in a given fractional ablative session. Fractional ablative devices must be used with caution on the face, where wound healing is slower and likelihood of scarring is higher.

VASCULAR LASERS

Vascular lasers target cutaneous vasculature based on the theory of selective thermolysis developed by Anderson and Parrish in 1983.[9] Rather than treating the entire full thickness of the skin, the wavelengths emitted by such lasers are preferentially absorbed by the chromophore oxyhemoglobin, and to a lesser extent, deoxyhemoglobin and methemoglobin. Heat transferred by laser light to the oxyhemoglobin is then dissipated to the vessel wall, which is consequently damaged. Absorption peaks for oxyhemoglobin include those at 410–429, 541, 577, and 700–1,200 nm. Ideal vascular lasers would emit at one of these peaks without concurrent absorption with melanin, which can happen at the shorter wavelengths.

The thermal relaxation time (TRT) is the time in which a chromophore, or laser target, loses to its surroundings half of the heat generated by the incident laser pulse. The ideal laser pulse duration for a particular chromophore approximates but does not exceed the TRT. If the pulse duration is longer than the TRT, structures peripheral to the chromophore may be injured, and if the pulse duration is much shorter, clinical effectiveness may be impaired, or in the case of some vascular lasers, vessels may be ruptured with attendant bruising. The TRT and hence the ideal pulse duration of a vascular laser is relatively short if the target is small, like a minute capillary or diffuse erythema, and longer if the target is a larger caliber vessel.

Early vascular lasers, including the argon laser (488, 514 nm), the copper vapor laser (578 nm), and the krypton (568 nm) were effective at heating oxyhemoglobin, but were not very selective, and frequently caused scarring or hypopigmentation. The pulsed-dye laser, developed in the early 1980s, was the first highly selective cutaneous vascular laser. The initial wavelength was 577 nm, and this was followed by devices that emitted at 585 nm, and then 595 nm, for progressively greater penetration depth, eventually exceeding 1 mm. Shorter pulse duration treatments with this device elicit purpura, which can be disfiguring and persist for 1–2 weeks.

Another selective vascular laser is the potassium-titanyl-phosphate (KTP; 532 nm) laser, or a frequency doubled neodymium-doped yttrium aluminum garnet (Nd:YAG) laser. Traditionally, this had a small 1–2 mm spot size for tracing individual telangiectatic vessels, but more recent devices allow treatment of a range of vascular lesions with much larger spot sizes. The 532 nm wavelength is also absorbed by melanin and needs to be used with care in darker skinned patients.

Near infrared laser wavelengths (700–1,200 nm) penetrate more deeply into the skin and are not highly absorbed by melanin. Lasers in this range can be useful for treatment of deeper vascular lesions and patients with ethnic skin. The most commonly used vascular device in this category is the Nd:YAG laser (1,064 nm). Since light at this wavelength is not as highly absorbed by hemoglobin, high fluences are needed to achieve the desired effect. This in turn can lead to inadvertent and unwanted bulk heating of water in the tissues, followed by necrosis and scar. To avoid such outcomes, adequate epidermal and superficial dermal cooling is essential during laser use.

HAIR REMOVAL LASERS

Laser hair removal entails selective treatment of the pigmented hair follicles, with melanin in the hair shaft being the chromophore.[10-13] However, targeting the hair follicle melanin alone can result in only temporarily hair loss, through induction of catagen. Long-term or permanent hair removal requires that the follicular stem cells in the bulge and dermal papilla of the hair unit be targeted. For this to occur, heat has to diffuse from the chromophore, melanin, to the preferred target, the adjacent stem cell reservoir. A longer pulse duration is needed for this to occur.

Devices used for hair removal include the ruby laser (694 nm), as well as the more commonly used alexandrite (755 nm), diode (810 nm), and Nd:YAG lasers. Comparative trials have shown that the diode is the most effective for hair removal, followed by the alexandrite, ruby, and Nd:YAG, in descending order. While the Nd:YAG works less well to remove hair, its longer wavelength is less absorbed by melanin and hence less likely to induce pigmentary abnormalities in dark-skinned patients. At every wavelength, higher fluences tend to be more effective.

Q-SWITCHED AND PICOSECOND LASERS

Tattoo pigment is an exogenous particulate material that can be removed from the skin through the use of selective lasers.[14-19] Two mechanisms may be operative. First, based on its photothermal effects, laser light absorbed selectively by a pigment chromophore of a particular color can shatter the pigment particle into smaller pieces, thus speeding its phagocytosis and clearance. As per the theory of selective thermolysis, the laser pulse duration in this case must not exceed the TRT. Second, laser energy also has photoacoustic effects. Specifically, light falling on a tattoo creates acoustic waves within the targeted pigment particle, thereby mechanically rupturing it.

In the 1980s, Q-switched lasers with pulse durations of 5–100 nm were shown to be effective for treating tattoos and other pigmentary disorders. But particles comprising tattoo pigments are usually 100 nm in width, which implies a TRT of less than 10 ns. Hence lasers with even shorter pulse durations would appear likely to be more effective for tattoo removal. This observation has led during recent years to the commercial launch of picosecond-domain lasers.

INTENSE PULSED LIGHT

Intense pulsed light (IPL) devices, pioneered in the early 1990s, are not lasers but bright flash lamps that generate noncoherent light of many colors.[20,21] The emission spectrum of traditional IPL devices is from below 500 nm to above 1,200 nm. High pass filters can be used to exclude light below a certain wavelength in order to restrict the wavelengths seen by the skin to those suitable for targeting the designated chromophore. Filters may also be chosen based on the body site, including the optical characteristics of the overlying skin and the depth of the relevant chromophore. In this way, IPL devices can be made to mimic lasers of particular wavelengths. Fluence, pulse duration, and cooling parameters are adjustable on some newer IPL devices. IPL hand pieces usually convey light through a rectangular crystal, which may be coupled to the skin through a transparent gel that allows light to be transmitted evenly while protecting against burns.

Intense pulsed light devices are routinely used to treat vascular lesions, pigmentation, photo damage, and unwanted hair. They are often preferred for skin rejuvenation in patients with both vascular and pigmentary complaints, as they are better suited to address multiple issues simultaneously than lasers, which may be optimized for a single chromophore. On the other hand, the complexity of the emission spectra of IPLs means that they must be used with caution to avoid overtreatment of a particular chromophore. Otherwise, adverse events, such as persistent erythema, crusting, blistering, burns, and hyperpigmentation, may manifest.

Newer IPL devices are faster than older ones and may calibrate after each use to account for aging of the bulb. Recent devices also produce square pulse beams, which allow for even and consistent illumination without initial peaks. Tissue trauma leading to bruising and late pulse attenuation that decreases effectiveness is thus avoided. Smaller spot sizes of just a few millimeters are also now available to make it easier to treat curved surfaces.

RADIOFREQUENCY

The skin effects of radiofrequency (RF) energy do not entail selective thermolysis of particular chromophores but rather heating of water.[22-26] This makes RF relatively color-blind, and suitable for treatment of ethnic skin types. RF entails an oscillating electrical current that stimulates molecular and ionic collisions, thereby creating heat. The specific biological effects are contingent on the depth of tissue treated, the frequency employed, and the method of superficial skin cooling. As expected, longer RF wavelengths penetrate more deeply. RF treatments can be adapted to preferentially heat, fat or water by selecting the electric field accordingly. In dermatology, treatments are typically optimized for either dermal skin tightening or subcutaneous adipose reduction. Medical treatments with RF are in the range between 3 kHz and 24 GHz, an RF band that is reserved for industrial, scientific, and medical applications.

Radiofrequency devices can be monopolar, bipolar, or unipolar. There are also combination devices, as well as those that fractionally treat a small portion of the skin. Monopolar devices typically have a single electrode and a grounding pad on the skin, and energy travels between the electrode and the ground. In general, monopolar RF devices offer the deepest energy penetration. Bipolar RF is delivered through a pair of electrodes, a negative and a positive pole, between which the RF energy travels. Typically effective within a few millimeters of the skin surface, bipolar devices are said to have a depth of penetration that is half of the distance between the electrodes. A variant of bipolar RF is insertional fractional RF, in which multiple pairs of electrodes, or bipolar needles, are mechanically introduced into the skin to be treated. Unipolar RF is comprised of a single electrode from which an omnidirectional RF field emanates without the need for a grounding pad.

ULTRASOUND

Ultrasound is a mechanical compression wave with a frequency higher than that detectable by the human ear (20 kHZ). Indications for therapeutic ultrasound in cutaneous medicine include skin tightening, fat reduction, and treatment of sweat glands. Ultrasound energy used for such indications is described by intensity (W/cm^2) and frequency (kHZ or MHz). As ultrasound enters the skin, it bounces off tissues or is absorbed. Higher frequency ultrasound waves are attenuated more rapidly and therefore penetrate less deeply.

Ultrasound used for fat reduction is of two types. One type is low intensity and low frequency mechanical ultrasound that works by generating a shock wave that causes cavitation, bubble formation, without generating much heat. The other is high frequency ultrasound (HIFU) with approximately 1 mm wavelengths. A 2 MHz such beam creates a zone of injury in the fat that is approximately 1 mm wide and 10 mm long. Both types of ultrasound used for fat reduction are focused, such that energy is delivered at the focal point deep in the subcutis, and the overlying epidermis and dermis are spared. Specifically, HIFU energies may exceed 1,000 W/cm^2 at the focal point but be only 1-3 W/cm^2 at the epidermal surface.

Microfocused ultrasound (MIFU) used for skin tightening delivers high energy ultrasound of >5 W/cm^2 to the skin surface at various frequencies in the megahertz range to induce thermal injury zones (TIZs) of approximately 1 mm^3. Tissue temperatures in excess of 60 degrees centigrade result in tissue necrosis, which is followed by neocollagenesis. Placement of numerous closely spaced TIZs at two or even three levels within the dermis may culminate in clinically significant tissue tightening at 60–90 days after treatment. Such ultrasound treatments have also been adapted for treatment of hyperhidrosis, which improves by destruction of the eccrine sweat glands in the axilla. Compared to thermal ultrasound for fat reduction, the intensity of MIFU per tissue volume treated is higher, and the focal points targeted are more superficially located in the skin.

CRYOLIPOLYSIS

Cryolipolysis is a noninvasive means for fat reduction.[27-30] The overlying skin is protected while transdermal cooling results in preferential destruction of fat cells. Subcutaneous fat is exposed to low but not freezing temperatures in order to trigger apoptotic cell death. Temperatures of approximately 10 degrees centigrade are maintained for 45–60 minutes per treatment area. Since adipocytes are more cold-sensitive than other skin tissues, localized fat injury is observed. Firm manual massage immediately posttreatment may facilitate rupture of affected adipocytes that have been partly crystallized. Nonviable fat cells are cleared by inflammation, which is observed within 3 days of treatment, and is at its maximum at 2 weeks. Elevated blood lipids are not detected during this process. Subsequent treatments can be performed at 2–3 months intervals to target remaining fat.

The cooling apparatus includes vacuum suction that is used to place and position cooling panels on the skin. A measure known as cooling intensity factor (mW/cm^2) denotes the rate of heat removal per unit volume. Since the cooling process has anesthetic properties, no additional anesthesia is required with treatment. Posttreatment, paresthesias may persist for a few weeks before resolving completely, and very rarely, instead of apoptosis, fat cells are stimulated to grow (paradoxical fat hypertrophy).

PHOTODYNAMIC THERAPY

Topical photodynamic therapy is a paired combination intervention in which a nontoxic photosensitizing dye and a visible light source are applied to the skin surface to target a susceptible oxygen-containing tissue.[31-33] The ensuing photochemical reaction creates reactive oxygen species that damage cells. The most common photosensitizer used for PDT is 5-aminolevulinic acid (5-ALA), which is sufficiently small for transepidermal penetration. 5-ALA is converted via the heme synthetic pathway to protoporphyrin IX (PPIX). PPIX accumulates in target tissues, notably sebaceous glands and hyperproliferative keratinocytes, until light irradiation mediates necrosis and apoptosis of the same.

While its absorption peak is at 410 nm, PPIX is also activated by other wavelengths, including 505, 540, 585 and 635 nm light. Numerous artificial illumination sources, including lasers as well as narrow- and broad-band lights, are therefore sufficient to initiate PDT. Natural ambient light and daylight can also be used. When the goal is amelioration of acne by targeting sebaceous glands, deeper penetrating red light is normally chosen. Actinic keratoses are adequately treated with blue light (Soret band).

REFERENCES

1. Aslam A, Alster TS. Evolution of laser skin resurfacing: from scanning to fractional technology. Dermatol Surg. 2014;40(11):1163-72.
2. Pozner JN, DiBernardo BE. Laser resurfacing: full field and fractional. Clin Plast Surg. 2016;43(3):515-25.
3. Narins RS, Tope WD, Pope K, Ross EV. Overtreatment effects associated with a radiofrequency tissue-tightening device: rare, preventable, and correctable with subcision and autologous fat transfer. Dermatol Surg. 2006; 32(1):115-24.
4. Alam M, Hsu TS, Dover JS, Wrone DA, Arndt KA. Nonablative laser and light treatments: histology and tissue effects--a review. Lasers Surg Med. 2003;33(1):30-9.
5. Farshidi D, Hovenic W, Zachary C. Erbium:yttrium aluminum garnet ablative laser resurfacing for skin tightening. Dermatol Surg. 2014;40(Suppl 12):S152-6.
6. Kauvar AN. Fractional nonablative laser resurfacing: is there a skin tightening effect? Dermatol Surg. 2014;40(Suppl 12):S157-63.
7. Metelitsa AI, Alster TS. Fractionated laser skin resurfacing treatment complications: a review. Dermatol Surg. 2010;36(3):299-306.
8. Carniol PJ, Hamilton MM, Carniol ET. Current status of fractional laser resurfacing. JAMA Facial Plast Surg. 2015;17(5):360-6.
9. Garden BC, Garden JM, Goldberg DJ. Light-based devices in the treatment of cutaneous vascular lesions: An updated review. J Cosmet Dermatol. 2017;16(3):296-302.
10. Gan SD, Graber EM. Laser hair removal: a review. Dermatol Surg. 2013;39(6):823-38.
11. Haedersdal M, Beerwerth F, Nash JF. Laser and intense pulsed light hair removal technologies: from professional to home use. Br J Dermatol. 2011;165(Suppl 3):31-6.
12. Ibrahimi OA, Avram MM, Hanke CW, Kilmer SL, Anderson RR. Laser hair removal. Dermatol Ther. 2011;24(1): 94-107.
13. Sadighha A, Mohaghegh Zahed G. Meta-analysis of hair removal laser trials. Lasers Med Sci. 2009;24(1):21-5.
14. Choudhary S, Elsaie ML, Leiva A, Nouri K. Lasers for tattoo removal: a review. Lasers Med Sci. 2010;25(5):619-27.
15. Forbat E, Al-Niaimi F. The use of picosecond lasers beyond tattoos. J Cosmet Laser Ther. 2016;18(6):345-7.
16. Hsu VM, Aldahan AS, Mlacker S, Shah W, Nouri K. The picosecond laser for tattoo removal. Lasers Med Sci. 2016;31(8):1733-7.
17. Levin MK, Ng E, Bae YS, Brauer JA, Geronemus RG. Treatment of pigmentary disorders in patients with skin of color with a novel 755 nm picosecond, Q-switched ruby, and Q-switched Nd:YAG nanosecond lasers: a retrospective photographic review. Lasers Surg Med. 2016;48(2):181-7.
18. Mariwalla K, Dover JS. The use of lasers for decorative tattoo removal. Skin Therapy Lett. 2006;11(5):8-11.
19. Reiter O, Atzmony L, Akerman L, Levi A, Kershenovich R, Lapidoth M, et al. Picosecond lasers for tattoo removal: a systematic review. Lasers Med Sci. 2016;31(7): 1397-405.
20. Li D, Lin SD, Cheng B. Intense pulsed light: from the past to the future. Photomed Laser Surg. 2016;34(10): 435-47.
21. DiBernardo BE, Pozner JN. Intense pulsed light therapy for skin rejuvenation. Clin Plast Surg. 2016;43(3): 535-40.
22. Carruthers J, Fabi S, Weiss R. Monopolar radiofrequency for skin tightening: our experience and a review of the literature. Dermatol Surg. 2014;40(Suppl 12):S168-73.
23. Simmons BJ, Griffith RD, Falto-Aizpurua LA, Nouri K. Use of radiofrequency in cosmetic dermatology: focus on

nonablative treatment of acne scars. Clin Cosmet Investig Dermatol. 2014; 7:335-9.
24. Dong J, Amir Y, Goldenberg G. Advances in minimally invasive and noninvasive treatments for submental fat. Cutis. 2017;99(1):20-3.
25. Duncan D. Megasessions: efficacy of fewer, longer treatment sessions for fat reduction in noninvasive body contouring using a radiofrequency based device. J Drugs Dermatol. 2017;16(5):478-80.
26. Hayre N, Palm M, Jenkin P. A clinical evaluation of a next generation, non-invasive, selective radiofrequency, hands-free, body-shaping device. J Drugs Dermatol. 2016;15(12):1557-61.
27. Derrick CD, Shridharani SM, Broyles JM. The safety and efficacy of cryolipolysis: a systematic review of available literature. Aesthet Surg J. 2015;35(7):830-6.
28. Thomas WW, Bloom JD. Neck contouring and treatment of submental adiposity. J Drugs Dermatol. 2017;16(1):54-7.
29. Friedmann DP. A review of the aesthetic treatment of abdominal subcutaneous adipose tissue: background, implications, and therapeutic options. Dermatol Surg. 2015;41(1):18-34.
30. Kennedy J, Verne S, Griffith R, Falto-Aizpurua L, Nouri K. Noninvasive subcutaneous fat reduction: a review. J Eur Acad Dermatol Venereol. 2015;29(9):1679-88.
31. Babilas P, Karrer S, Sidoroff A, Landthaler M, Szeimies RM. Photodynamic therapy in dermatology--an update. Photodermatol Photoimmunol Photomed. 2005;21(3):142-9.
32. Boen M, Brownell J, Patel P, Tsoukas MM. The role of photodynamic therapy in acne: an evidence-based review. Am J Clin Dermatol. 2017;18(3):311-21.
33. Wen X, Li Y, Hamblin MR. Photodynamic therapy in dermatology beyond non-melanoma cancer: An update. Photodiagnosis Photodyn Ther. 2017;19:140-52.

4

CHAPTER

Home-use Dermatological Devices: Principles and Applications

J Frank Nash, Frank Beerwerth

INTRODUCTION

The dermatological community has been at the forefront in advancing energy-based treatments for medical and cosmetic benefits. A number of these treatments are transitioning from the physician's office to direct use by consumers. For example, devices used to accelerate or prevent hair growth and treatments for acne and aging skin, populate the home-use market. The democratization of energy-based technologies is anchored in a set of principles including ease of use that requires no special training, an understandable mode of action leading to noticeable benefits with few adverse events, and consumer affordability. Using randomized controlled clinical trial (RCT) data as the "gold standard" for evaluating home-use devices, light based hair removal has proven efficacy with an acceptable adverse event profile. The success of light-based hair removal devices in the home-use market is attributable, in part, to the understood mode of action, i.e., selective photothermolysis, delivering meaningful light energy. Light-based hair growth using low-level light therapy (LLLT) has RCTs demonstrating efficacy with limited side effects, although the mode of action is not completely understood. Acne treatment using blue light, which kills bacteria responsible for such lesions, has not been fully established as efficacious or exceeding that of conventional chemistries available over-the-counter, e.g., benzoyl peroxide. Finally, among the multitude of devices sold as treatments for aging skin, published RCTs are lacking. A limited number of devices, based on fractional photothermolysis mode of action, have reported benefits but the adverse effects seem to be a limitation. The future for refinement and improving existing technologies together with the prospect of greater affordability, demonstrated efficacy, i.e., RCT, and the potential migration of "new" treatments from physician to consumer, make the home-use device market attractive.

BACKGROUND

The size of global home-use beauty device market, e.g., cleansing, hair removal, aging skin, etc., was estimated to be 1.7 billion dollars in 2015 with an annual growth of 10–20%. The American Society for Dermatological Surgery (ASDS) reported that more than 2.7 million procedures were performed by dermatologists using lasers, light and energy-based devices in 2014. Given the estimated size of this market and future growth potential, together with the number of procedures currently being done in professional settings, it is not surprising that manufacturers and ambitious entrepreneurs are looking to take advantage of this seemingly favorable environment by introducing energy-based devices that may not require oversight by a skilled profession and provide some cosmetic benefits. However, as such availability spreads, it is probable that consumer dissatisfaction will rise for many reasons including lack of meaningful results, adverse events or both. As new treatments/technologies migrate from the physician's office to consumers, dermatologists will be most knowledgeable of the risks and benefits. To this end, understanding the status of the home-use market in terms of treatments and technologies is critical for dermatologists as well as other health care providers in their role as trusted advisors to patients/consumers.

The focus of this overview will be on energy-based devices used directly by consumers currently available for hair and skin benefits beyond cleansing. There are recent reviews that provide supplemental details, particularly related to the evidence supportive of efficacy and adverse events of such home-use technologies.[1-5]

PRINCIPLES GOVERNING ENERGY-BASED DEVICES FOR HOME USE

To better understand advances in the home-use dermatological device market, it is useful to consider the relationship between the delivery of energy, i.e., "dose", duration, frequency of administration, and the associated biological effects at the treatment site, i.e., skin/hair follicle. This relationship, depicted in **Figure 1**, is divided arbitrarily into four categories based on energy in the electromagnetic radiation spectrum and exposure time. For this example, the form in which the energy is delivered, e.g., light, ultrasound, radiofrequency, etc., is

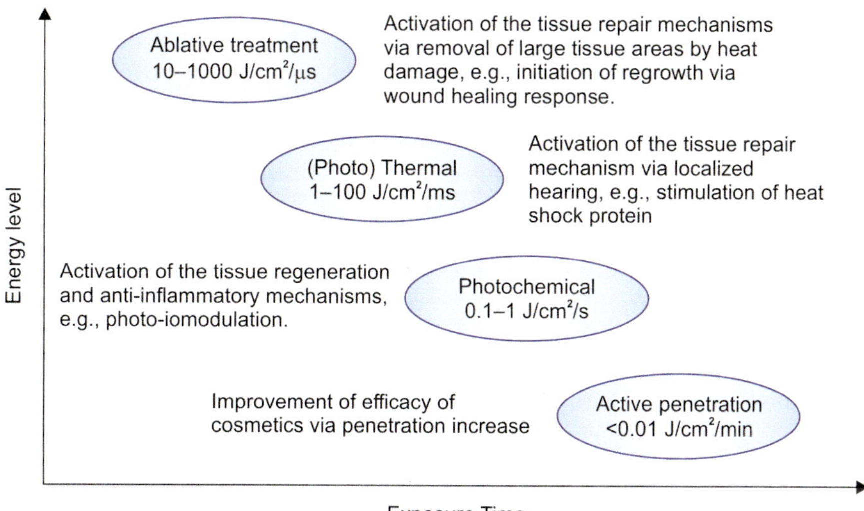

FIG. 1: Hypothetical relationship between energy level and exposure time.

unimportant. These categories—(1) Ablative treatments, (2) Photothermal, and (3) Photochemical, are a continuum rather than isolated, discrete silos, and may be operative proceeding left to right, i.e., low energy is not ablative while ablative may have photothermal and/or photochemical consequences. A fourth area, active skin penetration of exogenously applied chemicals attributed to very low energy, will not be discussed.

Skin exposure to high energy often in the context of resurfacing or body contouring requires a skilled medical professional to oversee patient selection, treatment site, amount of energy applied, adjunctive therapies, e.g., skin cooling, and after-care.[6-8] To date, such treatments are administered under clinically controlled conditions with, in some cases, an extended recovery time of several days requiring oversight and evaluation by a trained professional. Further, to deliver this energy, devices are often large and complex with multiple, operator-defined settings. It is clear that, at present and for the foreseeable future, such devices delivering high energy in ultra-short duration will unlikely be available for home use.

As the energy delivered to skin is reduced, photothermal and photochemical mechanisms predominate, both of which are operative over a wide energy range and represent the most common mode of action in current home-use device treatments. Photothermal effects in the skin are based primarily on the theory of selective photothermolysis in which the energy is absorbed by a chromophore and converted to heat resulting in the desired effect such as reduction in hair growth, disappearance of vascular lesions, tattoo removal or improvement in skin color.[9-11] The heat generated can be localized or "bulk" depending on the device specifications, e.g., fractional versus nonfractional, and targeted chromophore, e.g., melanin, hemoglobin or water. The generation of heat at the site of treatment can range from temperatures that denature protein to those producing mild discomfort. In the case of home-use devices, energy that produces widespread protein denaturation may not be deemed as "safe" without medical supervision. As such, energy delivered from home-use devices where selective or bulk heating is the mode of action must be designed to minimize adverse events, especially "burns", i.e., worst-case scenario, and pain, while still producing the desired outcome.

Examples of devices acting solely by a photochemical mode of action or photobiomodulation are used for hair growth and other alleged benefits such as wound healing and skin rejuvenation.[12-14] The energy used in photobiomodulation is most notably from low-level light (laser) therapy or LLLT which is, generally speaking, very low fluences of blue or red light. While the energy from such home-use photobiomodulation devices is without adverse consequences in skin, there is a questionable benefit for many such treatments.

A summary of the technologies used in home-use devices and their established/potential benefits are provided in **Table 1**. At present, intense pulsed light (IPL) and LLLT make up the majority of home-use devices with hair removal the most established treatment. There are multiple "benefit areas" presented individually, i.e., wrinkle reduction, age spots, skin tone, sagging, and pore size reduction, that could comprise a broader category of "skin rejuvenation". Presently, there are limited data supportive of the efficacy of such skin rejuvenation treatments. Finally, body contouring including body fat reduction and treatment of cellulite are increasingly popular targets with little or no data supportive of their efficacy with home-use devices.

TABLE 1: Summary of potential treatment benefits and the energy form used in home-use devices.

Benefit area	Energy form			
	Light			Radiofrequency
	Laser	Intense pulsed light (IPL)	Low-level light therapy (LLLT)	
Hair removal				
Hair growth				
Acne				
Wrinkle reduction				
Pore size reduction				
Age spots				
Skin tone				
Sagging skin				
Body fat reduction				
Cellulite				

Color Code: Good evidence | Some evidence | No evidence

DEVICE/TECHNOLOGY MIGRATION FROM PHYSICIAN-ASSISTED TO HOME USE

Without question, energy-based treatments have become part of the standard of care in dermatological offices. Medical doctors and nursing staff receive training in the use of such devices and based on their area of specialty likely have countless hours of practical experience. Importantly, treatment is based on careful patient evaluation and selection where the risk-to-benefit ratio is carefully considered. The goal is to deliver the desired outcome while minimizing adverse events, some of which could be permanent. Following a period of professional practice where device parameters, e.g., energy level, duration of treatment, etc., become established, such treatments may be administered by untrained personnel. At this point, device prototypes with appropriate safety interlocks may be developed and introduced into consumer testing and possibly marketed after a period of learning and refinement. This is an oversimplification of the democratization of professional devices, i.e., the process of making the professional device/treatment available to everyone. Importantly, this iterative scenario is expected to continue as treatments become more familiar and technology advances making such devices smaller, more user-friendly, safe/efficacious, and less expensive.

The path from skilled professional service/device to home-use is depicted in **Figure 2.** In this construct, the trained professional uses expert judgment and experience to guide decisions including what and when to treat followed by the selection of device/technology and suitable parameters. On the other side and for conservative reasons, it is assumed the consumer has limited knowledge regarding the technology and therefore selection of a device, effectiveness and individual suitability. For the manufacturer, the passageway between professional and consumer is based largely

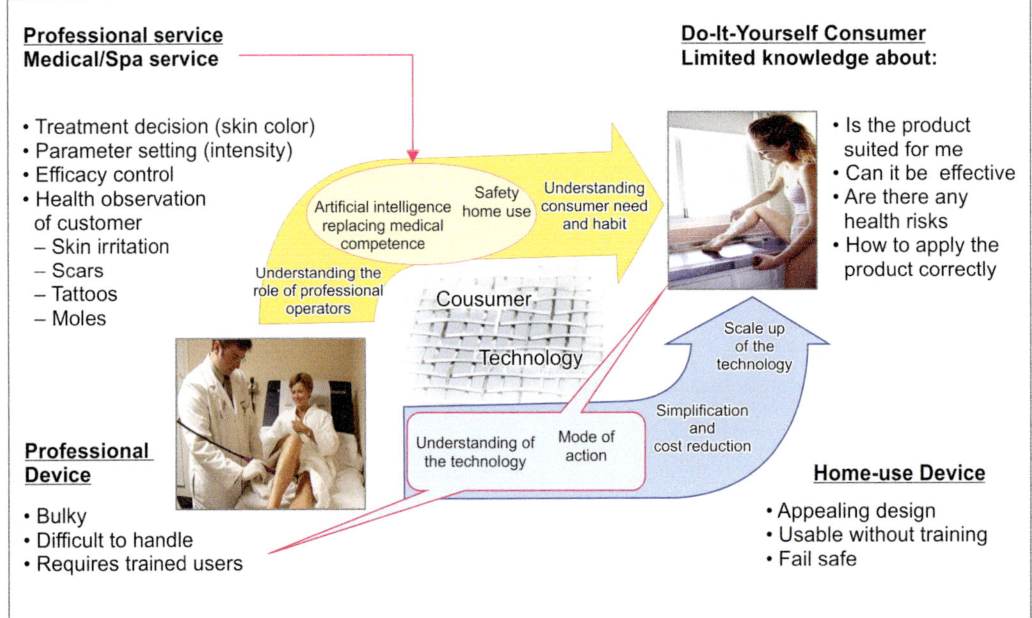

FIG. 2: Democratization of devices from professional administration to home use.

on understanding the technology and mode of action. The reasons include:

- *Device design:*
  - Safety features can be engineered into the device, e.g., pigmentometer or contact sensor, to minimize adverse events when used by unskilled consumer.
  - Esthetic qualities and usability can be designed with user input, e.g., human factors data.
- *Manufacturing:*
  - Simplification, cost reduction, and scale-up are best achieved when the technology and mode of action are known, and engineering can be directed and optimized with minimal impact on efficacy and safety.

In the end, the movement of energy-based treatments from physician's office into the hands of the consumer is dependent on the safety and efficacy of such devices when there is no oversight in the use and foreseeable misuse. This is an evolutionary process shaped by numerous variables including consumer demand and desires, technology advances, and competition. This is most evident in hair removal device segment where light-based devices have become faster, lighter and more elegant in their design since first introduced several years earlier.

REGULATORY AND SAFETY CONSIDERATIONS FOR HOME-USE DEVICES

The regulatory framework for energy-based devices used for cosmetic benefits such as skin rejuvenation, acne and hair removal or growth, varies from country to country. For example, in the United States, the Food and Drug Administration (FDA) regulates such technology as a "medical device" which requires a certain degree of premarket review and approval before selling to consumers. While this is true for other parts of the world, e.g., South Korea, Canada, it is not universal and independent of the technology and potential benefits. Regardless, it is the responsibility of the manufacturer to ensure devices are safe for consumer use.

Devices and the technology within, e.g., laser, radiofrequency, etc., are subject to "standards" that have been written by experts in fields such as engineering, health physics, and occupational health. The preeminent organization responsible for electrotechnology standards is the International Electrotechnical Commission (IEC), a nonprofit, nongovernmental international body which publishes requirements covering an immense range of items from home appliances to fiber optics to solar panels used for heating water or generating electricity. The regulatory classification, e.g., medical device or household appliance, will partly determine which standards are applicable. In most cases, devices are evaluated by independent National/International recognized testing laboratories, e.g., Intertek, UL, to ensure compliance with relevant standards. There are labels that appear on devices that designate such certification.

Device standards are not in place to explicitly protect consumers but, in effect do so. For example, exposure limits/thresholds to protect the eyes from light emitted by lasers are used for classification which ultimately impacts if such a device can be marketed to consumers or requires personal protective equipment, e.g., safety glasses. The threshold-based classification of lasers is based on calculations of retinal damage and independent of the end-user, i.e., laboratory versus industrial versus home-use. Such standards are updated by IEC committees and working groups.[15] As well, there are other groups such as International Organization for Standardization (ISO) which helps to develop quality systems for the manufacturing of devices. For example, ISO standards for "biocompatibility" are in place such that the material used to construct a home-use device is suited for the parts of the human body it touches. Likewise, the software, electrical circuitry and certain safety interlock systems are evaluated and certified according to specific standards. Finally, there are ISO standards that systematize "quality assurance" throughout the entire manufacturing process, including post-market surveillance. Collectively, these rules are in place to ensure the device will be safe for consumer use within the universe of possible environments.

Beyond standards, there is the need for ensuring that exposure to the energy emitted by the device has an acceptable adverse event profile. In most cases, this is part of the product risk assessment evaluating the foreseeable use of such technology. For example, understanding the interaction between light and skin at various wavelengths and fluences is critical when evaluating the safety profile and predicting possible adverse events.[16-18] The expected adverse event profile of a given technology, e.g., laser hair removal, nonablative fractional skin rejuvenation, is often based on what has been reported from professional use.[17,19-21] As well, mandatory adverse event reporting such as the FDA Manufacturer and User Facility Device Experience (MAUDE) provide "safety signals" from in-market exposure which together with premarket evaluations can be used to confirm the suitability of a given device.[22] Finally, in the case of light-based hair removal, there are guidelines on "best practices",[23] which may serve as a principle-based approach for other home-use treatment benefits.

HOME-USE DEVICE TREATMENTS

Hair Removal

Hair removal and growth reduction by light energy are based on thermal effects on hair follicles by selective photothermolysis.

Mode of Action

As stated, laser/light hair removal is based on the theory of photothermolysis.[24] Light energy of the appropriate wavelength and pulse duration is preferentially absorbed by melanin, the target chromophore, which is concentrated in the hair follicle. The hair and the tissue immediately surrounding it are heated to temperatures that stimulate denaturing of proteins in the hair follicle cells and stem cells in the bulge area. Unlike professional hair removal where the light intensity causes the tissue of the hair follicle to undergo necrosis, after home-use treatments the hair follicle is exposed to lower fluence of light which produces a transition from the anagen phase to the catagen. This results in the loss of the treated hair and delays or inhibits the growth of new hair. Due to the fact that the light is absorbed by the melanin, only hair/hair follicles containing melanin can be effectively treated. Blonde, red and white hair respond poorly or not at all to light-based hair growth reduction procedures.

Hair follicles contain greatest concentrations of melanin during the anagen phase. As such, hair in catagen and telogen phases respond weakly to the light treatment. Moreover, in either professional or home-use settings, multiple treatments are required to get to a "hair free" state because hair growth in humans is not synchronized. Further, because home-use devices use lower fluence and act by converting hair from anagen to catagen, users must treat areas of the skin continuous in order to keep the hair from growing.

Technology

As stated, selective photothermolysis is the mode of action and, as such, the technology used for generation of the light should provide the selectivity to stimulate only the hair follicle and bulge area and keep the rest of the skin tissue unaffected. There are two parameters of the light source that assure such selectivity, namely the proper selection of the wavelength or wavelength range and the duration of the light pulse.

Wavelengths used for selective photothermolysis are in the range of 600–1,100 nm. Within this wavelength range, light energy absorption by melanin is high, while absorption by tissue water and blood hemoglobin is low. In the dermis, melanin is present in the hair shaft and follicle only. Therefore, the heating effect is limited to the hair and by heat conduction to its immediate surroundings. The pulse duration should not be much longer than the thermal relaxation time of hair follicles, i.e., 10–60 ms, otherwise too much heat will be conducted to the tissue surrounding the hair and cause injury. Pulse durations of 20–150 ms are expected to provide optimal results.

To achieve the desired stimulation of the hair follicles, the fluence of the light should be in the range of 2–10 J/cm^2 for home-use devices, which is significantly lower than the typical fluence used for permanent hair removal of commercial professional devices, i.e., up to 100 J/cm^2.[25] To generate a light pulse with the intensity between 2 and 10 J/cm^2, most current home-use devices use Xenon arc flash bulbs, i.e., IPL. Treatment areas of known devices are in the range between 50 and 600 mm^2. The whole area is treated at once by an expanded laser light beam or IPL beam. With some systems, the treatment area is scanned by a laser beam of 3–8 mm diameter.

Efficacy and Safety

Thaysen-Petersen et al.[1] and more recently Hession et al.[2] reviewed the efficacy and safety of home-use light-based hair removal devices. Thaysen-Petersen reported one controlled (CT) and six uncontrolled trials (UCTs). No randomized controlled trials (RCT) were recognized at this time. The best evidence for hair removal efficacy was found for IPL devices (three devices, one CT, five UCTs) and some evidence for laser devices (one diode laser, one UCT). Importantly, there was evidence in support of short-term hair removal efficacy of currently available home-use light-based hair removal devices.[1]

Since the review of Thaysen-Petersen, a study by Wheeland reported "permanent" hair removal with 810 nm diode in CT of 13 subjects up to 1 year after treatment.[26] As well, Thaysen-Petersen et al.[27] reported an RCT for hair removal for a home-use device. In this study, 36 women randomized to no treatment up to 8 treatments with 810 nm diode laser in axillary region. Sustained usage of low-fluence laser induced a stable reduction of growing hair counts, thickness, and color. The reduction was reversible, and hairs regrew beyond baseline values after cessation of usage. Computer-aided image analysis was qualified for quantification of hair counts, thickness and color after laser epilation.[27]

The adverse event profile of home-use hair removal devices is consistent with that for professional devices and has been shown to be dependent on the melanin content in the skin.[28,29] As such, the darker the skin type, i.e., greater the concentration of melanin, the more likely adverse events might be observed. However, the current home-use hair removal devices are operated at relatively low fluences and the frequency and severity of adverse health effects appears to be tolerated by consumers. Moreover, the uses of onboard pigmentometers that adjust fluence have improved the safety profile of these devices. Nonetheless, it will be important to continue in-market monitoring of health effects not only those that might be anticipated, e.g., erythema, pigmentary changes, but also rare events, e.g., paradoxical or possibly low-fluence hair growth in darker skin types, urticaria, to ensure the safe use of such devices.

Hair Growth

Beside the wish of consumers to get rid of body hair, there is also a tremendous desire to increase hair growth on the scalp for people suffering from hair loss. For several years, laser and light emitting diode (LED) devices have been in the market claiming increase of hair growth.

Mode of Action

Treatment of hair loss with light goes back to 1968 when Endre Mester[30] detected increased hair growth by accident when he irradiated shaved mice with a 694 nm ruby laser. Since then several studies have been performed to understand the effect and to define an efficient treatment regimen. The hypothesized mode of action is based on photobiomodulation, previously referred to as low level light therapy (LLLT). It has been available for many years and been investigated with mixed levels of scientific enthusiasm.[4,5,31] The mode of action of LLLT or photobiomodulation to induce hair growth is not entirely understood. This fact makes the clinical findings difficult to understand. Nevertheless, the leading hypothesis is that exposure to light at the optimal wavelength increases the generation of ATP inside the mitochondria thus increasing the vitality of the irradiated cells.[32] The optimal wavelength of such a treatment is between 635 and 670 nm. The light intensity for the most favorable treatment outcome is in the range of ~10 mW delivering a total fluence of 1–10 J/cm^2. Higher fluence during single treatments will cause cell damage via generation of reactive oxygen species (ROS), which destroys the inner cell membrane and ultimately reverses the effect, i.e., no hair growth. A more detailed description of the mode of action can be found elsewhere.[14] Based on this hypothesis, treatment with light to increase hair growth can only work while thin and fine hair is still growing. Skin without terminal hair cannot be reactivated via photobiomodulation to grow hair.

Technology

For consumer use, there are generally two types of devices in the market, brush devices, and wearable helmets/hats. The technology of both devices is equivalent. An array of medium power laser diodes or LEDs with an output power of 0.5–10 mW each is arranged to irradiate the scalp. The brush-like devices have one or more rows of light emitters irradiating the scalp through or in between the teeth of the comb. To achieve the fluence required for efficient treatment the consumer uses the light comb 3–4 times a week for a duration of about 20 min. The helmet/hat devices improve the time-consuming light application and, in theory, improve compliance. The light emitter array is designed inside the helmet to irradiate the whole scalp at a time. Each light emitter typically generates lower light output power which is compensated by a higher number of emitters.

Efficacy and Safety

All home-use devices are designed to emit light with a radiance below the limit which is harmful for the eye. The devices are, therefore, inherently eye safe. Other safety risks, e.g., skin irritation, itching, etc., have not been identified for exposure to the red light. The efficacy of the devices has been demonstrated in several RCTs and some of the devices are sold in the US following FDA clearance. As reviewed by Zarei et al.[4] there are 5 RCTs among 12 clinical studies evaluating multiple devices that emitted red light, 635–685 nm, 5 mW power. In the 5 RCTs, improvements in overall hair regrowth, slowing hair loss, and thicker feeling hair were reported. Based on this review on all the available evidence about effect of LLLT in alopecia,[33] the FDA-cleared devices appear to be both safe and effective in patients with male and female pattern hair loss who did not respond or were not tolerant of standard hair-loss treatments. In an animal model of chemotherapy hair loss,[34] exposure to LLLT accelerates hair regrowth. This may be an important application of this technology for a compromised patient population.

In general, LLLT has very few adverse events reported from clinical studies. The skin response to such low fluences is minimal. The potential for ocular damage with currently marketed devices is negligible. It is possible with newer arrays and attempts to push the clinical response, such events, i.e., skin and eye effects, may emerge. Beyond hair growth, i.e., wound healing or skin rejuvenation, there is an absence of RCT and robust clinical studies to support efficacy.

Skin Rejuvenation/Wrinkle Reduction Around the Eye

This may be the area in which consumers are most desperate to have truly efficacious and tolerable (safe) treatment options for home-use. First, there are multiple benefit areas as summarized in **Box 1**. Fine/deep lines and wrinkles, pores, skin tone/age spots and sagginess are all common complaints. Second, there are countless topically applied cosmetic products that claim benefits treating one or more of these complaints with little or no evidence of a notable effect, except, perhaps for topical retinoids. Finally, the benefit of dermatological-based procedures using devices has made skin rejuvenation a fertile market and, as such, there exists a variety of home-use devices claiming benefits.

Technologies in the market include fractional laser, radiofrequency, photobiomodulation with red, green, and yellow light, and electrophoresis. The following text will concentrate on fractional laser and radiofrequency devices. Devices using photobiomodulation of any light color and

BOX 1: Benefits areas for devices.

- **Fine lines, wrinkles, and pores:** Reduced thickness of the dermis (reduction of collagen and elastin)
- **Deep wrinkles:**
  - Jowl lines, nasolabial fold: Reorganization of fat compartments in the face and thinning of skin
  - Neck wrinkles: Actinic elastosis (photo aging: accumulation of abnormal elastin in the dermis of the skin as a result of prolonged and excessive sun exposure)
- **Sagging:** Thinning skin with reduced content of elastin and collagen accompanied with re-organization of fat compartments in the face
- Skin tone homogeneity and age spots (Lentigines seniles/solares)
  Malfunction of melanocytes, over-generating melanin deposited close to the skin surface

electrophoresis are not part of the following due to the fact that RCT or controlled clinical studies with these technologies are largely unavailable and visible improvements of skin have not yet been demonstrated clinically.

Mode of Action

The mode of action for skin rejuvenation either in the professional or home-use setting makes use of the wound healing and heat shock response of the skin.[35-37] This skin response is initiated by ablative and nonablative thermolysis removing or damaging parts of the epidermis thermally via light, e.g., IPL, widened laser beams, or ultrasound and radiofrequency application. The skin reacts with the natural healing response of the body increasing the growth of fibroblasts and generating new collagen-rich tissue. The ablative technologies have been used in professional setting only, due to the severity of the skin wounds, long healing process and risk of infections. That changed in 2004 with the introduction of nonablative fractional technologies, e.g., fractional photothermolysis, by Manstein and colleagues.[38] This was a breakthrough which dramatically improved the treatment method by reducing significantly the infection risk, treatment pain, and recovery time.[37-39] Fractional technologies are treating only small spot-like sections of the face, in general about 5–20% of the skin surface, which is sufficient to initiate the intended regrowth of collagen in the dermis without producing widespread damage in the tissue. Home-use devices typically use lower energy and reduced treatment densities, i.e., only about 1% of the surface, compared to the professional devices.

Technology

There have been devices in the market for home-use utilizing nonablative factional photothermolysis. These devices generate laser light at a wavelength around 1,400 nm with medium power laser diodes. The light is focused to a spot with a diameter of around 100 μm just below the skin level. A scanner inside the device moves the focal spot in a line pattern for devices working in sliding motion and in a rectangular pattern for pick and place devices. The laser light at 1,400 nm is absorbed by the water in the skin. The tissue inside the beam profile is heated to a temperature sufficient to cause localized denaturation of the proteins and initiating the wound healing effect. Visible skin improvements can be identified with repeated application after about 3 months.

Radiofrequency (RF) devices generate a low-voltage high-frequency alternating current through the epidermis and dermis. The frequency is typically set to a value of 1 MHz, because the frequency defines the penetration depth of the current. With 1 MHz the penetration depth is optimal for reaching the targeted dermis. The alternating current heats up the skin below the device up to a temperature of 43–45°C. This causes a heat shock response of the skin,[40] which initiates a restructuring and growth of collagen leading to a skin tightening effect.

Both technologies cause some discomfort during the treatment and are therefore not yet widely spread and typically only used for small skin areas like for wrinkle reduction around the eye and the forehead.

Efficacy and Safety

There are no RCTs for either nonablative fractional or RF home-use devices. In one controlled clinical study, at total of 126 subjects, Pilot study $n = 36$; Pivotal study $n = 90$, subjects had daily treatments around the eyes for 4 weeks followed by twice/week for 4 weeks (Pilot) or 12 weeks (Pivotal) using 1,410 nm nonablative laser with 9 × 13 mm treatment window.[41] A blinded review of digital images and self-assessment were done. Self-applications by users demonstrated the utility of the device for home-use. Independent blinded review of clinical images confirmed the device's proficiency for improving periorbital wrinkles.

The home-use of radiofrequency device has not been reported in the literature. Professionally, this technology is used to treat skin laxity and rhytides although like other such treatments there is a need for RCTs.[42]

Presently, there are few studies systematically evaluating the tolerability and safety of skin rejuvenation technologies. By and large, the knowledge comes from clinical studies and reports presented at scientific meetings. There is a report by Richters et al.[43] that describes a subset of consumers treating the face, i.e., periorbital, with a nonablative fractional device who are sensitive to this treatment. The sensitive subjects report frequent discomfort when using the device compared to nonsensitive subjects. While this is only a single report, it raises an important point for all home-use devices, namely the response of subpopulations that may be refractory to the treatment or have exaggerated adverse event profiles. While either issue may be overcome, it is critical to address such findings to maintain consumer confidence.

Acne

Acne is a common skin disorder affecting millions of people worldwide. It is a multifactorial condition which presents as lesions, i.e., whiteheads, blackheads, inflamed pustules, resulting from: (1) an inflammatory response, (2) proliferation of *Propionibacterium acne* or *P. acnes*, (3) increased sebum production, and (4) cornification of the pilosebaceous duct.[44] Treatments generally target one or more of these events with the hope of preventing the appearance, speeding resolution of the lesion or both.

Mode of Action

Blue light has been reported to have bactericidal effects. *P. acnes* produces mainly coproporphyrin III, which has a very intense absorption spectrum peak at 415 nm and others around 625 nm and 805 nm, which are much lower. These could act as targets for a photodynamic reaction following irradiation with visible light in the blue or red/infrared spectrum. Due to the extremely effective cross-section of the blue light and as higher intensity blue light LEDs have become available and cost-effective in the last 10 years, there has been a significant growth in blue light research and devices. In vitro irradiation of *P. acnes* colonies with visible blue light has been shown to lead to photoexcitation of endogenous bacterial porphyrins, singlet oxygen production, and subsequent bacterial destruction.[45,46] In an animal model of acne, exposure to blue light was reported to reduce *P. acnes* and subsequent inflammation.[47]

Technology

There are two types of devices in the market for treating acne. Devices with xenon flash lamps for treatments of single acne lesions and blue LED (410 nm) devices for treating an area of up to 3 cm^2 at a time. Both technologies suffer from drawbacks of the technology, which limits use of the devices by the consumer.

The skin has very high absorption of the blue light, therefore the intensity of the light reaching the porphyrin and thus the *P. acnes* bacteria is low. Increase in the intensity of the light source is limited due to the heating of the skin by this absorption. Consequently, the treatment time to achieve the desired effect goes up to about 30 min for one full face treatment.

The flashlight devices target either the blue absorption band or the red/infrared absorption band. With each flash of the light source one acne lesion are irradiated. As such, treating all acne lesions, i.e., full face, has to be irradiated one after the other which also takes a significant amount of time. Thus, even when consumers see beneficial effects of the treatment, they may be unwilling to spend this amount of time every other day, particularly when conventional chemistries, i.e., salicylic acid or benzoyl peroxide, take much less time to administer.

Efficacy and Safety

In the Cochrane Database of Systematic Reviews, Barbaric et al. reviewed light therapies for acne in 2016. In this exhaustive and comprehensive review of light therapies in the treatment of acne, the authors concluded "High-quality evidence on the use of light therapies for people with acne is lacking".[3] This review of 71 studies with 4,211 participants including photodynamic therapies as randomized controlled trails carefully considered this complex landscape including self-assessment of outcomes. While such a conclusion is disappointing, it should not discourage further investigations which were recommended by Barbaric et al. and supported by the presumed mode of action and evidence of a small number of existing clinical studies.

There are two noteworthy RCTs evaluating the efficacy of home-use light based devices in the treatment of acne. Kwon et al. investigated the efficacy of 420 nm blue light and 660 nm red light for 2.5 minutes twice per day for 4 weeks in 35 patients with mild-to-moderate acne.[48] The authors report a significant decrease in both inflammatory and noninflammatory lesions 8 weeks after the final treatment. In the study by Ash et al., 41 adults with mild-to-moderate acne were treated with blue light, 220 J over 12.5 cm^2, every other day for 8 weeks.[49] Importantly, in this study, subjects used cleanser containing lactic, salicylic and glycolic acid, daily. There was a 50% reduction in inflammatory lesions, onset by week 3 of treatment reaching a maximum effectiveness at 8 and 12 weeks in the study. The authors concluded that non-thermal blue light in conjunction with cleansers can improve acne.

There are several clinical studies investigating the clinical efficacy of blue light using home-use devices.[50-52] In each case, an improvement in noninflammatory and inflammatory lesions was reported. As well, the adverse event profile reported was minimal and consistent with other nonprescription treatments.

CONCLUSION

There are many home-use devices marketed for treating a variety of hair and skin conditions. It is likely that this trend will continue and expand. Light-based hair removal is the most developed technology based on availability of devices and data supportive of efficacy and safety. The area of photobiomodulation and LLLT has gained "credibility" based on published RCTs showing efficacy. However, there remain several questions regarding the mode of action which hampers the widespread acceptance. For skin rejuvenation and acne treatment, there remains a paucity of data supporting benefit of such device technology, although it is likely that efforts in these areas will continue. The democratization of technologies from dermatological offices/clinics is anchored in fundamental principles of safety, first, followed closely by noticeable and measurable efficacy demonstrated in randomized controlled trials.

FUTURE DIRECTIONS

There are numerous opportunities and areas of investigation which are likely to develop on parallel tracks. In developed technologies of hair removal and growth, there is a need to better understand treatment regimens that maximize efficacy of such treatments. The current approach for light-based hair removal, i.e., once per week for 4–6 weeks, followed by monthly maintenance, is largely empirical following the approach used in clinical practice and demonstrated in clinical testing. However, dose-fractionation, threshold and frequency of application are largely unknown. While these may seem "academic" questions, in reality this knowledge will lead to safer and more effective treatments which could become the most prominent method to control hair growth. As well, treatment of blonde, red and white hair, male facial hair, and use by all skin types, i.e., including Fitzpatrick Skin Types V and VI, are areas of interest for home-use light-based hair removal.

A clear understanding of the mode of action of LLLT (photobiomodulation) and hair growth will help to improve current methods of delivery which are less than convenient at this point in time. Such an understanding may expand the use of LLLT beyond hair regrowth and perhaps fulfill the potential of this technology.

There are other forms of energy which one might expect to gravitate toward home use. Beyond radiofrequency, there are devices using high-focused ultrasound for full face skin rejuvenation. Again, such technologies seem to make it into consumers' hands with limited data available in the public domain.

It is conceivable that the biggest break-through in home-use devices is the cost, both to manufacturer and consumer. The improvement in LED technology makes for specific delivery of energy at a reduced cost and higher efficiency, i.e., reduction in heat loss. The reduced cost of home-use devices might make it likely that consumers will "take a chance" on a given technology. Such cost savings will, as well, bring more manufacturers into the fray which could mean more savings for consumers.

While it is intriguing to consider the universe of possibilities when it comes to home-use technologies, the reality is that regulatory safety and demonstrated efficacy are at the core of any device.

REFERENCES

1. Thaysen-Petersen D, Bjerring P, Dierickx C, Nash JF, Town G, Haedersdal M. A systematic review of light-based home-use devices for hair removal and considerations on human safety. J Eur Acad Dermatol Venereol. 2012;26:545-53.
2. Hession MT, Markova A, Graber EM. A review of hand-held, home-use cosmetic laser and light devices. Dermatol Surg. 2015;41:307-20.
3. Barbaric J, Abbott R, Posadzki P, Car M, Gunn LH, Layton AM, et al. Light therapies for acne. Cochrane Database Syst Rev. 2016;9(9): CD007917.
4. Zarei M, Wikramanayake TC, Falto-Aizpurua L, Schachner LA, Jimenez JJ. Low level laser therapy and hair regrowth: an evidence-based review. Lasers Med Sci. 2016;31:363-71.
5. Gupta AK, Foley KA. A critical assessment of the evidence for low-level laser therapy in the treatment of hair loss. Dermatol Surg. 2017; 43:188-97.
6. Geronemus RG. 2006. Fractional photothermolysis: current and future applications. Lasers Surg Med. 2006;38:169-76.
7. Nelson AA, Lask GP. Principles and practice of cutaneous laser and light therapy. Clin Plast Surg. 2011;38:427-36, vi.

8. Alexiades-Armenakas MR, Dover JS, Arndt KA. Fractional laser skin resurfacing. J Drug Dermatol. 2012;11:1274-87.
9. Anderson RR, Parrish JA. Selective photothermolysis: precise microsurgery by selective absorption of pulsed radiation. Science. 1983; 220:524-7.
10. Altshuler GB, Anderson RR, Manstein D, Zenzie HH, Smirnov MZ. Extended theory of selective photothermolysis. Lasers Surg Med. 2001;29(5):416-32.
11. Astner S, Anderson RR. Treating vascular lesions. Dermatol Ther. 2005;18:267-81.
12. Passarella S, Karu T. Absorption of monochromatic and narrow band radiation in the visible and near IR by both mitochondrial and non-mitochondrial photoacceptors results in photobiomodulation This paper is devoted to the memory of Prof. Lorenzo Bolognani who was one of the pioneers in the field of photobiomodulation. J Photochem Photobiol B. 2014;140:344-58.
13. Mignon C. Botchkareva NV, Uzunbajakava NE, Tobin DJ. Photobiomodulation devices for hair regrowth and wound healing: a therapy full of promise but a literature full of confusion. Experiment Dermatol. 2016;25:745-9.
14. Sawhney MK, Hamblin MR. Low-level laser (light) therapy for cosmetics and dermatology. In: Handbook of Low-Level Laser Therapy. New York: Jenny Stanford Publishing; 2016.
15. Town G, Gorisch W. International progress in standards and regulation for light based home use devices. The World's Leading Conference on Laser Safety, ILSC 2013. Louisiana: International Laser Safety Conference; 2013. pp. 63-9.
16. Nash JF, Ward M, Ahluwalia GS. Dermal Safety of Laser and Light-Based Systems. In: Ahluwalia GS (Ed). Cosmetic Applications of Laser and Light-Based Systems. Norwich: William Andrew Inc.; 2009.
17. Wanner M, Sakamoto FH, Avram MM, Anderson RR. Immediate skin responses to laser and light treatments Warning endpoints: How to avoid side effects. J Am Acad Dermatol. 2016;74:807-19.
18. Wanner M, Sakamoto FH, Avram MM, Chan HH, Alam M, Tannous Z, et al. Immediate skin responses to laser and light treatments Therapeutic endpoints: How to obtain efficacy. J Am Acad Dermatol. 2016;74:821-33.
19. Wheeland RG. 1997. Laser-assisted hair removal. Dermatol Clin. 1997;15:469-77.
20. Graber EM, Tanzi EL, Alster TS. 2008. Side effects and complications of fractional laser photothermolysis: experience with 961 treatments. Dermatol Surg. 2008;34: 301-7.
21. Hwang YJ, Lee YN, Lee YW, Choe YB, Ahn KJ. Treatment of acne scars and wrinkles in Asian patients using carbon-dioxide fractional laser resurfacing: its effects on skin biophysical profiles. Ann Dermatol. 2013;25:445-53.
22. Tremaine AM, Avram MM. FDA MAUDE data on complications with lasers, light sources, and energy-based devices. Lasers Surg Med. 2015;47:133-40.
23. Town G, Ash C, Dierickx C, Fritz K, Bjerring P, Haedersdal M. Guidelines on the safety of light-based home-use hair removal devices from the European Society for Laser Dermatology. J Eur Acad Dermatol Venereol. 2012;26:799-811.
24. Lask G, Eckhouse S, Slatkine M, Waldman A, Kreindel M, Gottfried V. The role of laser and intense light sources in photo-epilation: a comparative evaluation. J Cutan Laser Ther. 1999;1:3-13.
25. Haedersdal M, Gotzsche PC. Laser and photoepilation for unwanted hair growth. Cochrane Database Syst Rev. 2006;CD004684.
26. Wheeland RG. Permanent hair reduction with a home-use diode laser: Safety and effectiveness 1 year after eight treatments. Lasers Surg Med. 2012;44:550-7.
27. Thaysen-Petersen D, Barbet-Pfeilsticker M, Beerwerth F, Nash JF, Philipsen PA, Staubach P, et al. Quantitative assessment of growing hair counts, thickness and colour during and after treatments with a low-fluence, home-device laser: a randomized controlled trial. British J Dermatol. 2015;172:151-9.
28. Thaysen-Petersen D, Lin JY, Nash J, Beerwerth F, Wulf HC, Philipsen PA, et al. The role of natural and UV-induced skin pigmentation on low-fluence IPL-induced side effects: a randomized controlled trial. Lasers Surg Med. 2014;46:104-11.
29. Thaysen-Petersen D, Erlendsson AM, Nash JF, Beerwerth F, Philipsen PA, Wulf HC, et al. Side effects from intense pulsed light: Importance of skin pigmentation, fluence level and ultraviolet radiation-A randomized controlled trial. Lasers Surg Med. 2017;49:88-96.
30. Mester E, Szende B, Gartner P. The effect of laser beams on the growth of hair in mice. Radiobiol Radiother (Berl). 1968;9:621-6.
31. Moskvin SV. Low-level laser therapy in Russia: history, science and practice. J Lasers Med Sci. 2017;8:56-65.
32. Karu TI. Mitochondrial signaling in mammalian cells activated by red and near-IR radiation. Photochem Photobiol. 2008;84:1091-9.
33. Afifi L, Maranda EL, Zarei M, Delcanto GM, Falto-Aizpurua L, Kluijfhout WP, et al. Low-level laser therapy as a treatment for androgenetic alopecia. Laser Surg Med. 2017;49(1):27-39.
34. Wikramanayake TC, Villasante AC, Mauro LM, Nouri K, Schachner LA, Perez CI, et al. Low-level laser treatment accelerated hair regrowth in a rat model of chemotherapy-induced alopecia (CIA). Lasers Med Sci. 2013;28:701-6.
35. Ross R, Odland G. Human wound repair. II. Inflammatory cells, epithelial-mesenchymal interrelations, and fibrogenesis. J Cell Biol. 1968; 39:152-68.

36. Laubach HJ, Tannous Z, Anderson RR, Manstein D. Skin responses to fractional photothermolysis. Lasers Surg Med. 2006;38:142-9.
37. Helbig D, Moebius A, Simon J.C, Paasch U. Nonablative skin rejuvenation devices and the role of heat shock protein 70: results of a human skin explant model. J Biomed Opt. 2010;15:038002.
38. Manstein D, Herron GS, Sink RK, Tanner H, Anderson RR. Fractional photothermolysis: a new concept for cutaneous remodeling using microscopic patterns of thermal injury. Lasers Surg Med. 2004;34:426-38.
39. Tierney EP, Kouba DJ, Hanke CW. Review of fractional photothermolysis: treatment indications and efficacy. Dermatol Surg. 2009;35: 1445-61.
40. Tanaka Y, Tsunemi Y, Kawashima M, Tatewaki N, Nishida H. Treatment of skin laxity using multisource, phase-controlled radiofrequency in Asians: visualized 3-dimensional skin tightening results and increase in elastin density shown through histologic investigation. Dermatol Surg. 2014;40:756-62.
41. Leyden J, Stephens TJ, Herndon JH. 2012. Multicenter clinical trial of a home-Use nonablative fractional laser device for wrinkle reduction. J Am Acad Dermatol. 2012;67:975-84.
42. Lolis MS, Goldberg DJ. Radiofrequency in cosmetic dermatology: a review. Dermatol Surg. 2012;38:1765-76.
43. Richters RJ, Hoogedoorn L, Uzunbajakava NE, Janssen LD, Tom Nuijs AM, van Erp PE. Clinical, biophysical, immunohistochemical, and in vivo reflectance confocal microscopy evaluation of the response of subjects with sensitive skin to home-use fractional non-ablative photothermolysis device. Lasers Surg Med. 2016;48: 474-82.
44. Suh DH, Kwon HH. 2015. What's new in the physiopathology of acne? Br J Dermatol, 2015; 172(Suppl 1):13-9.
45. Ashkenazi H, Malik Z, Harth Y, Nitzan Y. Eradication of *Propionibacterium acnes* by its endogenic porphyrins after illumination with high intensity blue light. FEMS Immunol Med Microbiol. 2003;35:17-24.
46. Park YD, Lee KS. The effect of blue light on *Propionibacterium acnes* and the expression of inflammatory cytokines in HaCaT cells. Korean J Dermatol. 2009;47:1213-9.
47. Fan X, Xing YZ, Liu LH, Liu C, Wang DD, Yang RY, et al. Effects of 420-nm intense pulsed light in an acne animal model. J Eur Acad Dermatol Venereol. 2013;27(9):1168-71.
48. Kwon HH, Lee JB, Yoon JY, Park SY, Ryu HH, Park BM, el al. The clinical and histological effect of home-use, combination blue-red LED phototherapy for mild-to-moderate acne vulgaris in Korean patients: a double-blind, randomized controlled trial. Br J Dermatol. 2013;168;1088-94.
49. Ash C, Harrison A, Drew S, Whittall R. A randomized controlled study for the treatment of acne vulgaris using high-intensity 414 nm solid state diode arrays. J Cosmet Laser Ther. 2015;17:170-6.
50. Sadick NS, Laver Z, Laver L. Treatment of mild-to-moderate acne vulgaris using a combined light and heat energy device: home-use clinical study. J Cosmet Laser Ther. 2010;2:276-83.
51. Gold MH, Sensing W, Biron JA. Clinical efficacy of home-use blue-light therapy for mild-to moderate acne. J Cosmet Laser Ther. 2011;13:308-14.
52. Wheeland RG, Koreck A. Safety and effectiveness of a new blue light device for the self-treatment of mild-to-moderate acne. J Clin Aesthet Dermatol. 2012;5:25-31.

5

CHAPTER

Clinical Endpoints

Girish C Mohan, Molly Wanner

INTRODUCTION

Lasers are commonly used to treat a variety of conditions in dermatology. These devices typically induce immediate observable responses when treating the skin. These immediate laser-tissue reactions are referred to as clinical "endpoints" and are thought to be an indicator of treatment response. Depending on the type of laser and the target of the laser, different clinical endpoints may be seen. In this chapter, we will cover the desired, therapeutic endpoints that should be seen when treating skin with a variety of lasers, as well as the undesired, warning endpoints that practitioners should seek to avoid.[1,2]

Most of the lasers used in dermatology are directed at specific light-absorbing targets or chromophores, based on the theory of selective photothermolysis.[3,4] By using different wavelengths of light, different chromophores are selected. When the pulse of light from a laser source reaches the chromophore, heat is delivered. The target receives thermal energy, and this is ultimately what produces a reaction in the chromophore which is seen in the skin clinically as an endpoint. Generally, the pulse duration should be about equal or less than the time needed for a target to cool, called the thermal relaxation time. Chapter 2 discusses the mechanisms underlying selective photothermolysis in greater detail.

It should be noted however, that achieving a therapeutic endpoint does not guarantee the absence of adverse effects. Additionally, if the desired endpoint is not apparent, increase of fluence may not always be the solution, as many factors including pulse duration, skin type, and health of the patient can influence the laser-tissue reaction. Generally, setting the laser at the lowest fluence possible to achieve the therapeutic endpoint in absence of warning endpoints is recommended. Skin response endpoints are important to use because variation in skin pigmentation and sensitivity exists among patients and because calibration and output accuracy of devices can change over time. Awareness and careful observation for warning endpoints can minimize potential side effects from laser therapy.

ENDPOINTS IN TREATING VASCULAR LESIONS

The utilization of lasers and intense pulsed light (IPL) for vascular lesions is broad-ranging and includes telangiectasias, port-wine stains (capillary malformations), cherry angiomas and venous lakes. For the treatment of vascular lesions to be successful, pulses of light must be preferentially absorbed by oxyhemoglobin or deoxyhemoglobin. As the hemoglobin is thermally denatured, its iron atom becomes oxidized, and damage of vessel walls ensues. Lasers often used for treatment of vascular lesions include 532 nm KTP lasers, 585–595 nm pulsed dye lasers (PDLs), or near-infrared lasers (755 nm alexandrite, 800–810 nm diode lasers, 1,064 nm Nd:YAG).

When treating telangiectasias of any cause, including those seen in rosacea or telangiectasia as a result of photoaging, the desired therapeutic endpoints are either transient vessel darkening or vessel disappearance (**Fig. 1**). In addition to the lasers mentioned above, IPL can be used in this clinical scenario. Notably, treating to achieve purpura is not necessary here.[5] Thus, longer pulse durations are used when treating telangiectasia, typically from 10 to 50 ms.[6] Two different mechanisms lead to the clinical endpoints here. Transient vessel darkening is a product of the formation of methemoglobin when the iron atom of hemoglobin becomes oxidized. Immediate vessel disappearance occurs with higher fluences due to a photothermal effect that leads to contraction of blood plasma and collagen denaturation of the vessel wall from the delivered thermal energy and ultimately, clearing of blood from the vessel lumen which manifests clinically as vessel disappearance.[7] These same two endpoints are desired when treating spider veins with 1,064 nm Nd:YAG lasers (**Figs. 2A** to **C**).[8,9]

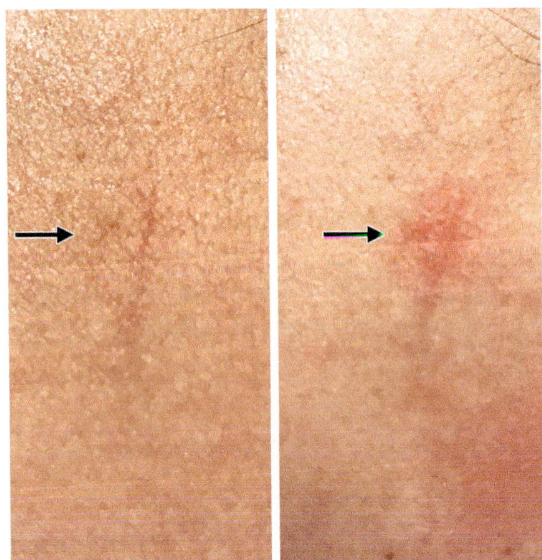

FIG. 1: Facial telangiectasia before and after treatment with PDL. Note the desired therapeutic endpoint of immediate vessel disappearance.

Cherry angiomas require a different therapeutic endpoint. The desired endpoint with these vascular lesions is the development of purpura. Vascular lasers with a short pulse duration are typically used to achieve this. The thermal energy delivered to the angioma, results in intravascular coagulation which leads to the appearance of purpura.[11] Similarly, venous lakes respond well to long pulsed (30 ms) diode lasers and 1,064 nm lasers with purpura of the venous lake. During treatments of venous lakes, sometimes a dull "pop" can be heard due to the creation of a steam bubble in the treatment area (**Figs. 3A** to **C**).[10,11]

Port-wine stains (capillary malformations) require the endpoint of purpura for effective treatment.[12-14] The thermal energy from the PDL causes blood to leak out of the damaged vessel walls, prompting the development of dark red-purple purpura.[15] Regions of persistent perfusion do exist even in areas that have developed purpura, and as such, purpura does not guarantee a complete clinical response and eradication of the port-wine stain.[16] Additionally it is important to ensure uniform purpuric response in the treated area, as creating an "egg-crate" pattern of purpura is not adequate. Typical PDL settings utilize a 7–10 mm spot size, with a fluence of 6–11 J/cm^2, and pulse duration of 0.4–3 ms. Of note, if the treating provider

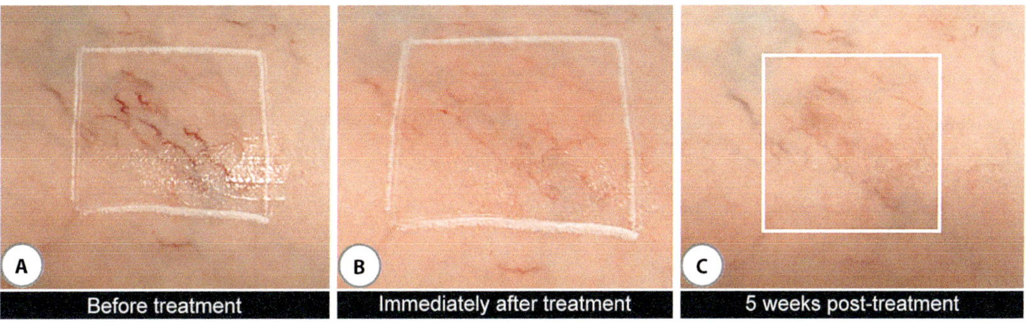

FIGS. 2A TO C: Leg spider veins treated with long pulsed 1064 nm Nd:YAG laser. Immediate vessel disappearance is the desired endpoint. 5 weeks posttreatment, the vessels are improved.

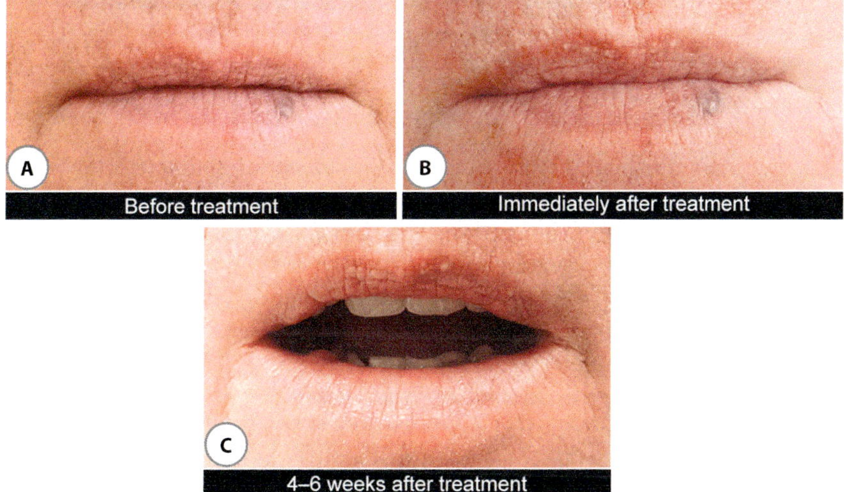

FIGS. 3A TO C: Venous lake treated with 810 nm diode laser with contact cooling. The desired endpoint is purpura.

is unable to achieve purpura with these settings, it may be prudent to pursue additional evaluation of the patient. For example, a mixed lymphatic malformation containing low levels of hemoglobin can be disguised clinically as a port-wine stain, or the patient may be anemic (and thus have low circulating hemoglobin, the chromophore of interest). Patients should be counseled that the purpura often darkens over the first 1–2 days posttreatment, with resolution over 7–14 days. If using the 755 nm alexandrite laser to penetrate deeper into hypertrophic stains or "resistant" stains, the correct endpoint is slightly different than that required by PDL: The lowest fluence that *subtly* causes purpura should be used. There is a narrow therapeutic window, since higher energies may cause ulcerations and scarring. Additionally, purpura of these lasers tends to be more blue-purple in color (**Figs. 4A** and **B**).[17,18]

Clinicians should be aware of a warning endpoint that is specific to lasers targeting the vasculature. If an metallic-gray

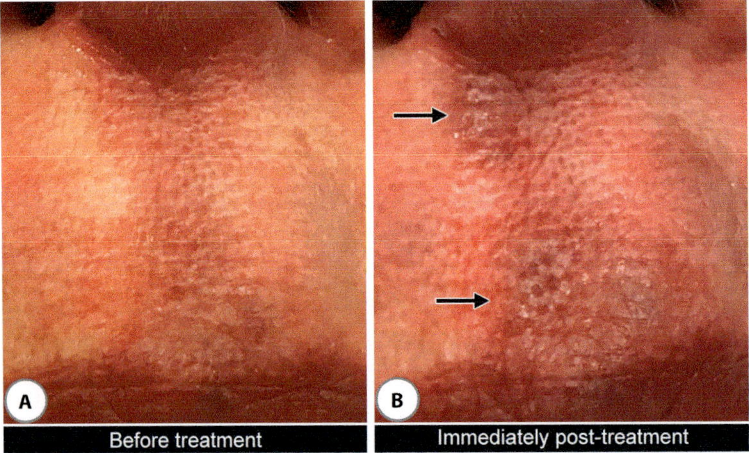

FIGS. 4A AND B: A port-wine stain treated with long pulsed 755 nm alexandrite laser (8 mm spot size, 60 J/cm^2, 3 ms pulse duration, DCD 60/40) before and immediately after treatment. Note the desired endpoint: A subtle uniform purpuric response in the treated area.

blanching of the vascular lesion treated is observed, this can indicate there has been overheating of the vessels with propagation of thermal energy into the surrounding dermis.[18] This can then progress to necrosis, ulceration, and scarring. If a gray discoloration is seen is seen, laser parameters should be adjusted. Only physicians with adequate laser experience and training should use 755 nm alexandrite lasers to treat vascular lesions due to their narrow therapeutic window.

ENDPOINTS IN TREATING PIGMENTED LESIONS

Therapeutic endpoints in treatment of benign lentigines vary with the type of laser device used. Use of lasers such as Q-switched 532, 694 and 755-nm devices operating at picosecond and nanosecond pulses with fluences ranging from 2 to 6 J/cm^2, elicits a desired endpoint of immediate whitening of the pigmented lesion. This whitening occurs because melanosomes are targeted and ruptured, cavitating and releasing gas bubbles into tissue.[19-24] The whitening fades over 3–20 minutes after the bubbles dissipate. Use of Q-switched picosecond or Q-switched 532 nm elicits the same immediate whitening, but also may elicit purpura or petechiae because hemoglobin is also absorbed at these wavelength (**Figs. 5A** and **B**).[25]

Long pulsed (millisecond) lasers or IPL can also treat lentigines, but the therapeutic endpoint in contrast is subtle darkening of the pigmented lesion, sometimes followed by erythema around the treatment area minutes later.[26-31] The darkening is a result of inducing necrotic pigmented cells in the epidermis, which continue to darken over the course of several days, after which the cells desquamate, leading to eradication of the pigmented lesion.[32] As such, PDL can be utilized; in this case, diascopy through a transparent window is the key, as firm pressure on the pigmented lesion will temporarily force blood out of the dermal vessels and remove hemoglobin as a competing target.[33] Thus, the lentigo will be isolated. As mentioned, the desired endpoint is subtle darkening or ash-gray color change of the pigmented lesion, usually apparent in minutes. These longer pulsed devices carry with them a lower risk of

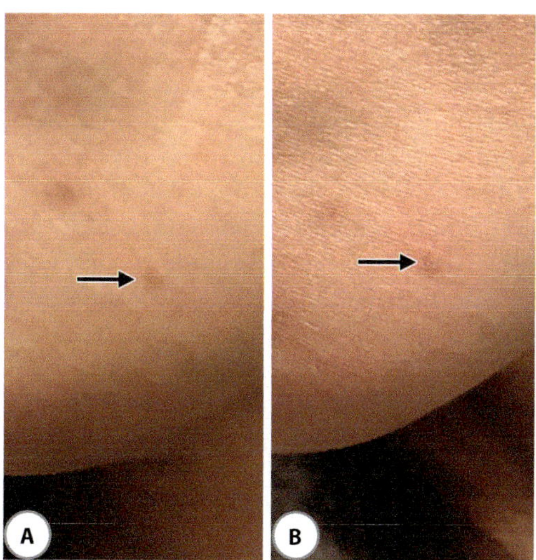

FIGS. 5A AND B: Lentigo—before and immediately after treatment with a Q-switched 755 nm laser. The desired endpoint is immediate whitening of the treatment area.

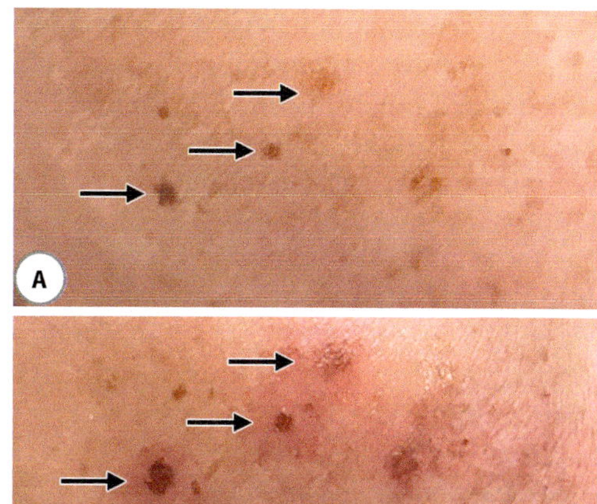

FIGS. 6A AND B: Lentigines treated with PDL (595 nm, no DCD, 1.5 ms, 9 J/cm^2), before and several minutes later. The immediate endpoint is subtle darkening of the lentigines. Erythema is present, but is not the desired endpoint. The erythema becomes more pronounced as time passes.

postinflammatory hyperpigmentation than picosecond and Q-switched lasers, especially when used in those with darker skin tones, such as Asian patients (**Figs. 6A** and **B**).[33]

The exception to treating pigmented lesions in Asian patients is Nevus of Ota (a type of dermal melanocytosis); in this setting, the appropriate choices are Q-switched lasers or picosecond 1064 nm lasers, which provide immediate dermal whitening of the lesional skin after treatment, with subsequent edema and erythema expected.[19,34,35] Purpura may also be incidentally seen.

With the use of picosecond Q-switched lasers, there is a specific warning endpoint to be wary of: chrysiasis. Using Q-switched lasers on a patient who has been treated at any time with gold causes immediate, gray-blue discoloration, termed chrysiasis. One way to preempt this is to obtain a thorough history of gold use in the patient before treatment, including using the drug name "aurothiomalate" (contains gold). Another useful pearl is to deliver a test pulse in a hidden area in any patient with a history of rheumatoid arthritis, to make certain there are no signs of chrysiasis.[36]

ENDPOINTS IN LASER HAIR REMOVAL

Laser hair removal employs melanin as the target in the hair follicle, ultimately causing irreversible damage to stem cells in the hair bulge, without damaging the overlying epidermis. Commonly used light sources include 694 nm ruby, 755 nm alexandrite, 810 nm diode, and 1,064 nm Nd:YAG lasers, at pulse durations of 3–100 ms. The IPL may also be used. Using longer pulse durations in that range will allow for thermal energy to propagate from the pigmented hair shaft to the nonpigmented stem cells and ultimately cause the requisite damage to these cells to initiate permanent hair loss. Shorter pulse durations are suitable for finer, thinner hairs.

The desired endpoint in laser hair removal, is the development of perifollicular erythema and edema a few minutes after treatment, which is correlated microscopically with an eosinophilic inflammatory reaction in response to injury of the hair follicle.[37-40] This endpoint is most easily observed in patients with lighter skin; in those with darker skin, side-lighting may be needed to observe this reaction (**Figs. 7A** and **B**). Vaporization or charring of actual intact hair shaft may occur but is neither a reliable nor a necessary endpoint to achieve permanent hair removal.[41]

There may be vaporization or charring of visible hair shafts, but there should be no such response in the skin. One must also remember to remove char from the window of the laser, or a burn to the skin could result. When a piece of charred hair adheres to a contact window device, energy is absorbed strongly by the charred tissue at each ensuing pulse and can subsequently cause a "stamping" burn pattern with each pulse.[1] The simple solution to avoid this is to clean the window before treatment and frequently during treatment, especially if charring of the hair shaft is seen.

ENDPOINTS IN TATTOO REMOVAL

Immediate dermal whitening in the tattoo-containing skin is the desired therapeutic endpoint when utilizing Q-switched or picosecond lasers for tattoo removal.[42-46] After the laser hits the tattoo pigment, small gas bubbles form in the dermis, causing the scatter of light and a white appearance; the tattoo itself may be raised by about 1 millimeter due to the volume of the gas bubbles engendered. The ensuing scatter of light may interfere with the efficacy of the laser itself, if a second pass is attempted over the immediate whitening; waiting about 20 minutes before the additional pass was shown in one study to be beneficial.[47] In successful tattoo removal, the pigment particles that are released by the delivery of thermal energy, are then shed in scale crust, taken away by an inflammatory response and/or repackaged into various dermal cells.[42,48,49]

It is important to note that tattoo removal should not be attempted by use of long pulsed (millisecond) laser, as there is a greater risk of diffusion of thermal energy into the dermis and subsequent scarring, because long pulse

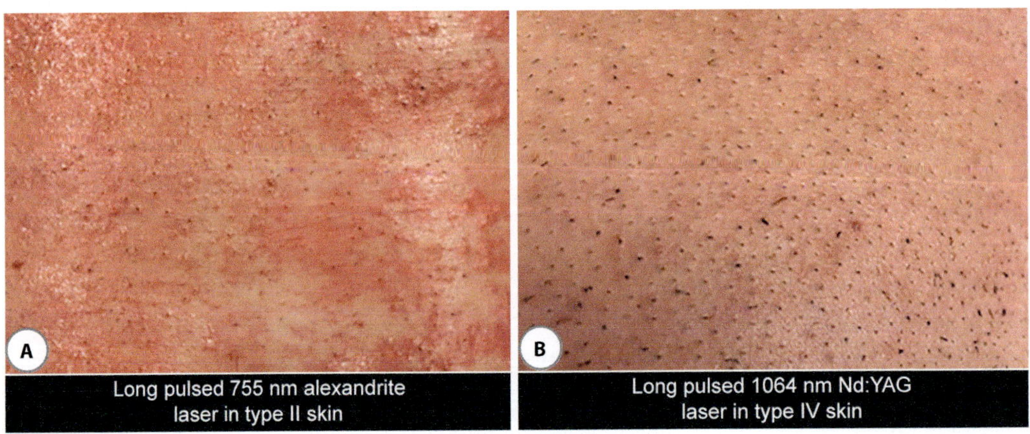

FIGS. 7A AND B: A few minutes after laser hair removal treatment. Note the development of perifollicular erythema and edema easily observed in the patient with lighter skin. In darker skin, perifollicular edema is present, but erythema is more difficult to appreciate.

durations exceed the thermal relaxation time of free ink particles as well as the cells that contain ink particles.[50]

Tattoo ink darkening is a warning end point to be aware of when performing tattoo removal with Q-switched and picosecond lasers on inks containing red iron oxide, or white titanium dioxide.[51,52] Treating these tattoos causes the reduction of ferric oxide to ferrous oxide, which manifests as immediate darkening of the tattoo ink, which is irreversible. Common tattoo colors where this is a risk are pink, rose and other reddish colors.[53]

NONSPECIFIC ENDPOINTS

Fractional nonablative and ablative lasers emit wavelengths absorbed by water. As water is present ubiquitously in the skin, these wavelengths of light are not absorbed by other specific chromophores. Thus, there are no specific therapeutic endpoints seen in use of fractionated nonablative or ablative lasers. Small white or dark dots may be seen that correspond to microthermal zones in fractionated lasers, and bleeding and oozing of edema can occur after using ablative lasers.[2]

WARNING ENDPOINTS IN ANY SELECTIVE PHOTOTHERMOLYSIS DEVICE

There are a variety of warning endpoints that have the potential to occur with use of any laser device that utilizes the process of selective photothermolysis, regardless of the attempted treatment administered.

One such sign is the Nikolsky sign, representative of keratinocyte necrosis, with subsequent separation of the epidermis and dermis when lateral pressure is applied to the skin. This appears within 5 minutes post-treatment[54] and can lead to eventual blister and ulcer formation, plus increased risk of infection, hyperpigmentation and scarring. This warning endpoint can occur without any other detectable sign of a first or second-degree burn, although the patient may report strong pain during treatment. The Nikolsky sign is most likely to occur in treatment of tan or pigmented skin, with use of high fluences, when pulse stacking, or when failing to adequately cool the skin during treatment. Checking for this warning endpoint is highly recommended.

Another warning endpoint is the development of the "half-moon sign" or a crescent-shaped pattern of skin injury. This can occur as a result of misalignment of the cryogen spray or the laser beam, or simply because the laser device is not being placed perpendicular to the cutaneous surface by the operator. Arcuate hyper or hypopigmentation can result. If aligned correctly, however, cryogen (actively cooling the skin) during laser treatment can reduce pain, and decrease the risk of skin burn, allowing use of higher fluences. However, excessive duration of cryogen spray (>100 ms) can quite literally freeze the skin, manifesting as a frosty-white color change, that can persist for several seconds and lead to dyspigmentation or scarring.[55-57]

Another dangerous warning endpoint is sometimes referred to as the "pucker sign". When type 1 collagen in the dermis (the most common type of collagen in the dermis) is heated above 70 degrees Celsius, there is denaturation of collagen and skin contraction, leading to a puckered appearance, with skin tension lines forming a radial pattern around the center of the site of injury.[58] There may also be firmness and elevation of the damaged cutaneous area. When a practitioner notices this sign, she or he should be aware that there has been significant thermal injury to the dermis. Of note, after the final pass of ablative laser resurfacing or ablative fractional laser therapy, mild shrinkage of the treatment area may be acceptable, but for any treatment using selective photothermolysis, the "pucker sign" indicates dermal damage and constitutes danger. Perhaps the most common scenario in which this warning endpoint is seen is when IPL is inappropriately used as a means of tattoo removal; pulse duration of IPL is too long for this use, leading to overheating of the surrounding tissue (**Fig. 8**).[59]

Charring is yet another warning endpoint that should be avoided. If energy continues to be directed at tissue where most of the water has already been removed, partial combustion can occur, manifesting as surface tissue charring with a thin layer of black or dark brown carbon adhered to the skin surface (**Figs. 9A** to **C**).[1] Lastly burns or stamping burns should be avoided.[2]

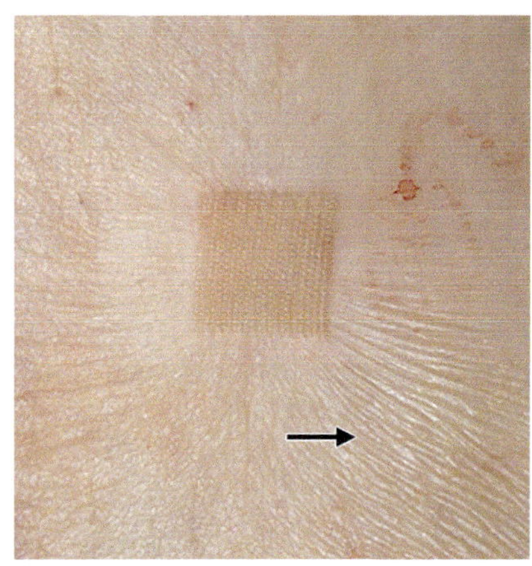

FIG. 8: The Pucker sign: Wrinkling around area of treatment. Although considered normal in ablative laser, this should not be seen in treatments utilizing selective photothermolysis.

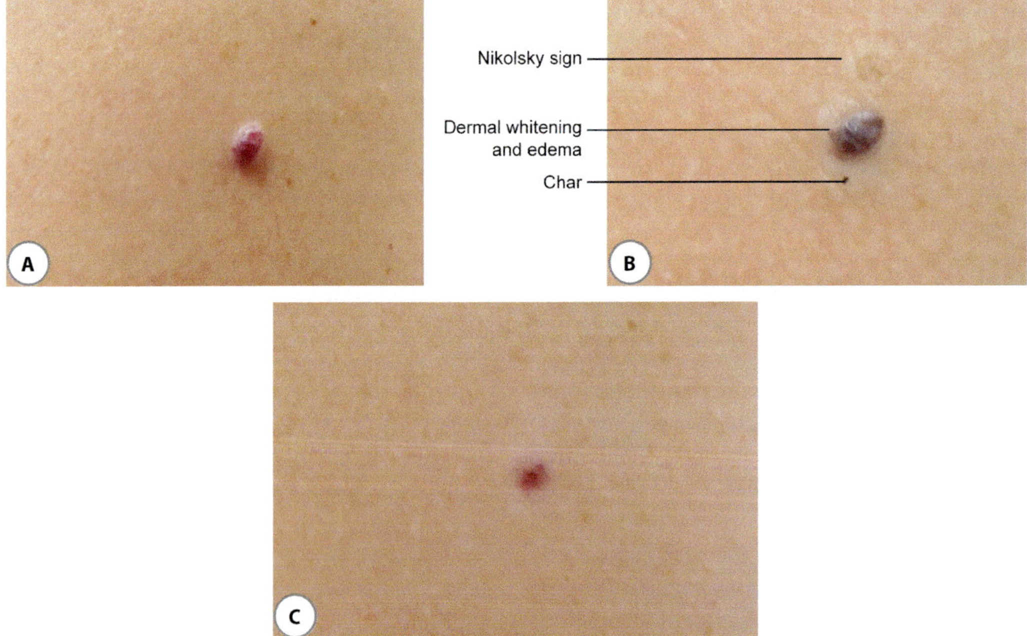

FIGS. 9A TO C: Angioma before (A), immediately after (B), and 8 weeks after (C) treatment with an 810-nm diode laser. (B) There was inadequate compression with the laser's sapphire tip. The angioma was cooled appropriately and displays the desired endpoint of purpura. However, in the areas that were not cooled, there is the Nikolsky sign, dermal whitening and edema, and charring of the skin. These endpoints should not be seen when treating vascular lesions. (C) Residual hypopigmentation is seen at 8 weeks after treatment and has persisted over 2 years after treatment.

As described in this chapter, immediate changes in the skin after treatment with certain lasers, can serve as markers for therapeutic efficacy or ominous signs of warning. Ultimately, these clinical endpoints are the most important factor in appropriate use of lasers, even more important than the "dosimetry" and numerical settings for each laser. We strongly recommend use of skin response endpoints to individualize treatment to a great range of patients who inevitably will have variations in skin pigmentation and skin sensitivity.

REFERENCES

1. Wanner M, Sakamoto FH, Avram MM, Anderson RR. Immediate skin responses to laser and light treatments - warning endpoints: how to avoid side effects. J Am Acad Dermatol. 2016;74(5):807-19.
2. Wanner M, Sakamoto FH, Avram MM, Chan HH, Alam M, Tannous Z, et al. Immediate skin responses to laser and light treatments - warning endpoints: how to obtain efficacy. J Am Acad Dermatol. 2016;74(5):821-33.
3. Anderson RR, Parrish JA. Microvasculature can be selectively damaged using dye lasers: a basic theory and experimental evidence in human skin. Lasers Surg Med. 1981;1:263-76.
4. Anderson RR, Parrish JA. Selective photothermolysis: precise microsurgery by selective absorption of pulsed radiation. Science. 1983; 220:524-7.
5. Iyer S, Fitzpatrick RE. Long-pulsed dye laser treatment for facial telangiectasias and erythema: evaluation of a single purpuric pass versus multiple subpurpuric passes. Dermatol Surg. 2005;31:898-903.
6. Astner S, Anderson RR. Treating vascular lesions. Dermatol Ther. 2005;18:267-81.
7. Suthamjariya K, Farinelli WA, Koh W, Anderson RR. Mechanisms of microvascular response to laser pulses. J Invest Dermatol. 2004;122:518-25.
8. Trelles MA, Allones I, Alvarez J, Vélez M, Martín-Vázquez M, Trelles OR, et al. The 800-nm diode laser in the treatment of leg veins: assessment at 6 months. J Am Acad Dermatol. 2006;54:282-9.
9. Eremia S, Li C, Umar SH. A side-by-side comparative study of 1064 nm Nd:YAG, 810 nm diode and 755 nm alexandrite lasers for treatment of 0.3-3 mm leg veins. Dermatol Surg. 2002;28:224-30.
10. Wall TL, Grassi AM, Avram MM. Clearance of multiple venous lakes with an 800-nm diode laser: a novel approach. Dermatol Surg. 2007; 33:100-3.
11. Aghassi D, Anderson RR, Gonzalez S. Time-sequence histologic imaging of laser-treated cherry angiomas with in vivo confocal microscopy. J Am Acad Dermatol. 2000;43:37-41.
12. Garden JM, Polla LL, Tan OT. The treatment of port-wine stains by the pulsed dye laser. Analysis of pulse duration and long-term therapy. Arch Dermatol. 1988;124:889-96.
13. Asahina A, Watanabe T, Kishi A, Hattori N, Shirai A, Kagami S, et al. Evaluation of the treatment of port-wine stains with the 595-nm long pulsed dye laser: a large prospective study in adult Japanese patients. J Am Acad Dermatol. 2006;54:487-93.
14. Morelli JG, Tan OT, Garden J, Margolis R, Seki Y, Boll J, et al. Tunable dye laser (577 nm) treatment of port wine stains. Lasers Surg Med. 1986;6:94-9.
15. Suthamjariya K, Farinelli WA, Koh W, Anderson RR. Mechanisms of microvascular response to laser pulses. J Invest Dermatol. 2004;122:518-25.
16. Huang YC, Ringold TL, Nelson JS, Choi B. Noninvasive blood flow imaging for real-time feedback during laser therapy of port wine stain birthmarks. Lasers Surg Med. 2008;40:167-73.
17. Yang MU, Yaroslavsky AN, Farinelli WA, Flotte TJ, Rius-Diaz F, Tsao SS, et al. Long-pulsed neodymium:yttrium-aluminum-garnet laser treatment for port-wine stains. J Am Acad Dermatol. 2005;52:480-90.
18. Izikson L, Anderson RR. Treatment endpoints for resistant port wine stains with a 755 nm laser J Cosmet Laser Ther. 2009;11:52-5.
19. Anderson RR, Margolis RJ, Watenabe S, Flotte T, Hruza GJ, Dover JS. Selective photothermolysis of cutaneous pigmentation by Q-switched Nd: YAG laser pulses at 1064, 532, and 355 nm. J Invest Dermatol. 1989;93:28-32.
20. Dover JS, Margolis RJ, Polla LL, Watanabe S, Hruza GJ, Parrish JA, et al. Pigmented guinea pig skin irradiated with Q-switched ruby laser pulses. Morphologic and histologic findings. Arch Dermatol. 1989;125:43-9.
21. Polla LL, Margolis RJ, Dover JS, Whitaker D, Murphy GF, Jacques SL, et al. Melanosomes are a primary target of Q-switched ruby laser irradiation in guinea pig skin. J Invest Dermatol. 1987;89:281-6.
22. Hruza GJ, Dover JS, Flotte TJ, Goetschkes M, Watanabe S, Anderson RR. Q-switched ruby laser irradiation of normal human skin. Histologic and ultrastructural findings. Arch Dermatol. 1991;127:1799-805.

23. Watanabe S, Takahashi H. Treatment of nevus of Ota with the Q-switched ruby laser. N Engl J Med. 1994;331:1745-50.
24. Taylor CR, Anderson RR. Treatment of benign pigmented epidermal lesions by Q-switched ruby laser. Int J Dermatol. 1993;32:908-12.
25. Kilmer SL, Wheeland RG, Goldberg DJ, Anderson RR. Treatment of epidermal pigmented lesions with the frequency-doubled Q-switched Nd:YAG laser. A controlled, single-impact, dose-response, multicenter trial. Arch Dermatol. 1994;130:1515-9.
26. Chan HH, Fung WK, Ying SY, Kono T. An in vivo trial comparing the use of different types of 532 nm Nd:YAG lasers in the treatment of facial lentigines in Oriental patients Dermatol Surg. 2000;26:743-9.
27. Chan HH, Ying SY, Ho WS, Kono T, King WW. An in vivo trial comparing the clinical efficacy and complications of Q-switched 755 nm alexandrite and Q-switched 1064 nm Nd:YAG lasers in the treatment of nevus of Ota. Dermatol Surg. 2000;26:919-22.
28. Alster TS. Complete elimination of large cafe-au-lait birthmarks by the 510-nm pulsed dye laser. Plast Reconstr Surg. 1995;96:1660-4.
29. Trafeli JP, Kwan JM, Meehan KJ, Domankevitz Y, Gilbert S, Malomo K, et al. Use of a long-pulse alexandrite laser in the treatment of superficial pigmented lesions. Dermatol Surg. 2007;33:1477-82.
30. Wang CC, Sue YM, Yang CH, Chen CK. A comparison of Q-switched alexandrite laser and intense pulsed light for the treatment of freckles and lentigines in Asian persons: a randomized, physician-blinded, split-face comparative trial. J Am Acad Dermatol. 2006;54:804-10.
31. Kono T, Sakurai H, Groff WF, Chan HH, Takeuchi M, Yamaki T, et al. Comparison study of a traditional pulsed dye laser versus a long-pulsed dye laser in the treatment of early childhood hemangiomas. Lasers Surg Med. 2006;38:112-5.
32. Yamashita T, Negishi K, Hariya T, Yanai M, likura T, Wakamatsu S. In vivo microscopic approaches for facial melanocytic lesions after quality-switched ruby laser therapy: time-sequential imaging of melanin and melanocytes of solar lentigo in Asian skin. Dermatol Surg. 2010;36:1138-47.
33. Kono T, Manstein D, Chan HH, Nozaki M, Anderson RR. Q-switched ruby versus long-pulsed dye laser delivered with compression for treatment of facial lentigines in Asians Lasers Surg Med. 2006;38:94-7.
34. Chan HH, Kono T. Nevus of Ota: clinical aspects and management. Skinmed. 2003;2:89-96.
35. Taylor CR, Flotte TJ, Gange RW, Anderson RR. Treatment of nevus of Ota by Q-switched ruby laser. J Am Acad Dermatol. 1994;30:743-51.
36. Trotter MJ, Tron VA, Hollingdale J, Rivers JK. Localized chrysiasis induced by laser therapy. Arch Dermatol. 1995;131:1411-4.
37. Grossman MC, Dierickx C, Farinelli W, Flotte T, Anderson RR. Damage to hair follicles by normal-mode ruby laser pulses. J Am Acad Dermatol. 1996;35:889-94.
38. Baugh WP, Trafeli JP, Barnette DJ Jr, Ross EV. Hair reduction using a scanning 800 nm diode laser. Dermatol Surg. 2001;27:358-64.
39. Ross EV, Cooke LM, Timko AL, Overstreet KA, Graham BS, Barnette DJ. Treatment of pseudofolliculitis barbae in skin types IV, V, and VI with a long-pulsed neodymium:yttrium aluminum garnet laser. J Am Acad Dermatol. 2002;47: 263-70.
40. Lask G, Elman M, Slatkine M, Waldman A, Rozenberg Z. Laser-assisted hair removal by selective photothermolysis. Preliminary results. Dermatol Surg. 1997;23:737-9.
41. Nanni CA, Alster TS. Optimizing treatment parameters for hair removal using a topical carbon-based solution and 1064-nm Q-switched neodymium:YAG laser energy. Arch Dermatol. 1997; 133:1546-9.
42. Taylor CR, Anderson RR, Gange RW, Michaud NA, Flotte TJ. Light and electron microscopic analysis of tattoos treated by Q-switched ruby laser. J Invest Dermatol. 1991;97:131-6.
43. Taylor CR, Gange RW, Dover JS, Flotte TJ, Gonzalez E, Michaud N, et al. Treatment of tattoos by Q-switched ruby laser. A dose-response study. Arch Dermatol. 1990;126(7):893-9.
44. Izikson L, Farinelli W, Sakamoto F, Tannous Z, Anderson RR. Safety and effectiveness of black tattoo clearance in a pig model after a single treatment with a novel 758 nm 500 picosecond laser: a pilot study. Lasers Surg Med. 2010;42: 640-6.
45. Kilmer SL, Anderson RR. Clinical use of the Q-switched ruby and the Q-switched Nd:YAG (1064 nm and 532 nm) lasers for treatment of tattoos. J Dermatol Surg Oncol. 1993;19:330-8.
46. Saedi N, Metelitsa A, Petrell K, Arndt KA, Dover JS. Treatment of tattoos with a picosecond alexandrite laser: a prospective trial. Arch Dermatol. 2012;148:1360-3.
47. Kossida T, Rigopoulos D, Katsambas A, Anderson RR. Optimal tattoo removal in a single laser session based on the method of repeated exposures. J Am Acad Dermatol. 2011;66:271-7.
48. Kilmer SL, Lee MS, Grevelink JM, Flotte TJ, Anderson RR. The Q-switched Nd:YAG laser effectively treats tattoos. A controlled, dose-response study. Arch Dermatol. 1993;129:971-8.
49. Ferguson JE, Andrew SM, Jones CJ, August PJ. The Q-switched neodymium:YAG laser and tattoos: a microscopic analysis of laser-tattoo interactions. Br J Dermatol. 1997;137:405-10.

50. Sakamoto FH, Avram M, Anderson RR. Laser and other energy technologies principles and skin interactions. In: Bolognia JL, Jorizzo JJ, SchafferJV (Eds). Dermatology, 3rd edition. New York: Elsevier Saunders; 2012. pp. 2251-9.
51. Anderson RR, Geronemus R, Kilmer SL, Farinelli W, Fitzpatrick RE. Cosmetic tattoo ink darkening. A complication of Q-switched and pulsed-laser treatment. Arch Dermatol. 1993;129:1010-4.
52. Ross EV, Yashar S, Michaud N, Fitzpatrick R, Geronemus R, Tope WD, et al. Tattoo darkening and nonresponse after laser treatment: a possible role for titanium dioxide. Arch Dermatol. 2001;137(1):33-7.
53. Ortiz AE, Alster TS. Rising concern over cosmetic tattoos. Dermatol Surg. 2011;38:424-9.
54. Arndt KA, Feingold DS. The sign of Pyotr Vasilyewich Nikolsky. N Engl J Med. 1970;282: 1154-5.
55. Cho SB, Lee SJ, Kang JM, Kim YK, Lee JH. Formation of arcuate crusted lesions after non-ablative 1450-nm diode laser treatment equipped with a dynamic cooling device. J Cosmet Laser Ther. 2010;12:124-5.
56. Datrice N, Ramirez-San-Juan J, Zhang R, Meshkinpour A, Aguilar G, Nelson JS, et al. Cutaneous effects of cryogen spray cooling on in vivo human skin. Dermatol Surg. 2006;32:1007-12.
57. Lee SJ, ParkSG, Kang JM, Kim YK, Kim DM. Cryogen-induced arcuate shaped hyperpigmentation by dynamic cooling device. J Eur Acad Dermatol Venereol. 2008;22:883-4.
58. Gevorkian SG, Allahverdyan AE, Gevorgyan DS, Simonian AL. Thermal (in) stability of type I collagen fibrils. Phys Rev Lett. 2009;102:048101.
59. Wenzel S, Landthaler M, Bäumler W. Recurring mistakes in tattoo removal. A case series. Dermatology. 2009;218:164-7.

6 CHAPTER

Laser Safety

Saami Khalifian, Sandy S Tsao

INTRODUCTION

Recent advances in laser technology have facilitated successful treatment of a wide array of dermatologic issues with relative ease. Cosmetic issues, medical conditions, and congenital defects can often be improved with a low risk of side effects or adverse outcomes, which has demonstrated superiority over prior treatment modalities.[1] However, this improved armamentarium to treat pigmented and vascular lesions, scars, tattoos, wrinkles, and hypertrichosis does pose significant risks, if handled improperly.

Laser practitioners should have a thorough understanding of laser science and consider potential complications to prioritize patient and personnel safety and improve outcomes. This includes appropriate patient selection, screening for potential patient risk factors, proper preoperative preparation, knowledge of relevant anatomy, use of correct technique, understanding the principles of laser safety, and selection of appropriate laser devices and settings based on patient demographics and intended target endpoints.[2] Although laser manufacturers have installed preset guidelines for most laser devices in the treatment of specific conditions, this does not ensure safety or efficacy. Therefore, knowledge of therapeutic and warning clinical endpoints is critical in guiding management and improving outcomes while concurrently minimizing the risk of side effects.[3,4] Policies for laser procedures, training, and credentialing should be established and strictly adhered to by personnel.

PRETREATMENT EVALUATION

Patient Selection and Screening for Risk Factors

Laser safety begins with the pretreatment evaluation of the patient. Screening for risk factors that may predispose the patient to unnecessary risk can often be gleaned from a thorough history, and if risk factors exist, a plan should be formulated to mitigate or eliminate potential hazards. If potential risks cannot be modified or eliminated, consideration should be given to abandoning laser therapy as an intervention.

Relevant historical elements include a history of viral infections, in particular herpes simplex virus (HSV) and bacterial skin infections.[1] Laser and light treatment, especially ablative laser treatment, may reactivate a pre-existing viral infection. Patients with a history of HSV or bacterial skin infections may require prophylactic antiviral medications or antibiotics, respectively.[5] Patients with an active viral or bacterial infection should not be treated with a laser to avoid the spread of infection. Given that laser surgery may cause significant thermal damage, it is important to note whether patients have a history of hypertrophic scarring or keloid formation. In the appropriate context, this may represent a contraindication to laser therapy.[6]

A medication history is an essential part of the pretreatment evaluation. Certain medications may interfere with laser treatment and result in difficult-to-correct pigmentary alterations. Gold particle-containing medications, e.g., are a contraindication to treatment with Q-switched lasers as they may cause grayish discoloration known as chrysiasis.[7] This risk persists throughout the lifetime of the patient. Other relevant medications include blood thinners, which may increase the risk of purpura and bleeding, photosensitizing agents, and isotretinoin. Although recent evidence suggests that laser therapy during isotretinoin use is safe, the issue remains controversial and most centers do not perform certain laser procedures until the patient has been off isotretinoin for several weeks to months.[8]

Most lasers and light sources utilize selective photothermolysis to destroy specific light-absorbing targets (e.g., pigmented cells, tattoo ink, and vascular structures) without damaging surrounding structures.[9-11] This allows for targeted treatment, while limiting potential side effects. Treating patients with tanned skin can often compromise the specificity of this, especially when the target chromophore is melanin, as is the case for treatment of pigmented lesions and hair removal.[2,5,12] Laser treatment of tanned skin significantly increases the risk of transient or permanent pigmentary changes or thermal burns.[8] Therefore, patients should practice strict sun avoidance prior to laser or light therapy, as well as for several weeks after treatment to minimize the risk of postinflammatory hyperpigmentation. Laser treatment of patients with an active tan should be avoided and treatment postponed until the tan fully resolves.

Laser Selection

Important determinants in selecting the appropriate laser settings include the target structure, chromophore, and patient's skin phototype.[9,11] This requires a thorough understanding of the relevant anatomy of the target structure, its depth in the skin, the chromophore that corresponds to it, and the level of risk associated with the use of a particular laser in a given skin phototype. Each of these points will inform the laser practitioner on the selection of appropriate laser parameters including the wavelength, pulse duration, fluence, and spot size. Specific chromophores include hemoglobin for vascular lesions, exogenous inks for tattoo removal, melanin for pigmented cells and hair follicles, fat and water for rhytids and photoaging. Knowledge of the absorption spectrum of each chromophore, including absorption peaks and overlap with other chromophores will allow for the most selective laser wavelength.

Choice of laser wavelength must correspond to the appropriate chromophore and must penetrate the skin to the appropriate depth of the target. The greater the wavelength, the greater the depth of light penetration. Pulse duration is related to the thermal relaxation time of the target structure, and in broad terms, shorter pulse durations will deliver the same energy to the target in a shorter period of time compared to a longer pulse duration, resulting in greater targeted injury, e.g., nanosecond or picosecond range pulse duration for tattoo ink particles versus millisecond range for terminal hair follicles.[13] With spot size, a larger spot size will penetrate more deeply into the skin while a smaller spot size will affect structures that are more superficial. Although manufacturers often preinstall guidelines for fluence based on clinical scenarios, the laser surgeon should instead understand and utilize therapeutic clinical endpoints to modulate the fluence.[4] In patients with darker skin phototypes, it is generally advisable to utilize lasers with longer wavelengths, longer pulse durations, efficient epidermal cooling, and lower fluence with uptitration of the fluence based on the expected clinical endpoint.[14]

Informed Consent

A thorough explanation of possible side effects and risks should be discussed with patients prior to treatment. Risk factors vary based on the specific laser used and target structure, but generally include transient or permanent pigment alterations, bruising/purpura, infection, pain, erythema, edema, urticaria, paradoxical hypertrichosis, acneiform eruptions, thermal burns, ulceration, vesiculation, scarring, ineffective treatment, inhalation of biohazardous materials, ocular injury, and blindness.[12,15] Other risks include Koebnerization of certain diseases, reactivation of diseases such as vitiligo or other autoimmune disorders, pigmentary changes to nevi, with the latter potentially complicating future melanoma screening and management. Patients should also be counseled that often more than one treatment is required to achieve a satisfactory response and that maintenance treatments may be expected to maintain a desired treatment endpoint. Written patient consent and preoperative photographs should be obtained.

PREOPERATIVE PREPARATION

The majority of lasers will illicit pain in most patients and this is further modulated by the anatomic site, target structure, and fluence delivered. To mitigate this, it may be appropriate to apply a topical anesthetic, e.g., lidocaine and/or prilocaine, up to 1 hour before the procedure under occlusion. Notably, topical anesthetics also pose some risk to the patient, as application of lidocaine or prilocaine to large body surface areas may result in systemic absorption with resultant vertigo, tinnitus, paresthesias, cardiac arrhythmias, methemoglobinemia, or seizures.[16-18] Topical application should be limited to small treatment regions and applied in-office to allow for patient monitoring. It is important to be cautious with topical anesthesia around the orbit and avoid contact of topical anesthesia with the eye. In addition, topical anesthesia can increase the penetration of topicals used in laser and light treatments, such as aminolevulinic acid and such combinations should be approached with consideration and care.

If skin is to be cleansed or prepped before laser surgery, care should be taken to avoid the use of flammable liquids near the target site or to ensure that they are dried before firing the laser. Interaction of the laser with alcohol, chlorhexidine, or other iodophor-containing solutions that are still wet on the skin can result in a burn and represent a fire hazard.[19] Patients should remove makeup and other cosmetic products that are within the target treatment area, as these may also represent a flammability risk. The greatest fire risk with laser use is the presence of oxygen. Oxygen concentrations greater than room air (>25%) pose an increased laser induced fire risk. The treatment suite should be equipped with a fire extinguisher, all sources of flammable gas or oxygen tanks should be removed from the laser room and flammable drapes should be avoided. Though carbon dioxide laser and erbium-doped yttrium aluminum garnet (Er:YAG) lasers pose the greatest risk of fire ignition, any laser use can result in a fire risk.[13] Laser ignition of endotracheal tubes and oil based lubricants has been reported. Avoidance of use of plastic endotracheal tubes and supplemental oxygen is recommended when possible. When utilized, supplemental oxygen should be kept to the lowest oxygen concentration possible when performing facial laser treatments. Wrapping the endotracheal tube with aluminum foil or wet gauze, as well as placing wet drapes around the face and neck and treatment regions reduces the risk of laser fires. Furthermore, the room should be cooled to prevent the laser from overheating. Electrical hazards can be minimized by installing electrical outlets designed for each laser device which have been installed by a competent biomechanical engineer or laser technician and equipped with appropriate safeguards, including grounding and automatic shut-off mechanisms.

Ocular injury can occur from direct or indirect laser exposure and the consequences may be devastating. The universal use of protective eyewear for the patient, laser surgeon, and all individuals in the treatment room is mandatory. The use of protective eyewear is specifically designated for the wavelength of a given laser device, and has a rated optical density at various wavelengths. In most instances, an optical density of ≥5 at the laser's specific wavelength is sufficient to prevent ocular injury.[14] The level of ocular injury is related to the specific laser wavelength used, with corneal injury induced by long wavelengths, corneal and/or lens injury from midrange infrared wavelengths, and retinal injury from short wavelengths (i.e., near-infrared and visible range).[19] The greatest risk of blindness is from Q-switched or picosecond near infrared lasers.[13]

The use of lasers inside the bony orbit should be avoided, especially those with longer wavelengths, as they may penetrate through the eyelid and result in ocular damage. Corneal eyeshields are recommended when performing periorbital laser treatments. There are a variety of plastic and metal corneal eyeshields available to provide ocular protection. Metal protective eyeshields are preferred over plastic eyeshields, as plastic eyeshields have an increased risk of thermal damage, resulting in a possible melting or igniting of the shield. The eyeshield should be lined with a layer of ophthalmic lubricating ointment prior to placement and care taken in the placement and removal of an eyeshield in order to avoid a corneal abrasion (**Figs. 1A** to **D**).

Metal instruments should be covered with black tape to minimize reflected laser light. "Laser in use" warning signs should be prominently placed outside the entrance of each laser room to avoid bystander injury. In addition, the laser room should be free of uncovered windows and hanging mirrors, which pose additional risks to the room's occupants as reflection of the laser energy may also lead to injury.[2] Indeed, all that is required is for 1% of the laser's beam to be reflected into the eye from a mirror, glass, or other shiny metal or plastic object to cause blindness.[13]

Laser Operation

Some forms of laser treatment may create a biohazardous plume when tissue is vaporized. Practitioners should utilize smoke evacuators and filtration systems and laser surgical masks, where appropriate. Laser hair removal, e.g., is associated with release of at least 20 known environmental toxins and over a dozen carcinogens in the laser plume with

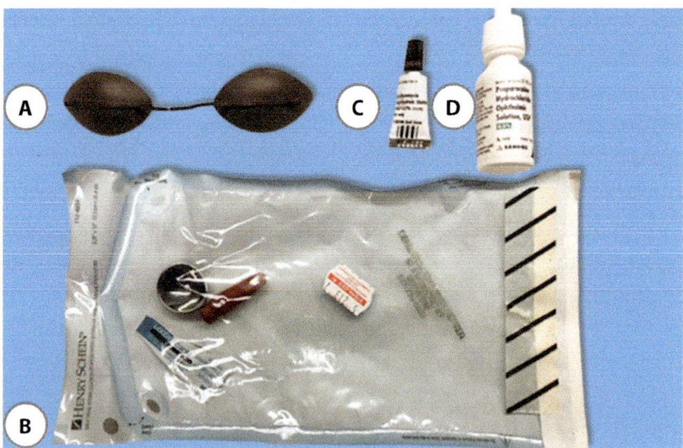

FIGS. 1A TO D: (A) Metal eye shield for use over the eye. The eye shield is placed over the eyelids. (B) Metal eye shield that is inserted over the eye and under the eyelid. This type of eye shield is crucial for treatment of the eyelid and for treatment near the eye. (C) Erythromycin Ophthalmic Ointment is used to coat the metal eye shield that is inserted under the eyelid. (D) Proparacaine Hydrochloride Ophthalmic solution is placed in the eye to numb the area prior to insertion of the metal eye shield.

a 26-fold increase over ambient air levels of the same chemicals.[20] Notably, even when an evacuator was used in this study, there was still an eightfold increase over ambient air levels of the aforementioned chemicals, highlighting the importance of using a surgical mask together with an evacuator. Correct placement of the evacuator tip within 1 cm of the laser during treatment maximizes plume removal.

Efficient skin cooling is critical to prevent complications such as vesiculation, ulceration, burns, and postinflammatory hyperpigmentation, especially in patients with darker skin phototypes.[21] Most laser devices today utilize pretreatment cooling, such as dynamic cooling with a cryogen spray or built-in contact cooling. Older devices may employ forced cold air. If no cooling device exists, the application of a cool gel applied directly to the target site should be considered. Epidermal cooling facilitates the use of higher fluences to achieve target therapeutic endpoints with minimal surrounding thermal damage.

Therapeutic Clinical Endpoints

Therapeutic clinical endpoints are unique for each laser device and indication, and should be used to guide the delivery of safe and effective laser therapy.[4] Treatment endpoints are further modulated by the fluence, pulse duration, and the patient skin phototype. Generally, employing the most conservative settings necessary to achieve a therapeutic endpoint should be followed. Performing a laser test site to determine a therapeutic endpoint is recommended in clinical situations where an expected endpoint is unknown or when the laser surgeon is seeking to up-titrate the fluence.[3,5] Adjustments should be made to the laser parameters until the target therapeutic endpoints are achieved, while keeping a close watch for warning endpoints that may be delayed up to 5 minutes or more after the laser pulse.[3,4]

The use of therapeutic endpoints allows for the optimization of treatment for each individual patient, as differences in skin type, sensitivity, and device output preclude a "one-size-fits-all" approach to laser therapy.[22-30] It should be noted, however, that achievement of a desired clinical endpoint does not necessarily safeguard against all side effects. Endpoints have been reviewed in depth, elsewhere in this book.

Warning Endpoints

Several important warning endpoints exist that represent the development of early complications and portend poor outcomes. The Nikolsky sign, i.e., epidermal detachment with lateral pressure on the skin, represents epidermal necrosis and usually manifests within 5 minutes.[3] This is usually followed by vesiculation, ulceration, and increased risk of scarring and pigmentary alterations. Patients may report unusually strong pain during treatment, which should alert the laser surgeon to examine the skin for this finding. Common scenarios where this warning endpoint is more likely to occur include laser pulse stacking, lack of appropriate skin cooling, use of high energy settings, or treatment of pigmented or tanned skin with intense pulsed light (IPL), visible light, or near-infrared laser devices.[3]

Dermal injury results from denaturation of collagen and manifests in different ways.[31] Skin shrinkage or contraction with the laser pulse may only exhibit subtle elevation and firmness of the skin, which may sometimes be difficult to appreciate.[3] In some instances the skin may pucker with radial skin surface lines pointing towards the target site, and this is a concerning warning sign that should cause the laser surgeon to stop. Notably, some amount of shrinkage is desired in ablative laser treatments.[32-34] However, there should never be unintended tissue ablation when a nonablative treatment is being performed as this represents a thermal burn and also increases the risk of tissue splatter towards the practitioner creating an additional biohazardous risk.[3] Studies of aerosolized tissue splatter fragments have been reported to contain human immunodeficiency virus (HIV) and human papillomavirus (HPV) viral particles, as well as a host of other microbial entities.[35-40] The use of safety goggles to prevent splatter of material into the eyes when performing ablative laser treatments is recommended.

Excessive energy applied to target tissue by ablative resurfacing lasers can vaporize the skin's water content, and cause thermal injury that may lead to deep dermal thermal injury.[3] Treatment of vascular lesions with inappropriately high fluences with near-infrared lasers, e.g., alexandrite, diode, or neodymium-doped yttrium aluminum garnet (Nd:YAG) 1,064 nm lasers, may lead to immediate gray blanching of the skin representing excessive dermal thermal injury.[41]

Effective epidermal cooling facilitates the use of higher laser fluences; however, cooling device malfunction or inappropriate use of cooling may also cause unintended side effects. If the cooling device is too aggressive, e.g., excessive cryogen spray, the patient may develop a freeze injury with white frost on the skin surface that lasts more than a few seconds.[3,42] Thermal burns on the other hand can occur with ineffective epidermal cooling. There are several warning signs associated with second or third degree burns including deep red erythema, severe pain, vesiculation, erosions, ulceration, and tissue splatter, which may later develop into scarring, pigmentary alterations, and infection.[3] An immediate skin burn may occur from poor skin contact with cold-window devices and can be corrected with proper technique by the laser operator. Hair or tissue present on the contact window may also cause an epidermal "stamping" burn, which can be avoided by cleaning the contact window. Finally, misalignment or poor application of the laser handpiece can lead to an arcuate pattern of epidermal injury.

The use of a Q-switched laser in a patient with a history of gold-intake at any point in their lifetime is likely to result in chrysiasis; an immediate bluish-gray darkening of the skin that is potentially permanent.[43] Similarly, if a patient develops immediate darkening of their tattoo after the use of Q-switched laser, this represents a warning endpoint that may not be reversible even with subsequent laser treatment.[44-46]

Control Measures

Regulations for laser safety and standards are set forth by several different organizations in the United States; however, none are strictly enforced and only about a dozen states have laser regulations, which mostly exempt physician-operated medical lasers.[14] The American National Standards Institute (ANSI) has created a regulatory document, ANSI Z136.3, which is the most frequently used guideline in the United States healthcare system to govern laser safety in medicine.[47] Yet, the standards in this document are voluntary and the onus is on the laser physician and/or institution to adopt and enforce these guidelines.

A variety of control measures exist to ensure laser safety, some of which are built-into the device, while others may be enforced by the health care facility or outside inspection agencies. Built-in engineering controls are developed by the device manufacturer to comply with Food and Drug Administration (FDA) standards, and include on-indicator light and sound, emergency disable switch, protected footswitch, standby mode, and a variety of other safety mechanisms.[19] Procedural control measures are typically enforced by the healthcare facility or hospital and include controlled access to the laser suite, visibly posted signage to signify the use of a laser device, use of personal protective equipment, testing and calibration of laser devices, and elimination of flammability, reflective, or electrical hazards from the operating room (**Fig. 2**).[19] Administrative control measures may occasionally be reviewed by outside inspection agencies, e.g., Occupational Safety and Health Administration, and include appointment of a laser safety officer, training for all individuals that work with laser devices, documentation of laser use, and development of a technical management and audit program.[19]

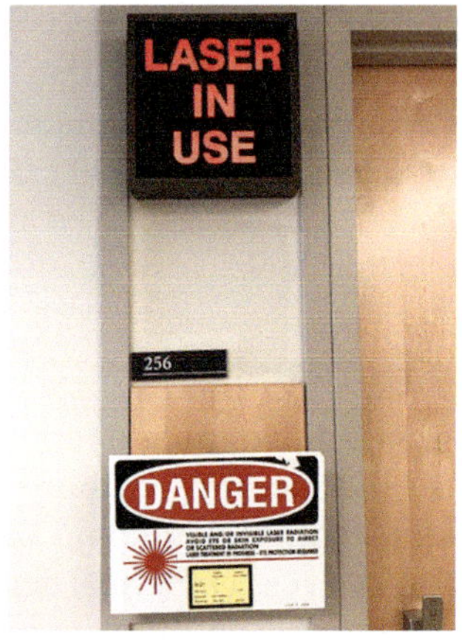

FIG. 2: Laser warning signs should be placed outside of any room with energy based devices.

CONCLUSION

Laser therapy has revolutionized laser surgery in the last few decades and has facilitated improved aesthetic outcomes with minimal to no morbidity or side effects when used properly. Appropriate use of laser devices begins with a thorough history and screening for risk factors, as patient selection may represent the most important step in ensuring safe and effective laser therapy. Selection of the correct laser is based on the target lesion and patient demographics, including skin type and medical history. While device manufacturers often have preloaded laser parameters built into the device, the laser surgeon should not rely on these settings as differences in patient sensitivity, skin type, and device calibration can result in poor outcomes if the practitioner does not know what to look for. Instead, management should be guided by desired therapeutic clinical endpoints with a vigilant watch for warning endpoints to appropriately titrate the laser settings. The use of personal protective equipment is mandatory but a myriad of other potential hazards and risks exist that practitioners must be aware of including biohazardous plume and tissue splatter; electrical, reflective, and flammability hazards; as well as risks associated with topical anesthetic use to name a few. Indeed, laser safety begins and ends with the laser operator. Physician competency is critical in the understanding and employment of laser biophysics and laser tissue interactions to ensure the safety of the laser operator, patient, and all staff.

REFERENCES

1. Tanzi EL, Lupton JR, Alster TS. Lasers in dermatology: four decades of progress. J Am Acad Dermatol. 2003;49(1):1-31.
2. Ibrahimi OA, Avram MM, Hanke CW, Kilmer SL, Anderson RR. Laser hair removal. Dermatol Ther. 2011;24(1):94-107.
3. Wanner M, Sakamoto FH, Avram MM, Anderson RR. Immediate skin responses to laser and light treatments: Warning endpoints: How to avoid side effects. J Am Acad Dermatol. 2016;74(5):807-19.
4. Wanner M, Sakamoto FH, Avram MM, Chan HH, Alam M, Tannous Z, et al. Immediate skin responses to laser and light treatments: Therapeutic endpoints: How to obtain efficacy. J Am Acad Dermatol. 2016;74(5):821-33.
5. Wanner M. Laser hair removal. Dermatol Ther. 2005;18(3):209-16.
6. Dierickx CC. Hair removal by lasers and intense pulsed light sources. Dermatol Clin. 2002;20(1):135-46.
7. Dierickx CC, Grossman MC. Chapter 4-Laser hair removal. In: Goldberg DJ, editor. Lasers and lights. 2005;2:61-6.
8. Gan SD, Graber EM. Laser hair removal: a review. Dermatol Surg. 2013;39(6):823-38.
9. Anderson RR, Parrish JA. Selective photothermolysis: precise microsurgery by selective absorption of pulsed radiation. Science. 1983;220(4596):524-7.
10. Hruza GJ, Geronemus RG, Dover JS, Arndt KA. Lasers in dermatology-1993. Arch Dermatol. 1993;129(8):1026-35.
11. Altshuler GB, Anderson RR, Manstein D, Zenzie HH, Smirnov MZ. Extended theory of selective photothermolysis. Lasers Surg Med. 2001;29(5):416-32.
12. Paasch U, Schwandt A, Seeber N, Kautz G, Grunewald S, Haedersdal M. New lasers and light sources-old and new risks? J Dtsch Dermatol Ges. 2017;15(5):487-96.
13. Sakamoto FH, Avram MM, Anderson RR. Lasers and other energy technologies—principles and skin interactions. In: Bolognia JL, Jorizzo JL, Schaffer JV, editors. Dermatol Surg. United Kingdom. Mosby. 2012:2251-60.
14. Lolis M, Dunbar SW, Goldberg DJ, Hansen TJ, MacFarlane DF. Patient safety in procedural dermatology: Part II. Safety related to cosmetic procedures. J Am Acad Dermatol. 2015;73(1):15-24.
15. Goldberg D. Laser complications: hair removal. J Cosmet Laser Ther. 2006;8(4):197-202.
16. Fox M, Helfrich Y, Kang S. Other topical medications. In: Bolognia JL, Jorizzo JL, Schaffer JV, eds. Dermatology. 3rd Ed. Philadelphia: Elsevier Limited. New York. 2012: 2153-64.
17. Friedman PM, Mafong EA, Friedman ES, Geronemus RG. Topical anesthetics update: EMLA and beyond. Dermatol Surg. 2001;27(12):1019-26.
18. Koay J, Orengo I. Application of local anesthetics in dermatologic surgery. Dermatol Surg. 2002;28(2):143-8.
19. Smalley PJ. Laser safety: Risks, hazards, and control measures. Laser Ther. 2011;20(2):95-106.
20. Chuang GS, Farinelli W, Christiani DC, Herrick RF, Lee NCY, Avram MM. Gaseous and particulate content of laser hair removal plume. JAMA Dermatol. 2016;152(12):1320-6.
21. Zenzie HH, Altshuler GB, Smirnov MZ, Anderson RR. Evaluation of cooling methods for laser dermatology. Lasers Surg Med. 2000;26(2):130-44.
22. Galadari I. Comparative evaluation of different hair removal lasers in skin types IV, V, and VI. Int J Dermatol. 2003;42(1):68-70.
23. Nanni CA, Alster TS. Laser-assisted hair removal: side effects of Q-switched Nd:YAG, long-pulsed ruby, and alexandrite lasers. J Am Acad Dermatol. 1999;41(2 Pt 1):165-71.
24. Lask G, Elman M, Slatkine M, Waldman A, Rozenberg Z. Laser-assisted hair removal by selective photothermolysis. Preliminary results. Dermatol Surg. 1997;23(9):737-9.
25. Alster TS. Complete elimination of large cafe-au-lait birthmarks by the 510-nm pulsed dye laser. Plast Reconstr Surg. 1995;96(7):1660-4.
26. Wang CC, Sue YM, Yang CH, Chen CK. A comparison of Q-switched alexandrite laser and intense pulsed light for the treatment of freckles and lentigines in Asian persons:

a randomized, physician-blinded, split-face comparative trial. J Am Acad Dermatol. 2006;54(5):804-10.

27. Trafeli JP, Kwan JM, Meehan KJ, et al. Use of a long-pulse alexandrite laser in the treatment of superficial pigmented lesions. Dermatol Surg. 2007;33(12):1477-82.
28. Wenzel S, Landthaler M, Baumler W. Recurring mistakes in tattoo removal. A case series. Dermatology. 2009;218(2):164-7.
29. Laubach HJ, Tannous Z, Anderson RR, Manstein D. Skin responses to fractional photothermolysis. Lasers Surg Med. 2006;38(2):142-9.
30. Dierickx CC, Khatri KA, Tannous ZS, Childs JJ, Cohen RH, Erofeev A, et al. Micro-fractional ablative skin resurfacing with two novel erbium laser systems. Lasers Surg Med. 2008;40(2):113-23.
31. Gevorkian SG, Allahverdyan AE, Gevorgyan DS, Simonian AL. Thermal (in) stability of type I collagen fibrils. Phys Rev Lett. 2009;102(4):048101.
32. Hantash BM, Bedi VP, Chan KF, Zachary CB. Ex vivo histological characterization of a novel ablative fractional resurfacing device. Lasers Surg Med. 2007;39(2): 87-95.
33. Chapas AM, Brightman L, Sukal S, Hale E, Daniel D, Bernstein LJ, et al. Successful treatment of acneiform scarring with CO_2 ablative fractional resurfacing. Lasers Surg Med. 2008;40(6):381-6.
34. Tierney EP, Hanke CW, Watkins L. Treatment of lower eyelid rhytids and laxity with ablative fractionated carbon-dioxide laser resurfacing: Case series and review of the literature. J Am Acad Dermatol. 2011;64(4):730-40.
35. Garden JM, O'Banion MK, Shelnitz LS, Pinski KS, Bakus AD, Reichmann ME, et al. Papillomavirus in the vapor of carbon dioxide laser-treated verrucae. JAMA. 1988;259(8):1199-202.
36. Sawchuk WS, Weber PJ, Lowy DR, Dzubow LM. Infectious papillomavirus in the vapor of warts treated with carbon dioxide laser or electrocoagulation: detection and protection. J Am Acad Dermatol. 1989;21(1): 41-9.
37. Baggish MS, Poliesz BJ, Joret D, Williamson P, Refai A. Presence of human immunodeficiency virus DNA in laser smoke. Lasers Surg Med. 1991;11(3):197-203.
38. Gloster HM, Roenigk RK. Risk of acquiring human papillomavirus from the plume produced by the carbon dioxide laser in the treatment of warts. J Am Acad Dermatol. 1995;32(3):436-41.
39. Capizzi PJ, Clay RP, Battey MJ. Microbiologic activity in laser resurfacing plume and debris. Lasers Surg Med. 1998;23(3):172-4.
40. Pay AD, Kenealy JM. Laser transmission through membranes using the Q-switched Nd: YAG laser. Lasers Surg Med. 1999;24(1):48-54.
41. Izikson L, Anderson RR. Treatment endpoints for resistant port wine stains with a 755 nm laser. J Cosmet Laser Ther. 2009;11(1):52-5.
42. Datrice N, Ramirez-San-Juan J, Zhang R, Meshkinpour A, Aguilar G, Nelson JS, et al. Cutaneous effects of cryogen spray cooling on in vivo human skin. Dermatol Surg. 2006;32(8):1007-12.
43. Trotter MJ, Tron VA, Hollingdale J, Rivers JK. Localized chrysiasis induced by laser therapy. Arch Dermatol. 1995;131(12):1411-4.
44. Anderson RR, Geronemus R, Kilmer SL, Farinelli W, Fitzpatrick RE. Cosmetic tattoo ink darkening: A complication of Q-switched and pulsed-laser treatment. Arch Dermatol. 1993;129(8):1010-4.
45. Ross EV, Yashar S, Michaud N, Fitzpatrick R, Geronemus R, Tope WD, et al. Tattoo darkening and nonresponse after laser treatment: a possible role for titanium dioxide. Arch Dermatol. 2001;137(1):33-7.
46. Kirby W, Kaur RR, Desai A. Paradoxical darkening and removal of pink tattoo ink. J Cosmet Dermatol. 2010;9(2):149-51.
47. US Department of Labor. Occupational Safety and Health Administration. OSHA Technical Manual, Section III, Chapter 6. [online] Available from https://www.osha.gov/dts/osta/otm/otm_iii/otm_iii_6.html [Last accessed March, 2021].

2 SECTION

VASCULAR

7

CHAPTER

Pediatric Vascular Lesions

Jennifer Lynn Goodrich, J Stuart Nelson

INTRODUCTION

Evaluation and treatment of vascular lesions and malformations entails a multidisciplinary approach. There has been a dramatic shift in treatment paradigm, steering away from a watchful waiting approach and taking a more hands-on and early intervention approach for the majority of malformations. The 2014 updated International Society for the Study of Vascular Anomalies (ISSVA) classification of vascular anomalies (**Table 1**) has allowed us to biologically differentiate the various malformations and tailor better treatment on an individual patient basis.[1] Vascular lesions can be divided into vascular tumors (infantile hemangioma, congenital hemangioma (CH), and kaposiform hemangioma) and vascular malformations (VM) [capillary/port wine stain (PWS), venous malformation, lymphatic malformation (LM), and arteriovenous malformation (AVM)]. The main focus of this chapter is on laser treatments for the various vascular lesions.

TABLE 1: Abbreviated classification of vascular anomalies, modified from International Society for the Study of Vascular Anomalies (ISSVA) 2014.[1]

Vascular anomalies	
Vascular tumors	**Vascular malformations**
Infantile hemangioma or proliferative hemangioma of infancy	Capillary vascular malformation or port wine stain (PWS)
Congenital Hemangioma: • Rapidly involuting congenital hemangioma (RICH) • Noninvoluting congenital hemangioma (NICH)	Venous malformation
Tufted hemangioma	Arteriovenous malformation
Kaposiform hemangioendothelioma (KHE)	Lymphatic malformation
Cherry angioma	
Pyogenic granuloma	

LIGHT INTERACTION WITH HUMAN SKIN

Selective photothermolysis is the theory that describes how light energy is used to target a specific light-absorbing chromophore residing at a particular depth within human skin while not injuring normal adjacent structures. Target selectivity is based upon each chromophore's preferential absorption of a light at a specific wavelength(s). Moreover, in order to maximize the spatial confinement of heat, the use of a laser with pulse duration on the order of the thermal relaxation time (t_r) of the target chromophore is needed: t_r is defined as the time required for the heat generated by the absorption of energy within the target chromophore to cool to 50% of the original value immediately after the laser pulse. During longer laser exposures a more generalized heating, and less spatial selectivity, is produced and results in nonspecific thermal damage to adjacent structures. However, if the laser pulse is suitably brief, the energy is invested in the target chromophore before thermal diffusion extends out of the exposure field.[2] A barrier to successful treatment in the past has been the inability to achieve high enough energy densities to cause vascular injury due to collateral damage to the epidermis. All of the lasers and other light sources used to treat vascular lesions have some absorption by epidermal melanin, which varies based on wavelength. For many vascular lesions, the threshold for epidermal damage following laser treatment is lower than that for permanent vascular damage.[3] Uncontrolled heating of epidermal melanin can result in scarring or dyspigmentation, or damage to other melanin containing structures in human skin, such as hair which can lead to alopecia. With the advent of "dynamic" or cryogen spray cooling (CSC)[4] and other cooling modalities, the epidermis is selectively cooled prior to laser exposure without affecting the temperature of the deeper target structures. This allows for a larger safety margin, permitting higher energy densities to be used to clear the vascular lesion while minimizing injury to the epidermis.[4]

DEVICES USED TO TREAT VASCULAR LESIONS

Lasers that are utilized in the treatment of VM are briefly described here. Additional information regarding each laser used in that specific malformation will be addressed in the sections below as applicable. **Table 2** highlights the various lasers and their specific wavelengths.

The pulsed dye laser (PDL) has become the major workhorse for vascular lesions. PDL, which is a yellow light at a wavelength of 577–595 nm, specifically targets hemoglobin. Light is preferentially absorbed by hemoglobin in the blood vessels where, after

TABLE 2: Specific devices used for vascular lesions and their wavelengths and epidermal cooling mechanisms.

Device	Wavelength (nm)	Epidermal cooling mechanism
PDL	577–595	Cryogen spray and air cooling
Alexandrite	755	Cryogen spray
Diode	800–940	Contact cooling
Nd:YAG	1,064	Cryogen spray and contact cooling
KTP	532	Contact cooling
Intense pulsed light (IPL)	390–1,200	Contact cooling
Carbon dioxide (CO_2)	10,600	Air cooling

(KTP: potassium titanyl phosphate; Nd:YAG: neodymium-doped-yttrium aluminum garnet; PDL: pulsed dye laser)

being converted to heat, causes vessel wall necrosis which ultimately leads to lightening and clearance of the vascular lesion. Current PDLs emit wavelengths ranging from 585 to 595 nm with pulse widths ranging from 0.45 to 40 ms. Spot sizes can vary from 3 to 15 mm in diameter. Maximal energy densities of 60 J/cm^2 are available, depending on the spot size. With the variable pulse durations, the physician can choose the clinical endpoint to be purpura or erythema depending on the lesion to be treated. Due to the rupturing of blood vessels when shorter laser pulse durations are used to treat lesions with smaller blood vessel diameters, purpura is oftentimes observed. When longer laser pulse durations are used to treat lesions featuring larger blood vessel diameters, no purpura is observed.

The long-pulsed millisecond domain alexandrite laser produces red light at a wavelength of 755 nm, which specifically targets deoxyhemoglobin. The long-pulsed millisecond alexandrite laser has pulse durations varying from 3 to 40 ms. Spot sizes are available from 6 to 18 mm, and maximal energy densities of 100 J/cm^2. Because there is much less optical scattering at 755 nm, as compared to 577–595 nm, light from the alexandrite laser has a much deeper penetration than the PDL and is useful for treatment of thicker, more hypertrophic vascular lesions, and those resistant to PDL.

The solid-state semi-conductor diode lasers are small, compact, portable, efficient light sources. Diode lasers produce near-infrared light in the range of 800–980 nm. Because of their relatively long wavelengths, diode lasers penetrate much deeper into human skin than visible yellow and green light sources. Therefore, diode lasers are generally used when vessels deep with the skin are to be targeted.

The long-pulsed millisecond domain neodymium-doped: yttrium-aluminum-garnet (Nd:YAG) laser produces photons at a wavelength of 1,064 nm that are poorly absorbed by hemoglobin, melanin, and water. Pulse durations may range up to 300 ms and energy densities up to 900 J/cm^2. Spot sizes range from 3 to 10 mm. Light from the Nd:YAG laser has a penetration of 4–6 mm into the skin, which results in a large volume of coagulated tissue under the skin surface. Due to its depth of penetration, there is increased risk for scar formation and collateral damage to surrounding structures. Due to its very low absorption by melanin, the Nd:YAG laser is frequently used in darker skinned individuals.

Potassium titanyl phosphate (KTP) laser is a frequency-doubled Nd:YAG laser at a wavelength of 532 nm. The KTP laser produces a green light, which is preferentially absorbed by hemoglobin. It is Food and Drug Administration (FDA) approved for many of the same applications as the PDL; however, due to its shorter wavelength, it has higher absorption by melanin, as compared to the PDL, and, as such, should be used with caution in patients with darker skin phototypes. The KTP laser has pulse durations from 1 to 150 ms, energy densities up to 20 J/cm^2, and spot sizes up to 10 mm.

Intense pulsed light (IPL) is not, in fact, a laser. Whereas all the aforementioned lasers produce monochromatic light at a single wavelength, the IPL produces light between 515 and 1,000 nm. Cutoff filters within the system limit the spectrum of light to the desired wavelengths for the treatment of vascular lesions. The larger spot size allows for the efficient treatment of larger areas for extensive lesions.

Carbon dioxide (CO_2) laser produces light at a wavelength of 10,600 nm. It is preferentially absorbed by water. The CO_2 laser is used for ablative procedures, resurfacing of skin and scars, and superficial tissue coagulation.

HEMANGIOMAS

Proliferative Hemangiomas of Infancy

Epidemiology: Infantile hemangiomas are the most common benign soft tissue tumor of infancy affecting 5–10% of newborns and up to 30% of premature deliveries.[5] Risks factors associated with infantile hemangiomas include Caucasian race, female gender, prematurity, multiple births, low birth weight, and in women who undergo chorionic villous sampling (CVS).[6] Often times the hemangioma is not identifiable at birth, but there may be a precursor lesion that is noted.[7]

While most hemangiomas occur sporadically, there can be a family history with an associated genetic component.[8] Hemangiomas can be classified into superficial (contained within the papillary dermis), deep (in the reticular dermis or subcutaneous tissue), and mixed or compound (combination of both). The majority of hemangiomas present as a single lesion, but up to 20% of patients may have >1 lesion.[8] When an infant has >5 cutaneous hemangiomas, they are at increased risk for having visceral hemangiomas; further imaging should be done to rule out visceral involvement, with liver being the most common.[9]

There is a strong association between hemangiomas in a "beard distribution" and hemangiomas of the airway, specifically subglottic area.[10] More than half of patients with laryngeal hemangiomas will have cervicofacial hemangiomas, but the opposite is not true.

Histopathology: Infantile hemangiomas are true tumors, which undergo both angiogenesis, growth of new vessels from existing vessels, and de-novo vasculogenesis, with creation of new blood vessels from stem cells of placental origin within the hemangioma.[11] Infantile hemangiomas are comprised of multipotent stem cells, immature endothelial cells, pericytes, dendritic cells, and mesenchymal cells.[12] These tumors express vascular endothelial growth factor (VEGF). Unlike the other vascular tumors, only the proliferative hemangiomas of infancy will express glucose transporter protein isoform-1 (GLUT-1), and as such, it can be used as a diagnostic tool, if the diagnosis is not obvious. The metastatic niche theory is based on evidence that the placenta, or possibly chorangiomas within the placenta, secrete substances that prepare the hemangioma sites for implantation. The approximately 9 month growth phase followed by stabilization and involution also supports this hypothesis.[13]

Usually, imaging is not necessary for diagnosis; however, in uncertain cases or for deeper hemangiomas, an ultrasound may be used which would show a solid mass with increased flow. Additionally, magnetic resonance imaging (MRI) characteristics include enhancement on T2-weighted images with likely serpiginous internal flow voids which represent the arterial feeder.[14]

Natural history: The natural history of an infantile hemangioma is rapid proliferation phase until 6–9 months of age. During this phase, the vessels are disorganized and immature.[15] Rapid proliferation of endothelial cells is observed during this phase.[16] Following the proliferative phase is a resting phase that takes years to complete. During this phase, the vessels mature and enlarge, but reduce in number.[17] Finally, the third phase, or involution phase, occurs over several years during which time the blood vessels degenerate into residual fibrofatty tissue.

Complications/special considerations: Although the great majority of proliferative hemangiomas of infancy follow a benign course, some may develop complications. Ulceration is the most common complication, occurring up to 10% of all patients.[8] While ulcerations may lead to infection, the feared sequelae is scarring, which is caused by the ulceration and not the treatment.[16] Spontaneous bleeding is a very rare complication, usually seen in patients with multiple hemangiomas or Kasabach-Merritt Syndrome (KMS), which is discussed below.

Treatment: The goals of treatment are to stop the growth of the hemangioma, shrink the hemangioma, and prevent or stop complications. Historically, it was recommended to pursue a watchful waiting course for the majority of all infantile hemangiomas because of their natural course to self-involute. The exception to this recommendation was for areas which would impose significant morbidity/mortality if not treated: Periocular (amblyopia and increased pressure of globe), perioral (feeding difficulties and interference with speech), periauricular (deformation of cartilage), perianal (difficulty with defecation and increased likelihood of ulceration), perigenital (impairment of voiding and increased likelihood of ulceration), and lesions which could impinge on the airway. If no intervention is taken, 25–40% of pediatric facial hemangiomas result in a poor cosmetic outcome.[18] In part because of the unacceptable outcomes for patients who underwent no intervention, the current approach to the clinical management of hemangiomas is to initiate therapies sooner, during the proliferative phase, for all lesions, if parents desire; to hasten recovery; reduce complications and mitigate posthemangioma sequelae (fibrofatty tissue).

Ames and Sykes[19] have reviewed the literature and provided a thorough review of the medical management of infantile hemangiomas, which is beyond the scope of this chapter. The reader is referred to their work for comprehensive review, but a few of the popular treatments are mentioned below as they are often used in combination with laser therapy.

Leaute-Labreze et al. first reported in 2008 that the use of propranolol led to the rapid involution and regression of infantile hemangiomas.[20] Obstructive hypertrophic cardiomyopathy developed in infants with massive head and neck hemangiomas due to high doses of systemic steroids. A French cardiologist serendipitously prescribed propranolol which led to the rapid involution of infantile hemangiomas. A rapid response, namely decreased lesion size and fading, was noted within 24 hours of propranolol treatment being initiated. Since that time, several large series and numerous case reports have proven oral propranolol to be a safe and effective therapy for the treatment of infantile hemangiomas. With the recognition of propranolol as an effective and safe treatment for infantile hemangiomas, it has become the primary medical treatment, surpassing oral steroids as the initial therapy. The exact mechanism by which propranolol induces regression of the hemangioma remains incompletely understood although there are several postulations such as: (1) vasoconstriction due to inhibition of beta-adrenergic receptors, (2) reduced VEGF expression inhibiting angiogenesis and vasculogenesis, and (3) allowing apoptosis by blocking beta-adrenergic receptors.[19] In 2013, a consensus statement was released to assist providers in treating patients with propranolol.[21] Most providers target dose range in between 1 and 3 mg/kg/day, divided two or three times a day.[21] The majority of patients can be treated as outpatients, but inpatient initiation is recommended for premature infants and those younger than 8 weeks. For an infantile hemangioma in the proliferative stage, treatment is continued until the child is between 9 and 15 months of age and is then tapered slowly, over weeks to months, to prevent rebound tachycardia. Generally, weaning occurs over 25% of the time that the infant was on oral propranolol. Dosing should be suspended for illness or poor oral intake, given the risk of masking hypoglycemia. Remarkably, cardiac side effects such as hypotension (<0.5%) and bradycardia (<0.1%) have been extremely rare for infants on oral propranolol.[22] Other side effects, such as sleep disturbance (10%), hypoglycemia (<0.5%), and bronchospasm (3%), are more common, generally mild and well tolerated.

For patients with smaller and more superficial hemangiomas, topical timolol, a nonselective beta-blocker, is an excellent alternative. The use of topical timolol for infantile hemangiomas was first described in 2010.[23] Topical timolol comes in both an ophthalmic drop formulation as well as a 0.5% gel forming substrate, with preference given to gel forming substrate. The safety profile of topical timolol is excellent and it should be considered in infants whose hemangiomas warrant treatment but systemic treatments are either not wanted or are contraindicated. According to one study,[24] topical timolol is most effective when used in superficial hemangiomas <100 mm^3 with a diameter <11 mm. For smaller periorbital lesions that do not pose immediate complications, timolol is the ideal treatment. However, topical timolol is not the treatment of choice for ulcerated or deep hemangiomas and is neither effective nor fast enough for lesions which pose a possible functional issue for the infant. It is not currently understood how topical application of the beta-blocker causes clearance of superficial infantile hemangiomas.

As mentioned above, due to the success and improved side effect profile of oral propranolol and topical timolol, oral glucocorticosteroids have become second-line treatment for infants with resistant hemangiomas or for those not tolerating beta-blocker treatment.

Laser treatments are particularly effective for treatment of infantile hemangiomas, with the PDL being the primary work horse. The PDL is ideally suited for superficial lesions, <3 mm thick, which are flat and smooth. Treatments should begin as early as possible at intervals of 2–3 weeks. Low energy densities should be used (<7 J/cm^2) with short pulse durations (0.45–1.5 ms) with large spot sizes. Epidermal cooling is essential as is eye protection for patient as well as providers in the room. Another main indication for treatment of infantile hemangioma with PDL is presence of ulceration because of their inhibitory effect on the growth of the hemangioma, which allows for re-epithelialization.[17,18]

Laser treatments can safely be used with both oral (**Figs. 1A** and **B**) and topical (**Figs. 2A** and **B**) beta blockers. A recent study suggested that combined PDL and beta blocker therapy work synergistically to slow the growth of the hemangioma as well as speed up the involution process.[25] Using PDL and propranolol concurrently has been shown to improve clearance rates and hasten time to clearance as well as reduce cumulative propranolol dose.[26] The exact mechanism of this synergy has not been elucidated, but the results comparing concomitant PDL and propranolol versus delayed PDL with propranolol versus propranolol alone favor the concomitant group.

The PDL is also effective in treating residual telangiectasias associated with involuted hemangiomas. One retrospective study showed 50–75% improvement in color of hemangioma in all patients.[27] Finally, the fractionated CO_2 laser can be very useful to treat any residual skin atrophy by stimulating dermal collagen neogenesis.

Surgical excision of hemangiomas is generally performed during involution and is typically reserved for: (1) hemangiomas located in airway, periorbital, nasal, perioral, and periauricular regions; (2) those that

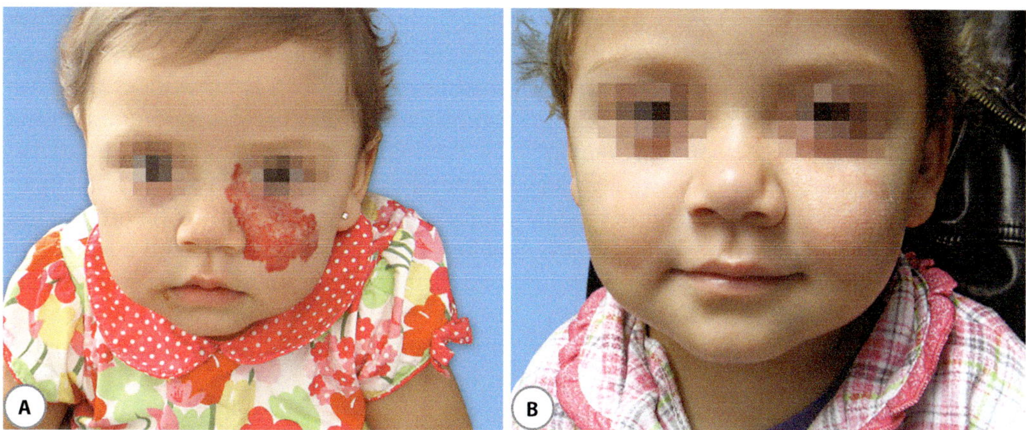

FIGS. 1A AND B: Hemangioma treated by combined oral propranolol and pulsed dye laser; (A) Pretreatment and (B) Posttreatment.

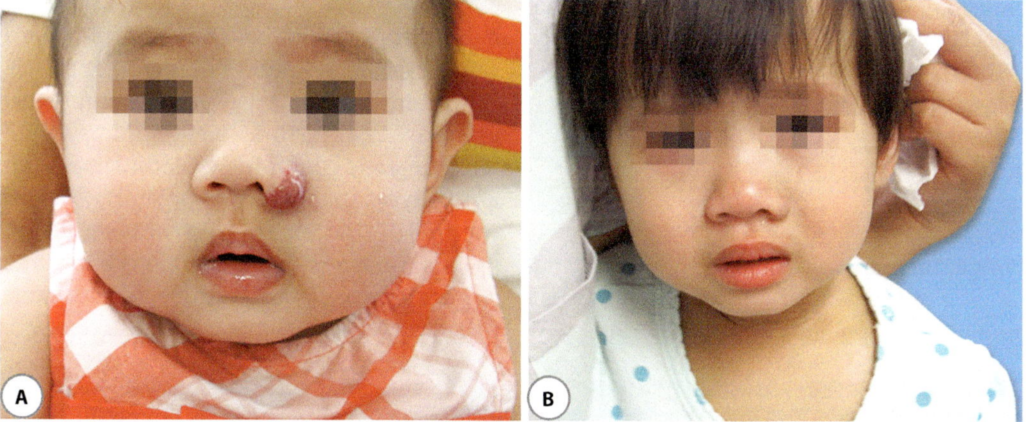

FIGS. 2A AND B: Hemangioma treated by combined topical timolol and pulsed dye laser; (A) Pretreatment and (B) Posttreatment.

impose a threat to the child's health; and (3) removal of remnant fibrofatty tissue after involution. Due to the potential for scarring and bleeding, surgical excision is usually not the main treatment of choice. Oftentimes, hemangiomas undergo embolization prior to surgical excision to limit bleeding risk.[28]

Phaces

Patients with extensive segmental facial hemangiomas may have associated arterial, central nervous system, and ophthalmic abnormalities.[29] The acronym PHACES (posterior fossa anomalies, hemangiomas, arterial anomalies, coarctation of aorta and cardiac defects, eye abnormalities, sternal clefting and supraumbilical raphe) has been given to the following constellation of findings:

- Posterior fossa malformations (e.g., Dandy-Walker malformation)
- Hemangiomas
- Arterial anomalies
- Coarctation of aorta and cardiac defects (e.g., aneurysm)

- Eye abnormalities (e.g., congenital cataract, microphthalmia, and abnormal retinal vessels)
- Sternal clefts or supraumbilical raphes

Infants with large facial segmental hemangiomas >20 cm² have an approximately 30% risk of PHACES. Those infants require urgent MRI/magnetic resonance angiography (MRA) of the head, neck and aortic arch, echocardiogram, and ophthalmological examination. PHACES is more common in females and >50% are affected by neurologic disorders (seizures, stroke, and developmental delay).[30] These hemangiomas are at more risk for ulceration and scarring.[31] The most common extracutaneous manifestation is brain malformations (71%).[31] Hemangiomas in association with PHACE have been successfully treated by combined oral propranolol and PDL (**Figs. 3A** and **B**).

Congenital Hemangiomas (RICH/NICH)

Congenital hemangiomas are clinically and histologically different than the more common infantile hemangioma. They compromise 3% of all hemangiomas seen in infancy.[32] CH are present at full size at birth and do not undergo further expansion. CH are subdivided into rapidly involuting congenital hemangioma (RICH) and noninvoluting congenital hemangioma (NICH).[33] At birth, RICH can appear as a violaceous mass with radiating veins, a telangiectatic mass with a pale halo, or a firm pink to violaceous plaque. RICH lesions generally involute by 12–24 months of age, with residual thin skin with associated prominent veins, without much fibrofatty tissue. Because they rapidly involute, usually no therapy is warranted for RICH lesions. There may be residual atrophic dermal changes, residual redundant skin, dysplastic veins, hyperpigmentation, or an anemic halo left behind after resolution. Each of these issues can be treated by surgical or laser therapy.

Noninvoluting congenital hemangiomas are present at birth as well circumscribed telangiectatic pink-blue-violet masses with a pale halo that grow proportionally with the infant. Rather than involuting, these lesions worsen with age and do not involute spontaneously and require subsequent treatment. Laser treatment, surgical removal,

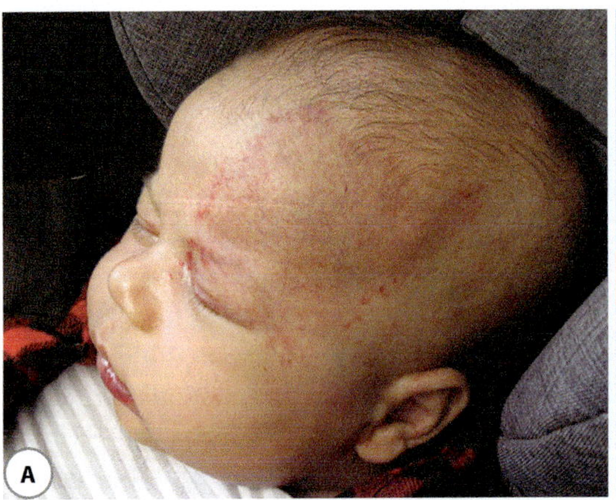

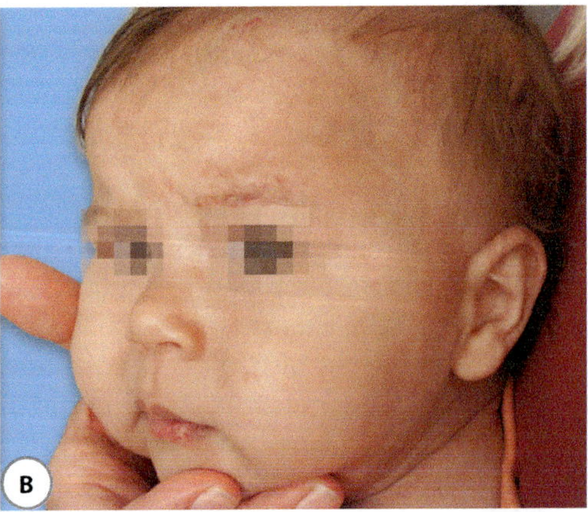

(PDL: pulsed dye laser; PHACES: posterior fossa anomalies, hemangiomas, arterial anomalies, coarctation of aorta and cardiac defects, eye abnormalities, sternal clefting and supraumbilical raphe)

FIGS. 3A AND B: Segmental hemangioma in association with PHACES treated by combined oral propranolol and PDL; (A) Pretreatment and (B) Posttreatment.

and sclerotherapy are the most frequently used therapies for NICH. Surgical removal should be proceeded by vascular imaging and embolization performed prior to excision in cases where large feeding vessels or high-flow are identified. Laser treatment options are similar to those presented under infantile hemangiomas.

Kaposiform Hemangioendothelioma/ Tufted Angioma

Kaposiform hemangioendothelioma (KHE) and tufted angioma (TA) are rare, locally aggressive infiltrative vascular neoplasm affecting 0.7–0.9/100,000 births.[34] KHE has a predilection for extremities, followed by head and neck, chest, and retroperitoneum. KHE often presents in infancy and can be confused with infantile hemangiomas although these two can be differentiated based on histology and natural history. Unlike infantile hemangiomas, KHE is an aggressive infiltrative tumor which often crosses tissue planes invading the underlying fascia, muscle, and bone. Also unlike infantile hemangiomas, KHE does not spontaneously regress. TA is thought to represent a more benign superficial variant of KHE. These lesions present early in life as bright red mottled patches or plaques, sometimes with papules, on the neck, shoulders, and trunk. They grow slowly by lateral extension but do not generally become invasive or infiltrative. This growth can last for months to years. Eventually, these lesions stabilize and may then persist, or rarely they may involute leaving a residual fibrotic tissue which can be excised by surgical excision without leaving substantial deformity.

Approximately 70% of patients with KHE and TA will have KMS, which is a consumptive coagulopathy caused by intralesional platelet trapping, leading to thrombocytopenia.[35,36] Due to local invasion, compression of vital organs or bleeding due to KMS, patients with KHE have a 20–30% mortality rate.[34,36]

Treatment options for KHE and TA include: corticosteroids, vincristine, intravascular embolization, and surgery, but due to risks of embolization and surgery, medical therapies are favored.[34] At the time of this publication, sirolimus, a potent inhibitor of mechanistic target of rapamycin (mTOR), which is involved in many cellular regulatory effects on antitumor and immunosuppressive activity including vascular growth, is showing promise as a therapy for those patients who fail steroids.[34] Currently, there is no role for lasers in the treatment of KHE or TA.

Cherry Angioma

Cherry angiomas are the most common acquired vascular proliferation of the skin.[37] They are benign skin growths, 1–5 mm in size, which are red, dome-shaped lesions, typically on trunk, or upper extremities. These lesions tend to increase in number as the patient ages but may also present during pregnancy, climate changes, and exposure to chemicals.[38] Pathology shows a true capillary hemangioma, formed by numerous newly formed capillaries with narrow lumens and prominent epithelial cells arranged in a lobular pattern in the papillary dermis.[38] The PDL and KTP lasers are both very effective for clearing cherry angiomas, usually in a single treatment session. Recurrences are unusual. Other treatment options include curettage or electrosurgery.

Pyogenic Granuloma

Pyogenic granulomas are benign vascular lesions, most commonly presenting in the head and neck and upper trunk regions of children and young adults. In 2014, the ISSVA recognized pyogenic granulomas as a benign vascular lesion.[1] The lesions tend to grow rapidly into a solitary red nodule.

The lesions are extremely friable and the most common reason for presentation is profuse, recurrent bleeding from incidental trauma. While the exact etiology of the lesion is not well known, trauma, hormonal changes, chronic skin irritation, and pre-existing vascular lesions have all been suggested as possible sources.[39] Treatment for these vascular lesions includes: shave excision, electrocautery, cryotherapy and lasers, including PDL, Nd:YAG, and CO_2.[40]

VASCULAR MALFORMATIONS

Vascular malformations are vascular lesions which are present at birth, do not regress, and grow with the patient. These lesions are divided into low-flow (venous, lymphatic, and capillary) and high-flow (AVM). VM show no cellular proliferation but progressive dilation of abnormal channels.[32] Each VM is reviewed below.

CAPILLARY VASCULAR MALFORMATION (PORT-WINE STAIN)

Capillary VM, or PWS, is a vascular lesion characterized by ectatic vessels within the cutaneous superficial vascular plexus of the papillary and reticular dermis.[41] Distinct from some hemangiomas, these lesions are always present at birth. PWS have equal gender distribution and affect 0.3–0.5% of all births.[42] While there can be a family history, the majority of the lesions are sporadic. Upon presentation, the vascular lesion is usually pink and flat. This lesion will grow with the patient and become darker, raised, irregularly surfaced, and may develop associated nodules.[41,43] By the fifth decade, almost two-thirds of patients will experience nodules and hypertrophy, with risk of spontaneous bleeding and pyogenic granuloma.[43] As over 40% of PWS develop on the face, intervention is sought early due to potential of social awkwardness and teasing.[43]

The cause and origin of PWS remains incompletely understood. It is believed that PWS develop within the first 2–8 weeks of gestation. The most likely hypothesis for the development of PWS is the deficiency or absence of surrounding neurons regulating blood flow through the ectatic postcapillary venules. As a result, the blood vessels are unable to constrict normally and remain permanently dilated.

Historically, PWS were treated with excision and skin grafting, cryotherapy, ionizing radiation, dermabrasion, and tattooing with unencouraging results.[41] As such, lasers targeting vascular chromophores have become the treatment of choice for PWS. In PWS, the target vessels are between 10 and 500 mm in diameter, located in the papillary and reticular dermis.[44] To minimize collateral damage, the pulse duration should be less than or equal to the target's t_r which in the case of PWS is 0.45–10 ms.[2]

Ideally, treatment for PWS should begin as early as possible. Early intervention is not only safe but also more effective with higher likelihood of clearance of PWS.[41] As mentioned above, the PWS will grow with the patient so the malformation is smallest during infancy. Treating a smaller lesion has a higher likelihood of achieving clearance as compared to a larger lesion.[45,46] Additionally, there are a number of key "optical" advantages to beginning laser treatment at the earliest possible age. In as much as infant's skin contains less melanin, more energy is delivered to the target chromophore (hemoglobin) without loss of energy to melanin containing structures (epidermis/hair). Infantile skin also contains much less dermal collagen and, therefore, less optical scattering which allows more laser light to penetrate deeper into the dermis. PWS blood vessels in infants are smaller and, therefore, an easier target for selective

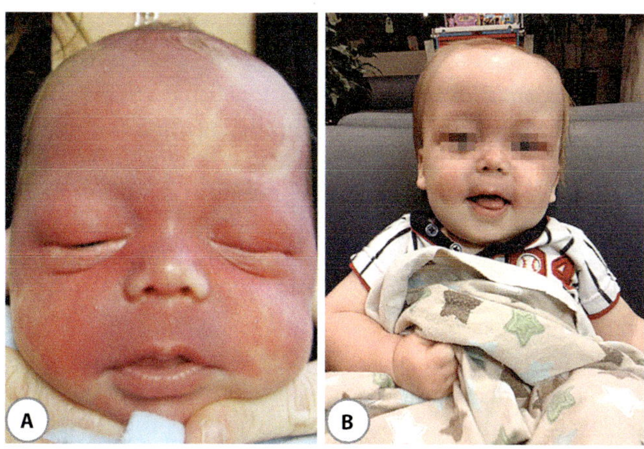

FIGS. 4A AND B: Capillary vascular malformation treated by pulsed dye laser; (A) Pretreatment and (B) Posttreatment.

photothermolysis to destroy. Finally, there is no shielding of deeper blood vessels in the skin by large and dilated blood vessels in the superficial layers of the skin. For all of the above reasons, most medical specialists agree that it is critical to begin treatment of PWS as early as possible and to maintain treatment in order to prevent the development of vascular nodules and hypertrophy in later years (**Figs. 4A** and **B**).

Pulsed dye laser treatment for PWS in infants has been used safely in children as young as 1 week old and at treatment intervals ranging from every 2 to 4 weeks with improved clearance rates in children following the 2-weeks protocol.[43] Pulse durations range from 0.45 to 40 ms with common spot sizes 10–12 mm and common initial energy densities of 8–9 J/cm^2.[47] Because of the range in size of the blood vessels in PWS, it is necessary to treat with several different pulse durations to target the vessels of different sizes, with longer pulse durations targeting the larger and deeper blood vessels. It is imperative to always ensure the patient's eyes are protected either with laser aids, if the PWS and PDL treatments are not near the eyes, or laser-safe metal corneal shields if the PWS and PDL treatments are periocular. PDL has an excellent safety profile for photo skin types 1–3, with increased chance of scarring and postinflammatory hyperpigmentation (PIH) in phototypes 4–5.[48] The size and color of the lesion, location, and hypertrophy are all characteristics of a PWS which can affect the efficacy of the laser treatment with smaller, lighter lesions located on periorbital area, lateral facial cheeks, chest, and proximal arms showing the best response.[49] Although PDL is the current initial treatment of choice for PWS, 20–30% of all patients show resistance so additional lasers may need to be utilized.[50]

The KTP laser can also be used to treat PWS. However, due to its shorter wavelength at 532 nm, the KTP laser has higher absorption by melanin, as compared to the PDL, and as such, should be used with caution in patients with darker skin phototypes.[51]

Alexandrite lasers with a wavelength of 755 nm have also been shown effective in resistant PWS, due to their deeper penetration.[52] Additionally, Nd:YAG lasers have found a niche in resistant PWS and those PWS with vascular nodules. Because the Nd:YAG laser is poorly absorbed by water, it can penetrate tissue to a depth of 4–5 mm in human skin. As it passes through the tissue, it emits heat and can coagulate down to a depth of 7–10 mm.[53] Because of its deeper penetration and low absorption by melanin, the Nd:YAG is appropriate for both resistant/nodular PWS as well as in patients with phototype 5–6 skin.[54] However, because higher fluences are necessary, there is an increased risk of scarring and permanent pigment changes.[55]

Side effects from laser treatment for PWS include redness, swelling, and ecchymosis. PWS are usually treated at settings which cause purpura, which regresses over 1–2 weeks. Blistering and ulceration are uncommon and should be treated aggressively with petroleum jelly and moist bandages to prevent scarring. Alopecia is possible when treating pigmented, hair-bearing areas. Likewise permanent skin changes both hypo- and hyperpigmentation are possible. Effective cooling, selecting the appropriate laser wavelength, conservative fluences, and pretreatment sun protection will all help to protect skin from pigment changes. Injury to the eye is a serious and rare complication, as such, it is required practice to cover eyes with laser approved goggles/stickers and even inserting a metallic contact lens into the eye when periocular facial lesions are treated by laser.

Sturge-Weber syndrome (SWS): There are two syndromes associated with a specific pattern of PWS presentation which merit mentioning. The first is SWS: Facial PWS, vascular involvement of leptomeninges, possible glaucoma of ipsilateral eye, possible seizures, and mental retardation.[56] When a PWS occurs in the V1 dermatome, 7–28% of patients will have SWS and 10% of patients will have glaucoma so evaluation by an ophthalmologist is necessary. Suspicion for possible SWS based on location of PWS should prompt an MRI which is the screening tool of choice.[47] However, it should be noted that a MRI may be negative for SWS in infants <1 year of age. More recently, serial electroencephalograms have been demonstrated to be more sensitive to SWS in young infants.[57] These patients may still undergo PDL treatment for their PWS, but it is imperative to have them screened by appropriate professions for possible glaucoma and cerebral manifestations.[47]

Several studies, including a systemic review, support safety profile of treating Kasabach-Merritt phenomenon and other VM, namely PWS, venous malformations and LM, with oral and/or topical sirolimus with significant clinical improvement, if not complete clearance. Sirolimus inhibits mTOR, a serine-threonine kinase, which is involved in cell growth/proliferation, angiogenesis, and lymphangiogenesis. Sirolimus can be used in conjunction with PDL to improve efficacy of treatment.

Klippel-Trénaunay syndrome (KTS): KTS includes a unilateral upper or lower extremity PWS with associated tissue and bony hypertrophy, evidence of venous insufficiency, lymphedema, and phleboliths.[58] As with SWS, an MRI is diagnostic and the associated PWS is treatable with PDL.

VENOUS MALFORMATIONS

Venous malformations are the most common of all VM and are present at birth but may not present until later in life. They are low-flow lesions which usually present as a soft, bluish, compressible mass which enlarges with Valsalva maneuver. These lesions tend to span multiple tissue planes. Diagnosis is confirmed with T2-weighted MRI showing hyperintense serpiginous lesions with phleboliths.[14] Venous malformations have irregular collections of venous channels with flat endothelium and scant mural smooth muscle.[32] Venous blood from normal vessels enters the malformation but does not find an easy exit, leading to expansion and stasis of blood, which predisposes to calcifications and clots.

Observation of venous malformations is a reasonable treatment option for small lesions which do not cause functional or cosmetic concerns. Daily aspirin has been shown to reduce thrombotic events and the pain associated with these events.[59]

For small venous malformations, percutaneous sclerotherapy is considered first. The sclerosing agent causes endothelial damage, inflammation, thrombosis, and fibrosis with eventual destruction of the lesion. Sclerotherapy often needs to be repeated several times for effect and has limited damage to surrounding structures (nerves).[60,61] Predictive factors associated with improved outcome in venous malformations treated with sclerosing agents are: Female gender and lesions <5 cm.[62] Sclerosis of venous malformations typically does not result in complete resolution of the lesion but does have favorable outcomes when used by itself or in combination with surgery.[63]

Superficial lesions or the superficial component of a deep venous malformation can be treated with Nd:YAG or diode lasers.[64] Additionally, mucosal and aerodigestive venous malformations may be treated with the Nd:YAG or diode lasers, which target the purplish hue of the malformation very well.

Surgical excision is the only treatment modality that offers the possibility of complete resolution.[63] Surgery is often used in combination with other treatment modalities, such as sclerosis or laser. An algorithm has been developed to help guide treatment for venous malformations:[65]

- Laser therapy as first line treatment for superficial lesions confined to skin and for mucosal lesions;
- Surgical excision for failed laser treatment or for small, localized venous malformations involving deep tissues of head and neck; and
- Sclerotherapy for first-line treatment or as an adjunct to surgery for deeper and ill-defined lesions.

ARTERIOVENOUS MALFORMATIONS

Arteriovenous malformations are the only high-flow VM. These lesions tend to grow rapidly with a palpable thrill. MRI is the diagnostic modality of choice with many flow voids.[14] Histology shows beds of venules and arterioles intermixed with large-caliber arteries and veins.[14] These high-flow lesions have aberrant connections between arterioles and venules, bypassing the capillary bed, which causes recruitment of more vessels over time with associated local tissue destruction.[66] Many AVMs do not present until adulthood with rapid growth occurring during hormonal fluctuations.

The mainstay treatment is preoperative embolization followed by surgical resection of the mass and feeder vessel. Even despite surgical resection, there remains a high rate of recurrence. There is no role for laser therapy in treatment of AVM.

LYMPHATIC MALFORMATIONS

Lymphatic malformations previously called cystic hygromas or lymphangiomas) are low-flow lesions, presenting as a soft, compressible, and cystic lesion with chylous material. They result from maldevelopment of embryonic lymphatic channels which fail to drain into the venous system.[32] LM are classified as micro- or macrocystic, or mixed. Microcystic lesions are composed of single or multiple cysts <2 cm^3 and are usually found above the level of the mylohyoid muscle. Macrocystic lesions have multiloculated cysts >2 cm^3 and usually occur below the level of the mylohyoid muscle. The distinction between these two categories is important as certain treatment modalities are more effective for one category versus the other. Although they rarely spontaneously involute,[67] observation is a reasonable treatment options for LMs that are small, not causing functional, or cosmetic dysfunction.

Because LMs tend to invade local tissues and have ill-defined borders, surgical excision is sometimes incomplete and associated with recurrence.[63] Typically, focal, macrocystic lesions tend to respond well to surgical excision whereas the invasive nature of the microcystic lesions makes them less amenable to surgery.[63] Because of possibility of recurrence and surgical morbidity, sclerotherapy has become the primary treatment for LMs.[63] There are a variety of sclerosing agents: Ethanol, hypertonic saline, doxycycline, and acetic acid,[68] although OK-432 (Penicillin-killed *Streptococcus pyogenes*) is the most common. Macrocystic lesions respond very well to OK-432 with fewer complications as compared to surgery and with higher clearance rates; however, microcystic lesions do not respond to OK-432.[69]

Carbon dioxide lasers and radiofrequency ablative devices have also been used to treat the cutaneous component of LM (lymphangioma circumscriptum) but recurrence has been problematic, particular if the deeper component of the malformation is not concurrently treated.[70] More recently, the inhibitors of cyclic guanosine monophosphate-specific phosphodiesterase (PDE) type 5, such as sildenafil and tadalafil, have been demonstrated to lead the major improvement of some LMs.[71]

CONCLUSION

Although not prevalent, infantile hemangiomas are the most common pediatric soft tissue tumor, and as such, the reader should have an understanding of the treatment options for infantile hemangiomas as well as the remainder of the vascular lesions. Diagnosis and treatment truly involves a multidisciplinary team, often with concomitant treatment protocols. Laser treatment for pediatric VM whether as a single modality or as a multimodality approach is a safe and effective option for the majority of the vascular lesions, favoring initiating treatment at an early age. **Table 3** summarizes the vascular anomalies discussed and the recommended treatment options.[72,73]

TABLE 3: Summary of vascular anomaly with associated treatment options.

Vascular anomaly	Recommended treatment
Infantile hemangiomas	• Medical management with beta blockers: Oral propranolol or topical timolol • PDL can be used concomitantly with beta blockers • Surgical resection of fibrofatty remnant after involution
RICH	Laser versus surgery for any residual effects following involution
NICH	• PDL • Sclerotherapy • Sclerotherapy surgical excision
KHE/TA	• Medical management with corticosteroids, vincristine, or sirolimus • Embolization versus surgery
Cherry angioma	• PDL or KTP • Curettage • Electrosurgery

Cont'd...

Cont'd...

Vascular anomaly	Recommended treatment
Pyogenic granuloma	• PDL, Nd:YAG, and CO_2 laser • Shave biopsy • Electrosurgery • Cryotherapy
Port wine stain	• PDL: Treatment of choice for infants/children • KTP: Less effective than PDL • Alexandrite: Used for resistant lesions • Nd:YAG for vascular nodules
Venous malformations	• Sclerotherapy: For small lesions • Laser (Nd:YAG or diode) for superficial or mucosal lesions • Surgical excision
Arteriovenous malformations	Preoperative embolization followed by surgical excision
Lymphatic malformations	• Sclerotherapy: More effective for macrocystic lesions • Sildenafil or tadalafil • Surgical excision • CO_2 laser for lymphangioma circumscriptum

(CO_2: carbon dioxide; KHE: kaposiform hemangioendothelioma; KTP: potassium titanyl phosphate; Nd:YAG: neodymium-doped:yttrium aluminum garnet; NICH: noninvoluting congenital hemangioma; PDL: pulsed dye laser; RICH: rapidly involuting congenital hemangioma; TA: tufted angiomas)

REFERENCES

1. ISSVA. (2014). Classification. [online] Available from https://www.issva.com/classification [Last accessed April, 2021].
2. Anderson RR, Parrish JA. Selective photothermolysis: precise microsurgery by selective absorption of pulsed radiation. Science. 1983;220(4596):524-7.
3. Nelson JS, Milner TE, Anvari B, Norvang LT, Tran NH, Tanenbaum BS, et al. Dynamic Cooling of the Epidermis During Laser Port Wine Stain Therapy. Lasers Surg Med. 1994:6S:48.
4. Nelson JS, Milner TE, Anvari B, Tanenbaum BS, Kimel S, Svaasand LO, et al. Dynamic epidermal cooling during pulsed laser treatment of port-wine stain. A new methodology with preliminary clinical evaluation. Arch Dermatol. 1995;131(6):695-700.
5. Kilcline C, Frieden IJ. Infantile hemangiomas: how common are they? A systematic review of the medical literature. Pediatr Dermatol. 2008;25(2):168-73.
6. Burton BK, Schulz CJ, Angle B, Burd LI. An increased incidence of hemangiomas in infants born following chorionic villus sampling (CVS). Prenat Diagn. 1995;15(3):209-14.
7. Tollefson MM, Frieden IJ. Early growth of infantile hemangiomas: What parent's photographs tell us. Pediatrics. 2012;130(2):e314-20.
8. Margileth AM, Museles M. Cutaneous hemangiomas in children: diagnosis and conservative management. JAMA. 1965;194(5):523-6.
9. Golitz LE, Rudikoff J, O'Meara OP. Diffuse neonatal hemangiomatosis. Pediatr Dermatol. 1986;3(2): 145-52.
10. Orlow SJ, Isakoff MS, Blei F. Increased risk of symptomatic hemangiomas of the airway in association with cutaneous hemangiomas in a "beard" distribution. J Pediatri. 1997;131(4):643-6.
11. Itinteang T, Withers AH, Davis PF, Tan ST. Biology of Infantile Hemangioma. Front Surg. 2014;1:38.
12. Janmohamed SR, Madern GC, de Laat PCJ, Oranje AP. Educational paper: pathogenesis of infantile hemangioma, an update 2014 (Part 1). Eur J Pediatr. 2015;174(1): 97-103.
13. Mihm MC Jr, Nelson JS. Hypothesis: the metastatic niche theory can elucidate infantile hemangioma development. J Cutan Pathol. 2010;37(1):83-7.
14. Tekes A, Koshy J, Kalayci TO, Puttgen K, Cohen B, Redett R, et al. S.E. Mitchell Vascular Anomalies Flow Chart (SEMVAFC): A Visual Pathway Combining Clinical and Imaging Findings for Classification of Soft-Tissue Vascular Anomalies. Clin Radiol. 2014;69(5):443-57.
15. Takahashi K, Mulliken JB, Kozakewich HP, Rogers RA, Folkman J, Ezekowitz RA. Cellular markers that distinguish

the phases of hemangioma during infancy and childhood. J Clin Invest. 1994;93(6):2357-64.

16. Dinehart SM, Kincannon J, Geronemus R. Hemangiomas: evaluation and treatment. Dermatol Surg. 2001;27(5): 475-85.
17. Finn MC, Glowacki J, Mulliken JB. Congenital Vascular Lesions: Clinical Application of a New Classification. J Pediatr Surg. 1983;18(6):894-900.
18. Batniji RK, Buckingham ED, Williams EF. An aesthetic approach to facial hemangiomas. Arch Facial Plast Surg. 2005;7(5):301-6.
19. Ames JA, Sykes JM. Current trends in medical management of infantile hemangioma. Curr Opin Otolaryngol Head and Neck Surg. 2015;23(4):286-91.
20. Leaute-Labreze C, de la Roque ED, Hubiche T, Boralevi F, Thambo JB, Taïeb A. Propranolol for severe hemangiomas of infancy. N Eng J Med. 2008;358(24):2649-51.
21. Drolet BA, Frommelt PC, Chamlin SL, Haggstrom A, Bauman NM, Chiu YE, et al. Initiation and use of propranolol for infantile hemangiomas: report of a consensus conference. Pediatrics. 2013;131(1):128-40.
22. Menezes MD, McCarter R, Greene EA, Bauman NM. Status of propranolol for treatment of infantile hemangioma and description of a randomized clinical trial. Ann Otol Rhinol Laryngol. 2011;120(10):686-95.
23. Guo S, Nina N. Topical Treatment for Capillary Hemangioma of the Eyelid Using Beta-Blocker Solution. Arch Ophthalmol. 2010;128(2):255-6.
24. Chan H, McKay C, Adams S. Wargon O. RTC of Timolol Maleate Gel for Superficial Infantile Hemangiomas in 5- to 24-week-olds. Pediatrics. 2013;131(6):1739-47.
25. Asilian A, Mokhtari F, Kamali AS, Abtahi-Naeini B, Nilforoushzadeh MA, Mostafaie S. Pulsed Dye Laser and Topical Timolol Gel versus Pulse Dye Laser in Treatment of Infantile Hemangioma: A Double-Blind Randomized Controlled Trial. Adv Biomed Res. 2015;4:257.
26. Reddy KK, Blei F, Brauer JA, Waner M, Anolik R, Bernstein L, et al. Retrospective Study of the Treatment of Infantile Hemangiomas Using a Combination of Propranolol and Pulsed Dye Laser. Dermatol Surg. 2013;39(6): 923-33.
27. Sajan JA, Tibesar R, Jabbour N, Lander T, Hilger P, Sidman J. Assessment of Pulsed-Dye Laser Therapy for Pediatric Cutaneous Vascular Anomalies. JAMA Facial Plast Surg. 2013;15(6):434-8.
28. Argenta LC, Bishop E, Cho KJ, Andrews AF, Coran AG. Complete Resolution of Life-Threatening Hemangioma by Embolization and Corticosteroids. Plast Reconstr Surg. 1982;70(6):739-44.
29. Frieden IJ, Reese V, Cohen D. PHACE syndrome: The association of posterior fossa brain malformations, hemangiomas, arterial anomalies, coarctation of the aorta and cardiac defects, and eye abnormalities. Arch Dermatol. 1996;132(3):307-11.
30. Burrows PE, Robertson RL, Mulliken JB, Beardsley DS, Chaloupka JC, Ezekowitz RA, et al. Cerebral vasculopathy and neurologic sequelae in infants with cervicofacial hemangioma: report of 8 patients. Radiology. 1998; 207(3):601-7.
31. Metry DW, Garzon MC, Drolet BA, Frommelt P, Haggstrom A, Hall J, et al. PHACE syndrome: current knowledge, future directions. Pediatr Dermatol. 2009;26(4):381-98.
32. Elluru RG. Cutaneous vascular lesions. Facial Plast Surg. 2013;21(1):111-26.
33. Berenguer B, Mulliken JB, Enjolras O, Boon LM, Wassef M, Josset P, et al. Rapidly involuting congenital hemangioma: clinical and histopathologic features. Pediatr Dev Pathol. 2003;6(6):495-510.
34. Alaqeel AM, Alfurayh NA, Alhedyani AA, Alajlan SM. Sirolimus for treatment of kaposiform hemangioendothelioma associated with Kasabach-Merritt phenomenon. JAAD Case Rep. 2016;2(6):457-61.
35. Reichel A, Hamm H, Wiegering V, Wiewrodt B, Neubauer H, Ernestus K, et al. "Kaposiform Hemangioendothelioma with Kasabach-Merritt Syndrome: Successful Treatment with Sirolimus. J Dtsch Dermatol Ges. 2017;15(3):329-31.
36. Liu XH, Li JY, Qu XH, Yan WL, Zhang L, Yang C, et al. Treatment of kaposiform hemangioendothelioma and tufted angioma. Int J Cancer. 2016;139(7):1658-66.
37. Murison AR, Sutherland JW, Williamson AM. De Morgan's Spots. Br Med J. 1947;1(4505):634-6.
38. Kim JH, Park HY, Ahn SK. Cherry Angiomas of the Scalp. Case Rep Dermatol. 2009;1(1):82-6.
39. Putra J, Rymeski B, Merrow AC, Dasgupta R, Gupta A. Four Cases of Pediatric Deep-Seated/Subcutaneous Pyogenic Granuloma: Review of the Literature and Differential Diagnosis. J Cutan Pathol. 2017;44(6):516-22.
40. Au S, Fancher W, Scribner J. Treatment of Pediatric Pyogenic Granuloma in a Functionally and Cosmetically Sensitive Area with the 1064 nm Nd:YAG Laser. Dermatol Online J. 2016;22(4):13030.
41. Chapas AM, Eickhorst K, Geronemus RG. Efficacy of Early Treatment of Facial Port Wine Stains in Newborns: A Review of 49 Cases. Lasers Surg Med. 2007;39(7):563-8.
42. Alper JC, Holmes LB. The Incidence and Significance of Birthmarks in a Cohort of 4,641 Newborns. Pediatr Dermatol. 1983;1(1):58-68.
43. Anolik R, Newlove T, Weiss ET, Brightman L, Hale EK, Karen JK, et al. Investigation into optimal treatment intervals of facial port wine stains using the pulsed dye laser. J Am Acad Dermatol. 2012;67(5):985-90.
44. Liu G, Jia W, Nelson JS, Chen Z. In vivo, high-resolution, three-dimensional imaging of port wine stain microvasculature in human skin. Lasers Surg Med. 2013;45(10):628-32.
45. Morelli JG, Weston WL, Huff JC, Yohn JJ. Initial lesion size as a predictive factor in determining the response of port-wine stains in children treated with pulsed dye laser. Arch Pediatr Adolesc Med. 1995;149(10):1142-4.

46. Nguyen CM, Yohn JJ, Huff C, Weston WL, Morelli JG. Facial Port Wine Stains in Childhood: Prediction of the Rate of Improvement as a Function of the Age of the Patient, Size and Location of the Port Wine Stain and the Number of Treatments with the Pulsed Dye (585nm) laser. Br J Dermatol. 1998;138(5):821-5.
47. Brightman LA, Geronemus RG, Reddy KK. Laser Treatment of Port-Wine Stains. Clin Cosmet Investig Dermatol. 2015;8:27-33.
48. Thajudheen CP, Jyothy K, Priyadarshini A. Treatment of Port-Wine Stains with Flash Lamp Pumped Pulsed Dye Laser on Indian Skin: a six Year Study. J Cutan Aesthet Surg. 2014;7(1):32-6.
49. Renfro L, Geronemus RG. Anatomical Differences of Port Wine Stains in Response to Treatment with the Pulsed Dye Laser. Arch Dermatol. 1993;129(2):182-8.
50. Savas JA, Ledon JA, Franca K, Chacon A, Nouri K. Pulsed Dye Laser-Resistant Port Wine Stains: Mechanisms of Resistance and Implications for Treatment. Br J Dermatol. 2013;168(5):941-53.
51. Becher GL, Cameron H, Moseley H. Treatment of Superficial Vascular Lesions with the KTP 532-nm Laser: Experience with 647 Patients. Lasers Med Sci. 2014;29(1):267-71.
52. Izikson L, Anderson RR. Treatment Endpoints for Resistant Port Wine Stains with a 755 nm Laser. J Cosmet Laser Ther. 2009;11(1):52-5.
53. Shapshay SM, David LM, Zeitels S. Neodymium-YAG Laser Photocoagulation of Hemangiomas of the Head and Neck. Laryngoscope. 1987;97(3 Pt 1):323-30.
54. Brauer JA, Geronemus RG. Single-Treatment Resolution of Vascular Blebs within Port Wine Stains Using a Novel 1,064nm neodymium-doped yttrium aluminum garnet Laser. Dermatol Surg. 2013;39(7):1113-5.
55. McGill DJ, MacLaren W, Mackay IR. A Direct Comparison of Pulsed Dye, Alexandrite, KTP and Nd:YAG Lasers and IPL in Patients with Previously Treated Capillary Malformations. Lasers Surg Med. 2008;40(6):390-8.
56. Shirley MD, Tang H, Gallione CJ, Baugher JD, Frelin LP, Cohen B, et al. Sturge-Weber Syndrome and Port Wine Stains Caused by Somatic Mutation in GNAQ. N Engl J Med. 2013;368(21):1971-9.
57. Ewen JB, Kossoff EH, Crone NE, Lin DDM, Lakshmanan BM, Ferenc LM, et al. Use of Quantitative EEG in Infants with Port-Wine Birthmark to Assess for Sturge-Weber Brain Involvement. Clin Neurophysiol. 2009;120(8):1433-40.
58. Lam SM, Williams EF. Practical Considerations in the Treatment of Capillary Vascular Malformations, or Port Wine Stains. Facial Plast Surg. 2004;20(1):71-6.
59. Buckmiller LM, Richter GT, Suen Y. Diagnosis and Management of Hemangiomas and Vascular Malformations of the Head and Neck. Oral Dis. 2010; 16(5):405-18.
60. Gurgacz S, Zamora L, Scott NA. Percutaneous Sclerotherapy for Vascular Malformations: a systemic review. Ann Vasc Surg. 2014;28(5):1335-49.
61. Colletti G, Valassina D, Bertossi D, Melchiorre F, Vercellio G, Brusati R. Contemporary Management of Vascular Malformations. J Oral Maxillofac Surg. 2014;72(3): 510-28.
62. Yun WS, Kim YW, Lee KB, Kim DI, Park KB, Kim KH, et al. "Predictors of Response to Percutaneous Ethanol Sclerotherapy (PES) in Patients with Venous Malformations: Analysis of Patient Self-Assessment and Imaging. J Vasc Surg. 2009;50(3):581-9.
63. Morgan P, Keller R, Patel K. Evidence-Based Management of Vascular Malformations. Facial Plast Surg. 2016;32(2):162-76.
64. Ulrich H, Baumler W, Hohenleutner U, Landthaler M. Neodymium-YAG Laser for Hemangiomas and Vascular Malformations-Long Term Results. J Dtsch Dermatol Ges. 2005;3(6):436-40.
65. Glade RS, Richter GT, James CA, Suen JY, Buckmiller LM. Diagnosis and management of pediatric cervicofacial venous malformations: retrospective review from a vascular anomalies center. Laryngoscope. 2010; 120(2):229-35.
66. Hoff SR, Rastatter JC, Richter GT. Head and Neck Vascular Lesions. Otolaryngol Clin North Am. 2015;48(1):29-45.
67. Zhou Q, Zheng JW, Mai HM, Luo QF, Fan XD, Su LX, et al. Treatment Guidelines of Lymphatic Malformations of the Head and Neck. Oral Oncol. 2011;47(12):1105-9.
68. Acevedo JL, Shah RK, Brietzke SE. Nonsurgical Therapies for Lymphangiomas: A Systematic Review. Otolaryngol Head Neck Surg. 2008;138(4):418-24.
69. Smith MC, Zimmerman MB, Burke DK, Bauman NM, Sato Y, Smith RJH. Efficacy and Safety of OK-432 Immunotherapy of Lymphatic Malformations. Laryngoscope. 2009;119(1):107-15.
70. Savas JA, Lendon J, Franca K, Chacon A, Zaiac M, Nouri K. Carbon Dioxide Laser for the Treatment of Microcystic Lymphatic Malformations (Lymphangioma Circumscriptum): A Systematic Review. Dermatolog Surg. 2013;39(8):1147-57.
71. Swetman GL, Berk DR, Vasanawala SS, Feinstein JA, Lane AT, Bruckner AL. Sildenafil for Severe Lymphatic Malformations. N Engl J Med. 2012;366:384-6.
72. Freixo C, Ferreira V, martins J, Almeida R, Caldeira D, Rosa M, et al. Efficacy and Safety of Sirolimus in the Treatment of Vascular Anomalies: A Systemic Review. J Vasc Surg. 2020;71(1):318-27.
73. Sandbank S, Molho-Pessach V, Farkas A, Barzilai A, Greenberger S. Oral and Topical Sirolimus for Vascular Anomalies: A Multicentre Study and Review. Acta Derm Venereol. 2019;99(11):990-6.

8

CHAPTER

Acquired Vascular Lesions

Hana Jeon, Roy G Geronemus

INTRODUCTION

Vascular lesions are one of the most common indications for using lasers in a clinical setting. Laser treatment of vascular lesions has also been one of the earliest applications of the theory of selective thermolysis in which the specific wavelength of light targets and destroys the chromophore without causing damage to the surrounding skin.[1]

Pretreatment Considerations

Prior to treating patients for vascular lesions, the clinician should discuss posttreatment expectations in detail. The pulsed dye laser (PDL) is one of the most commonly used vascular lasers, and when used at shorter pulse widths (0.45–3 ms) can cause purpura. The potential to bruise should be taken into consideration especially if the patient has an upcoming important work or social event. It should also be explained that additional treatments may be required to achieve the best possible clearance. The patient's prior treatment history can often be helpful in gauging the patient's prior experience with laser treatments and setting his or her expectations.

Potential discomfort during the treatment should be explained to the patient [e.g., "rubber band snaps" for the PDL and transient stinging sensation for the potassium titanyl phosphate (KTP) laser]. Depending on the patient's age and the individual pain tolerance, topical anesthesia could be considered to minimize discomfort. Potential transient side effects of erythema and edema should also be clearly explained. The patient's skin phototype is also an important consideration in any laser treatment. Patients with darker skin types tend to have a higher likelihood of postinflammatory hyperpigmentation or hypopigmentation, and such risk should be explained prior to treatment (**Box 1**).

Key Consultation Questions

A thorough medical history should be taken of patients presenting with vascular lesions

BOX 1: Pretreatment considerations.

- Timing of the treatment (potential for bruising should be considered)
- Setting patient expectations (possibility of requiring additional treatments and potential discomfort during the treatment)
- Prior treatment history (understanding the patient's prior experience with laser treatments)
- Skin phototype (potential for dyspigmentation)

to offer the most optimal and appropriate treatment options. Key consultation questions include the age of presentation, location(s), number of lesions, associated symptoms such as bleeding or pain, growth over time, prior treatment history, and any relevant medical conditions. The patient should also be interviewed for the presence of any active local infections as laser treatments should be avoided. Patients with skin conditions that Koebnerize such as vitiligo and psoriasis should be warned that the laser treatment may trigger a rash in the areas of treatment.

Diagnostic Tools

The use of polarized light can play a significant role in the evaluation and treatment of vascular lesions. Commercially available headlamps that combine the polarized light and magnification allow the clinician to visualize vessels that are not visible to naked eyes alone. In our experience, the use of polarized light has significantly improved accuracy and hence efficacy of vascular laser treatments.

On physical examination, the clinician can employ diascopy in which applied pressure with a finger or a glass slide blanches blood within vessels. This helps the clinician to distinguish vascular lesions from other types of erythematous lesions. The lesion will not blanch if the redness is due to blood that has extravasated into the skin (e.g., petechiae). Diascopy can be especially useful to identify the central feeder vessel in spider angiomas and to diagnose venous lakes, which are most often located on the mucosal lips and can otherwise be difficult to diagnose.

Dermoscopy, a noninvasive diagnostic tool that can be used to enhance visualization of skin lesions, can also be used to further aid the clinical diagnosis of vascular lesions. Cherry angiomas, for example, are composed of well-demarcated red or maroon lacunae when seen on a dermatoscope.[2] By recognizing the classic dermatoscopic findings of other erythematous lesions such as basal cell carcinomas or Bowen's disease, the clinician can arrive at the correct diagnosis and thus select the most appropriate treatment for the particular vascular lesion.

MANAGEMENT

Treatment Options

The PDL is the most specific laser for treating vascular lesions,[3] but many other options exist for laser treatment of vascular lesions (**Table 1**). The clinician needs to consider the characteristics of the vessels being treated so that the most optimal outcome can be achieved. Both the diameter and depth of vessels should guide the selection of the specific laser to be used for treatment. The wavelengths of 577 and 585 nm will target superficially located vessels in papillary dermis, whereas longer wavelengths will penetrate deeper and better target deeper vessels. Larger blood vessels have higher thermal relaxation times and require longer pulse durations. The neodymium-doped yttrium aluminum garnet (Nd:YAG) laser can successfully treat such vessels with larger diameters. In addition, lesions on the face and upper trunk tend to respond better than those on the lower trunk and legs.[4] Given that any potential complications on the legs can take longer to resolve when compared to upper body regions, a lower energy should be considered for the initial treatment.

Telangiectasias

Telangiectasias are manifestations of numerous dermatologic conditions such as rosacea, acne, overuse of topical corticosteroids, and scars. Many patients present with facial telangiectasias that result from chronic photodamage, and the PDL, KTP laser, and intense pulsed light (IPL) systems can be used to address this skin condition. The clinician

TABLE 1: Treatment options*.

Diagnosis	Clinical appearance	Laser	Wave-length	Skin phototypes	Settings	Clinical endpoint	Treatment interval	Treatment expectations	Medical considerations
Telangiectasia	0.1–1 mm diameter pink, red, or violaceous linear or arborizing macules or papules	KTP	532 nm	I–III	7–16 J/cm^2, 3–7 mm, 10–30 ms; purpuric settings (<3–6 ms) improve efficacy; when non-purpuric settings are chosen, pulse stacking at low fluences may improve efficacy	Blanching/ disappearance of vessel	4–6 weeks	Individual lesions typically resolve in 1–2 treatments; perinasal vessels are often more resistant or may not resolve; new telangiectasias commonly appear over time	Hereditary hemorrhagic telangiectasia, lupus erythematosus, systemic sclerosis (CREST syndrome), rosacea, hyper-estrogenic states, nevoid conditions, radiodermatitis, basal cell carcinoma, other conditions
Telangiectasia	"	PDL	585–595 nm	I–III	5–8 J/cm^2, 10–12 mm, 0.45–6 ms (Using Candela VBeam laser)	"	"	"	"
Telangiectasia	"	IPL	500–1,200 nm	I– III, cautious use in type IV	550–570 filter in lighter skin types; 2.5–5 ms double pulse, 25–45 J/cm^2, 10–30 ms delay; may treat through hole in opaque white paper to target desired area	Little to no purpura	"	Gradual improvement over multiple sessions, new telangiectasias commonly appear over time	"
Poikiloderma	Telangiectasia, hyperpigmentation, hypopigmentation, and atrophy; usually in sun-exposed skin of neck or chest	PDL	595 nm	I–III	5–7 J/cm^2, 7–10 mm spot size, 0.45–2 ms pulse width	Purpura	4–6 weeks	Gradual improvement over multiple sessions	Associated with extensive photodamage, occasionally with cutaneous T-cell lymphoma or dermatomyositis

Cont'd...

Cont'd...

Diagnosis	Clinical appearance	Laser	Wave-length	Skin phototypes	Settings	Clinical endpoint	Treatment interval	Treatment expectations	Medical considerations
Venous Lake	2–10 mm blue to purple macules or papules	KTP	532 nm	I–III	KTP: 7 J/cm^2, 4 mm, 14 ms	Purpura	4–6 weeks	Individual lesions typically resolve in 1–2 treatments	Associated with photodamage
Venous Lake	"	Nd:YAG	1,064 nm	I–VI	120–140 J/cm^2, 5–7 mm spot size, 0.45 ms pulse duration; pulse stacking may be required	Disappearance of the lesion	4–6 weeks	"	"
Spider angioma	Pink to red blanching papule	PDL	585–595 nm	I–III	6–8 J/cm^2; 7–10 mm spot size, 1.5 ms pulse width; May treat center through glass slide or glass contact cooling window, followed by feeding vessels	Disappearance of the lesion or purpura	4–6 weeks	Individual lesions typically resolve in 1–2 treatments	Hyperestrogenic states, pregnancy, and children
Cherry angioma	Cherry red dome-shaped papule	KTP	532 nm	I–III	7–16 J/cm^2, 3–7 mm, 10–30 ms	Purpura	4–6 weeks	Individual lesions typically resolve in 1–2 treatments	Associated with chronologic aging
Angiofibroma	1–1.0 cm flesh-colored papules	PDL	585–595 nm	I–III	7–8 J/cm^2, 7–10 mm spot size, 0.45–2 ms pulse width	Purpura	4–6 weeks	Individual lesions typically resolve in 1–2 treatments when treated with other modalities to address the papular component	Facial lesions associated with tuberous sclerosis
Reticular veins	Large blue to violaceous linear to tortuous macular to slightly raised vessels	Nd:YAG	1,064 nm	I–VI	125–150 J/cm^2, 5–7 mm spot, 75–100 ms	Disappearance of vessel	4–6 weeks	Individual lesions typically improve in 1–2 months	Consider ocular safety and risk of scarring when treating periorbital veins

*Note: Information provided in this table should be considered as suggestions only. All treatment parameters should be based on the treating physician's experience, patient presentation, and the specific device being used.

(CREST: calcinosis, Raynaud phenomenon, esophageal dysmotility, sclerodactyly, and telangiectasia; IPL: intense pulsed light; KTP: potassium-titanyl-phosphate; Nd:YAG: neodymium-doped yttrium aluminum garnet; PDL: pulsed dye laser)

Source: Adapted from Lasers and Related Technologies in Dermatology, McGraw-Hill.[20]

should look for optimal clinical endpoints (**Table 1**) and adjust the settings based on the reactions observed after the initial laser pulse. For telangiectasias treated with longer pulse durations, blanching of the vessels or a subtle change in color from red to purple should be expected. Epidermal whitening should be avoided to prevent an excessive delivery of thermal energy.

Short pulse durations (0.45–3 ms) of the PDL are effective for telangiectasias but create purpuric reactions. To minimize bruising, pulse stacking can be done by applying successive pulses with longer pulse durations (6–10 ms).[1] Because using longer pulse durations can be less effective than using shorter pulse durations, several approaches have been explored to achieve clearing without causing purpura. For example, a modified PDL with subpulses has shown to be effective without causing purpura (**Figs. 1A** and **B**).[5]

To avoid potential complications of dyspigmentation and scarring, various cooling methods such as cryogen spray cooling and forced cold air have been developed. Such cooling methods function to protect the epidermis during vascular laser treatments.[1] One must take special caution when treating the alae and alar grooves as these areas are prone to scarring especially with KTP laser (**Box 2**; **Figs. 2A** and **B**). Such complications can be avoided by using appropriate cooling methods and avoiding pulse stacking, particularly when using short pulse durations. In addition, using a lower energy and a longer pulse duration should be considered for darker skin type patients to avoid postinflammatory pigmentary changes. The long-pulsed 1,064-nm Nd:YAG laser can be used as an alternative laser for such individuals, though the absorption of hemoglobin will be much less than that of the PDL.

BOX 2: Tips for efficacy and safety (avoiding complications).

- Consider the diameter and depth of the vessels to select the appropriate laser
- Consider the patient's skin phototype to avoid potential complications of dyspigmentation (e.g., lower the fluence and select a laser with longer wavelength)
- Consider the locations of the lesions (e.g., better clearance on upper vs. lower parts of the body, higher risk of scarring on the alae of the nose and the alar grooves)

Poikiloderma of Civatte

Poikiloderma of Civatte is characterized by the following four changes in skin that result from chronic sun exposure: Hyperpigmentation, hypopigmentation, telangiectasia, and atrophy. The most common areas involved are the upper chest and the neck, sparing the submental region, which is a photoprotected area. The PDL has long been used to address the color changes present in poikiloderma safely on the thin skin of the neck due to its specific interaction with the hemoglobin.[6,7] In addition to the PDL, KTP, and IPL, fractionated ablative lasers and fractionated nonablative lasers can be used to improve poikiloderma. Fractionated ablative laser treatment performed for poikiloderma, for example, has been reported to improve telangiectasia, dyschromia, skin texture, and skin laxity with an average of 1.4 treatments.[8] However, ablative fractional lasers on the neck can cause scarring in unexperienced hands and should be used with caution.

Venous Lakes

Venous lakes are composed of dilated venules in the superficial dermis and most commonly found on the lips, as well as other areas of sun exposure such as the helix of the ears. They are violaceous compressible papules that are benign but can bleed. Due to their dark hue, the presence of the lesion can often cause

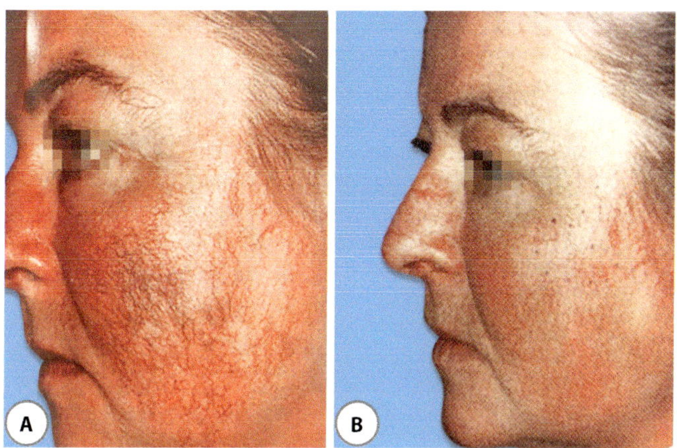

(PDL: pulsed dye laser)

FIGS. 1A AND B: Extensive facial telangiectasia before (A) and after (B) treatment with two sessions of 585-nm, 0.45 ms PDL treatments.

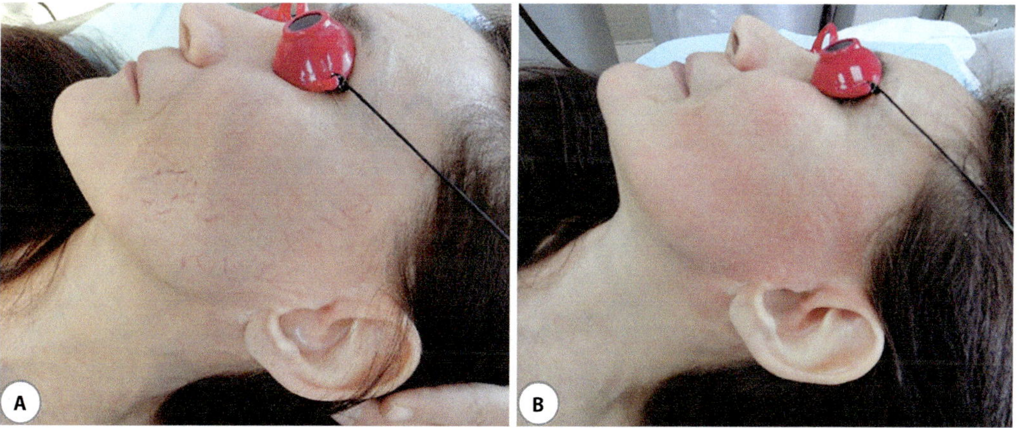

(KTP: potassium titanyl phosphate)

FIGS. 2A AND B: Facial telangiectasias before (A) and immediately after (B) treatment with a KTP laser. Resulting erythema and edema resolve within hours to days.

anxiety and distress, prompting patients to seek treatment. Electrocoagulation, excision, cryosurgery, and sclerotherapy have been used in the past but often result in scarring and recurrence. Multiple lasers can be used to treat venous lakes including KTP, Nd:YAG, and diode lasers (**Figs. 3A** and **B**). Many reports have shown that the long-pulsed Nd:YAG laser often requires only one treatment and minimizes scarring.[9,10] For example, a study involving 15 Chinese patients with venous lakes has shown that multi-wavelength lasers with the PDL and Nd:YAG laser can be used safely and effectively in patients with darker skin types when a low fluence of Nd:YAG (35–40 J/cm^2) is used with 10 ms.[11] Other options include a carbon dioxide (CO_2) (10,600 nm) laser and the argon (514 nm) laser, both of which have been reported to clear venous lakes, but are less efficacious

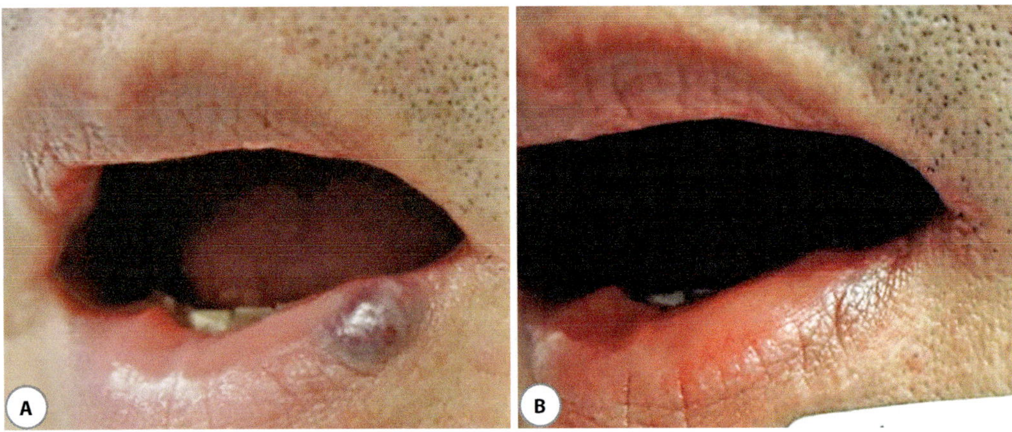

(KTP: potassium titanyl phosphate)

FIGS. 3A AND B: Venous lake before (A) and after (B) treatment with a KTP laser.

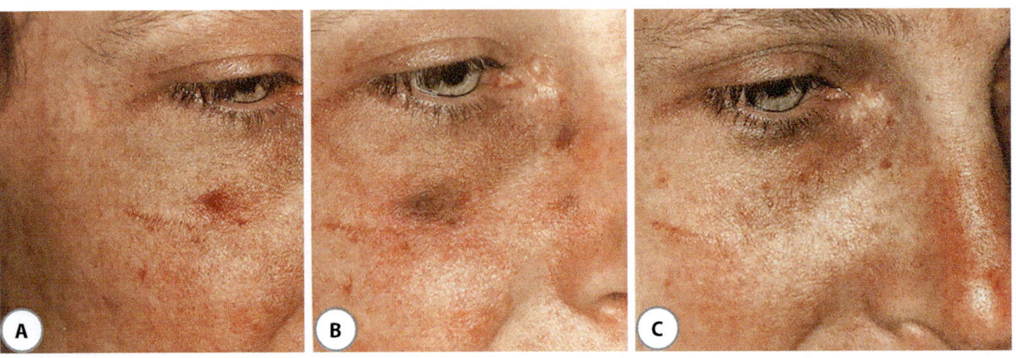

(PDL: pulsed dye laser)

FIGS. 4A TO C: (A) Spider angioma before and after treatment with a 585-nm PDL, 7.0J/cm^2. (B) Darkening of the treated area immediately after treatment. (C) Clearance 6 weeks after the treatment.

and less safe with possibility of scarring, when compared to the aforementioned lasers.[10]

Spider Angioma

Spider angiomas clinically present as easily blanchable erythematous papules that are raised at the center and have smaller attached radiating vessels (like a "spider"). They are often found on the face, neck, and chest of healthy individuals, but can be associated with liver disease. Multiple lesions are common with pregnancy and oral contraceptive pills. Electrosurgery or vascular lasers can be used, with the PDL or KTP laser often achieving a great response (**Figs. 4A** to **C**).[12] Spider angiomas usually resolve completely with one or two sessions with the PDL without complications.[13]

Cherry Angioma

Cherry angiomas are very common benign vascular skin lesions that occur with time. Clinically, they appear as bright red well-demarcated and symmetric papules. They can bleed with trauma (e.g., shaving) and can be treated with electrosurgery or shave removals, but these methods often result in scarring. Vascular lasers can be used easily and successfully to treat cherry angiomas, and are often superior as they tend to require fewer treatments with less side effects when compared to traditional methods such as hyfrecator.[14]. Although cherry angiomas are benign, having multiple lesions on the face can be distressful for patients and treating them has been shown to significantly reduce their psychological distress.[15] Vascular lasers are very effective to treat cherry angiomas, including PDL, KTP, and Nd:YAG lasers. In a study comparing the KTP laser and Nd:YAG laser for treatment of cherry angiomas, both were found to be effective, with Nd:YAG requiring fewer treatment sessions but a higher risk of scar formation.[16]

Angiofibromas

Angiofibromas are dome-shaped papules histologically composed of proliferated fibroblasts and dilated blood vessels. Numerous facial angiofibromas present classically in a number of conditions including tuberous sclerosis and Birt-Hogg-Dubé syndrome. They can be disfiguring for patients and invasive methods such as surgical excision and dermabrasion can result in recurrence, dyspigmentation, and scarring. Some reports support CO_2 laser ablation, but acknowledge that the side effects of recurrence and hyperpigmentation can occur.[17] A combination therapy using a PDL, an ablative fractional resurfacing laser, electrosurgery, and topical sirolimus 0.2% ointment has been reported to result in a significant improvement without complications.[18,19] This approach addresses the condition on multiple fronts; the PDL for increased vascularity, electrosurgery for debulking larger lesions, and AFR technology for using ablative wavelengths without scarring that are often associated with fully ablative lasers.

Reticular Veins

Reticular veins are large blue to violaceous vessels that can be linear or tortuous.[20] Patients often present with facial reticular veins and in particular periocular reticular veins. The 1,064 nm Nd:YAG laser is the laser of choice for these deep vessels (**Figs. 5** and **6**). Because relatively high fluences are required, appropriate epidermal cooling is especially important to avoid the risk of scarring. For the periocular reticular veins, care should be taken to protect the eyes with intraocular metal eyeshields.

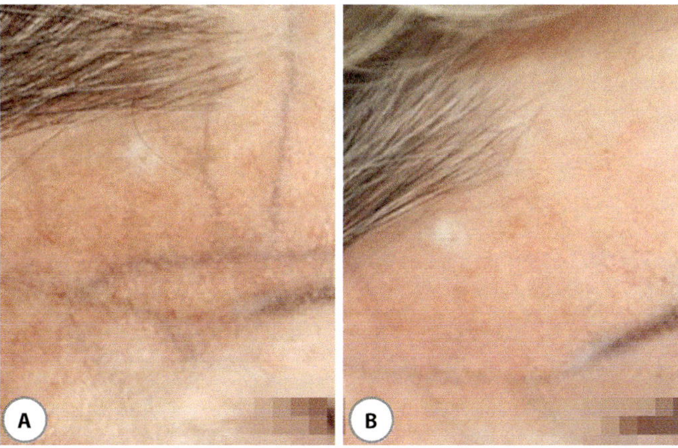

(Nd:YAG: neodymium-doped yttrium aluminum garnet)

FIGS. 5A AND B: Reticular veins on the temple and forehead before and after treatment with an Nd:YAG laser.

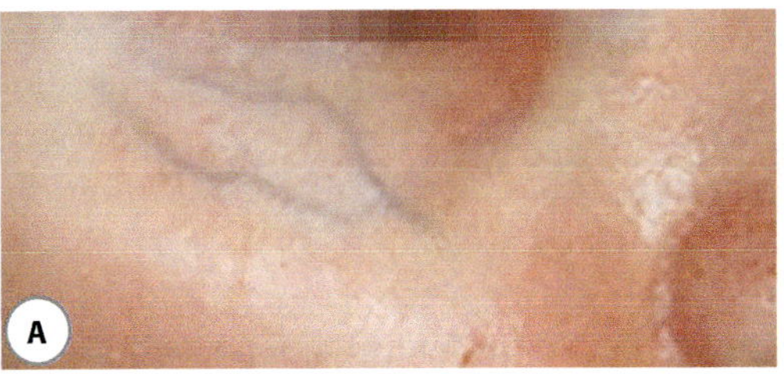

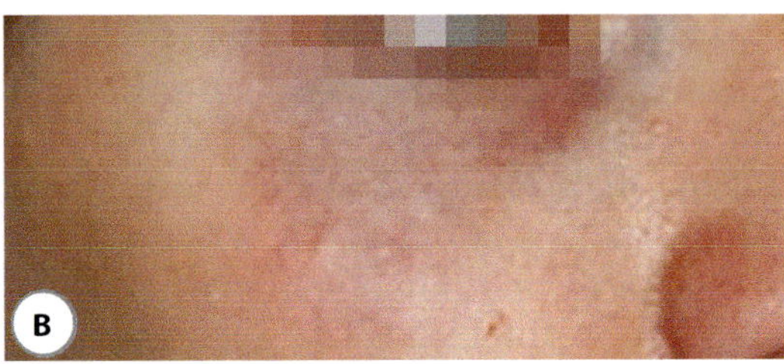

(Nd:YAG: neodymium-doped yttrium aluminum garnet)

FIGS. 6A AND B: Periocular reticular veins before and after treatment with an Nd:YAG laser.

CONCLUSION

When used appropriately, laser therapies can successfully and safely treat vascular lesions.

REFERENCES

1. Zachary CB, Rofagha R. Laser Therapy In: Bolognia J, Jorizzo JL, Schaffer JV, et al., (Eds). Dermatology. Elsevier, Philadelphia 2012:2263-6.
2. Argenziano G, Soyer HP, Chimenti S, Talamini R, Corona R, Sera F, et al. Dermoscopy of pigmented skin lesions: results of a consensus meeting via the Internet. J Am Acad Dermatol. 2003;48(5):679-93.
3. Ross BS, Levine VJ, Ashinoff R. Laser treatment of acquired vascular lesions. Dermatol Clin. 1997;15(3): 385-96.
4. Srinivas CR, Kumaresan M. Lasers for vascular lesions: standard guidelines of care. Indian J Dermatol Venereol Leprol. 2011;77(3):349-68.
5. Ross EV, Uebelhoer NS, Domankevitz Y. Use of a novel pulse dye laser for rapid single-pass purpura-free treatment of telangiectases. Dermatol Surg. 2007;33(12):1466-9.
6. Geronemus R. Poikiloderma of civatte. Arch Dermatol. 1990;126(4):547-8.
7. Wheeland RG, Applebaum J. Flashlamp-pumped pulsed dye laser therapy for poikiloderma of Civatte. J Dermatol Surg Oncol. 1990;16(1):12-6.
8. Tierney EP, Hanke CW. Treatment of Poikiloderma of Civatte with ablative fractional laser resurfacing: prospective study and review of the literature. J Drugs Dermatol. 2009;8(6):527-34.
9. John HE, Phen HS, Mahaffey PJ. Treatment of venous lesions of the lips and perioral area with a long-pulsed Nd:YAG laser. Br J Oral Maxillofac Surg. 2016;54(4): 376-8.
10. Mlacker S, Shah VV, Aldahan AS, McNamara CA, Kamath P, Nouri K. Laser and light-based treatments of venous lakes: a literature review. Lasers Med Sci. 2016;31(7):1511-9.
11. Yang J, Guo X, Tong X, Tao J. Treatment of venous lake with multiwavelength 595 and 1064 nm lasers in Asian Fitzpatrick skin type IV patients. Photodermatol Photoimmunol Photomed. 2017;33(5):267-70.
12. Becher GL, Cameron H, Moseley H. Treatment of superficial vascular lesions with the KTP 532-nm laser: experience with 647 patients. Lasers Med Sci. 2014;29(1):267-71.
13. Geronemus RG. Pulsed dye laser treatment of vascular lesions in children. J Dermatol Surg Oncol. 1993;19(4):303-10.
14. Dawn G, Gupta G. Comparison of potassium titanyl phosphate vascular laser and hyfrecator in the treatment of vascular spiders and cherry angiomas. Clin Exp Dermatol. 2003;28(6):581-3.
15. Gupta G, Bilsland D. A prospective study of the impact of laser treatment on vascular lesions. Br J Dermatol. 2000;143(2):356-9.
16. Pancar GS, Aydin F, Senturk N, Bek Y, Canturk MT, Turanli AY. Comparison of the 532-nm KTP and 1064-nm Nd:YAG lasers for the treatment of cherry angiomas. J Cosmet Laser Ther. 2011;13(4):138-41.
17. Ali FR, Mallipeddi R, Craythorne EE, Sheth N, Al-Niaimi F. Our experience of carbon dioxide laser ablation of angiofibromas: Case series and literature review. J Cosmet Laser Ther. 2016;18(7):372-5.
18. Bae-Harboe YS, Geronemus RG. Targeted topical and combination laser surgery for the treatment of angiofibromas. Lasers Surg Med. 2013;45(9):555-7.
19. Weiss ET, Geronemus RG. New technique using combined pulsed dye laser and fractional resurfacing for treating facial angiofibromas in tuberous sclerosis. Lasers Surg Med. 2010;42(5):357-60.
20. Reddy KK, Geronemus RG. Laser treatment of cutaneous vascular lesions. In: Lasers & Related Technologies in Dermatology, 1st ed, Geronemus RG (Ed). McGraw-Hill. New York. 2013.

9

CHAPTER

Leg Veins

Neil Sadick

INTRODUCTION

Treating leg veins is a common request from patients, as around 80% of the population is affected to some extent. To date, the gold standard of treatment has been sclerotherapy. However, there are situations where sclerotherapy is contraindicated, such as in patients with needle phobia, non-cannulizable microtelangiectasias, vessels that are refractory to conventional sclerotherapy or allergy to sclerosing agents. Laser therapy of leg veins is another treatment strategy that has proven valuable for these situations, and compared to sclerotherapy has a similar efficacy and safety profile.[1]

The efficacy of lasers and light sources for treating vascular lesions such as leg veins is based on the principle of selective photothermolysis. The target chromophore, deoxyhemoglobin, has three major absorption peaks at 418, 542, and 577 nm and optimal absorption is in the 577–600 nm range. The absorption of laser/light by the target chromophore results in its conversion to thermal energy, and ultimately to microvascular damage through photocoagulation and mechanical injury. When assessing laser/light treatment parameters, factors needed to be considered include pulse duration, spot size, fluence, vessel location and diameter, skin type, and age of patient.

TIPS FOR EFFICACY

Pulse Duration

To prevent nonselective damage of tissue peripheral to the vascular lesion, the pulse duration needs to be shorter than the thermal relaxation time (TRT) of the target. The greater the diameter of the vessel the higher the TRT, and thus the greater the pulse duration.

Spot Size

The larger the spot size, the greater the penetration and the shorter the treatment time. Large and deeper vessels though require a larger laser beam spot size for effective thermocoagulation. An important factor to consider, however, is that energy is dramatically increased when increasing spot size, so a conservative approach is recommended to minimize side effects such as swelling.[2]

Fluence

Darker vessels (purple/blue) absorb more energy than lighter ones (pink/red), and thus require less fluence. Fluence needs to be toggled in relation to the spot size, as smaller vessels treated with small spot size laser beam may require higher fluence for clinical results. Moreover, deeper vessels in the legs that are under intravascular pressure require higher fluences to achieve effective thermocoagulation.

Vessel Location

As legs veins are located deeper and contain more deoxyhemoglobin, the ideal treatment wavelengths lie between 800 and 1,200 nm. Superficial leg telangiectasias can respond effectively to shorter wavelengths (532–585 nm), the deeper vessels will require longer wavelengths and longer pulses widths.[3]

Skin Type

Treating leg veins in patients with darker skin types is feasible, however some important adjustments are required to avoid side effects such as hypopigmentation. As epidermal melanin also absorbs laser energy at the shorter wavelengths, darker skin types need to be treated with longer pulses, longer pulse intervals and higher fluences.[4]

Age of Patients

Treatment response of younger patients is better than that of the elderly as the veins are typically smaller, more superficial and their wound healing capacity is superior to that of the elderly.

PRETREATMENT CONSIDERATIONS AND CONSULTATION

Prior to performing any laser treatment, patients should undergo a thorough medical consultation where their medical history/current medications are documented, and a physical examination is performed. Treatment is contraindicated in patients with active local infections, diseases, and medical conditions such as unstable vitiligo, keloid and keloidal tendencies. Patients on isotretinoin, or on nonsteroidal anti-inflammatory drugs/anticoagulants should be warned that laser treatment may increase the risk of scarring and erythema, respectively. During the consultation, the course of lesions, possibility of natural involution, anticipated results, cost, need for multiple treatments, and possible postoperative complications need to be discussed. Use of sun protection, and minimizing sun exposure prior, and several weeks posttreatment, is recommended to reduce pigment-related problems.

During the physical examination, the physician should evaluate the type, location and size of the leg veins. With the patient in an upright position, patterns of telangiectasias, reticular veins, and varicose veins can be identified. Importantly, identification of the feeder is crucial during the preoperative assessment.[5] In addition, Duplex ultrasound of both the superficial and deep venous system might be desirable, as patients with telangiectasias may have some form of trunk varicose veins.[6] Noting the severity of telangiectasias is informative, as increasing severity has been significantly associated with increased reflux in the upper and lower great saphenous and femoral vein segments.[7] In these cases, treatment of the trunk varicose veins needs to precede any treatment, with procedures such as endovenous thermal ablation, (foam) sclerotherapy, and in severe cases surgery.

MANAGEMENT

The main lasers and light technologies used for leg veins are: 532 nm potassium titanyl phosphate (KTP) laser, 585–600 nm pulsed dye laser (PDL), 755 nm alexandrite laser, 1,064 nm neodymium yttrium-aluminum-garnet (Nd:YAG) laser, and various intense pulsed light sources (IPL).

Potassium Titanyl Phosphate Laser (532 nm)

The KTP laser is effective in the treatment of leg veins smaller than 1 mm in diameter, in patients with skin type I–III. Typically, veins are ablated after 1–2 treatments, and no improvement is observed with additional treatments.[8,9] Although in research studies a wide heterogeneity of laser settings are reported to be clinically effective, in the author's experience pulse durations 10–100 ms, spot sizes from 0.75 to 5 mm and fluences ranging from 12 to 38 J/cm^2 are optimal for veins 0.5–1.5 mm. Compared to other lasers, KTP is preferred by patients over both Nd:YAG and PDL, as it is not as painful or less likely to be associated with the development of purpura.[10]

Pulsed Dye Laser (585–600 nm)

Similar to the KTP laser, PDL lasers are effective for treating small lower extremity veins that are less than 1.5 mm in diameter in light skin type patients. Treatment parameters vary with pulse duration ranging from 0.45 to 40 ms, increasing depending on vessel size, but most authors use a short pulse duration (1.5 ms). Longer pulse durations are associated with less side effects such as erythema, and postinflammatory hyperpigmentation.[11,12] Fluence settings also vary from 10 to 15 J/cm^2, spot size 1–7 mm.[13] Compared to the KTP laser, PDL lasers are slightly more effective for small telangiectasias, but due to their side effect profile (burns, hyperpigmentations) they are not as popular with patients for leg vein treatment.

Alexandrite Laser (755 nm)

Alexandrite lasers emit light at a wavelength of 755 nm which corresponds to absorption by deoxygenated hemoglobin and melanin. These lasers are suitable for the treatment of veins larger than 0.5 mm, however longer pulse durations (< 3 ms pulse durations) need to be used for patients with skin type III or higher. For light skin types, the optimal fluence is 90 J/cm^2, and larger spot sizes (over 6 mm) generate more response.[14]

Nd:YAG (1,064 nm)

Due to their lower absorption in melanin, Nd:YAG lasers are safer to use in darker skin types, as they are less likely to cause pigmentary changes (**Figs. 1** and **2**). The longer wavelength penetrates deeper and can be used to treat veins from 0.3 to 3 mm in diameter. Although larger veins are typically treated by sclerotherapy, various studies have shown comparable efficacy when veins are treated with Nd:YAG laser or sclerotherapy.[15,16] However, due to the increased pain associated with the Nd:YAG lasers they are not preferred by patients, even though similar side effects (hyperpigmentation, telangiectatic matting) are seen after both treatments.[17,18]

Longer pulse durations (≥ 40 ms) are recommended when treating leg veins with Nd:YAG lasers, in order to minimize purpura and hemosiderin deposition.[19] According to the authors experience, spot sizes varying from 1.5 to 3 mm, radiant exposures varying from 250 to 600 J/cm^2 and pulse widths varying from 30 to 60 ms are recommended for optimal laser clearance.[20] Clinical results of leg vein treatment with the Nd:YAG are durable, and recurrence is infrequent.[21] It must be noted however that in the hands of inexperienced providers, there is a risk of ulceration using Nd:YAG for leg veins, particularly in patients with darker skin types.

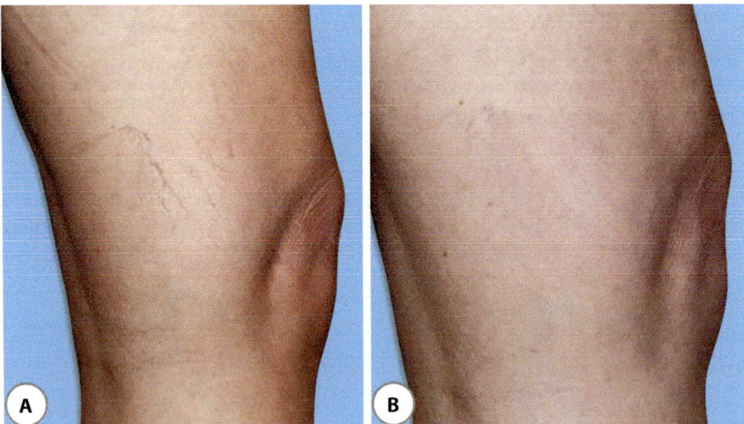

FIGS. 1A AND B: A 24-year-old female. Before and 6 months after two treatments with 1,064 nm (4–6 mm, 140–150 J/cm^2, 10–30 ms, 5–8°C).

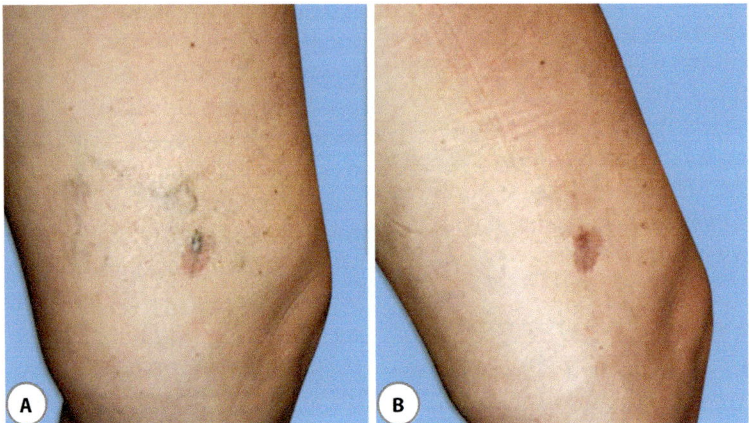

FIGS. 2A AND B: A 40-year-old female. Before and 2 months after treatment with 1,064 nm (5 mm, 100–180 J/cm^2, 10–40 ms, 5°C).

Intense-pulsed Light (IPL)

Intense pulsed light sources emit light from 515 to 1,200 nm, and can be used to treat leg veins with the use of filters (550 and 570 nm). They are most effective for superficial, red telangiectasias <1 mm in diameter in fair-skin individuals. Due to the concomitant absorption by melanin, they are not usually used for treating leg veins, however small vessels have been shown to be effectively cleared, with no recurrence or side effects.[22]

COMPLICATIONS

Complications from treating leg veins with lasers are mild and typically self-resolving. Common local reactions associated with laser therapy include pain, redness, swelling, bruising, and itching. These are transient and usually resolve quickly. More significant adverse reactions include telangiectatic matting, pigmentation changes, hyperpigmentation, hypopigmentation, ulceration, thrombophlebitis, and scarring.

Pain is associated with longer wavelength lasers, but the use of topical anesthetics or cooling can minimize discomfort. Purpura and ecchymosis are due to vessel wall rupture resulting in leakage of blood into the surrounding tissue. These reactions are most likely to occur with short pulsed laser treatments (e.g., PDL) and usually occur within minutes of treatment. Posttreatment bruising is a significant drawback for the alexandrite and long PDL lasers.

In patients with darker skin types, pigmentary changes may occur after treatment but they usually resolve within 4–6 months. Careful use, reducing the laser fluence by 20% is advised for areas such as the ankles, due to the thinness of the dermis. Patients experiencing severe inflammation post-laser may be treated with fluticasone propionate cream 0.05% (twice daily for 7 days). In cases of skin ulceration or wounding, management is done with moist dressing or occlusive hydrocolloid dressings. These are left on the ulcer for 2–3 days followed by gentle debridement of necrotic tissue to facilitate re-epithelialization. Thrombosis has been reported in the superficial veins following laser therapy. It may take up to 6 weeks to resolve but rarely has sequelae.

CONCLUSION

Several lasers are available for treating leg veins, with a good clinical efficacy and safety profile. New trend in laser treatment strategy include the use of nonuniform pulse sequence, dual-wavelength modalities, pulse stacking, multiple pass laser treatment and combination of laser therapy with sclerotherapy or radiofrequency.

REFERENCES

1. Schmults CD. Laser treatment of vascular lesions. Dermatol Clin. 2005;23(4):745-55.
2. Srinivas CR, Kumaresan M. Lasers for vascular lesions: standard guidelines of care. Indian J Dermatol Venereol Leprol. 2011;77(3):349-68.
3. Bucci J, Goldberg D. Past, present, and future: vascular lasers/light devices. J Cosmet Laser Ther. 2006;8(3):149-53.
4. Anderson RR, Parrish JA. The optics of human skin. J Invest Dermatol. 1981;77(1):13-9.
5. Somjen GM. Anatomy of the superficial venous system. Dermatol Surg. 1995;21(1):35-45.
6. Ruckley CV, Evans CJ, Allan PL, Lee AJ, Fowkes FG. Telangiectasia in the Edinburgh Vein Study: epidemiology and association with trunk varices and symptoms. Eur J Vasc Endovasc Surg. 2008;36(6):719-24.
7. Ruckley CV, Allan PL, Evans CJ, Lee AJ, Fowkes FG. Telangiectasia and venous reflux in the Edinburgh Vein Study. Phlebology. 2012;27(6):297-302.
8. Fournier N, Brisot D, Mordon S. Treatment of leg telangiectases with a 532 nm KTP laser in multipulse mode. Dermatol Surg. 2002;28(7):564-71.
9. West TB, Alster TS. Comparison of the long-pulse dye (590-595 nm) and KTP (532 nm) lasers in the treatment of facial and leg telangiectasias. Dermatol Surg. 1998;24(2):221-6.
10. Woo WK, Jasim ZF, Handley JM. 532-nm Nd:YAG and 595-nm pulsed dye laser treatment of leg telangiectasia using ultralong pulse duration. Dermatol Surg. 2003;29(12):1176-180.
11. Hsia J, Lowery JA, Zelickson B. Treatment of leg telangiectasia using a long-pulse dye laser at 595 nm. Lasers Surg Med. 1997;20(1):1-5.
12. Reichert D. Evaluation of the long-pulse dye laser for the treatment of leg telangiectasias. Dermatol Surg. 1998;24(7):737-40.
13. Alora MB, Stern RS, Arndt KA, Dover JS. Comparison of the 595 nm long-pulse (1.5 msec) and ultralong-pulse (4 msec) lasers in the treatment of leg veins. Dermatol Surg. 1999;25(6):445-9.
14. Ross EV, Meehan KJ, Gilbert S, Domankevitz Y. Optimal pulse durations for the treatment of leg telangiectasias with an alexandrite laser. Lasers Surg Med. 2009;41(2): 104-9.
15. Coles CM, Werner RS, Zelickson BD. Comparative pilot study evaluating the treatment of leg veins with a long pulse ND:YAG laser and sclerotherapy. Lasers Surg Med. 2002;30(2):154-9.
16. Levy JL, Elbahr C, Jouve E, Mordon S. Comparison and sequential study of long pulsed Nd:YAG 1,064 nm laser and sclerotherapy in leg telangiectasias treatment. Lasers Surg Med. 2004;34(3):273-6.

17. Omura NE, Dover JS, Arndt KA, Kauvar AN. Treatment of reticular leg veins with a 1064 nm long-pulsed Nd:YAG laser. J Am Acad Dermatol. 2003;48(1):76-81.
18. Rogachefsky AS, Silapunt S, Goldberg DJ. Nd:YAG laser (1064 nm) irradiation for lower extremity telangiectases and small reticular veins: efficacy as measured by vessel color and size. Dermatol Surg. 2002;28(3):220-3.
19. Parlette EC, Groff WF, Kinshella MJ, Domankevitz Y, O'Neill J, Ross EV. Optimal pulse durations for the treatment of leg telangiectasias with a neodymium YAG laser. Lasers Surg Med. 2006;38(2):98-105.
20. Sadick NS. Laser treatment with a 1064-nm laser for lower extremity class I-III veins employing variable spots and pulse width parameters. Dermatol Surg. 2003;29(9):916-9.
21. Sadick NS. Long-term results with a multiple synchronized-pulse 1064 nm Nd:YAG laser for the treatment of leg venulectasias and reticular veins. Dermatol Surg. 2001;27(4):365-9.
22. Goldman MP, Eckhouse S. Photothermal sclerosis of leg veins. ESC Medical Systems, LTD Photoderm VL Cooperative Study Group. Dermatol Surg. 1996;22(4):323-30.

3 SECTION

HAIR

10

CHAPTER

Energy-based Hair Removal

Saami Khalifian, Christine Caroline Dierickx

INTRODUCTION

Energy-based hair removal (EBHR) is the most commonly performed procedure in the world with nearly 1 million procedures performed per year by healthcare providers.[1,2] In addition to removal of unwanted hair for cosmetic reasons, there are a number of medical conditions that respond to EBHR including pseudofolliculitis barbae (PFB), pilonidal sinus disease, and hidradenitis suppurativa.[3] A variety of energy-based devices are now available for photoepilation and the continued advances in the field have facilitated improved outcomes in a wide array of clinical scenarios. One of the goals of EBHR is to destroy follicle stem cells in the bulge region of the hair follicle without damaging the surrounding skin.[4,5] This is achieved through the process of selective photothermolysis, which posits that thermal injury can be confined to a target structure by choosing energy-based device parameters that are based on the optical and thermal properties of the target itself.[6] Adjustments to the energy-based device parameters can affect the target structures. An important concept to increase the selectivity of the thermal damage is to select a pulse duration that is equal to or slightly shorter than the thermal relaxation time of the target, which for the hair follicle is approximately 10–100 ms depending on the thickness of the terminal hair shaft.[7] In practice, however, the chromophore in EBHR and the desired target stem cells are not identical; therefore, a slightly longer pulse duration is used for EBHR because heat must diffuse from the follicle to the amelanotic stem cells in order to achieve optimal results.[8-12] Generally, longer pulse durations are used for thicker hair and shorter pulse durations are used for thinner hair with greater efficacy achieved at higher fluences.[13]

The target chromophore in EBHR is melanin found in the terminal hair shaft and matrix. Small amounts of melanin are also found throughout the epidermis with increasing concentration of melanin found in the epidermis of darker skinned patients. Melanin absorbs optical radiation from wavelengths 400 to 1,200 nm; however, other chromophores, such as hemoglobin or water, can interfere with the absorption of optical radiation at the low and high end of this spectrum, which may lead to off-target effects. Therefore, the best energy-based devices for photoepilation fall between 600 and 1,100 nm. This region is a more selective part of the electromagnetic spectrum for melanin and reduces off-target damage due to absorption by hemoglobin or water.[12] Accordingly, the diode and alexandrite lasers achieve the best treatment responses for EBHR, followed by intense pulsed light (IPL) and neodymium-doped yttrium aluminum garnet (Nd:YAG), although any wavelength can achieve excellent outcomes with appropriate fluences.[14]

PRETREATMENT CONSIDERATIONS

Energy-based hair removal has excellent success rates when used properly in the appropriate candidates. Nevertheless, setting realistic expectations with patients is a critical aspect of the pretreatment evaluation, as EBHR requires multiple treatments to achieve complete and long-term eradication of all unwanted hair, and some patients, such as those with hirsutism, may require ongoing maintenance therapy. In appropriate candidates, approximately 80–90% of individuals achieve a good response and long-term hair reduction, with an expected 25% hair loss per treatment; yet, patients should be made aware that their results may differ.[12,15] Selection of inappropriate candidates or wrong energy-based device parameters will be unlikely to yield such excellent response rates.

Patient selection and education are key to successful EBHR. The ideal candidate for EBHR is an individual with light skin and dark hair, as the contrast between the epidermal and hair follicle melanin is greatest in these patients; however, patients of all skin types can be safely treated, albeit with differential efficacy across skin phototypes. Successful treatment depends on selecting the appropriate device for the appropriate patient and is further dictated by skin color, hair thickness, hair color, and choice of energy-based device parameters. Hirsutism or hypertrichosis due to an underlying endocrine disorder, such as polycystic ovarian syndrome, is also pertinent as it is more difficult to achieve permanent, complete hair loss in these patients. They should be screened for an underlying endocrine disorder and treatment in conjunction with medical management is recommended.[16,17]

Light hair is unlikely to undergo permanent hair reduction and is generally treated poorly by all energy-based device modalities.[15,18-22] Removal of blonde, gray, red, or white hair is usually unsuccessful as the target chromophore, melanin, is decreased in lighter color hair or absent in white hairs.

The location of the treated area is also an important consideration. Melanin is present in different structures of the eyes. Energy-based devices designed for hair removal, can therefore cause significant eye hazards such as uveitis, iritis, or permanent ocular injury, especially to the retina, which contains the highest density of melanin in the body. Therefore, we do not recommend treating the bony orbit, including the zygoma, the glabella, or eyebrows due to the risk of permanent blindness.[12,23-29]

Perhaps the most important concept of EBHR is to not treat patients with tanned skin as this increases the risk for epidermal damage, which can result in burns and permanent pigmentary changes.[18] Sun avoidance should be stressed to patients and they should be encouraged to wear broad-spectrum sunscreens for 1–3 months before and after EBHR. Patients should also avoid tanning immediately after EBHR to avoid postinflammatory hyperpigmentation.

Pigmented lesions and tattoos should likewise be avoided. When treating areas close to tattoos, caution should be taken to avoid a possible color change or scar injury after treatment with energy-based device or IPL at the site.[30,31] Exposure of melanin-containing skin lesions, especially congenital melanocytic nevi and dysplastic nevi to red or near infrared light should be avoided because of the risk of burn and potential scarring. Moreover, there has been a report of the appearance of clinically atypical nevi when nevus cells were treated in areas previously treated for hair removal. This should be kept in mind, especially in patients with a history of dysplastic nevi or with a personal or family history of malignant melanoma.[32] It is therefore advisable to avoid treating skin for hair removal when melanocytic nevi are present in this area.

KEY CONSULTATIVE QUESTIONS

The patient encounter should include a thorough screening for historical elements that may increase the risks associated with EBHR. These include a history of herpes simplex virus (HSV), prior staphylococcal infections, immunodeficiency, and hypertrophic or keloid scarring.[10,12] A history of HSV near the treatment site is notable because the photothermal insult from the energy-based device can lead to reactivation of the virus leading some to recommend prophylactic antiviral therapy the day before EBHR;[10] however, prophylactic antiviral therapy is not widely agreed to be necessary.[33]

A medication history is another essential consultative question. Some medications or drugs may increase the risk of bruising, e.g., aspirin or other anticoagulants; however, these are not a contraindication to therapy.[34] EBHR during isotretinoin therapy is controversial, with recent evidence suggesting it may be safe; nevertheless, most centers generally advise a washout period of six months, and some authors recommend waiting up to a year.[35,36] Certain medications may cause hypertrichosis or hirsutism as a side effect of their use, including minoxidil, testosterone, phenytoin, cyclosporine, and glucocorticoids among others, and these should be noted before initiation of EBHR.[16]

Pragmatically, it is important to have a discussion with patients regarding the surface area that can realistically be treated in a single session. Other key discussion points include the number of treatments needed and the interval between treatments. There is also the risk of facial paradoxical hypertrichosis, which has been reported most commonly in Middle Eastern, Mediterranean, and South Asian women, particularly after treatment of vellus hairs of the lateral cheeks and chin (**Figs. 1A** and **B**).[12,37-42] The mechanism of paradoxical hypertrichosis remains unclear, but it is speculated that subtherapeutic thermal injury may induce activation of the hair cycle.

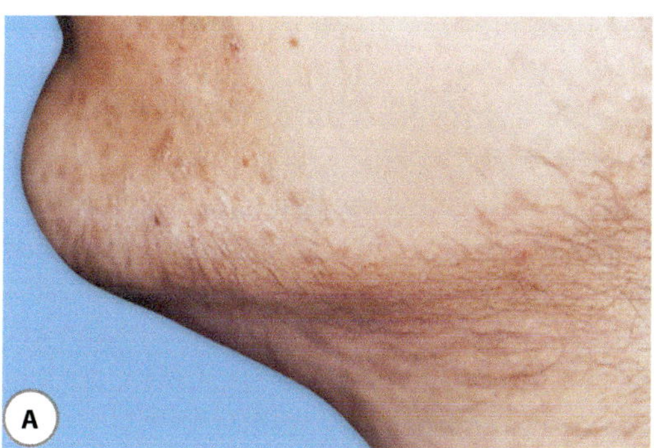

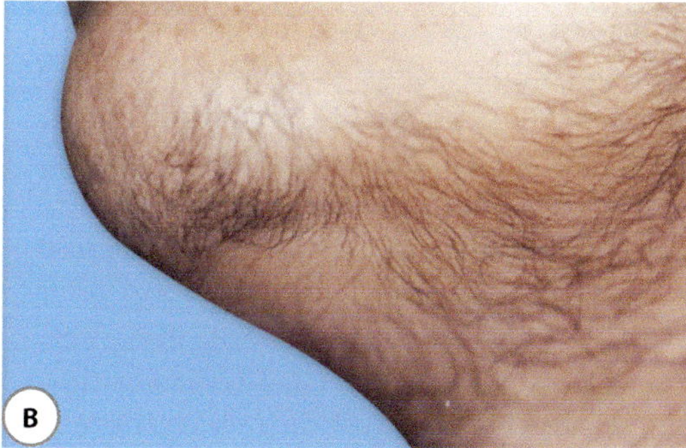

FIGS. 1A AND B: Paradoxical hypertrichosis.

MANAGEMENT OPTIONS

Treatment

Although manufacturers often have preloaded settings built into the energy-based device to guide treatment parameters, these do not ensure safety or efficacy due to differences in patient sensitivity, skin type, device calibration, and energy output.[43] Instead, the energy-based device surgeon should seek to achieve the desired therapeutic endpoint of perifollicular erythema and edema.[33] In darker skin patients, perifollicular edema is easier to appreciate than erythema.

Test spots in an inconspicuous area are advisable to accurately determine the appropriate fluence.[12] Starting at the lowest possible fluence to achieve the desired endpoint is recommended. If at any time, warning endpoints are seen (see endpoint chapter in this book), fluence shoulder be lowered. It should be noted, however, that test spots are not always predictive.

Treatments are typically spaced four to eight weeks apart, but there is no disadvantage to longer intervals between treatments despite limited evidence to suggest slightly greater efficacy with shorter intervals.[20,44] In clinical practice, prolonged treatment intervals have not resulted in suboptimal outcomes.

The key to successful EBHR is absorption of light by the hair shaft and follicle, which can be compromised by hair that remains on the surface of the skin. It is essential that the external hair shaft is removed prior to photoepilation, preferably by shaving, as hair left on the surface of the skin will absorb the energy-based device's energy and can induce a cutaneous thermal burn. Patients should avoid other modalities of hair removal prior to EBHR such as waxing, plucking, threading, or electrolysis for at least 2–3 weeks as they disturb the follicle and hair shaft thereby preventing successful photoepilation.[10] It is also acceptable to bleach unwanted hair before EBHR as this preserves the hair shaft. Immediately before the procedure, the skin should be cleansed thoroughly and any make-up, creams, or topical cosmetic products should be removed.

Finally, patients should be informed that some people find EBHR to be uncomfortable if performed without a topical anesthetic. This should come as no surprise given that the mechanism of hair removal is most commonly via photothermal destruction through local heating. The degree of discomfort is modulated by patient-specific characteristics, such as the density of hairs and anatomic location of hair removal, as well as the energy density delivered by the energy-based device, with higher fluences causing greater discomfort. Topical anesthetics, e.g., lidocaine and/or prilocaine, can be applied under occlusion up to one hour before EBHR to help minimize discomfort. It is important to utilize safe practices with topical anesthetics, as they also pose some risk to the patient. Application of lidocaine or prilocaine to large body surface areas may result in systemic absorption with resultant vertigo, tinnitus, paresthesias, cardiac arrhythmias, methemoglobinemia, and seizures.[45-47]

Treatment Options

Safe and effective treatment of patients with dark hair and skin phototypes I–III can be readily achieved with multiple different energy-based device types. The long-pulsed ruby (694 nm) was the first to be described in this context, and subsequent studies with the long-pulsed alexandrite (755 nm), long-pulsed diode (800-810 nm), long-pulsed Nd:YAG (1,064 nm) and IPL have all shown similar efficacy in comparative studies.[48-52]

The long-pulsed ruby (694 nm) has demonstrated long-term reduction in hair density since the mid-1990s, first reported by Grossman et al., in skin types I–III with dark hair.[53-55] In the original study, 13 patients were treated on the back or thighs with fluence ranging between 20 and 60 J/cm^2 with a 6 mm spot size, and demonstrated delayed hair growth at 1 and 3 months follow-up and with no further significant change in hair counts 6 months, 1 year, and 2 years after laser exposure. The laser-induced alopecia correlated histologically with miniaturized, vellus-like hair follicles.[53-55] Since then, multiple studies have demonstrated effective photoepilation (with some technique modifications including fluence, pulse duration, and spot size) yielding 20–60% hair reduction after a single treatment, and nearly 80% after multiple treatments.[8,18,34,53-55] A multicenter trial with over 180 patients demonstrated the safety and efficacy of the ruby energy-based device resulting in nearly 80% hair loss in the majority of patients after an average of four treatments with fluence ranging from 10 to 60 J/cm^2.[56]

The long-pulsed alexandrite (755 nm) is theoretically safer than the ruby in darker skin types.[8] Indeed, multiple studies have shown that the alexandrite is both safe and effective in skin phototypes I–III, as well as in darker phototypes IV–VI with appropriate parameters and cooling.[8,19,44,50-52,57-66] The evidence supporting the efficacy for the long-pulsed alexandrite laser is demonstrated in a randomized controlled trial by Davoudi et al. in patients with phototypes III–IV skin treated with fluences of 20 or 40 J/cm^2, 1.5 millisecond pulse duration, with four treatments at 8-week intervals demonstrated a 76–84% hair reduction at 18 months after the last treatment.[67] Multiple other studies have consistently demonstrated nearly 80% reduction of hair at fluences usually in the 20–40 J/cm^2 range, with differential efficacy again noted in some studies based on anatomical site.[57,63,66,67]

The semiconductor diode (800–810 nm) energy-based device has been used extensively for EBHR with multiple studies demonstrating safety and efficacy (**Figs. 2A** and **B**) comparable to the ruby and alexandrite energy-based devices.[12,13,20,68-70] In fact, due to its longer wavelength, the diode is theoretically safer for darker phototypes than both the ruby and alexandrite, but still sufficiently absorbed by melanin to make it effective for EBHR.[68-70] The adjustable pulse duration and contact-cooling of the diode further improves its safety

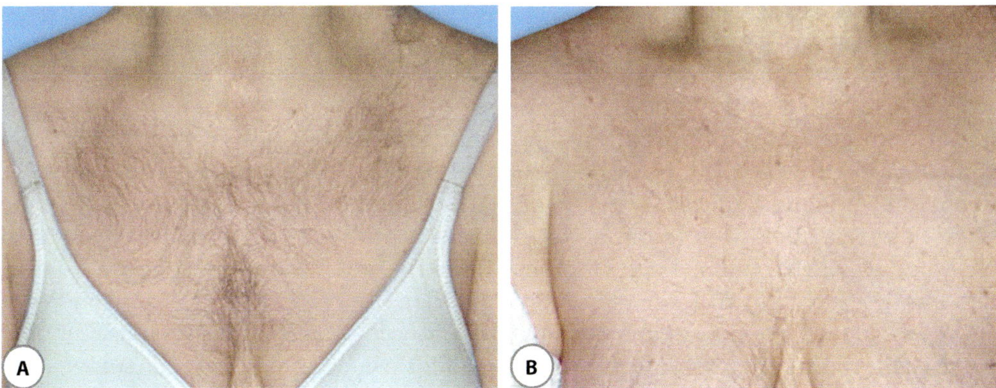

FIGS. 2A AND B: Effective hair removal 1.5 years after third treatment with a 800 nm diode laser.

profile in darker patients; however, caution is still mandatory when treating skin type VI.[71] Overall, studies have reported approximately 40% hair reduction after one or two treatments with fluences of 15–40 J/ cm^2, pulse duration of 5–30 ms, 9-mm spot size, and long follow-up times.[69,70] After four treatments with similar parameters, another study reported an 84% hair reduction with 12 months follow-up.[49]

The long-pulsed Nd:YAG (1,064 nm) is considered to be the safest energy-based device for hair removal in darker skin phototypes.[59] In depth description of the efficacy and safety of this laser is discussed in the section "skin of color considerations" in this chapter.

Intense pulsed light sources emit non-coherent, polychromatic light at wavelengths ranging from 550 to 1,200 nm, although various cutoff filters can be used to limit the range of wavelengths to target particular chromophores, such as melanin.[2] IPLs can be used in darker skin phototypes only with the use of cutoff filters to allow emission in the infrared spectrum.[12] Data regarding the efficacy of IPL is mixed, with multiple studies demonstrating good results,[72-75] including 60% reduction at 3 months after a single treatment,[75] 54% reduction at 6 months after a single treatment,[73] and 75% or greater reduction after several treatments.[75-77] On the other hand, two studies comparing IPL versus either the Nd:YAG[78] or the long-pulsed alexandrite[79] both demonstrated that the IPL was inferior for hair epilation.

Removal of light and white hairs has been attempted with combined bipolar radiofrequency and pulsed light-based devices and has shown modest success at removal of light hairs. An attempt to remove white hairs, especially when combined with a topical photosensitizer such as topical aminolevulinic acid, showed low success rates and did not achieve stable reductions over time.[80,81]

A prospective, multicenter study examined hair reduction in the axillae after treatment with a noninvasive microwave energy device. In this study, fifty-six adult subjects were enrolled and treated with the device in 1 or 2 treatment sessions 3 months apart at various energy levels, and followed for 12 months. An average total underarm hair reduction of approximately 70% for both light and dark hair was obtained with mild transient post-treatment effects such as localized edema, discomfort, and bruising. This clinical study provides evidence for safe and stable axillary hair reduction that lasted through the year of follow-up.[22]

Skin cooling is critical to achieving higher fluences sufficient for efficacious depilation with minimal off-target epidermal damage.[82] Multiple modalities exist for skin cooling but all function through the primary mechanism of creating a heat sink thereby removing heat from the skin surface. The use of a cold gel applied directly to the skin at the interface between the energy-based device and skin surface is the least effective mechanism, as it only passively extracts heat and cannot further cool the skin. Forced cold air can provide skin cooling before, during, and after energy-based device pulse discharge; however, most EBHR devices now utilize built-in contact cooling or cryogen spray.[2] Treatments with longer pulse durations, i.e., over 10 ms, generally are better served by contact cooling, which provides skin cooling before, during, and after an energy-based device pulse.[2] Treatments with shorter pulse durations, i.e., 5 ms or less, often utilize cryogen liquid spray, which is a dynamic cooling process that precools the skin with a brief pulse of cryogen spray immediately before energy-based device discharge and can also deliver a second spray after the energy-based device pulse for post-cooling.[2] Unfortunately, cryogen spray cannot be utilized during the energy-based device pulse because it interferes with the energy-based device.

Proper technique by the energy-based device operator is critical in achieving excellent outcomes and minimizing risk of complications. Correct technique of energy based device pulses, such as avoidance of pulse stacking and ensuring complete contact of the device tip with the skin surface, can decrease the risk of complications. However, minor overlap is recommended as zones of untreated hairs will result if the pulses are completely nonoverlapping.

Post-procedure, patients can expect to have perifollicular edema and erythema for up to 2 days (**Fig. 3**), and could be given ice or topical corticosteroids immediately after treatment to decrease swelling and discomfort. If epidermal injury has occurred, an antibiotic ointment should be prescribed and patients should avoid using make up on injured skin. Furthermore, patients may experience hair cast shedding during the first 1–2 weeks after EBHR, which may be confused with hair growth.[2] Patients should be advised that after each treatment, one may experience a transient initial period of total hair loss in the treatment field, and that decreasing partial regrowth is expected to occur after each subsequent treatment. Finally, strict sun protection with sunscreen, protective clothing, and sun avoidance should be stressed to patients as tanning after EBHR can cause pigmentary disturbances and will interfere with the safety and efficacy of the next EBHR session.

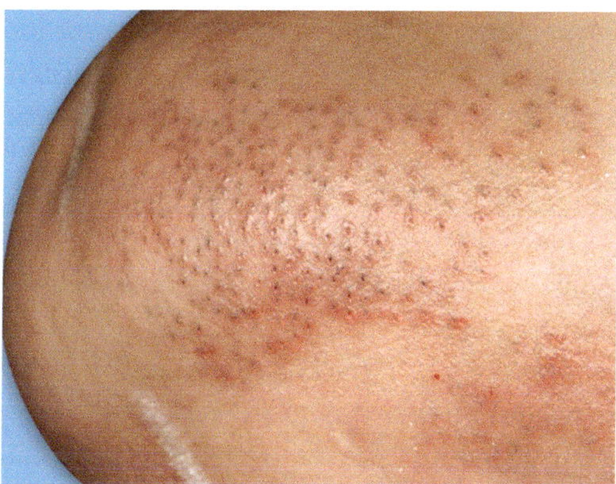

FIG. 3: Perifollicular erythema and edema immediately after energy-based hair removal (EBHR).

Skin of Color Considerations

Patients with darker skin are more difficult to treat, as they are at greater risk for complications due to the greater melanin content in their epidermis. Specifically, the energy-based device is unable to differentiate between follicular and epidermal melanin, which puts the epidermis at risk of absorbing the energy-based devices energy, thereby increasing the potential for off-target damage.[9] This lack of contrast between epidermal and follicular melanin is the underpinning that makes dark skinned patients more challenging to treat.

Strategies to successfully treat patients with darker phototypes include selection of an energy-based device with a longer wavelength. Perhaps the most important strategy after selection of the correct wavelength is the utilization of aggressive cooling systems to protect against thermal damage.[12] The safety profile is further increased by increasing the pulse duration, which targets and heats the hair follicle more efficiently than the skin, thereby mitigating the risk of epidermal injury. [11,83]

The long-pulsed Nd:YAG (1,064 nm) is considered to be the safest energy-based device for hair removal in darker skin phototypes.[59] Clinical studies have demonstrated fewer side effects for the Nd:YAG in patients with skin phototypes IV–VI when compared with the alexandrite and diode energy-based device, with good long-term efficacy data.[2,59] Galadari et al demonstrated a 35% hair reduction at 1 year after six treatments (30–120 J/cm^2, 9.5 ms pulse duration, 5 mm spot size) compared with the diode and alexandrite, which showed a 40% hair reduction during the same interval [both energy-based devices used 20–40 J/cm^2, 40 ms pulse duration, 9 mm spot size (diode) and 10 mm spot size (alexandrite)].[59] Notably, hair reduction up to 70–90% at one year has been reported for facial, leg, and axillary hair after three treatments with the Nd:YAG (40–50 J/cm^2, pulse duration 50 ms, 5 mm spot size),[84] while another study achieved approximately 50% hair reduction in dark-skinned patients at six months after three treatments [fluence 30-60 J/cm^2, spot size 10 mm, pulse duration 20 ms (type III/IV skin), and 30 ms (type V/VI skin)][85]. In the majority of studies with Nd:YAG, side effects of fibrosis and scarring were not seen, and transient pigmentary alterations rarely occurred except in photo-exposed sites, lasting for several weeks.[12]

The Nd:YAG has also demonstrated benefit in the treatment of PFB in skin types IV–VI. A study evaluating various fluences in the treatment of PFB including 50, 80, and 100 J/cm^2 found that most patients did best at the 50 and 80 J/cm^2 range, as more side effects were noted at the highest fluence.[86,87] After a single treatment, patients had significant reduction in PFB lesions, and this treatment is considered safe if done at the correct fluence with adequate skin cooling. Treatment of PFB in type V and VI skin may also be achieved with the diode, although side effects occurred in type VI skin.

Several studies have demonstrated the safety and efficacy of the long-pulsed alexandrite in patients with skin type IV, although this energy-based device should be used with caution or avoided in skin types V and VI due to the higher incidence of adverse events.[58,59] In a large cohort of Asian patients with skin types III–V, the long-pulsed alexandrite energy-based device achieved 55% hair reduction after three treatments with 9 months of follow-up (fluence 16–24 J/cm^2, 40 ms pulse duration, 12.5 mm spot size).[88] No patients experienced permanent pigmentary changes or scarring, although folliculitis, crusting, and transient pigmentary changes did occur.

The diode energy-based device can also be safely used in skin types IV and V, and although it has been reported safe in skin type VI, it is not frequently used in this population. A study in patients with skin types V and VI achieved 75–90% hair reduction, albeit after 8–10 treatments (fluence 10 J/cm^2, pulse duration 30 ms).[89] The use of long pulse durations, at least 30 ms or higher, along with a contact cooling device is recommended, as longer pulse durations allow the epidermis to have additional cooling time. Similar rates of transient pigmentary alterations were noted after the diode compared to the alexandrite, with time to resolution of approximately 3 months in one study.[49,50]

In summary, the Nd:YAG is the safest for darker skin types IV–VI, the alexandrite can be safely used in skin types III and IV, and the diode can be used in skin types IV or V, but should generally be avoided in type VI skin. Epidermal cooling is crucial for darker skin types and longer pulse durations with contact cooling devices further increase the safety profile. As a result, thicker, coarser hair is likely to respond better due to the need for longer pulse durations. The removal of fine, thin hair in dark-skinned patients remains a challenge as shorter pulse durations need to be used that also increase the risk of pigment alterations.

COMPLICATIONS

It is important for patients to understand that some side effects are common and should be expected, including minor pain, erythema, perifollicular edema, and shedding of dead hairs. These are transient and do not constitute complications (**Fig. 3**).

The incidence of adverse cutaneous effects after EBHR is associated with selection of inappropriate wavelength, pulse duration, and fluence, or inefficient epidermal cooling, or treating tanned skin.[90] The most common complication is pigmentary alteration, including hypo- and hyperpigmentation, which may occur despite appropriate energy-based device setting selections.[2] This is usually transient and resolves over 3–4 months although is rarely permanent in some patients, especially those with darker skin types. Sun-protected sites tend to develop complications less frequently than sun-exposed sites.[16]

Less common side effects include blistering, infections (bacterial or viral), or textural changes; reported but rare complications are reticulate erythema (**Fig. 4**),[91] purpura,[33] induction or aggravation of acne or folliculitis,[92] and delayed urticaria.[93] However, it is also possible for patients to experience more concerning side effects including thermal burns, permanent scarring, or blindness.[92]

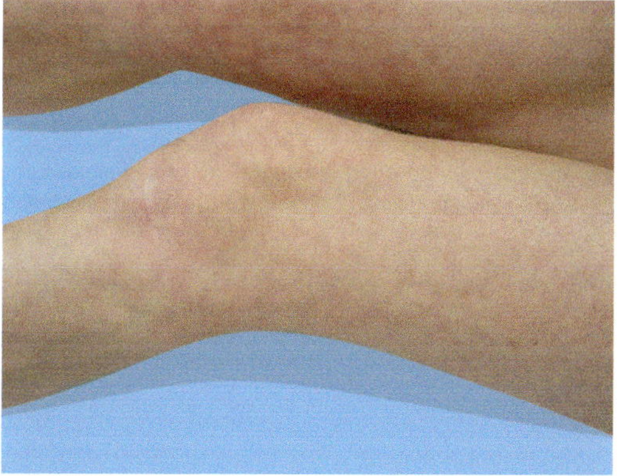

FIG. 4: Reticulate erythema after energy-based hair removal (EBHR).

Interestingly, there are few case reports of Koebnerization of certain diseases including reactive perforating collagenosis, lichen planus, vitiligo, and psoriasis after EBHR.[94,95] Patients with vitiligo and psoriasis should be warned for the risk of Köebner phenomenon after laser treatment.[95-97]

The risks of EBHR extend beyond tissue damage from the energy-based device pulse itself. A recent study identified over 300 chemical compounds released into the air when hair was vaporized with EBHR.[98,99] Of these compounds, over a dozen were known or suspected carcinogens and over 20 were known environmental toxins, each with strong absorption peaks as measured by gas chromatography-mass spectrometry, with a more than 26-fold increase in particulate count compared to baseline ambient levels. The presence of an evacuator close to the site of EBHR decreased these levels to 8-fold higher than baseline ambient levels highlighting the need for further personal protective equipment. Therefore, both evacuators and surgical masks should be utilized to decrease the inhalation of biohazardous materials that are produced during EBHR.

The risk of destruction of the melanin content in pre-existing nevi, or the induction of inflammatory or pigmentary changes in nevi, may lead to increased rates of biopsies, with difficulty in accurately evaluating histologic atypia. This may have undue consequences for the patient in the management of their pigmented lesions due to concern for malignant transformation. Therefore, we recommend avoiding EBHR around nevi wherever possible.

Finally, it is important to note that EBHR was found to be the most commonly litigated energy-based device procedure, with non-physician operators accounting for a disproportionately large number of cases.[100] As the number of EBHR procedures has increased over the last 15 years, so too has the number of legal claims related to their use, with mean indemnity payments that exceed the average reported payments across all other specialties. Therefore, providers should have a thorough understanding of the pretreatment considerations, key consultative questions, treatment options and parameters, complications and their treatments to safely provide the highest quality of patient care (**Boxes 1** to **3**).

BOX 1: Key points regarding pretreatment considerations and key consultative questions.

- Set realistic expectations for the patient
- Treatment intervals are 4–6 weeks apart
- Patients should shave their unwanted hair prior to EBHR. Other methods of hair removal should be avoided
- Sun avoidance is essential and tanned patients should not undergo EBHR
- Patients with light skin and dark hair are the best candidates
- A history of HSV or bacterial skin infections, a history of polycystic ovary syndrome or other hormonal abnormalities, thorough medication history, and history of hypertrophic or keloid scarring are important determinants of the EBHR treatment algorithm
- Ocular damage is a major risk of EBHR and all individuals in the treatment room should wear wavelength-specific safety goggles

(EBHR: energy-based hair removal; HSV: herpes simplex virus)

BOX 2: Management options.

- Overall, alexandrite and diode achieve the best treatment responses, although any wavelength can achieve satisfactory results with appropriate fluence and cooling
- Patients with skin phototypes I–III are effectively treated with long-pulsed ruby (694 nm), long-pulsed alexandrite (755 nm), long-pulsed diode (810 nm), and IPL, with similar efficacy across these modalities
- Patients with phototypes IV–VI are more challenging to treat. The long-pulsed Nd:YAG is the safest energy-based device for dark-skinned patients, however, is less effective at a given fluence compared to the other energy-based devices
- With aggressive epidermal cooling, the alexandrite and diode may be safely used in some darker skin types
- Both the diode and Nd:YAG have demonstrated efficacy in the treatment of pseudofolliculitis barbae

(IPL: intense pulsed light; Nd:YAG: neodymium-doped yttrium aluminum garnet)

BOX 3: Tips for safety and efficacy.

- Better efficacy is achieved at higher fluence
- Avoid using dark marker on the skin as this may be absorbed by the laser
- Patients with psoriasis and vitiligo should be warned about the Koebner phenomenon possibly occurring with EBHR
- Axillary hair tends to respond well to EBHR and is well tolerated
- For men, the beard area, chest, abdomen, and back tend to respond well but can be quite uncomfortable due to the density of hair at those sites. Likewise, bony areas such as the ankles also tend to be more sensitive
- The groin and perianal area respond well to treatment but due to the increased pigment in this region, longer wavelengths should be selected for treatment
- Do not treat near the periocular rim as this increased the risk of ocular injury
- Epidermal injury can be avoided by increasing cooling, increasing the pulse duration, and/or decreasing the fluence

(EBHR: energy-based hair removal)

CONCLUSION

Energy-based hair removal is a safe and effective modality for long-term hair removal, with numerous energy-based devices available that can remove hair in all skin phototypes. It is critical for providers to possess a detailed understanding of each energy-based device's properties to individualize and optimize treatment for the patient. Furthermore, the energy-based device surgeon should seek to achieve desired therapeutic endpoints of perifollicular erythema and edema to guide management, rather than to rely on manufacturer settings. EBHR in light-skinned patients has shown similar results with the ruby, alexandrite, and diode energy-based devices, as well as with IPL, while in patients with darker skin types the long-pulsed Nd:YAG is likely the safest option. Unfortunately, EBHR of patients with light hair remains a challenge that has yet to be overcome. While complications from EBHR are relatively rare, they can occur. Adjusting the energy-based device settings to appropriate parameters for patients based on their skin type and providing efficient epidermal cooling to prevent thermal injury to the skin can avoid most complications.

REFERENCES

1. Jalian HR, Jalian CA, Avram MM. Common causes of injury and legal action in laser surgery. JAMA Dermatol. 2013;149(2):188-93.
2. Ibrahimi OA, Avram MM, Hanke CW, Kilmer SL, Anderson RR. Laser hair removal. Dermatol Ther. 2011;24(1):94-107.
3. Koch D, Pratsou P, Szczecinska W, Lanigan S, Abdullah A. The diverse application of laser hair removal therapy: A tertiary laser unit's experience with less common indications and a literature overview. Lasers Med Sci. 2015;30(1):453-67.
4. Sun TT, Cotsarelis G, Lavker RM. Hair follicular stem cells: the bulge-activation hypothesis. J Invest Dermatol. 1991;96(5):77S-8S.
5. Olsen EA. Methods of hair removal. J Am Acad Dermatol. 1999;40(2 Pt 1):143-55.
6. Anderson RR, Parrish JA. Selective photothermolysis: precise microsurgery by selective absorption of pulsed radiation. Science. 1983;220(4596):524-7.
7. Hruza GJ, Geronemus RG, Dover JS, Arndt KA. Lasers in dermatology-1993. Arch Dermatol. 1993;129(8):1026-35.
8. Tanzi EL, Lupton JR, Alster TS. Lasers in dermatology: four decades of progress. J Am Acad Dermatol. 2003;49(1):1-31.

9. Ross EV, Ladin Z, Kreindel M, Dierickx C. Theoretical considerations in laser hair removal. Dermatol Clin. 1999;17(2):333-55,viii.
10. Dierickx CC. Hair removal by lasers and intense pulsed light sources. Dermatol Clin. 2002;20(1):135-46.
11. Altshuler GB, Anderson RR, Manstein D, Zenzie HH, Smirnov MZ. Extended theory of selective photothermolysis. Lasers Surg Med. 2001;29(5):416-32.
12. Wanner M. Laser hair removal. Dermatol Ther. 2005;18(3):209-16.
13. Campos VB, Dierickx CC, Farinelli WA, Lin TY, Manuskiatti W, Anderson RR. Hair removal with an 800-nm pulsed diode laser. J Am Acad Dermatol. 2000;43(3):442-7.
14. Haedersdal M, Wulf HC. Evidence-based review of hair removal using lasers and light sources. J Eur Acad Dermatol Venereol. 2006;20(1):9-20.
15. Dierickx CC, Grossman MC. Laser hair removal. In: Goldberg DJ (Ed). Laser and Lights, vol. 2. China: Elsevier Saunders; 2005. pp. 61-76
16. Gan SD, Graber EM. Laser hair removal: a review. Dermatol Surg. 2013;39(6):823-38.
17. Haedersdal M, Haak CS. Hair removal. Curr Probl Dermatol. 2011;42:111-21.
18. Williams R, Havoonjian H, Isagholian K, Menaker G, Moy R. A clinical study of hair removal using the long-pulsed ruby laser. Dermatol Surg. 1998;24(8):837-42.
19. Nanni CA, Alster TS. Long-pulsed alexandrite laser-assisted hair removal at 5, 10, and 20 millisecond pulse durations. Lasers Surg Med. 1999;24(5):332-7.
20. Bouzari N, Tabatabai H, Abbasi Z, Firooz A, Dowlati Y. Hair removal using an 800-nm diode laser: comparison at different treatment intervals of 45, 60, and 90 days. Int J Dermatol. 2005;44(1):50-3.
21. Lorenz S, Brunnberg S, Landthaler M, Hohenleutner U. Hair removal with the long pulsed Nd:YAG laser: a prospective study with one year follow-up. Lasers Surg Med. 2002;30(2):127-34.
22. Brauer JA, Neckman JP, Zelickson B, Vasily DB, Geronemus RG. A Prospective Study of Axillary Hair Reduction in Patients Treated With Microwave Technology. Dermatol Surg. 2017;43(4):558-65.
23. Shulman S, Bichler I. Ocular complications of laser-assisted eyebrow epilation. Eye (Lond). 2009;23(4):982-3.
24. Sheikh A, Hodge W, Coupland S. Diode laser-induced uveitis and visual field defect. Ophthalmic Plast Reconstr Surg. 2007;23(4):321-3.
25. Lee WW, Murdock J, Albini TA, O'Brien TP, Levine ML. Ocular damage secondary to intense pulse light therapy to the face. Ophthalmic Plast Reconstr Surg. 2011;27(4):263-5.
26. Le Jeune M, Autie M, Monnet D, Brezin AP. Ocular complications after laser epilation of eyebrows. Eur J Dermatol. 2007;17(6):553-4.
27. Herbold TM, Busse H, Uhlig CE. Bilateral cataract and corectopia after laser eyebrow [corrected] epilation. Ophthalmology. 2005;112(9):1634-5.
28. Halkiadakis I, Skouriotis S, Stefanaki C, Patsea E, Papakonstatndinou D, Amariotakis A, et al. Iris atrophy and posterior synechiae as a complication of eyebrow laser epilation. J Am Acad Dermatol. 2007;57(2 Suppl):S4-5.
29. Carrim ZI, Chohan AW, Devlin HC. Iris damage and acute pigment dispersion following photo-epilation. Eye (Lond). 2006;20(12):1486-8.
30. Riml S, Larcher L, Grohmann M, Kompatscher P. Second-degree burn within a tattoo after intense-pulsed-light epilation. Photodermatol Photoimmunol Photomed. 2013;29(4):218-20.
31. Kluger N, Hakimi S, Del Giudice P. Keloid occurring in a tattoo after laser hair removal. Acta Derm Venereol. 2009;89(3):334-5.
32. Soden CE, Smith K, Skelton H. Histologic features seen in changing nevi after therapy with an 810 nm pulsed diode laser for hair removal in patients with dysplastic nevi. Int J Dermatol. 2001;40(8):500-4.
33. Nanni CA, Alster TS. Laser-assisted hair removal: side effects of Q-switched Nd:YAG, long-pulsed ruby, and alexandrite lasers. J Am Acad Dermatol. 1999;41(2 Pt 1):165-71.
34. Williams RM, Christian MM, Moy RL. Hair removal using the long-pulsed ruby laser. Dermatol Clin. 1999;17(2):367-72.
35. Waldman A, Bolotin D, Arndt KA, Dover JS, Geronemus RG, Chapas A, et al. ASDS Guidelines Task Force: Consensus Recommendations Regarding the Safety of Lasers, Dermabrasion, Chemical Peels, Energy Devices, and Skin Surgery During and After Isotretinoin Use. Dermatol Surg. 2017;43(10):1249-62.
36. Spring LK, Krakowski AC, Alam M, Bhatia A, Brauer J, Cohen J, et al. Isotretinoin and Timing of Procedural Interventions: A Systematic Review with Consensus Recommendations. JAMA Dermatol. 2017;153(8):802-9.
37. Moreno-Arias G, Castelo-Branco C, Ferrando J. Paradoxical effect after IPL photoepilation. Dermatol Surg. 2002;28(11):1013-6.

38. Bernstein EF. Hair growth induced by diode laser treatment. Dermatol Surg. 2005;31(5):584-6.
39. Willey A, Torrontegui J, Azpiazu J, Landa N. Hair stimulation following laser and intense pulsed light photo-epilation: review of 543 cases and ways to manage it. Lasers Surg Med. 2007;39(4):297-301.
40. Desai S, Mahmoud BH, Bhatia AC, Hamzavi IH. Paradoxical hypertrichosis after laser therapy: a review. Dermatol Surg. 2010; 36(3):291-8.
41. Lolis MS, Marmur ES. Paradoxical hypertrichosis after laser therapy: a review. Dermatol Surg. 2010:36(3):291-8.
42. Alajlan A, Shapiro J, Rivers JK, MacDonald N, Wiggin J, Lui H. Paradoxical hypertrichosis after laser epilation. J Am Acad Dermatol. 2005;53(1):85-8.
43. Wanner M, Sakamoto FH, Avram MM, Chan HH, Alam M, Tannous Z, et al. Immediate skin responses to laser and light treatments: Therapeutic endpoints: How to obtain efficacy. J Am Acad Dermatol. 2016;74(5):821-33.
44. Lloyd JR, Mirkov M. Long-term evaluation of the long-pulsed alexandrite laser for the removal of bikini hair at shortened treatment intervals. Dermatol Surg. 2000;26(7):633-7.
45. Fox M, Helfrich Y, Kang S. Other Topical Medications. In: Bolognia JL, Jorizzo JL, Schaffer JV, eds. Dermatology. 3rd ed. New York: Elsevier Limited. 2012:2153-64.
46. Friedman PM, Mafong EA, Friedman ES, Geronemus RG. Topical anesthetics update: EMLA and beyond. Dermatol Surg. 2001;27(12):1019-26.
47. Koay J, Orengo I. Application of local anesthetics in dermatologic surgery. Dermatol Surg. 2002;28(2):143-8.
48. Bouzari N, Tabatabai H, Abbasi Z, Firooz A, Dowlati Y. Laser hair removal: comparison of long-pulsed Nd:YAG, long-pulsed alexandrite, and long-pulsed diode lasers. Dermatol Surg. 2004;30(4 Pt 1):498-502.
49. Eremia S, Li C, Newman N. Laser hair removal with alexandrite versus diode laser using four treatment sessions: 1-year results. Dermatol Surg. 2001;27(11):925-9.
50. Handrick C, Alster TS. Comparison of long-pulsed diode and long-pulsed alexandrite lasers for hair removal: a long-term clinical and histologic study. Dermatol Surg. 2001;27(7):622-6.
51. Alster TS. Prolonged clinical experience with laser assisted hair removal: a clinical comparison of systems. Surg Medicine. 1999;11:14-5.
52. Nanni CA, Alster TS. A practical review Laser of laser-assisted hair removal using the Q-switched Nd:YAG, long-pulsed ruby, and long-pulsed alexandrite lasers. Dermatol Surg. 1998;24(12):1399-405.
53. Grossman MC, Dierickx C, Farinelli W, Flotte T, Anderson RR. Damage to hair follicles by normal-mode ruby laser pulses. J Am Acad Dermatol 1996;35(6):889-94.
54. Dierickx C. Laser-assisted hair removal: state of the art. Dermatol Ther. 2001;13(1):80-9.
55. Dierickx CC, Grossman MC, Farinelli WA, Anderson RR. Permanent hair removal by normal-mode ruby laser. Arch Dermatol. 1998;134(7):837-42.
56. Goldberg DJ. Laser hair removal. Dermatol Clin. 2002;20(3):561-7.
57. Eremia S, Li CY, Umar SH, Newman N. Laser hair removal: long-term results with a 755 nm alexandrite laser. Dermatol Surg. 2001;27(11):920-4.
58. Garcia C, Alamoudi H, Nakib M, Zimmo S. Alexandrite laser hair removal is safe for Fitzpatrick skin types IV-VI. Dermatol Surg. 2000;26(2):130-4.
59. Galadari I. Comparative evaluation of different hair removal lasers in skin types IV, V, and VI. Int J Dermatol. 2003;42(1):68-70.
60. Connolly C, Paolini L. Study reveals successful removal of unwanted hair with LPIR laser. Cosmet Dermatol. 1997;10(12):38-40.
61. McDaniel DH, Lord J, Ash K, Newman J, Zukowski M. Laser hair removal: a review and report on the use of the long-pulsed alexandrite laser for hair reduction of the upper lip, leg, back, and bikini region. Dermatol Surg. 1999;25(6):425-30.
62. Eliezri Y. Fifteen month clinical trial of hair removal with Alexandrite laser. Lasers Surg Med. 1998;10(Suppl):200.
63. Finkel B, Eliezri YD, Waldman A, Slatkine M. Pulsed alexandrite laser technology for noninvasive hair removal. J Clin Laser Med Surg. 1997;15(5):225-9.
64. Goldberg DJ, Ahkami R. Evaluation comparing multiple treatments with a 2-msec and 10-msec alexandrite laser for hair removal. Lasers Surg Med. 1999;25(3):223-8.
65. Touma DJ, Rohrer TE. Persistent hair loss 60 months after a single treatment with a 3-millisecond alexandrite (755 nm) laser. J Am Acad Dermatol. 2004;50(2):324-5.
66. Gorgu M, Aslan G, Akoz T, Erdogan B. Comparison of alexandrite laser and electrolysis for hair removal. Dermatol Surg. 2000;26(1):37-41.
67. Davoudi SM, Behnia F, Gorouhi F, Keshavarz S, Nassiri Kashani M, Rashighi Firoozabadi M, et al. Comparison of long-pulsed alexandrite and Nd:YAG lasers, individually and in combination, for leg hair reduction: an assessor-blinded, randomized trial with 18 months of follow-up. Arch Dermatol. 2008;144(10):1323-7.

68. Dierickx CC, Grossman MC, Farinelli WA, Anderson RR. Hair removal by a pulsed, infrared laser system. Lasers Surg Med. 1998;10(Suppl):198.
69. Lou WW, Quintana AT, Geronemus RG, Grossman MC. Prospective study of hair reduction by diode laser (800 nm) with long-term follow-up. Dermatol Surg. 2000;26(5):428-32.
70. Baugh WP, Trafeli JP, Barnette DJ Jr, Ross EV. Hair reduction using a scanning 800 nm diode laser. Dermatol Surg. 2001;27(4):358-64.
71. Smith EP, Winstanley D, Ross EV. Modified superlong pulse 810 nm diode laser in the treatment of pseudofolliculitis barbae in skin types V and VI. Dermatol Surg. 2005;31(3):297-301.
72. Raulin C, Greve B, Grema H. IPL technology: a review. Lasers Surg Med. 2003;32(2):78-87.
73. Weiss RA, Weiss MA, Marwaha S, Harrington AC. Hair removal with a non-coherent filtered flashlamp intense pulsed light source. Lasers Surg Med. 1999;24(2):128-32.
74. Sadick NS, Shea CR, Burchette JL Jr, Prieto VG. High-intensity flashlamp photoepilation: a clinical, histological, and mechanistic study in human skin. Arch Dermatol. 1999;135(6):668-76.
75. Gold MH, Bell MW, Foster TD, Street S. One-year follow-up using an intense pulsed light source for long-term hair removal. J Cutan Laser Ther. 1999;1(3):167-71.
76. Troilius A, Troilius C. Hair removal with a second generation broad spectrum intense pulsed light source-a long-term follow-up. J Cutan Laser Ther. 1999;1(3):173-8.
77. Schroeter CA, Raulin C, Thurlimann W, Reineke T, De Potter C, Neumann HA. Hair removal in 40 hirsute women with an intense laser-like light source. Eur J Dermatol. 1999;9(5):374-9.
78. Goh CL. Comparative study on a single treatment response to long pulse Nd:YAG lasers and intense pulse light therapy for hair removal on skin type IV to VI-is longer wavelengths lasers preferred over shorter wavelengths lights for assisted hair removal. J Dermatolog Treat. 2003;14(4):243-7.
79. McGill DJ, Hutchison C, McKenzie E, McSherry E, Mackay IR. A randomised, split-face comparison of facial hair removal with the alexandrite laser and intense pulsed light system. Lasers Surg Med. 2007;39(10):767-72.
80. Goldberg DJ, Marmur ES, Hussain M. Treatment of terminal and vellus non-pigmented hairs with an optical/bipolar radiofrequency energy source-with and without pre-treatment using topical aminolevulinic acid. J Cosmet Laser Ther. 2005;7(1):25-8.
81. Sadick NS, Shaoul J. Hair removal using a combination of conducted radiofrequency and optical energies-an 18-month follow-up. J Cosmet Laser Ther. 2004;6(1):21-6.
82. Zenzie HH, Altshuler GB, Smirnov MZ, Anderson RR. Evaluation of cooling methods for laser dermatology. Lasers Surg Med. 2000;26(2):130-44.
83. Ash K, Lord J, Newman J, McDaniel DH. Hair removal using a long-pulsed alexandrite laser. Dermatol Clin. 1999;17(2):387-99.
84. Alster TS, Bryan H, Williams CM. Long-pulsed Nd:YAG laser-assisted hair removal in pigmented skin: a clinical and histological evaluation. Arch Dermatol. 2001;137(7):885-9.
85. Tanzi EL, Alster TS. Long-pulsed 1064-nm Nd:YAG laser-assisted hair removal in all skin types. Dermatol Surg. 2004;30(1):13-7.
86. Ross EV, Cooke LM, Timko AL, Overstreet KA, Graham BS, Barnette DJ. Treatment of pseudofolliculitis barbae in skin types IV, V, and VI with a long-pulsed neodymium:yttrium aluminum garnet laser. J Am Acad Dermatol. 2002;47(2):263-70.
87. Kauvar AN. Treatment of pseudofolliculitis with a pulsed infrared laser. Arch Dermatol. 2000;136(11):1343-6.
88. Hussain M, Polnikorn N, Goldberg DJ. Laser-assisted hair removal in Asian skin: efficacy, complications, and the effect of single versus multiple treatments. Dermatol Surg. 2003;29(3):249-54.
89. Greppi I. Diode laser hair removal of the black patient. Lasers Surg Med. 2001;28(2):150-5.
90. Tierney EP, Goldberg DJ. Laser hair removal pearls. J Cosmet Laser Ther. 2008;10(1):17-23.
91. Lapidoth M, Shafirstein G, Ben Amitai D, Hodak E, Waner M, David M. Reticulate erythema following diode laser-assisted hair removal: a new side effect of a common procedure. J Am Acad Dermatol. 2004;51(5):774-7.
92. Goldberg D. Laser complications: hair removal. J Cosmet Laser Ther. 2006;8(4):197-202.
93. Landa N, Corrons N, Zabalza I, Azpiazu JL Urticaria induced by laser epilation: a clinical and histopathological study with extended follow-up in 36 patients. Lasers Surg Med. 2012;44(5):384-9.

94. Wimmershoff MB, Hohenleutner U, Landthaler M. Isomorphic phenomenon: adverse effect after epilation with the long-pulsed ruby laser. Arch Dermatol. 2000;136(12):1570-1.
95. Doshi SN, Levy ML, Markus R. Koebnerization of reactive perforating collagenosis induced by laser hair removal. Lasers Surg Med. 2003;32(3):177-9.
96. Sellheyer K. Mechanisms of laser hair removal: could persistent photoepilation induce vitiligo or defects in wound repair? Dermatol Surg. 2007;33(9):1055-65.
97. Drosner M, Adatto M. Photo-epilation: guidelines for care from the European Society for Laser Dermatology (ESLD). J Cosmet Laser Ther. 2005;7(1):33-8.
98. Casey AS, Goldberg D. Guidelines for laser hair removal. J Cosmet Laser Ther. 2008;10(1):24-33.
99. Chuang GS, Farinelli W, Christiani DC, Herrick RF, Lee NC, Avram MM. Gaseous and Particulate Content of Laser Hair Removal Plume. JAMA Dermatol. 2016;152(12):1320-6.
100. Jalian HR, Jalian CA, Avram MM. Increased risk of litigation associated with laser surgery by nonphysician operators. JAMA Dermatol. 2014;150(4):407-11.

11

CHAPTER

Hair Transplantation for Women and Men

Marc R Avram

INTRODUCTION

Hair frames our face. It is one of the few physical attributes that we can control. The length, color, and style of our hair together reflect our personality to the world. Equally or more importantly, our hair style is often a reflection of how we perceive ourselves. The gradual *involuntary* loss of hair overtime by male and female pattern hair loss restricts how we can style our hair. As the hair loss continues, the natural frame around our face disappears. This alters our appearance to the world. Along with wrinkles and blemishes, hair loss is a sign of aging in our society. The psychological impact varies from mild to traumatic.[1]

Unfortunately, many men and women and their treating physicians are unaware of the safe and effective medical and surgical treatment options available to treat male and female pattern hair loss. Between medical and surgical therapy, the vast majority of patients can maintain or recreate a natural frame of hair around their face.

MEDICAL THERAPY

Minoxidil and finasteride are the only two Food and Drug Administration (FDA)-approved medications for male pattern hair loss (**Table 1**).

The majority of patients who use minoxidil and/or finasteride can slow, maintain, or regrow hair.[2,3] Both medications are more effective for patients with earlier stages of hair loss and are an excellent treatment option for patients losing hair, but who are not candidates for surgery. For patients that are surgical candidates, continuing medical treatment will often help increase the density of transplanted hair, slow down the rate of loss of existing hair, and increase the caliber of existing and transplanted hair. In addition these medications may help reduce a postsurgical telogen effluvium and maintain donor density.[4]

Compliance with the medications is the key to success. Since each medication affects the hair cycle, it can take 6–8 months for each one to begin to work.

Low level light therapy (LLLT) has been used for decades to treat a variety of medical conditions. Over the past few years, it has been used to treat female and male pattern hair loss. The mechanism of action is unknown. There are several studies that confirm the efficacy of LLLT for hair loss as a monotherapy and a positive synergistic affect to minoxidil.[5-8]

TABLE 1: FDA approved medical therapy and comparison of the only two FDA approved medications for male pattern hair loss.

	Finasteride	Minoxidil
Mechanism of action	5-alpha-reductase type II inhibitor blocking the conversion of testosterone to dihydrotestosterone	Unknown
Key to success	Emphasize maintenance over regrowth of hair and compliance for at least 6–8 months to see benefit	Emphasize maintenance over regrowth of hair and compliance 6–8 months to see benefit
Side effects	• 2–4% of men experience sexual dysfunction. This can be a short or long-term side effect. The long-term side effect is known as post-finasteride syndrome that patients should be made aware of • No allergic reactions, blood monitoring or drug interactions • Females should never handle or take this medication • All men should let their primary physician know that they are taking it when being screened for their PSA level	• Dryness and pruritus of the scalp. The introduction of a 5% foam in 2006 has greatly reduced these side effects • Rare allergic reaction
Clinical onset of action	6–8 months	6–8 months
Dose	1 mg qd (once a day) with or without food. If one day is skipped take usual 1 mg dose the next day	Apply the foam 1–2 times daily to frontal scalp and vertex of scalp

(FDA: Food and Drug Administration; PSA: prostate-specific antigen)

Platelet rich plasma therapy (PRP) has been a new treatment option for treating male and female pattern hair loss. It is not FDA approved and there are no long-term safety or well-designed studies confirming efficacy or side effects. There are numerous published clinical trials that do suggest a positive impact on male and female pattern hair loss.[9-12] Some fail to demonstrate any efficacy.[13] As with LLLT, PRP is currently being used as a monotherapy or in combination with finasteride, LLLT and/or minoxidil.

HAIR TRANSPLANTATION

Introduction

All patients undergoing a hair transplant should expect natural-appearing transplanted hair. A hair transplant is an outpatient procedure performed under local anesthesia. It is a procedure with a high physician and patient satisfaction with a low medical and surgical complication rates.

The average procedure takes 3-6 hours depending on the number of transplanted hairs. Patients may resume normal activities immediately, but should restrict heavy exercise for 3-7 days after surgery. The postoperative pain, if any, is restricted to the day of the procedure and a mild pain medication is adequate for relief. The patients usually do not feel any discomfort the day after the procedure. A short course of prednisone is given to prevent frontal edema. Typically, the only physical evidence of the procedure is the perifollicular crusting that remains for 6–8 days. Most patients return to work 2–3 days after the procedure without any negative cosmetic impact.

The Consult

As with all procedures, appropriate candidate selection and expectations are the key to success. Each consult begins with the patient's hair loss history, including any previous medical or surgical treatments. It is vital to examine the entire scalp to confirm the diagnosis of male or female pattern hair loss and examine the caliber and density of donor hair in the posterior scalp. The donor density and caliber of hair follicles will help determine the expected density from the procedure. Patients with below-average donor density and fine caliber hair will have natural but thin transplanted hair. Those with above-average density with wide caliber hair follicle can expect greater perceived density.

The extent and rate of hair loss varies from person to person. During the consult, the ongoing loss of existing pigmented terminal hair with or without surgery must be emphasized. The net density from a hair transplant is equal to how many follicles were transplanted minus the loss of existing hair. For all patients with existing pigmented terminal hair (overwhelming majority). It is essential to discuss the medical therapy in tandem with a surgical consult. The goal of patients is to have more hair, more density in the most natural way possible. Current surgical methods allow this. For maximum long-term density, successful medical therapy is important.

Elliptical donor harvesting and follicular unit extraction (FUE) are the state of the art donor harvesting techniques that should be discussed with patients during the consult. Both techniques ultimately create individual follicular units which is what is transplanted into the thinning scalp. Follicular units, when distributed appropriately, will create consistently natural appearing transplanted hair. The amount of donor hair available is still the rate-limiting factor in hair transplantation.

With elliptical donor harvesting, a 1–1.5 cm wide by 15–20 cm long strip of hair trimmed to a length of 1–2 mm. If a patient wears his/her hair longer than 1.5 cm, his/her existing hair will camouflage the sutures immediately with no evidence of a procedure having been performed. This is a huge practical advantage of elliptical donor harvesting over FUE which needs an extensive part of the donor region to be trimmed to 1–2 mm length to be performed (**Table 2**).

For elliptical donor harvesting, the patient is placed in the prone position and the area anesthetized with 1% lidocaine with epinephrine. Saline is added to the donor region. The saline helps to provide anesthesia, hemostasis, and reduces the transection of

TABLE 2: Advantages and disadvantages of donor harvesting techniques.

	Ellipse	Follicular unit extraction
Minimal transection of donor hair	Yes, with experienced surgical team	Variable depending on device and operator
Number of grafts safely harvested per procedure	1,500–2,000	1,500–2,000 depending on physician skill
• Time to harvest donor hair	15–20 min	1–2 h
• Visible donor scar with hair length > 1 cm long	No	No
• Visible donor scar with hair < 0.5 cm long	Yes	Yes
• Overall percentage of cases used	>50%	<50%

hair follicles by increasing turgor. The donor ellipse is created using number 10 blades on a surgical handle with 0.6–1.2 cm spacers in between the blades. The length of the donor strip is determined by the number of grafts required for the surgery. It is better to take longer rather than wider strips to reduce tension on the wound. The average patient has 60–85 follicular groupings per square centimeter.[14] As an example, a donor strip 12–14 cm long and 1 cm wide will create approximately 800–1,200 grafts.

Undermining is rarely needed to close the donor site. Either sutures or staples can be used to close the wound. They are removed 7–10 days after the procedure. The majority of donor scars are 1–3 mm wide and are of no physical or cosmetic significance.

Follicular unit extraction has become an increasingly popular method for removing donor hair over the past several years.It is the direct removal of individual follicular units either by 0.9–1.1 mm punches, or by mechanically assisted devices or robotically.[15-18] Transaction rates are comparable to donor elliptical harvesting.[19,20] It is well-suited for patients with shaved or closely cropped hair where the linear scar of a donor ellipse can be a cosmetic concern. In addition, some patients prefer FUE because no suture or staples are required. Each incision is 1 mm or less and heals in the 3–4 days making the procedure less invasive since the majority of surgical techniques in medicine have become minimally invasive resulting in less scarring and quicker recovery for patients. The primary practical disadvantage of FUE is the need to trim extensive amount of the donor to 1–2 mm in length. This makes the technique not feasible for the overwhelming majority of women and many men who are not concerned with a visible scar that will never be seen, unless they trim their hair very short.

By presenting both techniques to the patients during the consult and emphasizing that both will result in natural transplanted hair, patients and the physician can decide together which technique is best suited for them.

Hairline Design and Recipient Site Creation

Rather than considering the hairline to be a fixed boundary, it should be thought of as a natural transition zone of gradually increasing density from skin to terminal-hair-bearing skin. This ill-defined "feathering zone" is created by randomly placing, in an irregular pattern, 1–4 hair grafts along the newly created hairline.[21]

The level at which the hairline is created varies from individual to individual. It is important to look at each patient in a global, 360° view, before deciding where to place the hairline.

Male pattern hair loss is progressive but transplanted hair will grow long-term. Therefore, when viewing patients, surgeons must assume all patients will progress to complete hair loss with only transplanted hair remaining. This assumption allows transplanted hair to look equally natural 1 year and 20 years after surgery. For the majority of patients, to avoid future aesthetic complications the posterior hairline should be placed at the same plane as the frontal hairline. This will avoid "chasing" the ever expanding ring of hair loss on the vertex of the scalp with valuable donor grafts.

For women, their hairline is fixed and does not recede. A transplant adds density to a stable hairline.

Anesthesia and Recipient Site Creation

A combination of supraorbital/supratrochlear nerve blocks, field blocks, and local infiltration with 1% lidocaine is performed. Hemostasis is vital for good visibility when creating recipient sites and for graft placement. The epinephrine in the local anesthesia (placed into dermis not subcutaneous space) will create excellent hemostasis. The key for success in hemostasis is to place the lidocaine with epinephrine into the dermis not subcutaneous tissue to constrict the dermal vessels that produce the majority of bleeding intraoperatively.

Recipient sites should mimic the natural 30–45° angle of hair growth on the scalp. There are a variety of needles that are used to make sites large enough to place the 1–4 hair follicle grafts. Some of the most popular needles to make sites include number 19 and number 20 gauge needles and coronal angled grafting (CAG) needles. When making recipient sites, surgeons must be careful not to transect existing hair follicles. Some advocate using magnification to create recipient sites, in order to limit the loss of existing hair during surgery.[22] The key to success is to create recipient sites in a random, highly irregular pattern with 10–30 sites per square centimeter depending on the density of existing hair on the scalp.

Graft Placement and Postoperative Course

The grafts are placed by 2–3 surgical assistants using microvascular forceps (**Fig. 1**). The forceps pick up the 1–4 hair grafts by their perifollicular tissue, avoiding trauma to the hair follicles. Regular surgical forceps will not work. The placement of grafts into recipient sites is often the most challenging part of the procedure for both novice and experienced hair transplant teams. The chief challenges include hemostasis and "popping" of grafts from sites after they are placed. The "popping" of grafts is unpredictable from patient to patient. "Popping" of grafts is overcome by placing light pressure over a paced graft and holding it for 10–20 seconds with a moist saline-soaked Q-tip before placing the next graft.

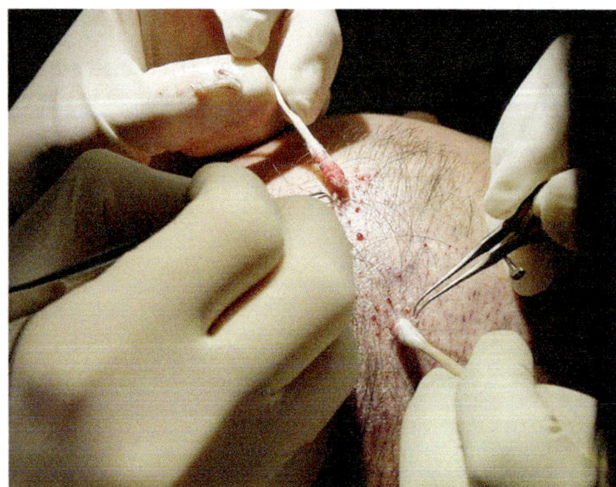

FIG. 1: Placing grafts.

The robot used in hair transplantation can currently remove follicular units, create recipient sites but cannot place grafts. Well-trained surgical assistants are still required to place transplanted hair.

Postoperative Course

Once all the grafts are placed, a dressing is applied overnight. The dressing helps protect the grafts from any unintended trauma as they heal. All patients are given a mild pain medication such as Tylenol number 3, and a short course of prednisone to prevent frontal edema. The next day the dressing is removed by the patient. They may shower but are told not to pick or rub off the perifollicular crusting that occurs around some grafts and lasts for 6–8 days. Patients may resume regular activities immediately, performing light exercise 3–4 days postoperatively and more strenuous exercise 7 days after surgery when the donor sutures are removed. The transplanted hair will begin to grow 3–6 months after the surgery and achieves its full cosmetic impact 9–15 months after the surgery (**Fig. 2** and **3**).

THE FUTURE

Hair transplantation creates consistently natural appearing hair for women and men.

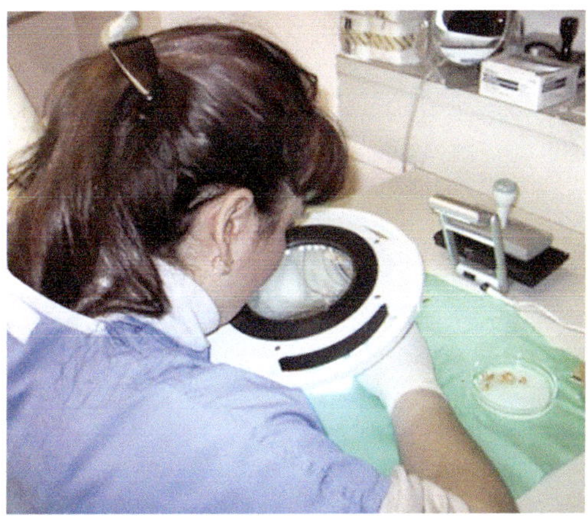

FIG. 2: Magnification helps visualize 1–4 hair bundles and minimize transection, when separating with surgical preparation blades.

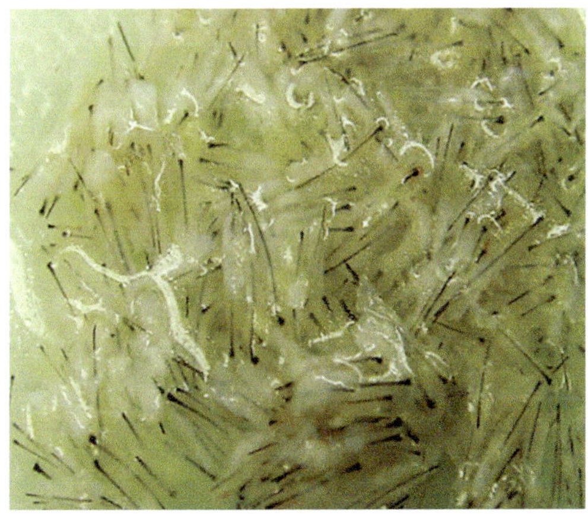

FIG. 3: 1–4 hair grafts in chilled saline.

The only limiting factor is the amount of donor hair available for each patient. The next leap will be cloning hair follicles. In the early 21st century, the claims on web sites regarding cloning hair are far more optimistic than the actual scientific progress. The amount of research in the area should allow hair to be cloned in the next several years. Future refinements with lasers and robotics will also allow an even more efficient procedure for patients and physicians.

REFERENCES

1. Ellis JA, Sinclair R, Harrap SB. Androgenetic alopecia: pathogenesis and potential for therapy. Expert Rev Mol Med. 2002;4(22):1-11.
2. Price VH, Menefee E, Sanchez M, Kaufman KD. Changes in hair weight in men with androgenetic alopecia after treatment with finasteride (1 mg daily): three- and 4-year results. J Am Acad Dermatol. 2006;5(1):71-4.
3. Roenigk HH, Berman MD. Topical 2% minoxidil with hair transplantation. Face. 1993;4:213-6.
4. Avram MR, Cole JP, Gandelman M, Haber R, Knudsen R, Leavitt MT, et al. The potential role of minoxidil in the hair transplantation setting. Dermatol Surg. 2002;28(10): 894-900.
5. Esmat SM, Hegazy RA, Gawdat HI, Abdel Hay RM, Allam RS, El Naggar R, et al. Low level light-minoxidil 5% combination versus either therapeutic modality alone in management of female patterned hair loss: A randomized controlled study. Lasers Surg Med. 2017;49(9):835-43.
6. Friedman S, Schnoor P. Novel Approach to treating androgenetic alopecia in females with photobiomodulation (low-level laser therapy). Dermatol Surg. 2017;43(6):856-67.
7. Zarei M, Wikramanayake TC, Falto-Aizpurua L, Schachner LA, Jimenez JJ. Low level laser therapy and hair regrowth: an evidence-based review. Lasers Med Sci. 2016;31(2):363-71
8. Jimenez JJ, Wikramanayake TC, Bergfield W, Hordinsky M, Hickman JG, Hamblin MR, Schachner LA. Efficacy and safety of a low level laser device in the treatment of male and female pattern hair loss: a multicenter, randomized, sham device controlled, double blind study. Am J Clin Dermatol. 2014;15(2):115-27.
9. Tawfik AA, Osman MAR. The effect of autologous activated platelet-rich plasma injection on female pattern hair loss: a randomized placebo-controlled study. J Cosmet Dermatol. 2018;17(1):47-53.
10. Giordano S, Romeo M, Lankinen P. Platelet rich plasma for androgenetic alopecia: Does it work? Evidence from meta analysis. J Cosmet Dermatol. 2017;16(3):374-81.
11. Sadick NS. New generation therapies for the treatment of hair loss in men. Dermatol Clin. 2018;36(1):63-7.
12. Singhal P, Agarwal S, Dhot PS, Sayal SK. Efficacy of platelet rich plasma in treatment of androgenetic alopecia. Asian J Transfus Sci. 2015;9(2):159-62.
13. Puig CJ, Reese R, Peters M. Double blind, placebo controlled pilot study on the use of platelet rich plasma in women with female androgenetic alopecia. Dermatol Surg. 2016;42(11):1243-7.
14. Jimenez F, Ruifernandez JM. Distribution of human hair in follicular units. A mathematical model for estimating the donor size in follicular unit transplantation. Dermatol Surg. 1999;25(4):294-8.

15. Rassman WR, Bernstein RM, McClellan R, Jones R, Worton E, Uyttendaele H. Follicular unit extraction: minimally invasive surgery for hair transplantation. Dermatol Surg. 2002;28(8):720-8.
16. Jimenez-Acosta F, Ponce-Rodriguez I. Follicular unit extraction for hair transplantation: an update. Actas Dermosifiliogr. 2017;108(6):532-7.
17. Zontos G, Williams KL Jr, Nikiforidis G. Minimizing injury to the donor area in follicular unit extraction (FUE) harvesting. J Cosmet Dermatol. 2017;16(1):61-9.
18. Harris JA. Follicular unit extraction. Facial Plast Surg Clin North Am. 2013;21(3):375-84.
19. Avram MR, Watkins SA. Robotic follicular unit extraction in hair transplantation. Dermatol Surg. 2014;40(12):1319-27.
20. Rose PT. Advances in hair restoration. Dermatol Clin. 2018;36(1):57-62.
21. Stough DB. Hair transplantation by the feathering zone technique. Am J Cosmet Surg. 1993;10:243-8.
22. Avram MR. Polarized light-emitting diode for optimal recipient site creation during hair transplant. Dermatol Surg. 2005;31:1124-7.

4 SECTION

PIGMENTARY DISORDERS AND TATTOOS

12

CHAPTER

Melasma and Postinflammatory Hyperpigmentation

Hao Feng, Arielle NB Kauvar

INTRODUCTION

Hyperpigmentation is a common complaint among patients seeking cosmetic consultations. Regardless of the underlying cause, hyperpigmentation contributes to both emotional and psychological distress for patients and have demonstrated to negatively impact the quality of life.[1] Melasma and postinflammatory hyperpigmentation (PIH) are characterized by asymptomatic, hyperpigmented macules and patches, and are two of the most common causes for hyperpigmentation. Like other pigmentary disorders, melasma and PIH are more common in darker skinned individuals with Fitzpatrick skin phototypes IV–VI,[1-3] but they can affect patients of all skin types. Treatment of both melasma and PIH can be challenging especially in darker skinned individuals and will likely require a combination of thera peutic modalities. In this chapter, we will discuss the etiology, clinical manifestation, pretreatment considerations, treatment options, and treatment efficacy for melasma and PIH (**Boxes 1** to **3**).

BACKGROUND

Melasma

Melasma is a common, acquired pigmentary skin disorder that affects millions of people worldwide and found most commonly in women with Fitzpatrick skin phototypes III–IV.[4-7] Reported prevalence ranges from 8.8 to 40% depending on the population composition.[4,8,9] In some populations,

BOX 1: Key points on pretreatment considerations.

- Thorough medical history, physical examination, and medications
- Evaluate the patient's skin phototype, extent, location, and cause of dyschromia
- Weigh the benefit of pigmentary improvement against the risk of posttreatment irritation and exacerbation of hyperpigmentation
- Discuss realistic expectations and counsel on the need for a series of treatments
- Assess ultraviolet and visible light protective behavior

BOX 2: Treatment options.

Melasma:

- *Topical agents:* Hydroquinone, tretinoin, adapalene, triple combination therapy, azelaic acid, tranexamic acid, ascorbic acid, kojic acid, licorice extract, mequinol, tazarotene, arbutin, deoxyarbutin, and soy
- *Chemical peels:* Glycolic acid, lactic acid, salicylic acid, Jessner solution, tretinoin, and Kligman–Willis formula
- *Lasers and light-based therapies:* 1064-nm Q-switched (QS) Nd:YAG, nonablative fractional laser, IPL, KTP, and pulsed dye laser
- *Sun protection:* Broad-spectrum sunscreen, avoiding sun at peak hours, and ultraviolet protective clothing

PIH:

- *Topical agents:* Hydroquinone, azelaic acid, tretinoin, tazarotene, adapalene, triple combination therapy, mequinol, kojic acid, arbutin, niacinamide, N-acetyl glucosamine, ascorbic acid, and licorice extract
- *Chemical peels:* Glycolic acid and lactic acid
- *Lasers and light-based therapies*: 578- and 511-nm copper bromide laser and light emitting diodes, IPLs, variable pulsed light, 694-nm QS ruby laser, 1064-nm QS Nd:YAG, fractional photothermolysis, and fractional carbon dioxide lasers
- *Sun protection:* Broad-spectrum sunscreen, avoiding sun at peak hours, and ultraviolet protective clothing

(IPL: intense pulsed light; KTP: potassium titanyl phosphate; Nd:YAG: neodymium-doped yttrium aluminum garnet; PIH: postinflammatory hyperpigmentation)

BOX 3: Tips for efficacy and safety.

- Ensure sufficient trial with topical bleaching agents and photoprotective measures
- Stay conservative with procedures that produce epidermal and dermal heating or damage, such as chemical peels, ablative lasers, and high energy pigment lasers, to minimize likelihood of post-treatment inflammation and PIH
- Consider utilizing topical steroid and bleaching cream before and after invasive procedures

(PIH: postinflammatory hyperpigmentation)

melasma may affect up to 50% of women.[10] The exact etiology of melasma remains unclear, but multiple factors are likely involved in its pathogenesis with a complex interplay of environmental, genetic, and hormonal factors. Although melasma was historically thought to be a hormonally driven disease in setting of contraceptive use and pregnancy, recent studies have shown that it is a chronic disorder that may last for decades. Reported risk factors for the development of melasma and increased melanogenesis include genetic predisposition, Fitzpatrick phototype III and IV skin, ultraviolet light exposure, thyroid disorders, cosmetics, phototoxic medications, pregnancy, and exogenous hormones.[4,6,11-13] Additionally, stem cell factor (SCF), a fibroblast derived chemical messenger that increases melanin synthesis, nerve growth factor (NGF) and vascular endothelial growth factor are all upregulated in lesional melasma skin.[4,14-17] Clinically, melasma most commonly presents as symmetrical hyperpigmented macules and patches on the face, especially the malar cheeks, lip region, chin, and forehead.[4,11] The patches may vary in color, ranging from light brown to dark brown.[4] Historically, the location of the pigment further divides melasma into epidermal, dermal, and mixed components although some histological studies how that most, if not all, of patients have some dermal component of the disease.[18,19] Histological studies have observed the presence of more biologically active melanocytes in affected melasma skin.[18,19]

Postinflammatory Hyperpigmentation

Postinflammatory hyperpigmentation is a form of acquired hypermelanosis that occurs after a variety of inflammatory skin conditions, such as trauma, acne vulgaris, cosmetic procedures, infections, and eczema.[20,21] While PIH may occur in all skin types, PIH in patients with darker skin phototypes typically occur with higher frequency, longer duration, and greater severity in addition to being more clinically apparent.[20,22,23] PIH results from either excessive melanin production or irregular distribution of melanin in the epidermis or dermis after cutaneous inflammation.[20,24] In epidermal hypermelanosis, inflammatory mediators cause a rise in melanocyte activity, with resulting increased production and transfer of melanin to surrounding keratinocytes.[20,24-27] In dermal hypermelanosis, inflammatory damage to basal keratinocytes causes melanin incontinence, which is subsequently engulfed by macrophages, forming melanophages in the upper dermis.[27-29] Clinically, PIH manifests as asymptomatic, irregularly shaped, hyperpigmented macules or patches at the site of the initial inflammatory process. Pigmentation at the epidermis will appear tan, brown, or dark brown clinically, while pigmentation at the dermis possesses a blue-gray appearance.[20,24] The two patterns may also coexist. Because of the location, dermal pigmentation may be permanent or resolve over a protracted period of time as compared to epidermal pigmentation. However, the course can often be unpredictable and unrelated to the site of injury, depth of injury, mode of injury, or postoperative care.

Pretreatment Considerations

A thorough medical history including medical conditions, current and previous medications, allergies, and results of prior treatments should be obtained at the initial consultation. Patients should be questioned about a history of systemic gold therapy (which is a risk factor for laser-induced chrysiasis when treating with nanosecond and picosecond lasers), herpes simplex virus in the treatment area (which can be reactivated with laser and light-based treatment), and a history of keloid formation, abnormal wound healing, and PIH. The patient's expectations, risk of post-treatment adverse reactions, and allowable downtime should be carefully considered and weighed when planning treatment and deciding between various modalities.

On physical examination, the clinician should evaluate the patient's skin phototype, extent, location, and cause of dyschromia. It is important that the clinician is confident about the diagnosis, especially if another provider is referring the patient. If there is any doubt, it is prudent to perform a biopsy to confirm diagnosis before treatment.

For patients with melasma and PIH, those with skin phototypes I–III tend to have a lower risk of recurrence after therapies that alter the skin barrier including chemical peels and laser therapy compared to those with skin phototypes IV–VI who tend to have higher risk of posttreatment inflammation, recurrence, and PIH.

It is important to emphasize the frequent application of broad-spectrum sunscreens and rigorous sun-protective habits in order to optimize treatment results and prevent further disease progression. Pre- and post-treatment with bleaching agents after invasive procedure could minimize post-treatment dyspigmentation and further optimize results, particularly in individuals with a tendency toward hyperpigmentation.

Discussing realistic expectation is also important, as the treatment is challenging for both melasma and PIH. Counseling prior to treatment should disclose that procedural treatments may not cure PIH and melasma, but lightening of the affected skin may occur after a series of treatments. Patients should also be counseled on the potential of recurrence, exacerbation, and rebound hyperpigmentation.

Key Consultation Questions

Some key consultation questions include:

- Are there underlying causes or trigger factors for the dyschromia? If so, have these causes been actively addressed?
- Could medications be causing the hyperpigmentation?
- Is the patient practicing strict photoprotection?
- What treatments have been performed to treat the discoloration and how did the patient respond?
- What are the patient's expectations for treatment?

Diagnostic Tools

The diagnosis of melasma is primarily clinical. Historically, lesions that did and did not enhance under a Wood's lamp implied increased epidermal and dermal melanin content respectively. Those with both enhancing and nonenhancing lesions under Wood's lamp were deemed to have mixed component. Histologic studies demonstrated the presence of melanin deposition in basal and suprabasal layers in the epidermal form, as compared to superficial and deep perivascular melanosomes in the dermal form.[19,30] However, recent studies have shown that Wood's lamp may not accurately detect dermal melanin in those with melasma.[18,19,30] The Melasma Area and Severity Index (MASI) score can serve as an objective assessment scoring system to grade the extent and severity of melasma.[2,31] Tristimulus reflectance colorimeters and narrow-band reflectance spectrophotometers can be useful in assessing dermal changes, but less useful for assessing epidermal pigmentation.[2,32,33]

The diagnosis of PIH is generally a clinical diagnosis based on medical history and physical examination. Laboratory tests and skin biopsies are often unnecessary. Skin biopsy of the pigmented lesion can help confirm the location of the increased melanin content and may also assist in establishing the underlying inflammatory trigger.[25] Melanin in the epidermis, but not in the dermis, will generally enhance with Wood's lamp although a mixed pattern can be observed.[34] For patients with PIH from acne, the postacne hyperpigmentation index provides quantification of severity and has been found to be reliable and validated against other measures.[2,31,33,35] Tristimulus reflectance colorimeters and narrow-band reflectance spectrophotometers may be useful for quantifying melanin content.[25,32,33]

MANAGEMENT

Treatment Options for Melasma

It is the authors' experience that patients with pigment limited to the epidermis respond quickly to simple interventions (i.e., sunscreen, hydroquinone, gentle exfoliation), but those with persistent or refractory melasma also have dermal pigment.

Multiple treatment options exist for melasma and can be divided into topical agents, chemical peels, lasers, and other light-based therapies.[11,36-38] A Cochrane systemic review of randomized controlled trials on melasma interventions concluded that there is no standard treatment for melasma, and the evidence supporting any particular intervention is weak.[36] The goals of all the treatments are to remove existing melanin pigmentation in the epidermis and dermis and to prevent further cutaneous melanin production. In difficult cases, especially involving dermal pigmentation, combining multiple modalities may be necessary to optimize outcomes.

Topical Agents

Strict sun protection including frequent and proper application of broad-spectrum sunscreen and avoidance of trigger factors are important in both preventing and treating melasma.[11,38] Broad-spectrum sunscreens have been shown to improve melasma,[39] and they should be utilized to protect all patients from both ultraviolet and visible light induced pigmentary changes.[40]

Most topical agents inhibit tyrosinase and interfere with melanogenesis. Hydroquinone is the best-studied and most effective topical agents for hyperpigmentation.[7] In a double-blind, placebo-controlled trial involving 48 patients with facial melasma, 38% of patients who used hydroquinone 4% achieved complete clinical response compared to only 8% in the placebo group.[41] The addition of broad-spectrum sunscreen enhances the efficacy of hydroquinone in a double blind study, 96.2% versus 80.7% of patients showing improvement with sunscreen versus vehicle.[42]

Topical retinoids, including tretinoin and adapalene, have some efficacy in treating melasma. The mechanism of action may involve inhibiting tyrosinase transcription, decreasing melanosome transfer, stimulating keratinocyte turnover, and permitting increased penetration of other active ingredients.[38,43] In a randomized, vehicle-controlled trial involving white women, 68% of patients treated with tretinoin rated improved or much improved as compared to 5% of patients treated with vehicle.[44] In a similar study with black female patients, 32% improvement in MASI scores was observed in the tretinoin group versus 10% improvement in the vehicle group.[31] Adapalene 0.1% has similar reduction in MASI scores compared to tretinoin 0.05% while more tolerable with fewer side effects.[45] Topical isotretinoin gel in combination with sunscreen did not demonstrate statistically significance in clinical improvement compared to sunscreen with vehicle in Thai patients.[46]

Triple combination topical agents consisting of hydroquinone, corticosteroid, and retinoid are highly effective, including the original Kligman-Willis formula which consist of hydroquinone 5%, tretinoin 0.1%, and dexamethasone 0.1%.[47] Other combination therapies that have also shown to be effective in melasma include combinations of hydroquinone 4%, tretinoin 0.05%, and fluocinolone acetonide 0.01%;[48-51] hydroquinone and retinoic acid;[52] hydroquinone and retinol;[53] and tretinoin, triamcinolone, hydroquinone, and ascorbic acid.[54] In addition to being more cost effective,[55] triple-combination therapy is more effective than hydroquinone 4% alone with 35% of subjects achieving subjective clearance in the combination group as compared to 5.1% in the hydroquinone-alone group.[56]

Azelaic acid is effective in treating melasma. In a randomized, double-blind, multicenter trial involving patients with Fitzpatrick skin phototypes IV–VI with at least moderate melasma, the azelaic acid 20% treatment group showed greater clinical improvement compared to vehicle group.[57] In comparison studies, azelaic acid 20% has similar efficacy as hydroquinone 4%[58] and greater efficacy than hydroquinone 2%.[59]

Tranexamic acid, a synthetic derivative of lysine and an anti-fibrinolytic agent, used orally or topically has recently emerged as a potential effective treatment for melasma.[60-69] Several systematic reviews and meta-analyses support the efficacy and safety of tranexamic acid, either alone or as an adjuvant to routine treatment modalities for melasma.[70-72]

Ascorbic acid may be a useful adjunctive therapy based on clinical evidence,[73,74] while kojic acid provides modest improvement with risk of irritation.[75,76] Licorice extract, which contains active ingredients of liquiritin and isoliquiritin, demonstrated effectiveness in a split-face trial.[77] Other topical agents used to treat melasma but lack specific studies and rigorous data include mequinol, tazarotene, arbutin, deoxyarbutin, and soy.[38]

Chemical Peels

Chemical peels may provide some modest benefit for the treatment of melasma with glycolic acid peels possessing the best evidence. Glycolic acid induces clinical improvement at a concentration of 52.5%, but not at lower concentrations in one study.[78] In another study involving 25 Asian Indian women, 50% glycolic acid facial peel once per month for three consecutive months after pretreating with sunscreen and glycolic acid 10% lotion nightly for 2 weeks demonstrated improvement in melasma with reduction in MASI score in 91% of patients.[79] In addition, glycolic acid may help further decrease MASI score when utilized as adjunctive therapy to other topical treatments including a modified Kligman–Willis formula (hydroquinone 5%, tretinoin 0.05%, and hydrocortisone 1%),[80] and combination therapy consisting of adapalene and azelaic acid.[81] Pretreatment with hydroquinone enhances the effect of glycolic acid,[82] but glycolic acid did not show additional benefit when used as an adjunctive therapy to hydroquinone in a split-face study, based on objective and subjective evaluations.[83]

Other chemical peels that have been studied include lactic acid, salicylic acid, Jessner solution, and tretinoin peels. Lactic acid peels provided some benefit in Fitzpatrick skin type IV patients with reduction of MASI scores by 57% without relapse at 6 months follow up.[84] In this split-face, nonrandomized, blinded trial, both Jessner solution and lactic acid peels showed similar reduction in MASI score.[84] In a small open study, salicylic acid was shown to have moderate to significant improvement in 6 patients with melasma, and only transient side effects of dyspigmentation and dryness without permanent pigmentary changes.[85] In a randomized, double-blind study comparing Jessner's solution peel and salicylic acid 30% peel, both had significant decrease in MASI scores with no significant differences between both group.[86] Salicylic acid 20–30% peels did not enhance the efficacy of hydroquinone 4% in a randomized controlled, split-face study.[87] Jessner solution peel and tretinoin peel are no more effective than glycolic acid peels.[88,89]

Lasers and Light-based Therapy

Many lasers and light based therapies have been studied and used for melasma and these include Q-switched (QS) lasers, ablative carbon dioxide and erbium-doped yttrium aluminium garnet (Er:YAG) lasers, ablative and nonablative fractional lasers, and intense pulsed light (IPL). They are best suited for patients with refractory melasma who failed topical treatment or chemical peels.

Although early studies with fractional resurfacing lasers demonstrated promising results for melasma,[90-92] subsequent studies with longer duration of follow up demonstrated a high incidence of recurrence and exacerbation of hyperpigmentation.[93-96] The depth of the pigment will need to be considered when choosing nonablative fractional lasers. Epidermal melasma is likely more responsive at 1,927-nm whereas dermal melasma is likely more sensitive to nonablative fractional treatments at 1,440-nm, 1,540-nm, and 1,550-nm wavelengths.[97]

Intense pulsed light, which produces noncoherent light emission ranging from 500- to 1,200-nm with millisecond pulse durations, provide only modest improvement in epidermal melasma. In a study of 89 Asian females with melasma unresponsive to topical therapy and chemical peels, mean MASI score decreased from 15.2 to 4.5.[98] Another study with Taiwanese women with phototype III–IV skin demonstrated additional reduction in pigmentation when IPL treatments were added to topical hydroquinone and broad-spectrum sunscreen.[99] The combination treatment of fractional QS ruby laser and IPL has also shown promise for managing melasma in Chinese patients.[100]

Q-switched lasers effectively target melanosomes and treat pigmented skin lesions, but when used at high fluences in melasma patients, produce a high incidence of hypopigmentation, hyperpigmentation, and rebound melasma.[11,101,102] QS ruby laser largely produced either no improvement or worsening of pigmentation in two studies.[102,103] Although Er:YAG laser showed improvement in melasma immediately after the procedure, all of the patients who had refractory melasma with Fitzpatrick skin phototype II–V eventually developed PIH despite systemic steroids.[104] Disappointing results were also obtained when combining ablative carbon dioxide and QS 755-nm alexandrite laser with a high incidence of posttreatment dyspigmentation.[105,106] Treating melasma with the QS 1064-nm neodymium-doped yttrium aluminum garnet (Nd:YAG) laser had shown some promising results but also carried risk of recurrence and dyspigmentation. Melasma clearance was observed after 10 weekly session in a study of 23 Korean patients,[107] and 67% of patients had >50% reduction in melasma in a study of 35 patients combining QS Nd:YAG and arbutin.[108] However, side effects of guttate hypopigmentation, hyperpigmentation, and even permanent depigmentation have been observed.[108-112] Kauvar studied the combination of low-fluence QS Nd:YAG laser, microdermabrasion, and topical hydroquinone in 27 patients with refractory melasma and skin phototype II–V, and found all subjects achieved at least a 50% improvement and >80% experienced >76% improvement without dyspigmentation or rebound melasma (**Figs. 1** and **2**).[112] Two passes of QS Nd:YAG laser are applied to the entire face in a painting technique using spot sizes of 5–7 mm with fluences of 1–2 J/cm^2 immediately after microdermabrasion. The skin is cooled with ice packs and a topical corticosteroid is applied. Physical block sunscreen is used immediately after treatment, and a melanin-suppressing topical regimen is begun 2 days later. The rationale for using very low fluence QS Nd:YAG laser is that melanophages can be disrupted with minimal thermal effects which may contribute to increased melanin production. Other studies have corroborated the benefit of low fluence QS Nd:YAG laser, especially in combination with melanogenesis-suppressing topical therapy for melasma with minimal risk of adverse events observed with higher fluences.[109,113-118] Adjunctive treatment with vascular lasers [i.e., potassium titanyl phosphate (KTP), pulsed dye laser] may provide additional improvement in melasma in those individuals who have a prominent telangiectatic component in lesional skin.[118,119]

Treatment Algorithm

In the authors' opinion, initial therapy should include strict sun protection (broad-spectrum

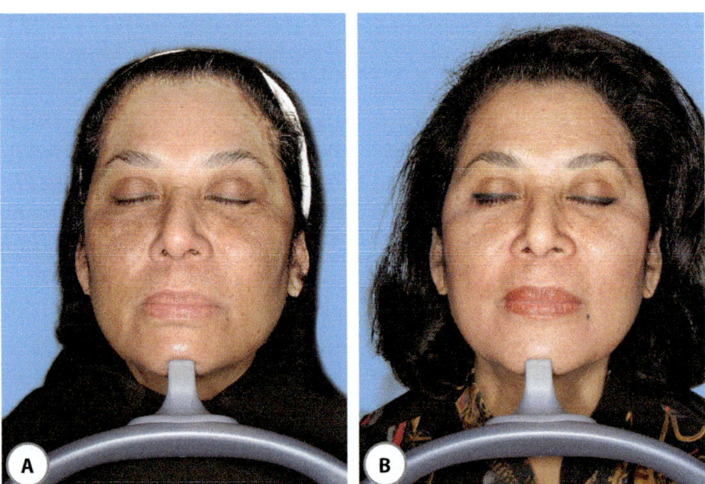

FIGS. 1A AND B: (A) Pretreatment; and (B) 3 months after one treatment with microdermabrasion, low fluence QSYL laser, and topical therapy with hydroquinone, tretinoin 0.5%, and broad spectrum sunscreen.

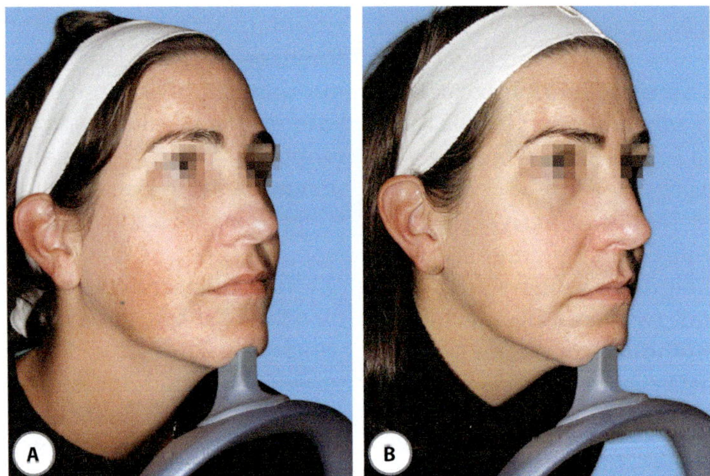

FIGS. 2A AND B: (A) Pretreatment; and (B) 6 months after three treatments with microdermabrasion, low fluence QSYL laser, and topical therapy with hydroquinone, tretinoin 0.5%, and broad spectrum sunscreen.

sunscreen, sun protective behavior, and clothing), topical hydroquinone, or topical triple combination cream that contains hydroquinone, corticosteroid, and tretinoin. After several months of treatment, tranexamic acid and superficial chemical peels, such as with glycolic acid, may be used adjunctively if patients do not respond to the above regimen. For refractory melasma, the clinician can consider adding low-density, low-fluence nonablative laser, or combination of microdermabrasion, topical bleaching cream, and very low fluence QS Nd:YAG. Maintenance therapy to preserve clinical improvement and prevent relapse may include sunscreen, hydroquinone 2%, triple combination cream, kojic acid, azelaic acid, and tranexamic acid, or a combination of these agents.

Treatment Options for Postinflammatory Hyperpigmentation

The initial management should address the underlying inflammatory process driving the PIH. Additionally, strict sun protection in addition to allowing passage of time can be a simple and effective method of treating PIH. In one study, 57% of patients with postacne PIH had spontaneous resolution by 40 weeks.[120] Behavioral modifications including avoidance of physical manipulation of the lesion can help prevent increased hyperpigmentation. For those who desire additional management of their PIH, a variety of safe and effective treatment options are available, including topical agents, chemical peels, laser treatments, and light-based therapy.

Topical Agents

Topical agents that inhibit tyrosinase, an enzyme that is critical in the conversion of tyrosine to melanin, reduce PIH. They are primarily used to treat epidermal pigmentation as deeper pigmentation are not responsive to topical medications.[121]

Hydroquinone is one of the most commonly used therapies at concentrations of 2–4%, although higher concentrations up to 10% are available, and may be effective for epidermal hypermelanosis. However, prolonged treatment periods of 6–12 months are often necessary.[122] The efficacy of hydroquinone in combination with other topical agents has been demonstrated in treating PIH. In an open label study, all patients demonstrated improvement with combination of hydroquinone 4%, glycolic acid 10%, vitamin C, vitamin E, and sunscreen based on both objective spectrometer reading and subjective physician and patient assessments.[123]

Topical retinoids are effective in treating PIH. Tretinoin may help reduce pigmentation through induction of desquamation and interruption of melanin synthesis by inhibiting tyrosinase transcription and dopachrome conversion factor.[25] In a 40-week randomized, double-blind, vehicle-controlled study involving 54 black subjects, 91% of tretinoin-treated patients had lighter or much lighter skin at the end of the study compared to 57% with vehicle.[120] Other retinoids have also been shown to be efficacious. Patients using adapalene 0.1% gel showed significant PIH improvement at weeks 4, 8, and 12.[124] In a double-blind, randomized, vehicle-controlled study of 74 acne patients, tazarotene 0.1% cream significantly reduced the overall disease activity and intensity and area of hyperpigmentation.[125]

Azelaic acid has shown promising results, but must be used for several months. In a 24-week, multicenter, double-blind study with 52 patients with skin phototypes IV–VI, azelaic acid resulted in significantly decreased pigment intensity based on investigator's scale and chromometer analysis and significantly greater global improvement.[57] Furthermore, the combination of hydroquinone 4% and retinol 0.15% was effective in decreasing lesion size, pigmentation, and disease severity.[53,126] Another study showed the combination of hydroquinone 4% and glycolic acid 2% with and without tretinoin 0.05% were effective in reducing PIH in patients with moderate to severe dyschromia and actinic photodamage.[127]

Because PIH is often difficult to treat, combination topical therapies may be used. In two phase III randomized, investigator-blinded, four arm studies involving nearly 800 patients with postacne PIH, triple combination therapy with hydroquinone 4%, tretinon 0.05%, and fluocinolone acetonide

0.01% was more effective than any of the comparators (hydroquinone + tretinoin, fluocinolone + hydroquinone, and fluocinolone + tretinoin).[128] Two studies of Asian subjects with PIH showed a combination of tretinoin, hydroquinone, and lactic acid were effective based on physician assessment.[129,130]

Other topical agents used in the treatment of PIH include mequinol, kojic acid, arbutin deoxyarbutin, niacinamide, N-acetyl glucosamine, ascorbic acid, licorice extracts of liquiritin and glabridin, and soy, although there is a lack of data and studies on their efficacy for treating PIH.[24]

Chemical Peels

Chemical peels reduce epidermal pigmentation by means of physical removal of epidermal cells that contain excessive melanin in patients of all skin phototypes. These are usually superficial peels that can be used alone or in combination with other lightening agents. Chemical peels should be used cautiously as they have the potential for irritation, thereby further contributing to PIH.

In a study with 19 black patients, glycolic acid peels provided additional PIH improvement when added to a topical regimen containing tretinoin, glycolic acid, and hydroquinone based on colorimetric analysis and the Hyperpigmentation Area and Severity Index.[131] Grime showed that superficial salicylic acid peels at concentration of 20–30% administered at 2-week intervals were effective and safe in patients with PIH and skin phototypes V and VI.[85]

Lasers and Light-based Therapy

Although topical-based therapies remain first-line treatment for PIH, lasers and light-based therapies that target melanin may also be effective. Modalities utilized to treat PIH include the combined 578- and 511-nm copper bromide laser and light emitting diodes,[132] IPLs,[133,134] variable pulsed light,[135] 694-nm QS ruby laser,[101,102,136] 1064-nm QS Nd:YAG,[137-142] fractional photothermolysis,[143-147] and fractional carbon dioxide lasers.[148] In a systemic review, the authors concluded that most studies were not methodologically rigorous with some studies showing no improvement or worsening of PIH after treatment.[21] QS Nd:YAG laser was the most extensively studied device and showed the most promising results, and to a lesser degree, IPL has shown some limited efficacy for treatment of PIH.[21]

Treatment Algorithm

Patients with PIH should be thoroughly evaluated for underlying cause of cutaneous inflammation, which should be treated aggressively. First-line therapy should consist of strict photoprotection in addition to either hydroquinone as solo agent or in combination with topical retinoid and mild corticosteroids. After 3–6 months, if clinical improvement has not been sufficiently achieved, additional topical therapies such as azelaic acid can be added. If topical therapy does not produce adequate clinical response, chemical peels and light-based therapies including lasers should be considered.

Treatment Efficacy

Treatment of PIH and melasma in Fitzpatrick skin phototype IV–VI patients is often difficult. Furthermore, treatment may cause irritation and further exacerbate hyperpigmentation. It is important that clinicians take preventative measures to identify patients at high risk for PIH, rapidly treat any underlying inflammatory diseases, and actively avoid unnecessary dermatologic and cosmetic procedures that may cause PIH. Furthermore, these patients must practice strict ultraviolet light protection.

When treating PIH in darker skinned individuals with laser therapy, devices with longer wavelengths such as the 1,064-nm Nd:YAG laser used at low fluences can provide greater margin of safety while achieving satisfactory response by avoiding targeting the patient's normal epidermal melanin.

COMPLICATIONS

All treatments have potential side effects, and these must be weighed against benefits of the treatment. Irritation, inflammation, and scarring from treatment may reduce the efficacy of treatment or even exacerbate the patient's existing hyperpigmentation and cosmetic appearance. Adverse effects such as skin irritation, peeling, burning, stinging, and PIH are common with topical agents.

Side effects of hydroquinone including irritant contact dermatitis, which may exacerbate PIH and necessitate therapy discontinuation, a halo of hypopigmentation around the treated area, and the idiosyncratic reaction of exogenous ochronosis with long-term use at high concentrations.[25,38,149,150] In general, the risk of exogenous ochronosis with hydroquinone 4% is minimal in the United States.[151-153] There have been concerns raised about the safety of hydroquinone based on a rodent study in which high doses were administered orally over prolonged time periods and resulted in the development of renal tubular cell adenomas, leukemia, and hepatocellular adenomas. No instances of cancer in humans have ever been attributed to hydroquinone, and the systemic absorption is no greater than that observed from common foods that contain hydroquinone.[154]

Chemical peels include risk of PIH, which is especially common in patients with darker skin types. Peels and other procedures that alter the epidermal barrier should be performed with extreme caution.[38,80,155]

Light-based therapies and lasers used at high energies or short wavelengths carry an increased risk of adverse effect secondary to deposition by epidermal melanin and may cause exacerbation in hyperpigmentation following treatment.[37] IPL can cause temporary erythema and edema, microcrust, and PIH.[98,99]

CONCLUSION

Dyspigmentation from melasma and PIH are cosmetically troubling for patients and frustrating for the treating physicians. Currently, there is no standard and single best therapy for patients, who often require long-term treatment with a combination of treatment agents and modalities. Based on current evidence, broad spectrum ultraviolet and visible light protection and topical lightening creams appear to be first line treatment for melasma and PIH, with chemical peels, lasers, and other light-based therapies as adjunctive therapies. Further studies are needed to investigate novel treatments and overcome many limitations with existing modalities for melasma and PIH, including lack of standardization in methodology, subject heterogeneity, variations in randomization and controls, and subjective endpoint grading. A better understanding of etiology along with well-designed prospective, randomized controlled trials would help with the development of more effective therapies and establishing treatment guidelines.

REFERENCES

1. Stratigos AJ, Katsambas AD. Optimal management of recalcitrant disorders of hyperpigmentation in dark-skinned patients. Am J Clin Dermatol. 2004;5(3):161-8.
2. Molinar VE, Taylor SC, Pandya AG. What's new in objective assessment and treatment of facial hyperpigmentation? Dermatol Clin. 2014;32(2):123-35.
3. Halder RM, Nootheti PK. Ethnic skin disorders overview. J Am Acad Dermatol. 2003;48(6 Suppl):S143-8.
4. Sheth VM, Pandya AG. Melasma: a comprehensive update: part I. J Am Acad Dermatol. 2011;65(4):689-97.
5. Zhou LL, Baibergenova A. Melasma: systematic review of the systemic treatments. Int J Dermatol. 2017;56(9):902-8.
6. Grimes PE. Melasma. Etiologic and therapeutic considerations. Arch Dermatol. 1995;131(12):1453-7.

7. Gupta AK, Gover MD, Nouri K, Taylor S. The treatment of melasma: a review of clinical trials. J Am Acad Dermatol. 2006;55(6):1048-65.
8. Werlinger KD, Guevara IL, Gonzalez CM, Rincón ET, Caetano R, Haley RW, et al. Prevalence of self-diagnosed melasma among premenopausal Latino women in Dallas and Fort Worth, Tex. Arch Dermatol. 2007;143(3): 424-5.
9. El-Essawi D, Musial JL, Hammad A, Lim HW. A survey of skin disease and skin-related issues in Arab Americans. J Am Acad Dermatol. 2007;56(6):933-8.
10. Rathore SP, Gupta S, Gupta V. Pattern and prevalence of physiological cutaneous changes in pregnancy: a study of 2000 antenatal women. Indian J Dermatol Venereol Leprol. 2011;77(3):402.
11. Kauvar ANB. The evolution of melasma therapy: targeting melanosomes using low-fluence Q-switched neodymium-doped yttrium aluminium garnet lasers. Semin Cutan Med Surg. 2012;31(2):126-32.
12. Goh CL, Dlova CN. A retrospective study on the clinical presentation and treatment outcome of melasma in a tertiary dermatological referral centre in Singapore. Singapore Med J. 1999;40(7):455-8.
13. Ortonne JP, Arellano I, Berneburg M, Cestari T, Chan H, Grimes P, et al. A global survey of the role of ultraviolet radiation and hormonal influences in the development of melasma. J Eur Acad Dermatol Venereol. 2009;23(11):1254-62.
14. Kang HY, Hwang JS, Lee JY, Ahn JH, Kim JY, Lee ES, et al. The dermal stem cell factor and c-kit are overexpressed in melasma. Br J Dermatol. 2006;154(6):1094-9.
15. Grichnik JM, Burch JA, Burchette J, Shea CR. The SCF/KIT pathway plays a critical role in the control of normal human melanocyte homeostasis. J Invest Dermatol. 1998;111(2):233-8.
16. Bak H, Lee HJ, Chang SE, Choi JH, Kim MN, Kim BJ. Increased expression of nerve growth factor receptor and neural endopeptidase in the lesional skin of melasma. Dermatol Surg. 2009;35(8):1244-50.
17. Kim EH, Kim YC, Lee ES, Kang HY. The vascular characteristics of melasma. J Dermatol Sci. 2007;46(2):111-6.
18. Kang WH, Yoon KH, Lee ES, Kim J, Lee KB, Yim H, et al. Melasma: histopathological characteristics in 56 Korean patients. Br J Dermatol. 2002;146(2):228-37.
19. Grimes PE, Yamada N, Bhawan J. Light microscopic, immunohistochemical, and ultrastructural alterations in patients with melasma. Am J Dermatopathol. 2005;27(2):96-101.
20. Davis EC, Callender VD. Postinflammatory hyperpigmentation: a review of the epidemiology, clinical features, and treatment options in skin of color. J Clin Aesthet Dermatol. 2010;3(7):20-31.
21. Agbai O, Hamzavi I, Jagdeo J. Laser Treatments for Postinflammatory Hyperpigmentation: A Systematic Review. JAMA Dermatol. 2017;153(2):199-206.
22. Halder RM, Grimes PE, McLaurin CI, Kress MA, Kenney JA Jr. Incidence of common dermatoses in a predominantly black dermatologic practice. Cutis. 1983;32(4):388-90.
23. Alexis AF, Sergay AB, Taylor SC. Common dermatologic disorders in skin of color: a comparative practice survey. Cutis. 2007;80(5):387-94.
24. Callender VD, St Surin-Lord S, Davis EC, Maclin M. Postinflammatory hyperpigmentation: etiologic and therapeutic considerations. Am J Clin Dermatol. 2011;12(2):87-99.
25. Taylor S, Grimes P, Lim J, Im S, Lui H. Postinflammatory hyperpigmentation. J Cutan Med Surg. 2009;13(4):183-91.
26. Ortonne JP. Retinoic acid and pigment cells: a review of in-vitro and in-vivo studies. Br J Dermatol. 1992;127 (Suppl 41):43-7.
27. Tomita Y, Maeda K, Tagami H. Melanocyte-stimulating properties of arachidonic acid metabolites: possible role in postinflammatory pigmentation. Pigment Cell Res. 1992;5(5 Pt 2):357-61.
28. Masu S, Seiji M. Pigmentary incontinence in fixed drug eruptions. Histologic and electron microscopic findings. J Am Acad Dermatol. 1983;8(4):525-32.
29. Nanni CA, Alster TS. Complications of carbon dioxide laser resurfacing. An evaluation of 500 patients. Dermatol Surg. 1998;24(3):315-20.
30. Sanchez NP, Pathak MA, Sato S, Fitzpatrick TB, Sanchez JL, Mihm MC Jr. Melasma: a clinical, light microscopic, ultrastructural, and immunofluorescence study. J Am Acad Dermatol. 1981;4(6):698-710.
31. Kimbrough-Green CK, Griffiths CE, Finkel LJ, Hamilton TA, Bulengo-Ransby SM, Ellis CN, et al. Topical retinoic acid (tretinoin) for melasma in black patients. A vehicle-controlled clinical trial. Arch Dermatol. 1994;130(6):727-33.
32. Clarys P, Alewaeters K, Lambrecht R, Barel AO. Skin color measurements: comparison between three instruments: the Chromameter(R), the DermaSpectrometer(R) and the Mexameter(R). Skin Res Technol. 2000;6(4):230-8.
33. Shriver MD, Parra EJ. Comparison of narrow-band reflectance spectroscopy and tristimulus colorimetry for measurements of skin and hair color in persons of different biological ancestry. Am J Phys Anthropol. 2000;112(1):17-27.
34. Katsambas AD, Stratigos AJ. Depigmenting and bleaching agents: coping with hyperpigmentation. Clin Dermatol. 2001;19(4):483-8.
35. Savory SA, Agim NG, Mao R, Peter S, Wang C, Maldonado G, et al. Reliability assessment and validation of the postacne hyperpigmentation index (PAHPI), a new instrument to

measure postinflammatory hyperpigmentation from acne vulgaris. J Am Acad Dermatol. 2014;70(1):108-14.

36. Jutley GS, Rajaratnam R, Halpern J, Salim A, Emmett C. Systematic review of randomized controlled trials on interventions for melasma: an abridged Cochrane review. J Am Acad Dermatol. 2014;70(2):369-73.
37. Rivas S, Pandya AG. Treatment of melasma with topical agents, peels and lasers: an evidence-based review. Am J Clin Dermatol. 2013;14(5):359-76.
38. Sheth VM, Pandya AG. Melasma: a comprehensive update: part II. J Am Acad Dermatol. 2011;65(4): 699-714.
39. Lakhdar H, Zouhair K, Khadir K, Essari A, Richard A, Seité S, et al. Evaluation of the effectiveness of a broad-spectrum sunscreen in the prevention of chloasma in pregnant women. J Eur Acad Dermatol Venereol. 2007;21(6):738-42.
40. Pathak MA, Riley FC, Fitzpatrick TB. Melanogenesis in human skin following exposure to long-wave ultraviolet and visible light. J Invest Dermatol. 1962;39:435-43.
41. Ennes S, Paschoalick R, Mota De Avelar Alchorne M. A double-blind, comparative, placebo-controlled study of the efficacy and tolerability of 4% hydroquinone as a depigmenting agent in melasma. J Dermatolog Treat. 2000;11(3):173-9.
42. Vazquez M, Sanchez JL. The efficacy of a broad-spectrum sunscreen in the treatment of melasma. Cutis. 1983;32(1):92, 95-6.
43. Ortonne JP. Retinoid therapy of pigmentary disorders. Dermatol Ther. 2006;19(5):280-8.
44. Griffiths CE, Finkel LJ, Ditre CM, Hamilton TA, Ellis CN, Voorhees JJ. Topical tretinoin (retinoic acid) improves melasma. A vehicle-controlled, clinical trial. Br J Dermatol. 1993;129(4):415-21.
45. Dogra S, Kanwar AJ, Parsad D. Adapalene in the treatment of melasma: a preliminary report. J Dermatol. 2002;29(8):539-40.
46. Leenutaphong V, Nettakul A, Rattanasuwon P. Topical isotretinoin for melasma in Thai patients: a vehicle-controlled clinical trial. J Med Assoc Thai. 1999;82(9):868-75.
47. Kligman AM, Willis I. A new formula for depigmenting human skin. Arch Dermatol. 1975;111(1):40-8.
48. Taylor SC, Torok H, Jones T, Lowe N, Rich P, Tschen E, et al. Efficacy and safety of a new triple-combination agent for the treatment of facial melasma. Cutis. 2003;72(1): 67-72.
49. Grimes P, Kelly AP, Torok H, Willis I. Community-based trial of a triple-combination agent for the treatment of facial melasma. Cutis. 2006;77(3):177-84.
50. Balkrishnan R, Kelly AP, McMichael A, Torok H. Improved quality of life with effective treatment of facial melasma: the pigment trial. J Drugs Dermatol. 2004;3(4):377-81.
51. Grimes PE, Bhawan J, Guevara IL, Colón LE, Johnson LA, Gottschalk RW, et al. Continuous therapy followed by a maintenance therapy regimen with a triple combination cream for melasma. J Am Acad Dermatol. 2010;62(6):962-7.
52. Pathak MA, Fitzpatrick TB, Kraus EW. Usefulness of retinoic acid in the treatment of melasma. J Am Acad Dermatol. 1986;15(4 Pt 2):894-9.
53. Grimes PE. A microsponge formulation of hydroquinone 4% and retinol 0.15% in the treatment of melasma and postinflammatory hyperpigmentation. Cutis. 2004;74(6):362-8.
54. Guevara IL, Pandya AG. Melasma treated with hydroquinone, tretinoin, and a fluorinated steroid. Int J Dermatol. 2001;40(3):212-5.
55. Cestari T, Adjadj L, Hux M, Shimizu MR, Rives VP. Cost-effectiveness of a fixed combination of hydroquinone/tretinoin/fluocinolone cream compared with hydroquinone alone in the treatment of melasma. J Drugs Dermatol. 2007;6(2):153-60.
56. Ferreira Cestari T, Hassun K, Sittart A, de Lourdes Viegas M. A comparison of triple combination cream and hydroquinone 4% cream for the treatment of moderate to severe facial melasma. J Cosmet Dermatol. 2007;6(1):36-9.
57. Lowe NJ, Rizk D, Grimes P, Billips M, Pincus S. Azelaic acid 20% cream in the treatment of facial hyperpigmentation in darker-skinned patients. Clin Ther. 1998; 20(5):945-59.
58. Balina LM, Graupe K. The treatment of melasma. 20% azelaic acid versus 4% hydroquinone cream. Int J Dermatol. 1991;30(12):893-5.
59. Verallo-Rowell VM, Verallo V, Graupe K, Lopez-Villafuerte L, Garcia-Lopez M. Double-blind comparison of azelaic acid and hydroquinone in the treatment of melasma. Acta Derm Venereol Suppl (Stockh). 1989;143:58-61.
60. Kim SJ, Park JY, Shibata T, Fujiwara R, Kang HY. Efficacy and possible mechanisms of topical tranexamic acid in melasma. Clin Exp Dermatol. 2016;41(5):480-5.
61. Na JI, Choi SY, Yang SH, Choi HR, Kang HY, Park KC. Effect of tranexamic acid on melasma: a clinical trial with histological evaluation. J Eur Acad Dermatol Venereol. 2013;27(8):1035-9.
62. Kanechorn Na Ayuthaya P, Niumphradit N, Manosroi A, Nakakes A. Topical 5% tranexamic acid for the treatment of melasma in Asians: a double-blind randomized controlled clinical trial. J Cosmet Laser Ther. 2012;14(3):150-4.
63. Tan AWM, Sen P, Chua SH, Goh BK. Oral tranexamic acid lightens refractory melasma. Australas J Dermatol. 2017;58(3):e105-8.
64. Lajevardi V, Ghayoumi A, Abedini R, Hosseini H, Goodarzi A, Akbari Z, et al. Comparison of the therapeutic efficacy and safety of combined oral tranexamic acid and topical

hydroquinone 4% treatment vs. topical hydroquinone 4% alone in melasma: a parallel-group, assessor- and analyst-blinded, randomized controlled trial with a short-term follow-up. J Cosmet Dermatol. 2017;16(2):235-42.

65. Lee HC, Thng TGS, Goh CL. Oral tranexamic acid (TA) in the treatment of melasma: A retrospective analysis. J Am Acad Dermatol. 2016;75(2):385-92.
66. Chung JY, Lee JH, Lee JH. Topical tranexamic acid as an adjuvant treatment in melasma: Side-by-side comparison clinical study. J Dermatolog Treat. 2016;27(4):373-7.
67. Li Y, Sun Q, He Z, Fu L, He C, Yan Y. Treatment of melasma with oral administration of compound tranexamic acid: a preliminary clinical trial. J Eur Acad Dermatol Venereol. 2014;28(3):393-4.
68. Karn D, Kc S, Amatya A, Razouria EA, Timalsina M. Oral tranexamic acid for the treatment of melasma. Kathmandu Univ Med J (KUMJ). 2012;10(40):40-3.
69. Lee JH, Park JG, Lim SH, Kim JY, Ahn KY, Kim MY, et al. Localized intradermal microinjection of tranexamic acid for treatment of melasma in Asian patients: a preliminary clinical trial. Dermatol Surg. 2006;32(5):626-31.
70. Kim HJ, Moon SH, Cho SH, Lee JD, Kim HS. Efficacy and Safety of Tranexamic Acid in Melasma: A Meta-analysis and Systematic Review. Acta Derm Venereol. 2017;97(7):776-81.
71. Perper M, Eber AE, Fayne R, Verne SH, Magno RJ, Cervantes J, et al. Tranexamic Acid in the Treatment of Melasma: A Review of the Literature. Am J Clin Dermatol. 2017;18(3):373-81.
72. Taraz M, Niknam S, Ehsani AH. Tranexamic acid in treatment of melasma: A comprehensive review of clinical studies. Dermatol Ther. 2017;30(3).
73. Choi YK, Rho YK, Yoo KH, Lim YY, Li K, Kim BJ, et al. Effects of vitamin C vs. multivitamin on melanogenesis: comparative study in vitro and in vivo. Int J Dermatol. 2010;49(2):218-26.
74. Espinal-Perez LE, Moncada B, Castanedo-Cazares JP. A double-blind randomized trial of 5% ascorbic acid vs. 4% hydroquinone in melasma. Int J Dermatol. 2004;43(8):604-7.
75. Lim JT. Treatment of melasma using kojic acid in a gel containing hydroquinone and glycolic acid. Dermatol Surg. 1999;25(4):282-4.
76. Garcia A, Fulton JE Jr. The combination of glycolic acid and hydroquinone or kojic acid for the treatment of melasma and related conditions. Dermatol Surg. 1996;22(5):443-7.
77. Amer M, Metwalli M. Topical liquiritin improves melasma. Int J Dermatol. 2000;39(4):299-301.
78. Gupta R, Mahajan B, Garg G. Chemical peeling—evaluation of glycolic acid in varying concentrations and time intervals. Indian J Dermatol Venereol Leprol. 2001;67(1):28-9.
79. Javaheri SM, Handa S, Kaur I, Kumar B. Safety and efficacy of glycolic acid facial peel in Indian women with melasma. Int J Dermatol. 2001;40(5):354-7.
80. Sarkar R, Kaur C, Bhalla M, Kanwar AJ. The combination of glycolic acid peels with a topical regimen in the treatment of melasma in dark-skinned patients: a comparative study. Dermatol Surg. 2002;28(9):828-32.
81. Erbil H, Sezer E, Tastan B, Arca E, Kurumlu Z. Efficacy and safety of serial glycolic acid peels and a topical regimen in the treatment of recalcitrant melasma. J Dermatol. 2007;34(1):25-30.
82. Garg VK, Sarkar R, Agarwal R. Comparative evaluation of beneficiary effects of priming agents (2% hydroquinone and 0.025% retinoic acid) in the treatment of melasma with glycolic acid peels. Dermatol Surg. 2008;34(8):1032-9.
83. Hurley ME, Guevara IL, Gonzales RM, Pandya AG. Efficacy of glycolic acid peels in the treatment of melasma. Arch Dermatol. 2002;138(12):1578-82.
84. Sharquie KE, Al-Tikreety MM, Al-Mashhadani SA. Lactic acid as a new therapeutic peeling agent in melasma. Dermatol Surg. 2005;31(2):149-54.
85. Grimes PE. The safety and efficacy of salicylic acid chemical peels in darker racial-ethnic groups. Dermatol Surg. 1999;25(1):18-22.
86. Ejaz A, Raza N, Iftikhar N, Muzzafar F. Comparison of 30% salicylic acid with Jessner's solution for superficial chemical peeling in epidermal melasma. J Coll Physicians Surg Pak. 2008;18(4):205-8.
87. Kodali S, Guevara IL, Carrigan CR, Daulat S, Blanco G, Boker A, et al. A prospective, randomized, split-face, controlled trial of salicylic acid peels in the treatment of melasma in Latin American women. J Am Acad Dermatol. 2010;63(6):1030-5.
88. Lawrence N, Cox SE, Brody HJ. Treatment of melasma with Jessner's solution versus glycolic acid: a comparison of clinical efficacy and evaluation of the predictive ability of Wood's light examination. J Am Acad Dermatol. 1997;36(4):589-93.
89. Khunger N, Sarkar R, Jain RK. Tretinoin peels versus glycolic acid peels in the treatment of Melasma in dark-skinned patients. Dermatol Surg. 2004;30(5):756-60.
90. Rokhsar CK, Fitzpatrick RE. The treatment of melasma with fractional photothermolysis: a pilot study. Dermatol Surg. 2005;31(12):1645-50.
91. Tannous ZS, Astner S. Utilizing fractional resurfacing in the treatment of therapy-resistant melasma. J Cosmet Laser Ther. 2005;7(1):39-43.
92. Katz TM, Glaich AS, Goldberg LH, Firoz BF, Dai T, Friedman PM. Treatment of melasma using fractional photothermolysis: a report of eight cases with long-term follow-up. Dermatol Surg. 2010;36(8):1273-80.

93. Kroon MW, Wind BS, Beek JF, van der Veen JP, Nieuweboer-Krobotová L, Bos JD, et al. Nonablative 1550-nm fractional laser therapy versus triple topical therapy for the treatment of melasma: a randomized controlled pilot study. J Am Acad Dermatol. 2011;64(3):516-23.
94. Wind BS, Kroon MW, Meesters AA, Beek JF, van der Veen JP, Nieuweboer-Krobotová L, et al. Non-ablative 1,550 nm fractional laser therapy versus triple topical therapy for the treatment of melasma: a randomized controlled split-face study. Lasers Surg Med. 2010;42(7):607-12.
95. Karsai S, Fischer T, Pohl L, Schmitt L, Buhck H, Jünger M, et al. Is non-ablative 1550-nm fractional photothermolysis an effective modality to treat melasma? Results from a prospective controlled single-blinded trial in 51 patients. J Eur Acad Dermatol Venereol. 2012;26(4):470-6.
96. Ho SGY, Yeung CK, Chan NPY, Shek SY, Chan HHL. A retrospective study of the management of Chinese melasma patients using a 1927 nm fractional thulium fiber laser. J Cosmet Laser Ther. 2013;15(4):200-6.
97. Trivedi MK, Yang FC, Cho BK. A review of laser and light therapy in melasma. Int J Womens Dermatol. 2017;3(1):11-20.
98. Li YH, Chen JZ, Wei HC, et al. Efficacy and safety of intense pulsed light in treatment of melasma in Chinese patients. Dermatol Surg. 2008;34(5):693-700.
99. Wang CC, Hui CY, Sue YM, Wong WR, Hong HS. Intense pulsed light for the treatment of refractory melasma in Asian persons. Dermatol Surg. 2004;30(9):1196-200.
100. Tong LG, Wu Y, Wang B, Xu XG, Tu HD, Chen HD, et al. Combination of fractional QSRL and IPL for melasma treatment in Chinese population. J Cosmet Laser Ther. 2017;19(1):13-7.
101. Kopera D, Hohenleutner U. Ruby laser treatment of melasma and postinflammatory hyperpigmentation. Dermatol Surg. 1995;21(11):994.
102. Taylor CR, Anderson RR. Ineffective treatment of refractory melasma and postinflammatory hyperpigmentation by Q-switched ruby laser. J Dermatol Surg Oncol. 1994;20(9):592-7.
103. Tse Y, Levine VJ, McClain SA, Ashinoff R. The removal of cutaneous pigmented lesions with the Q-switched ruby laser and the Q-switched neodymium: yttrium-aluminum-garnet laser. A comparative study. J Dermatol Surg Oncol. 1994;20(12):795-800.
104. Manaloto RM, Alster T. Erbium:YAG laser resurfacing for refractory melasma. Dermatol Surg. 1999;25(2):121-3.
105. Nouri K, Bowes L, Chartier T, Romagosa R, Spencer J. Combination treatment of melasma with pulsed CO_2 laser followed by Q-switched alexandrite laser: a pilot study. Dermatol Surg. 1999;25(6):494-7.
106. Angsuwarangsee S, Polnikorn N. Combined ultrapulse CO_2 laser and Q-switched alexandrite laser compared with Q-switched alexandrite laser alone for refractory melasma: split-face design. Dermatol Surg. 2003;29(1):59-64.
107. Suh KS, Sung JY, Roh HJ, Jeon YS, Kim YC, Kim ST. Efficacy of the 1064-nm Q-switched Nd:YAG laser in melasma. J Dermatolog Treat. 2011;22(4):233-8.
108. Polnikorn N. Treatment of refractory melasma with the MedLite C6 Q-switched Nd:YAG laser and alpha arbutin: a prospective study. J Cosmet Laser Ther. 2010;12(3):126-31.
109. Wattanakrai P, Mornchan R, Eimpunth S. Low-fluence Q-switched neodymium-doped yttrium aluminum garnet (1,064 nm) laser for the treatment of facial melasma in Asians. Dermatol Surg. 2010;36(1):76-87.
110. Chan NPY, Ho SGY, Shek SYN, Yeung CK, Chan HH. A case series of facial depigmentation associated with low fluence Q-switched 1,064 nm Nd:YAG laser for skin rejuvenation and melasma. Lasers Surg Med. 2010;42(8):712-9.
111. Kim T, Cho SB, Oh SH. Punctate leucoderma after 1,064-nm Q-switched neodymium-doped yttrium aluminum garnet laser with low-fluence therapy: is it melanocytopenic or melanopenic? Dermatol Surg. 2010;36(11):1790-1.
112. Kauvar ANB. Successful treatment of melasma using a combination of microdermabrasion and Q-switched Nd:YAG lasers. Lasers Surg Med. 2012;44(2):117-24.
113. Gokalp H, Akkaya AD, Oram Y. Long-term results in low-fluence 1064-nm Q-Switched Nd:YAG laser for melasma: Is it effective? J Cosmet Dermatol. 2016;15(4):420-6.
114. Yue B, Yang Q, Xu J, Lu Z. Efficacy and safety of fractional Q-switched 1064-nm neodymium-doped yttrium aluminum garnet laser in the treatment of melasma in Chinese patients. Lasers Med Sci. 2016;31(8):1657-63.
115. Hofbauer Parra CA, Careta MF, Valente NY, de Sanches Osorio NE, Torezan LA. Clinical and Histopathologic Assessment of Facial Melasma After Low-Fluence Q-Switched Neodymium-Doped Yttrium Aluminium Garnet Laser. Dermatol Surg. 2016;42(4):507-12.
116. Fabi SG, Friedmann DP, Niwa Massaki AB, Goldman MP. A randomized, split-face clinical trial of low-fluence Q-switched neodymium-doped yttrium aluminum garnet (1,064 nm) laser versus low-fluence Q-switched alexandrite laser (755 nm) for the treatment of facial melasma. Lasers Surg Med. 2014;46(7):531-7.
117. Lee MC, Chang CS, Huang YL, Chang SL, Chang CH, Lin YF, et al. Treatment of melasma with mixed parameters of 1,064-nm Q-switched Nd:YAG laser toning and an enhanced effect of ultrasonic application of vitamin C: a split-face study. Lasers Med Sci. 2015;30(1):159-63.
118. Na SY, Cho S, Lee JH. Intense Pulsed Light and Low-Fluence Q-Switched Nd:YAG Laser Treatment in Melasma Patients. Ann Dermatol. 2012;24(3):267-73.
119. Geddes ER, Stout AB, Friedman PM. Retrospective analysis of the treatment of melasma lesions exhibiting

increased vascularity with the 595-nm pulsed dye laser combined with the 1,927-nm fractional low-powered diode laser. Lasers Surg Med. 2017;49(1):20-26.
120. Bulengo-Ransby SM, Griffiths CE, Kimbrough-Green CK, Finkel LJ, Hamilton TA, Ellis CN, et al. Topical tretinoin (retinoic acid) therapy for hyperpigmented lesions caused by inflammation of the skin in black patients. N Engl J Med. 1993;328(20):1438-43.
121. Ruiz-Maldonado R, Orozco-Covarrubias ML. Postinflammatory hypopigmentation and hyperpigmentation. Semin Cutan Med Surg. 1997;16(1):36-43.
122. Nordlund JJ. Postinflammatory hyperpigmentation. Dermatol Clin. 1988;6(2):185-92.
123. Cook-Bolden FE. The efficacy and tolerability of a combination cream containing 4% hydroquinone in the treatment of postinflammatory hyperpigmentation in skin types IV-VI. Cosmetic Dermatol. 2004;17(3):149-55.
124. Jacyk WK, Mpofu P. Adapalene gel 0.1% for topical treatment of acne vulgaris in African patients. Cutis. 2001;68(4 Suppl):48-54.
125. Grimes P, Callender V. Tazarotene cream for postinflammatory hyperpigmentation and acne vulgaris in darker skin: a double-blind, randomized, vehicle-controlled study. Cutis. 2006;77(1):45-50.
126. Cook-Bolden FE, Hamilton SF. An open-label study of the efficacy and tolerability of microencapsulated hydroquinone 4% and retinol 0.15% with antioxidants for the treatment of hyperpigmentation. Cutis. 2008;81(4):365-71.
127. Swinyer LJ, Wortzman M. Study of hydroquinone USP 4%, 0.05% tretinoin, and in combination in UV-induced dyschromia with actinic photodamage. Cosmetic Dermatol. 2000;13:13-8.
128. Baumann L, Grimes P, Pandya AG. Triple combination cream is an effective treatment for post-inflammatory hyperpigmentation. Presented at the 65th Annual American Academy of Dermatology Conference. Washington, DC. 2007.
129. Yoshimura K, Harii K, Aoyama T, Shibuya F, Iga T. A new bleaching protocol for hyperpigmented skin lesions with a high concentration of all-trans retinoic acid aqueous gel. Aesthetic Plast Surg. 1999;23(4):285-91.
130. Yoshimura K, Harii K, Aoyama T, Iga T. Experience with a strong bleaching treatment for skin hyperpigmentation in Orientals. Plast Reconstr Surg. 2000;105(3):1097-108.
131. Burns RL, Prevost-Blank PL, Lawry MA, Lawry TB, Faria DT, Fivenson DP. Glycolic acid peels for postinflammatory hyperpigmentation in black patients. A comparative study. Dermatol Surg. 1997;23(3):171-4.
132. Park KY, Choi SY, Mun SK, Kim BJ, Kim MN. Combined treatment with 578-/511-nm copper bromide laser and light-emitting diodes for post-laser pigmentation: a report of two cases. Dermatol Ther. 2014;27(2):121-5.
133. Ho WS, Chan HH, Ying SY, Chan PC, Burd A, King WWK. Prospective study on the treatment of postburn hyperpigmentation by intense pulsed light. Lasers Surg Med. 2003;32(1):42-5.
134. Park JH, Kim JI, Kim WS. Treatment of Persistent Facial Postinflammatory Hyperpigmentation With Novel Pulse-in-Pulse Mode Intense Pulsed Light. Dermatol Surg. 2016;42(2):218-24.
135. Augustyniak A, Erkiert-Polguj A, Rotsztejn H. Variable pulsed light treatment of melasma and post-inflammatory hyperpigmentation-a pilot study. J Cosmet Laser Ther. 2015;17(1):15-9.
136. Mitra A, Yeung R, Sheehan-Dare R, Wilson CL. Lentiginous hyperpigmentation confined to resolved psoriatic plaques and treated with a Q-switched ruby laser. Clin Exp Dermatol. 2006;31(2):298-9.
137. Cho SB, Park SJ, Kim JS, Kim MJ, Bu TS. Treatment of post-inflammatory hyperpigmentation using 1064-nm Q-switched Nd:YAG laser with low fluence: report of three cases. J Eur Acad Dermatol Venereol. 2009;23(10):1206-7.
138. Kim S, Cho KH. Treatment of procedure-related post-inflammatory hyperpigmentation using 1064-nm Q-switched Nd:YAG laser with low fluence in Asian patients: report of five cases. J Cosmet Dermatol. 2010;9(4):302-6.
139. Kim S, Cho KH. Treatment of facial postinflammatory hyperpigmentation with facial acne in Asian patients using a Q-switched neodymium-doped yttrium aluminum garnet laser. Dermatol Surg. 2010;36(9):1374-80.
140. Ho SGY, Yeung CK, Chan NPY, Shek SY, Kono T, Chan HHL. A retrospective analysis of the management of acne post-inflammatory hyperpigmentation using topical treatment, laser treatment, or combination topical and laser treatments in oriental patients. Lasers Surg Med. 2011;43(1):1-7.
141. Zawar VP, Agarwal M, Vasudevan B. Treatment of Postinflammatory Pigmentation Due to Acne with Q-Switched Neodymium-Doped Yttrium Aluminum Garnet In 78 Indian Cases. J Cutan Aesthet Surg. 2015;8(4):222-6.
142. Lee YB, Park SM, Kim JW, Yu DS. Combination treatment of low-fluence Q-switched Nd:YAG laser and oral tranexamic acid for post-inflammatory hyperpigmentation due to allergic contact dermatitis to henna hair dye. J Cosmet Laser Ther. 2016;18(2):95-7.
143. Lee SJ, Chung WS, Lee JD, Kim HS. A patient with cupping-related post-inflammatory hyperpigmentation successfully treated with a 1,927 nm thulium fiber fractional laser. J Cosmet Laser Ther. 2014;16(2):66-8.
144. Katz TM, Goldberg LH, Firoz BF, Friedman PM. Fractional photothermolysis for the treatment of postinflammatory hyperpigmentation. Dermatol Surg. 2009;35(11):1844-8.

145. Cho SB, Lee SJ, Kang JM, Kim YK, Oh SH. Treatment of refractory arcuate hyperpigmentation using a fractional photothermolysis system. J Dermatolog Treat. 2010;21(2):107-8.
146. Rokhsar CK, Ciocon DH. Fractional photothermolysis for the treatment of postinflammatory hyperpigmentation after carbon dioxide laser resurfacing. Dermatol Surg. 2009;35(3):535-7.
147. Kroon MW, Wind BS, Meesters AA, Wolkerstorfer A, van der Veen JP, Bos JD, et al. Non-ablative 1550 nm fractional laser therapy not effective for erythema dyschromicum perstans and postinflammatory hyperpigmentation: a pilot study. J Dermatolog Treat. 2012;23(5):339-44.
148. Oram Y, Akkaya AD. Refractory Postinflammatory Hyperpigmentation Treated Fractional CO_2 Laser. J Clin Aesthet Dermatol. 2014;7(3):42-4.
149. Bhattar PA, Zawar VP, Godse KV, Patil SP, Nadkarni NJ, Gautam MM. Exogenous Ochronosis. Indian J Dermatol. 2015;60(6):537-43.
150. Levin CY, Maibach H. Exogenous ochronosis. An update on clinical features, causative agents and treatment options. Am J Clin Dermatol. 2001;2(4):213-7.
151. Nordlund JJ, Grimes PE, Ortonne JP. The safety of hydroquinone. J Eur Acad Dermatol Venereol. 2006;20(7):781-7.
152. Draelos ZD. Skin lightening preparations and the hydroquinone controversy. Dermatol Ther. 2007;20(5):308-13.
153. Lawrence N, Bligard CA, Reed R, Perret WJ. Exogenous ochronosis in the United States. J Am Acad Dermatol. 1988;18(5 Pt 2):1207-11.
154. Levitt J. The safety of hydroquinone: a dermatologist's response to the 2006 Federal Register. J Am Acad Dermatol. 2007;57(5):854-72.
155. Lim JT, Tham SN. Glycolic acid peels in the treatment of melasma among Asian women. Dermatol Surg. 1997;23(3):177-9.

13

CHAPTER

Pigmented Lesions

Wai Man Mandy Chan, Henry HL Chan

INTRODUCTION

The use of lasers to treat pigmented lesions was started by Leon Goldman, who used a ruby laser (694 nm) to treat skin lesions including nevi and tattoo in the 1960s.[1] Technological advances and understanding of Anderson and Parish's[2] theory of *selective photothermolysis* has revolutionized the applications of lasers in the treatment of pigmented lesions. The three key elements needed to achieve selective photothermolysis are: (1) Emitted laser wavelength should be highly absorbed by targeted structures; (2) Sufficient fluence should be provided to induce thermal damage in target; and (3) Duration of tissue exposure to laser should be short enough to inflict damage on target without heat diffusion to surrounding tissues. The most selective target heating is achieved when energy is deposited at a greater speed than rate of cooling of target structures.

PRETREATMENT CONSIDERATIONS (BOX 1)

Before a laser procedure, a thorough medical history should be taken, including medical conditions, medications, and history of drug allergy. It is important to illicit a clear medical history, as laser use in patients taking isotretinoin has shown to cause scarring and prolonged healing.[3] The cause is postulated to be the inhibition of collagenase but the exact etiology is unknown.[4] Laser treatment should be avoided within 6 months of isotretinoin usage, though this recommendation is controversial.[5] A history of vitiligo and gold injection treatment should also be elicited in the medical history. Patients with a history recurrent herpes simplex, antivirals such as acyclovir or valacyclovir prophylaxis should be prescribed.[6]

BOX 1: List of pretreatment considerations.

Pretreatment considerations:

- Obtain thorough medical history including history of recurrent herpes simplex and vitiligo
- Drug allergies
- History of oral isotretinoin or gold injection
- Patient counseling: Manage expectations, frequency of treatment, potential cost, and complications
- Set realistic expectations
- Obtain informed consent from patient
- Pre- and posttreatment photos
- Assess pigmented lesion and determine type of pigmented lesion
- Assess compliance to post-laser care

Patients should be counseled regarding treatment expectations, frequency of laser treatments, cost, and possible complications. In the treatment of some pigmented lesions, complete clearance may not be possible and realistic expectations must be conveyed to patients. Informed consent must be obtained, and pre- and posttreatment photos should be taken. Patients should be advised to avoid sun exposure after laser treatment, and to use a broad-spectrum SPF sunscreen of at least SPF 50 daily for at least 2 weeks. Post-procedure counseling, including wound care should be given.

KEY CONSULTATION QUESTIONS

Before embarking on laser treatment for a pigmented lesion, the physician must determine whether the lesion is benign or malignant. It is important not to mistake a melanoma for a benign pigmented lesion. The use of dermoscopy and reflectance confocal microscopy (RCM) can be used if in doubt. Any suspicious lesion should be biopsied before any treatment.

Benign pigmented lesions can be classified into epidermal and intradermal lesions. It is important to recognize location of the pigment in order to decide which wavelength to use. Absorption of melanin decreases as wavelength increases, and longer wavelengths penetrate deeper in the skin. Therefore, in darker skin type patients, a longer wavelength can be employed to minimize epidermal damage and the risk of PIH.

Pigmented lesions that respond well to laser therapy include: Lentigines, ephelides, nevus of Ota, nevus of Ito, and blue nevus. Other pigmented lesions such as café-au-lait macules (CALM), nevus spilus, Becker's nevus, melasma, congenital, and acquired nevus have varying response (**Box 2**). We have discussed the treatment of each of these pigmented lesions in **Table 1**.

BOX 2: Pigmented lesions amenable to laser treatment.

Epidermal:

- Lentigines
- Ephelides
- Café-au-lait macules
- Nevus spilus
- Becker's nevus
- Melasma

Dermal:

- Nevus of Ota
- Nevus of Ito
- Blue nevi
- Melanocytic nevi
- Post-inflammatory hyperpigmentation
- Tattoos

PIGMENTARY CONDITIONS

Epidermal Lesions

Lentigines (Figs. 1A and B)

Lentigines are benign brown hyperpigmented macules that occur in sun-exposed areas. Histological features include elongated rete ridges with increased melanocytes. They respond well to laser treatment and usually clear with 1–3 sessions. Lasers used to treat lentigines include frequency-doubled Q-switched (QS) Nd:YAG (neodymium-doped yttrium aluminum garnet) laser, Q-switched ruby laser (QSRL), alexandrite, Nd:YAG, picosecond (PS) lasers, and other pulsed visible-light lasers.

Recurrence of lentigines is common and the use of sunscreen is important. Complications include hyperpigmentation, particularly in dark-skinned individuals, and a test-area should be done before the treatment of multiple lesions.

In patients with multiple lentigines particularly if they start developing in infancy, one should raise a suspicion for LEOPARD

TABLE 1: Treatment of the pigmented lesions.

Treatment options (Suggested treatment parameters for pigmented lesions)			
Epidermal pigmented lesions	**Laser**	**Spot size**	**Fluence (J/cm^2)**
Lentigines and ephelides	Q-switch 532 nm	2 mm	0.6
	Picosecond 532 nm	4 mm	0.3–4
	Long-pulsed 532 KTP	3 mm (with cooling 10°C)	8.8–9.6, 2 ms
	Long-pulsed 595 nm	7 mm	11–13, 1.5 ms
Café-au-lait macules	Long-pulsed alexandrite	10	20–30, 3 ms
	Picosecond 532 nm	4	0.3–0.4
	Picosecond 755 nm alexandrite	2–3.5	2.08–6.37
Nevus spilus	Picosecond 755 nm alexandrite	3.5	2.08–3.49
Becker's nevus	LP alexandrite 755 nm	10	20–35
	PS 755 nm alexandrite	3.2	2.08–3.49
Dermal pigmented lesions			
Nevus of Ota and nevus of Ito	PS 755 nm alexandrite	2.3–3.8	1.75–4.80
Hori's nevus	PS 755 nm alexandrite	2.9–3.8	1.76–3.03
Melanocytic nevus (surgery remains first line treatment)	Nonablative fractional laser 1,550 nm		65–70
	LP 755 nm alexandrite	10	20–25
	QS 694 nm ruby	4	3–3.5
Tattoos	Nonablative fractional laser 1,550 nm		50–65 mJ
	Picosecond 1064 nm	4–8 mm	0.8–3.5
Red color	Picosecond 532 nm	4–8 mm	0.4–0.6
Orange color	Picosecond 532 nm	8 mm	0.4
Yellow color	Picosecond 532 nm	4–8 mm	0.4–0.6
Green color	PS 755 nm alexandrite	3.6 mm	1.96
Purple color	PS 755 nm alexandrite	3.5 mm	2.08
Brown color	PS 755 nm alexandrite	3.6 mm	1.96
Black color	PS 755 nm alexandrite	3.5–3.8 mm	1.76–2.08

syndrome caused by *PTPN11* or *RAF1* genes. If a patient has multiple brown macules on the lips, oral mucosa, or fingers then Peutz-Jeghers syndrome, caused by the mutation in serine/threonine kinase *STK11* gene, needs to be ruled out. It is important not to treat a lentigo maligna as a lentigo, and suspicious lesions must be biopsied before any laser treatment.

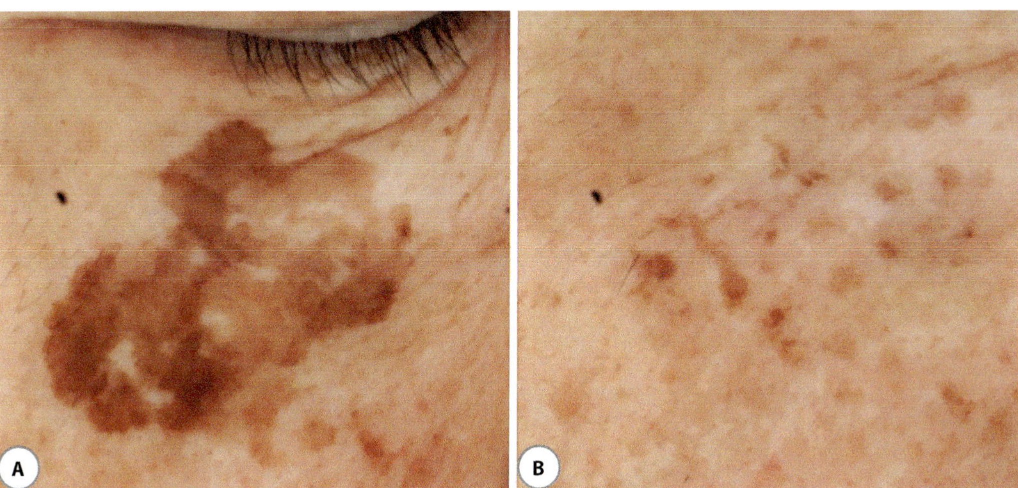

FIGS. 1A AND B: (A) Lentigines before laser treatment. (B) Near clearance of lentigines 3 months after two treatments with 532 nm Nd:YAG laser (0.3–0.4 J/cm^2 fluence, 2 Hz, 4 mm spot size, 750 ps).

Ephelides

Ephelides (freckles) are different from lentigines as they usually present in early childhood and on sun-exposed sites. Histological findings include increased melanin production in the basal layer with no elongated of rete ridges. Q-switched lasers[7,8] are effective and can be the treatment of choice especially for light-skinned patients. However for dark-skinned individuals, treatment with Q-switched lasers can cause excessive erythema and be associated with PIH lasting from 6 to 12 months. Intense pulsed light (IPL) source can be one of the most effective treatments among light-skinned patients.[9] For darker-skinned patients, the contrast between lesion and normal skin is less pronounced, therefore over treatment to foot-print appearance, or under treatment can occur, with minimal side effects. Long-pulsed (LP), small spot size lasers can be particularly applicable among dark-skinned patients with lower risk of PIH but requires multiple sessions.[10]

Café-au-lait Macules and Nevus Spilus

Café-au-lait macules are light to brown hyperpigmented lesions that are histologically characterized by increased melanin in the basal layer, with macromelanosomes seen in electron microscopy. CALM (**Figs. 2A** and **B**) may be benign or associated with certain genodermatosis such as neurofibromatosis.

Café-au-lait macules are difficult to treat, requiring multiple treatment sessions with high rate of recurrence. Q-switched lasers (532 nm Nd:YAG and ruby)[11,12] and the pulsed 510 nm[13] laser have limited success, and studies demonstrating complete removal without recurrence have been inconsistent.

Paradoxical darkening has been reported and the proposed mechanism is due the incomplete removal of follicular melanocytic component of the CALM. One option is to use LP alexandrite laser to also target the follicular component and in doing so, reduce the risk of recurrence. Our approach to the treatment of CALM is to divide the lesion into four quadrants and to test each area with four different lasers: LP Alex, QSRL, PS Alex, and PS 532 nm, and to proceed with subsequent sessions after assessing response of the four quadrants.

Recent report indicates that the morphological pattern of CALM can correlate to the

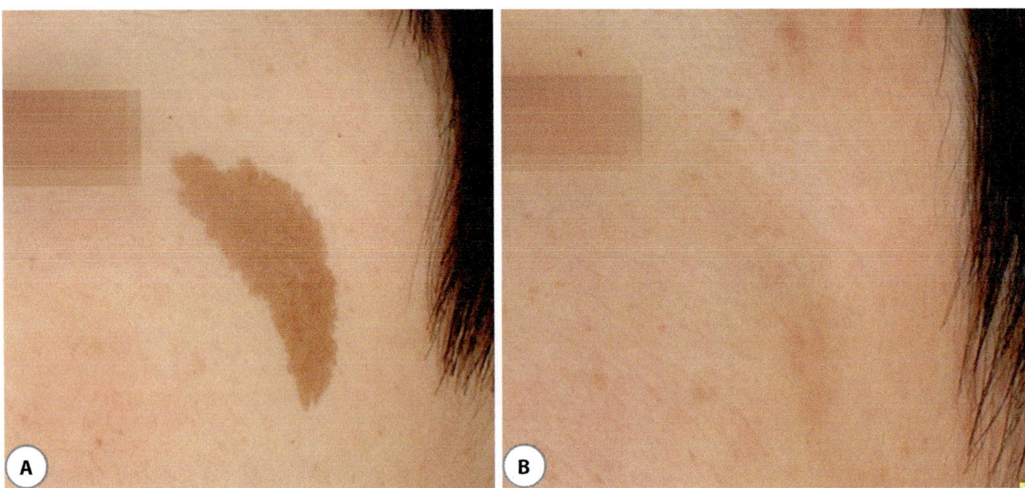

FIGS. 2A AND B: (A) Café-au-lait macules before laser treatment. (B) After 4 treatments with long-pulsed alexandrite laser (25–30 J/cm^2 fluence, 1.5 Hz, 10 mm).

clinical outcome, with a rigged ill-defined border being more responsive to laser treatment than compared to those with smooth and well-defined borders.[14] Although this is a clinical observation, it does allow for a degree of predictability in informing patients and managing their expectations in response to laser treatment.

Nevus Spilus

Nevus spilus are darker-pigmented macules or papules that lie within a CALM. Lasers used to treat CALM are also used to treat nevus spilus and these include PDL,[12] Erbium:YAG,[15] QS Nd:YAG, QSRL,[16] and PS Alex lasers (parameters: 2.08-3.49 J/cm^2 fluence, 2.5-5.0 Hz, 2.7-3.5 mm spot size).[17] Nevus spilus tends to respond better than the CALM portion.

Some cases of nevus spilus has been reported to transform into melanoma, therefore careful assessment and examination is required before treatment, and reassessment if lesion transforms overtime.[18]

Becker's Nevus

Becker's nevus is a unilateral large hairy hyperpigmented plaque, usually located on the shoulder of male adolescents. A biopsy reveals hyperkeratosis, papillomatosis, increased melanin, and an increase in hair follicles and smooth muscle. QS lasers, Erbium:YAG laser and 1,550 nm fractional erbium-doped fiber lasers have demonstrated improvement of the pigmentation in some patients.[19-21]

In the author's experience, the LP Alex 755-nm laser (20-35 J/cm^2, 10 mm spot size, 3 ms pulse duration) is used to target the pigment and surrounding hair follicles, with a 50% success rate after 4-8 treatments. Hypopigmentation can be an issue, which can respond very well to alternative treatment with nonablative fractional resurfacing with 1,927 nm thulium fiber laser.[22] PS 755-nm alexandrite laser device lasers have also been used with some success with parameters of 2.08-3.49 J/cm^2, 2.5 Hz, 3.2 mm spot size with fair response after three treatments.[16] Scarring and hyperpigmentation are possible side effects.

Dermal Pigmented Lesions

Nevus of Ota and Nevus of Ito

Nevus of Ota is a bluish-gray patch found in the trigeminal area of the face and sometimes involve the sclera at birth or early childhood, more commonly found in Asian females. It is a dermal melanocytic hamartoma and histological findings include spindle-shaped dendritic melanocytes in the dermis with increased fine granules of melanin.

Nevus of Ito is a bluish-gray patch found on the shoulder or upper arm in the area where the posterior supraclavicular and lateral brachial cutaneous nerves innervate. Histological features are the same as nevus of Ota.

The dermal melanocytes with abundant fine melanin granules are treated with QSRL,[23] QS Alex, QS Nd:YAG,[24] and PS Alex lasers (parameters: 1.75–4.80 J/cm^2 fluence, 2.5–5 Hz, 2.3–3.8 mm spot size) effectively with minimal adverse effects. Total of 4–8 treatment sessions are typically required and possible side effects include PIH, hypopigmentation, and recurrence of pigmentation. Among all the pigmentary conditions, PS lasers can be particularly useful, as the number of treatment sessions are found to be fewer, without any increase in complication. This poses distinct advantages especially among the children population, as sedation is often necessary (**Figs. 3A** and **B**).

Acquired Bilateral Nevus of Ota-like Macules or Hori's Nevus

Acquired bilateral nevus of Ota-like macules (ABNOM) or Hori's nevus, are bluish-brown-gray speckles found bilaterally over the face. Unlike nevus of Ota, they develop at around 20 years of age, and histological features include active melanin synthesizing dermal melanocytes in upper and deep reticular dermis.

Q-switched ruby laser, alexandrite, and Nd:YAG lasers have all been reported to be effective and once again PS lasers can be effective. The authors current clinical practices include PS Alex laser (parameters: 1.76–3.03 J/cm^2 fluence, 1.0–2.5 Hz, and 2.9–3.8 mm spot size), and patients are aware of risks of PIH and hypopigmentation which are usually temporary in nature.

Blue Nevi

Blue nevi are benign melanocytic lesions that present at blue-black papule or nodule in early childhood. Histologically rete ridges are clubbed and elongated, with poorly circumscribed nests of melanocytes at dermoepidermal junction that can extend deep into the dermis. The melanocytic nests

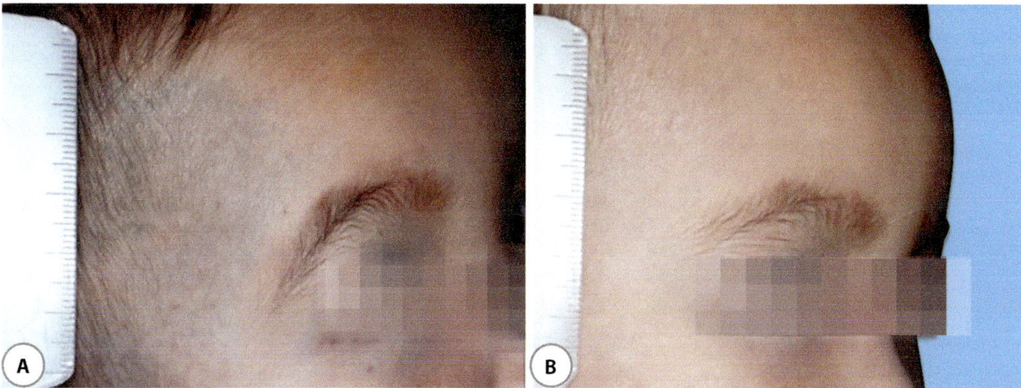

FIGS. 3A AND B: (A) Nevus of Ota before treatment. (B) Clearance with two treatments with picosecond alexandrite laser (2.08–2.49 J/cm^2 fluence, 2.5 Hz, 2.6–3.2 mm).

usually demonstrate maturation with descent into the dermis. QSRL has been used to treat blue nevi with clearance.[25] However, atypical blue nevi and malignant blue nevi exist and should be ruled out before any attempt of a laser treatment. Still, the treatment of choice for blue nevi and all melanocytic nevi is surgery, except in particular circumstances when surgery is not feasible.

Melanocytic Nevi

Melanocytic nevi are common and removal is often due to cosmetic reasons. Our approach to removing melanocytic nevi include ablative laser such as CO_2 and Erbium:YAG laser, or a longer pulse pigmented laser (LP 532 nm or ruby) to remove the epidermis, followed by multiple passes of QS laser (ruby/Alex/Nd:YAG). Parameters of LP Alex are 24–30 J/cm^2 fluence, 8–10 mm spot size without cooling followed by QSRL (parameters: 3–3.5 J/cm^2 fluence, and 4 mm spot size).

In congenital melanocytic nevi (**Figs. 4A to C**), as the surface area of treatment may be larger in some cases, we tend to use fractional resurfacing in conjunction with PS laser to prevent the risk of infection. Typical parameters for nonablative fractional laser are 1,550 nm, 65–70 mJ, level 11, 8 passes or for fractional CO_2 laser with a scanning mode 50 mJ, treatment level 8, 4 passes, followed by PS Alex laser (parameters: 1.26–3.49 J/cm^2 fluence, 5 Hz, 2.7–4.5 mm spot size).

The development of melanoma in treated congenital melanocytic nevi has been reported, and the clinician must always be aware of suspicious lesions, especially amelanotic melanoma developing on previously treated sites. It is important not to laser melanomas and any suspicious lesions must be biopsied. Again, the treatment of choice for all melanocytic nevi is surgery, except in particular circumstances when surgery is not feasible.

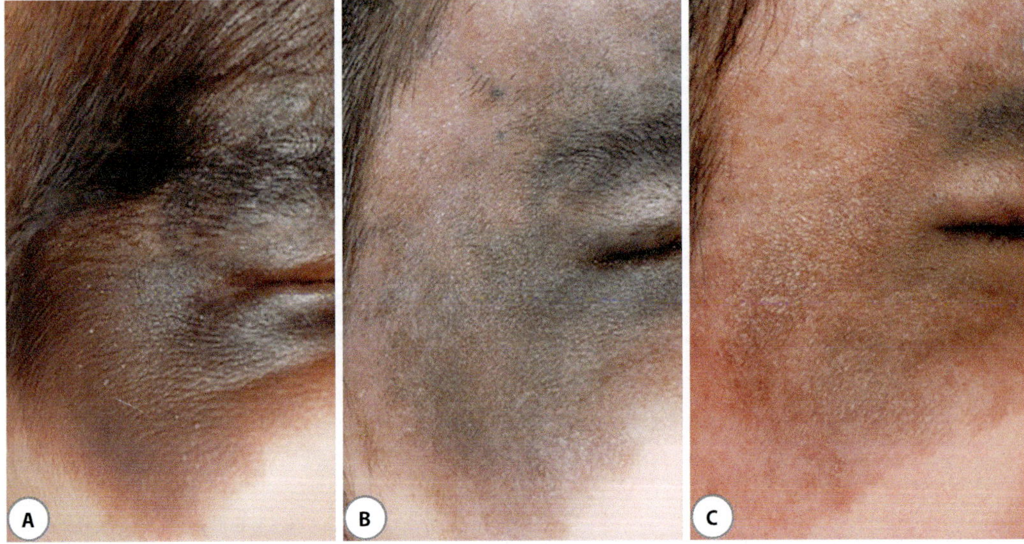

FIGS. 4A TO C: (A) Congenital melanocytic nevus before treatment. (B) After 6 treatments with picosecond 755 nm laser (0.87–6.37 J/cm^2 fluence, 10 Hz, 2.0–5.4 mm) combined with factional 1550 nm laser (60–70 mJ × 4, wind speed 5, total energy 0.43–0.99 kj, depth 1301–1359 u, passes 8, treatment level 9–11, total cover 26–32%, cover/pass 38–52 mtz/cm^2) (C) 6 weeks after 13 treatments.

Postinflammatory Hyperpigmentation

Postinflammatory hyperpigmentation can be a result from hemosiderin or melanin deposition. To avoid or minimize the risks of PIH, test spots should be used before treating a large area. As PIH may be a result of lasers, caution should be used when using lasers to treat PIH. Erbium-doped fiber laser,[26] QS Nd:YAG laser[27] has been used for the treatment of PIH, but caution is advised.

In our practice, we encourage the use of broad-band sunscreen, and topical bleaching agents such as hydroquinone 4%. Topical retinoids such as 0.025% tretinoin cream, vitamin C and E, and chemical peels are all used with varying success for PIH.

Laser toning can also be effective in the treatment of PIH. Typical laser parameters are QS 1,064 Nd:YAG (2.3-3.1 J/cm^2 fluence, 8 mm spot size, 3 passes) or PS Alex lasers fractionated hand-piece 6 mm spot size 0.57 J/cm^2, 3 to 4 passes.

Tattoos

Tattoos (**Figs. 5A** to **C**) are amenable to laser removal, but factors such as ink composition, color used, and technique of tattoo implantation affects the rate of success. Tattoo pigment can also contain heavy metals and salts such as lead, aluminum, cobalt, copper, iron, chromium, lead, and mercury, but with more governing and awareness, a shift to more organic pigments are made, although phototoxicity and allergic reactions can still occur. **Table 2** highlights the efficacies of lasers in tattoo removal based on the pigment. Complications include pain, PIH, partial removal, and rarely scarring (gunpowder or firework tattoos).

Picosecond laser has distinct advantages over nanosecond lasers given its greater degree of photomechanical effect, which allows for a more effective destruction without a greater risk of complication.[28] The addition of fractional laser can also be effective in the reduction of blister formation, a common complication that can be associated with PS laser.[29]

To further enhance treatment outcome the R20 method for tattoo removal (wait for 20 min for disappearance of the immediate whitening tissue response which correlates with laser induced stream pockets) before further laser treatment is based on the principle

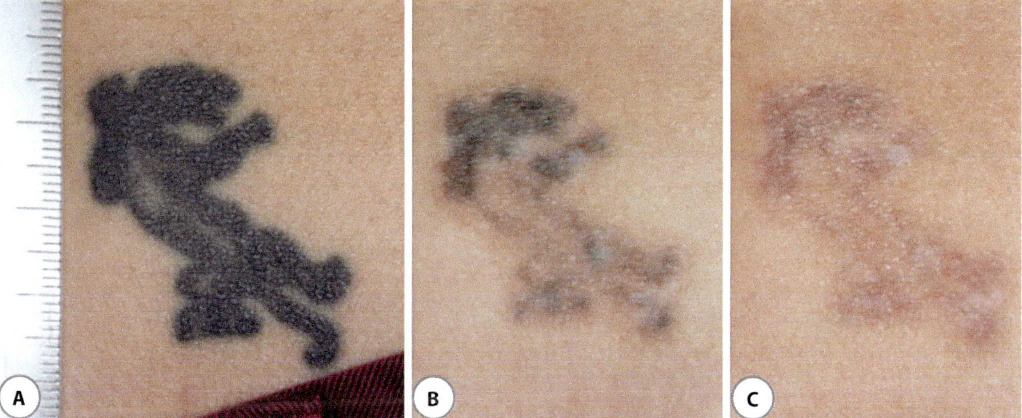

FIGS. 5A TO C: (A) Tattoo pigment pre-treatment. (B) After 6 treatments using picosecond 755 nm laser (1.96–3.49 J/cm^2 fluence, 2.5–5 Hz, 2.7–3.6 mm spot size); (C) 11 months after baseline, after 3 treatments with picosecond 1064 nm, (0.65–5.14 J/cm^2 fluence, 1–3 Hz, 3–5 mm spot size, 450 ps).

TABLE 2: Lasers for tattoo pigment removal.

	QS Ruby 694 nm (red light)	QS Alexandrite 755 nm (red light)	Qs Nd:YAG 532 (green light)	Pulse dye 510 nm (green light)	QS Nd:YAG 1064 nm
Blue-black	+	+	–	–	+
Red	–	–	+	+	–
Green	+	+	–	–	–
Yellow	–	–	+	+	–
Orange	–	–	+	+	–
Purple	–	–	+	+	–

BOX 3: Tips for efficacy and safety.

- Biopsy any suspicious lesions
- Test spots to be used prior to treating large areas
- Ensure adequate posttreatment care and patient adherence

of repeated exposure of laser light in a single session.[30] Kossida et al.[31] reported a higher efficacy of this method in tattoo clearance when compared to standard method at the end of 3 months (**Box 3**). The advantage of R20 method is a reduction in number of tattoo removal sessions, but a single session can take up to 3–4 hours, and increases the risk of blistering, scarring, and pigmentary alteration especially in darker skinned individuals.

To avoid the waiting time, Reddy et al.[32] reported the use of perfluorodecalin to reduce frosting immediately so laser can be used in quick succession without the 20-minute wait (R0 method), with results demonstrating equal effectiveness when compared to R20 method. As frosting is observed due to release of gas bubbles in the stratum corneum, perfluorodecalin is a liquid perfluorocarbon that absorbs the released gas, thus clearing the frosting within seconds, reducing the waiting time from 80 minutes to 5 minutes.[32] Apart from gas clearance, it saturates air spaces when applied, thus increasing the depth of penetration of laser,[30] and also thought to reduce collateral thermal tissue damage due to tissue compression owing to its high specific gravity.[33]

CONCLUSION

The use of lasers in the treatment of pigmented lesions continues to evolve as technology advances allowing for greater efficacy and minimal side effects. We stress the importance of making a correct diagnosis of the pigmented lesion before starting any laser treatment. Methods to avoid complications and treatment of PIH have been discussed.

REFERENCES

1. Goldman L, Wilson RG, Hornby P, Meyer RG. Radiation from a Q-switched ruby laser. Effect of repeated impacts of power output of 10 megawatts on a tattoo of man. J Invest Dermatol. 1965;44:69-71.
2. Anderson RR, Parrish JA. Selective photothermolysis: precise microsurgery by selective absorption of pulsed radiation. Science. 1983;220(4596):524-7.
3. Zachariae H. Delayed wound healing and keloid formation following argon laser treatment or dermabrasion during isotretinoin treatment. Br J Dermatol. 1988;118(5):703-6.
4. Khatri KA. Diode laser hair removal in patients undergoing isotretinoin therapy. Dermatol Surg. 2004;30(9):1205-7.

5. Spring LK, Krakowski AC, Alam M, Bhatia A, Brauer J, Cohen J, et al. Isotretinoin and timing of procedural interventions: a systematic review with consensus recommendations. JAMA Dermatol. 2017;153(8):802-9.
6. Nestor MS. Prophylaxis for and treatment of uncomplicated skin and skin structure infections in laser and cosmetic surgery. J Drugs Dermatol. 2005;4(6 Suppl):s20-5.
7. Jang KA, Chung EC, Choi JH, Sung KJ, Moon KC, Koh JK. Successful removal of freckles in Asian skin with a Q-switched alexandrite laser. Dermatol Surg. 2000;26(3):231-4.
8. Rashid T, Hussain I, Haider M, Haroon TS. Laser therapy of freckles and lentigines with quasi-continuous, frequency-doubled, Nd:YAG (532 nm) laser in Fitzpatrick skin type IV: a 24-month follow-up. J Cosmet Laser Ther. 2002;4(3-4):81-5.
9. Chan H. The use of lasers and intense pulsed light sources for the treatment of acquired pigmentary lesions in Asians. J Cosmet Laser Ther. 2003;5(3-4):198-200.
10. Ho SGY, Chan HHL. The Asian dermatologic patient: review of common pigmentary disorders and cutaneous diseases. Am J Clin Dermatol. 2009;10(3):153-68.
11. Levy JL, Mordon S, Pizzi-Anselme M. Treatment of individual cafe au lait macules with the Q-switched Nd:YAG: A clinicopathologic correlation. J Cutan Laser Ther. 1999;1(4):217-23.
12. Grossman MC, Anderson RR, Farinelli W, Flotte TJ, Grevelink JM. Treatment of café au lait macules with lasers: a clinicopathologic correlation. Arch Dermatol. 1995;131(12):1416-20.
13. Alster TS, Williams CM. Café-au-lait macule in type V skin: successful treatment with a 510 nm pulsed dye laser. J Am Acad Dermatol. 1995;33(6):1042-3.
14. Belkin DA, Neckman JP, Jeon H, Friedman P, Geronemus RG. Response to Laser Treatment of Café au Lait Macules based on morphologic features. JAMA Dermatol. 2017;153(11):1158-61.
15. Alora MB, Arndt KA. Treatment of a cafe-au-lait macule with the erbium: YAG laser. J Am Acad Dermatol. 2001;45(4):566-8.
16. Tse Y, Levine VJ, McClain SA, Ashinoff R. The removal of cutaneous pigmented lesions with the Q-switched ruby laser and the Q-switched neodymium: yttrium-aluminum-garnet laser: A comparative study. J Dermatol Surg Oncol. 1994;20(12):795-800.
17. Chan JC, Shek SY, Kono T, Yeung CK, Chan HH. A retrospective analysis on the management of pigmented lesions using a picosecond 755-nm alexandrite laser in Asians. Lasers Surg Med. 2016;48(1):23-9.
18. Borrego L, Santana JH, Baez O, Hernandez BH. Naevus spilus as a precursor of cutaneous melanoma: report of a case and literature review. Clin Exp Dermatol. 1994;19(6):515-7.
19. Nanni CA, Alster TS. Case Report: Treatment of a Becker's Nevus Using a 694-nm long-pulsed ruby laser. Dermatol Surg. 1998;24(9):1032-4.
20. Trelles MA, Allones I, Vélez M, Moreno-Arias GA. Becker's nevus: Erbium: YAG versus Q-switched neodimium: YAG? Lasers Surg Med. 2004;34(4):295-7.
21. Glaich AS, Goldberg LH, Dai T, Kunishige JH, Friedman PM. Fractional resurfacing: a new therapeutic modality for Becker's nevus. Arch Dermatol. 2007;143(12):1488-90.
22. Chan HH, Ho SG. Laser treatment of ethnic skin. Lasers and Lights E-Book: Procedures in Cosmetic Dermatology Series. Elsevier. 2017;1:125.
23. Goldberg DJ, Nychay SG. Q-switched ruby laser treatment of nevus of Ota. J Dermatol Surg Oncol. 1992;18(9):817-21.
24. Chan HH, Leung RS, Ying SY, Lai CF, Kono T, Chua JK, et al. A retrospective analysis of complications in the treatment of nevus of Ota with the Q-switched alexandrite and Q-switched Nd:YAG lasers. Dermatol Surg. 2000;26(11):1000-6.
25. Milgraum SS, Cohen ME, Auletta MJ. Treatment of blue nevi with the Q-switched ruby laser. J Am Acad Dermatol. 1995;32(2):307-10.
26. Polder KD, Landau JM, Vergilis-Kalner IJ, Goldberg LH, Friedman PM, Bruce S. Laser eradication of pigmented lesions: a review. Dermatol Surg. 2011;37(5):572-95.
27. Cho SB, Park SJ, Kim JS, Kim MJ, Bu TS. Treatment of post-inflammatory hyperpigmentation using 1064-nm Q-switched Nd:YAG laser with low fluence: report of three cases. J Eur Acad Dermatol Venereol. 2009;23(10):1206-7.
28. Ross V, Naseef G, Lin G, Kelly M, Michaud N, Flotte TJ, et al. Comparison of responses of tattoos to picosecond and nanosecond Q-switched neodymium: YAG lasers. Arch Dermatol. 1998;134(2):167-71.
29. Au S, Liolios AM, Goldman MP. Analysis of incidence of bulla formation after tattoo treatment using the combination of the picosecond Alexandrite laser and fractionated CO_2 ablation. Dermatol Surg. 2015;41(2):242-5.
30. Kossida T, Rigopoulos D, Katsambas A, Anderson RR. Optimal tattoo removal in a single laser session based on the method of repeated exposures. J Am Acad Dermatol. 2012;66(2):271-7.
31. Reddy KK, Brauer JA, Anolik R, Bernstein L, Brightman L, Hale E, et al. Topical perfluorodecalin resolves immediate whitening reactions and allows rapid effective multiple pass treatment of tattoos. Lasers Surg Med. 2013;45(2):76-80.
32. Zawar V, Sarda A, De A. Bindi tattoo on forehead: Success with modified R-20 technique using low fluence Q-switched Nd YAG laser: A case report. J Cutan Aesthet Surg. 2014;7(1):54-5.
33. Littlejohn GR, Gouveia JD, Edner C, Smirnoff N, Love J. Perfluorodecalin enhances in vivo confocal microscopy resolution of Arabidopsis thaliana mesophyll. New Phytol. 2010;186(4):1018-25.

14

CHAPTER

Tattoos

Kelly Stankiewicz, Suzanne Linsmeier Kilmer

INTRODUCTION

The history of modern day tattoo removal spans many decades, and in fact, tattoo removal is the first known cutaneous application for laser. In 1963, Dr Leon Goldman used a ruby laser for the removal of a tattoo, which resulted in scarring.[1,2] He subsequently used a Q-switched (QS) ruby laser with the report of a superior tissue response.[3,4] However, it was not until nearly three decades later that the concept was truly revisited and QS lasers were used regularly for tattoo removal. Prior to the regular use of QS lasers, tattoo removal was a nonselective and destructive procedure which aimed to replace the tattoo with scar. Options included excision, dermabrasion, salabrasion (abrasion of skin with table salt), and CO_2 laser resurfacing. The introduction of the theory of selective photothermolysis in 1983 provided an understanding of the physics of the laser-skin interaction, and tattoo removal began its progression to what we know today. Theory predicted that lasers with extremely short pulse durations were needed for the selective destruction of tattoo particles without causing surrounding damage.[5] First nanosecond, and now picosecond pulse durations are the standard for successful tattoo removal.

Like any cosmetic laser treatment, the consultation, including appropriate patient selection and counseling, is the most important step in the tattoo removal process. When evaluating a tattoo, the type of tattoo, the color of the tattoo, the location of the tattoo, and the patient's skin phototype should be taken into consideration. The medical and social history of the patient is also pertinent when considering tattoo removal and should be part of the consultation process.

Tattoos can be categorized into several subtypes: Professional, amateur, cosmetic, and traumatic. All can be removed with laser, but some pose more challenges than others. Professional tattoos have precisely placed ink particles residing in the lower papillary to mid-dermis[6] (**Fig. 1**). These particles are placed by the moving needle of a tattoo machine. Amateur tattoos have more haphazardly placed ink particles residing in all layers of skin and even into the fat. These particles are placed with make-shift devices, like handheld needles. A greater volume of ink found in professional tattoos make this type of tattoo more difficult to remove.[7] Similarly, tattoos placed over other tattoos, or "cover-ups", present a challenge due to the high quantity of ink in the skin and possible hidden ink colors

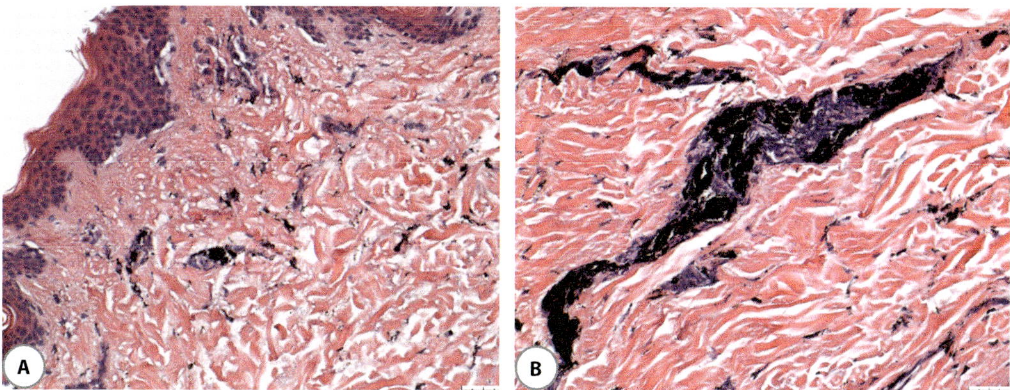

FIGS. 1A AND B: (A) In a professional tattoo, ink particles are placed in the lower papillary to mid-dermis. The ink particles are either extracellular or reside within fibroblasts and macrophages distributed perivascularly. The particle size ranges from 2-400 nanometers with smaller particles grouped into larger membrane-bound granules measuring 0.5-4.0 micrometers.[6] (B) A closer view reveals the predominately perivascular distribution of particles.

Courtesy: H. Ray Jalian.

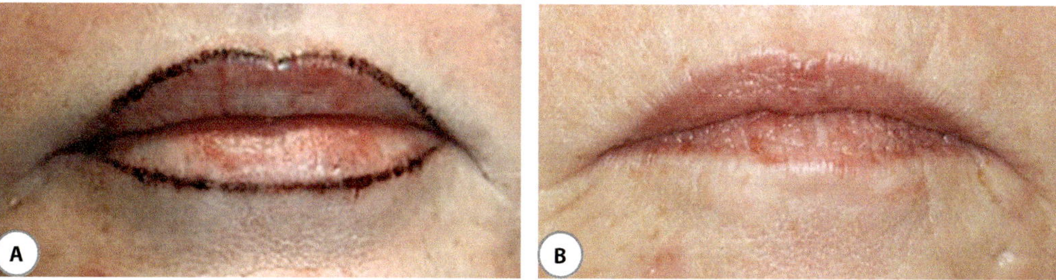

FIGS. 2A AND B: Immediate ink darkening in a cosmetic tattoo. (A) Immediately after laser treatment of a brown cosmetic tattoo with a QS alexandrite laser, the ink darkens. (B) Darkened ink was treated on the same day after waiting 20 minutes leading to complete resolution of ink on follow-up.

underneath that may not be responsive to the wavelength used.

Cosmetic tattooing is another form of professional tattoo that is increasingly popular. Using varying techniques, permanent makeup can be placed in areas of the face where makeup is usually found. Often, cosmetic tattoos are challenging to remove. The ink used in cosmetic tattoos is particularly susceptible to the phenomenon of immediate ink darkening. At the time of laser treatment, reduction of metal oxides turns ink black (**Fig. 2A**). Brown, white, beige, pink, and red cosmetic inks are vulnerable to this change. Although subsequent treatments with laser can usually remove darkened ink, failure to remove this ink has been reported.[8] Patients should be counseled of this risk. Separate from immediate ink darkening, some cosmetic inks, especially brown, can undergo multiple color changes with laser treatments.[9] To achieve varying shades of brown, the colors red, yellow, black, orange, green, and blue are used. Once the more responsive component of ink is removed, underlying hues are revealed that are often times more difficult to treat, like orange, green, or blue (**Fig. 3**). Subsequent treatment with the appropriate laser wavelengths are

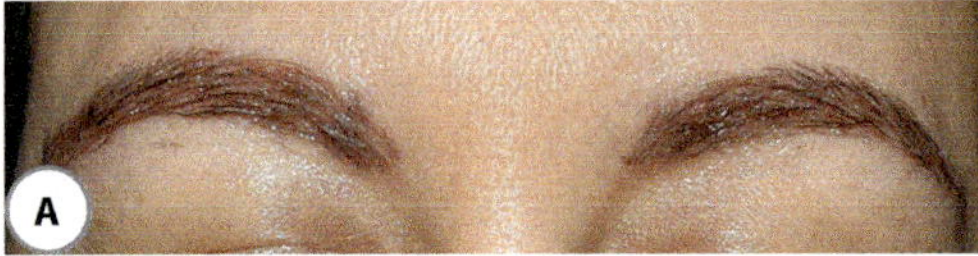

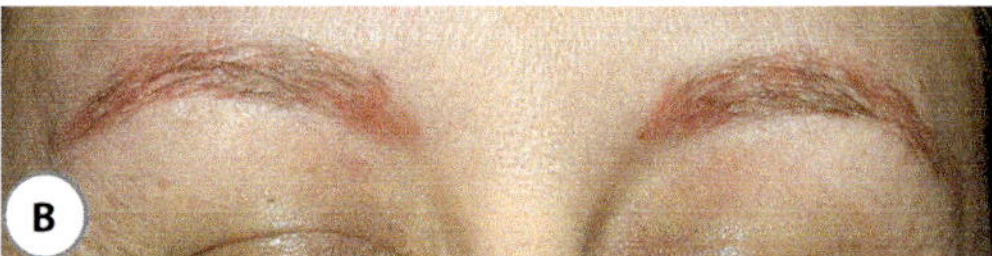

FIGS. 3A AND B: Color changes with treatment of cosmetic tattoo. (A) Brown ink was treated with a picosecond Nd:YAG laser to reveal a bright orange ink. (B) Orange ink revealed after picosecond Nd:YAG treatment was then removed with the picosecond frequency doubled Nd:YAG (532 nm) laser.

needed to complete the removal process. During the consultation process, patients should be counseled of the risk of multiple color changes of ink, including immediate ink darkening. These complications can increase the number of treatments needed and in some cases, create fixed changes. Because of multiple color changes of ink, cosmetic tattoo removal may require lasers with multiple wavelengths to complete the job.

Traumatic tattoos are caused by the inadvertent deposition of foreign material into the skin, such as asphalt or graphite. These tattoos are typically easy to treat. Tattoos from explosives like firework debris or gunpowder should be treated with caution. Combustion of these materials can cause scarring.[10]

Tattoo color also dictates the ease with which the tattoo can be removed. Some tattoo colors are more difficult to remove with current technology, including yellow, orange, and purple. Black and red are the easiest ink colors to remove. Green, blue, and blue-green are increasingly easier to remove with newer commercially available devices. Some colors, including white, brown, beige, and pink are very likely to immediately darken after laser treatment. Patients should be counseled about these limitations. Furthermore, skin phototype limits the wavelengths that can be used on the skin. Melanin is a chromophore that competes with tattoo particles for laser energy. Absorption of laser energy by melanin decreases with longer wavelengths. Treating darker skin types should be limited to longer wavelengths to prevent the unintended permanent loss of pigment or scarring.

TABLE 1: Pretreatment considerations.

Absolute contraindications	Relative contraindications
History of parenteral gold therapy	Recent sun exposure or tanned skin
	Psoriasis, lichen planus, vitiligo, or other Koebnerizing dermatosis
	Tattoo ink allergies

The number of treatments needed to completely remove a tattoo can never be accurately predicted. An average of 4–6 treatments is reported for amateur tattoos and 6–10 treatments for professional tattoos.[11] Although treatment numbers in excess of 20 are not unusual. Picosecond lasers can decrease number of treatments needed, but by precisely how much, is not yet known. In a large observational prospective cohort study spanning 15 years, tattoo characteristics more associated with difficult removal were: Large tattoo size (>30 cm^2), location on the legs and feet, tattoos on people who smoke, colors other than black or red, and dense ink.[12] Facial tattoos were the easiest to remove.

There are a few absolute and relative contraindications for tattoo removal and these conditions can be elucidated when taking a good medical history (**Table 1**). Treatment with parenteral gold therapy is the only absolute contraindication for the use of QS or picosecond lasers. Parenteral gold was primarily used as a treatment for rheumatoid arthritis or other autoimmune diseases. It has long since fallen out of favor, replaced by more efficacious, modern medications with more favorable side effect profiles. Nevertheless, history of treatment with gold salts is relevant as it is never cleared from the body and should prevent treatment with QS or picosecond lasers. When someone with history of treatment with gold is treated with a QS or picosecond laser, laser-induced chrysiasis occurs, creating a dark blue-black hyperpigmentation that is typically considered permanent.

History of vitiligo, or any Koebnerizing dermatosis like psoriasis, lichen planus, or necrobiosis lipoidica, can be precipitated by laser tattoo removal and is a relative contraindication. A complete skin history should be obtained prior to tattoo removal. Other relative contraindications include acutely tanned skin and allergic tattoos. Treating tanned skin can increase risk of temporary or permanent hypo- or hyper-pigmentation. Treatment of allergic tattoos with QS lasers has been reported to cause systemic hypersensitivity reactions, including anaphylaxis.[13] Allergic tattoos are raised and itchy, often times in areas limited to one particular color. Red is the most likely ink to cause allergy in the skin. Besides destructive treatments like full laser ablation, treatment with ablative or nonablative fractional lasers may be an option for these allergic tattoos.

MANAGEMENT

Laser tattoo removal requires very short laser pulses in the nanosecond or picosecond domain along with appropriate wavelength selection. By the theory of selective photo-thermolysis, laser pulses must be very short to match the small size of the targets for tattoo removal. These targets include fibroblasts and macrophages, tattoo particles and larger membrane-bound granules.[6] Due to the short pulse durations used, photomechanical effects, and not photothermal, predominate. Shock waves and subsequent cavitation are created as a result of sudden heating and thermal expansion and lead to the destruction of pigment containing cells and fragmentation of tattoo particles. Cavitation is the formation of bubbles within the dermis that translates into the whitening of the tattoo seen clinically after treatment. It is worth noting that short pulse durations do not permanently remove larger skin structures, like hair follicles.

There are two categories of laser with pulse durations appropriate for tattoo removal: QS lasers which operate in the nanosecond pulse duration range and picosecond lasers which are newer and more expensive technology. Theory predicts that picosecond lasers are superior to QS lasers for tattoo removal, but the current picosecond lasers are closer to nanosecond domains and data is still emerging to show how this translates clinically.[14,15]

Nanosecond versus Picosecond Lasers

There is currently no perfect comparative study between nanosecond and picosecond lasers. In vitro models and computer simulation show that when fluence is matched, the picosecond laser is more efficient at destroying small tattoo particles.[15,16] The same in vitro studies show that nanosecond and picosecond pulses are both very efficient at fragmenting large particles, unless the fluence is $<1\ J/cm^2$. Destruction of large particles dramatically decreases at $0.5\ J/cm^2$. Because darker and untreated tattoos have predominantly larger tattoo particles. This suggests that if low fluences are used, the tattoo is less likely to lighten. Low fluences are more likely to be used with picosecond lasers and this could be artificially shaping the perception of picosecond lasers. In clinical comparisons when fluence is matched, picosecond lasers outperform nanosecond lasers.[14,17,18] In one well-designed recent prospective study, picosecond pulses were not shown to be superior.[19] But, in this study, the fluences used for the picosecond laser were 30% lower than the fluences used for the nanosecond laser and improvement was graded on a quartile scale. Further clinical data is needed before we know exactly how much better picosecond lasers are at removing tattoos. Evidence and clinical experience prove that picosecond lasers are in fact more effective, especially for lighter, faded, and treatment resistant tattoos, which are usually comprised of smaller tattoo particles. This particularly holds true for picosecond pulses that are at least <100 picoseconds .

Wavelength Selection

The other critical variable in tattoo removal is proper wavelength selection. The current commercially available wavelengths for tattoo removal are: 532 nm (nanosecond and picosecond), 585 nm (nanosecond), 650 nm (nanosecond), 670 nm (picosecond), 694 nm (nanosecond), 755 nm (nanosecond and picosecond), 785 nm (picosecond), and 1,064 nm (nanosecond and picosecond) (**Box 1**). The laser wavelength selected for removal should match the predicted maximum absorption for each ink color. Using color theory, ink best absorbs light at the wavelength of its complimentary color. This has been proven in vitro. For instance, green ink absorbs red light the best, red ink absorbs green light the best, blue ink absorbs yellow light the best, and so on.[20] Laser wavelengths can be selected to exploit this relationship for maximum ink clearance (**Table 2**). Black ink absorbs all wavelengths of light, and is therefore the easiest ink color to remove. Orange and yellow inks are difficult to remove because they absorb light in the shortest wavelengths of visible light that do not correspond to commercially available lasers.

When selecting the laser wavelength for tattoo removal, skin phototype must also be considered. Melanin is a chromophore that strongly absorbs shorter wavelengths of light, with absorption decreasing at increasing wavelengths. Therefore, darker skin types cannot be safely treated with shorter wavelengths. This becomes a problem for treatment of red ink on dark skin, for instance. The safest laser for treatment of darker skin types is the neodymium-doped yttrium aluminum garnet (Nd:YAG) (1,064 nm) laser.

BOX 1: Tips for safety and efficacy.

- Tattoos should only be treated with very short pulse duration lasers (nanosecond and picosecond domain lasers)
- The lowest effective fluence should be chosen to achieve the desired endpoint, which is immediate whitening
- The largest spot size allowed by the laser should be used to maximize depth of penetration
- The laser wavelength chosen should match the maximum absorption of the tattoo ink
- If immediate ink darkening is anticipated, a small test area should be treated and assessed for subsequent lightening
- Consider repeat treatments on the same day (R20 method), particularly if immediate darkening is seen
- Perfluorodecalin (PFD) patches can aid in more rapid repeat treatments and can help with resistant ink as PFD is an optical clearing agent
- Patients should be instructed that the aftercare is as important for a good result as the treatment itself. The tattoo should be covered with vaseline and a bandage, and the bandage should be changed daily until the area is healed

Enhancing Ink Clearance

In addition to the introduction of picosecond lasers and new wavelengths, there have been several attempts to enhance clearance of tattoos in the last decade. One of those

TABLE 2: Ink color and wavelength selection.

Ink color	Measured maximum absorption[20]	Laser selection	Treatment notes
Red	500–570 nm	532 nm	Most likely to cause adverse inflammatory reactions
Orange	420–540 nm	532 nm	
Yellow	470–485 nm	532 nm	
Green	570–800 nm	694 nm 755 nm	
Blue	590–770 nm	630 nm 694 nm 755 nm	
Violet	500–570 nm	532 nm 630 nm	Can cause inflammatory reactions
Black	600–800 nm	694 nm 755 nm 1064 nm	
Brown	410–550 nm	532 nm 694 nm 755 nm 1064 nm	Immediate ink darkening
White	790 nm	532 nm 755 nm	Immediate Ink darkening
Flesh	None	532 nm	Immediate ink darkening

advancements is the multipass treatment of tattoos. In the same treatment session, once the immediate whitening of a tattoo resolves, it is treated again with 1-3 more passes. The whitening takes about 20 minutes to resolve, and therefore this technique was named "R20", which is short for repeat exposures with a 20 minute delay. On subsequent passes, the tattoo does not whiten as it does on the first pass. The original study introducing the R20 method showed a marked improvement, with 61% of tattoos completely removed in one treatment session when treated with four passes done 20 minutes apart.[21] These results have not yet been duplicated, but it does appear that R20 can improve the clearance of tattoos (**Fig. 4**).[22,23] R20 may have the greatest utility in treating inks that have undergone immediate pigment darkening, like cosmetic tattoos. Once the ink has darkened, a multipass technique may be able to clear the darkened ink in one treatment session (**Fig. 2B**).

To eliminate the need to wait 20 minutes between passes, perfluorodecalin (PFD) alone or embedded in silicone patches can be used to dissolve the cavitation bubbles and facilitate faster, more efficient multipass treatments.[22,24] Aside from facilitating a rapid multipass treatment, PFD in silicone patches may have additional benefits for tattoo removal. PFD is an optical clearing agent that allows laser energy to penetrate deeper into

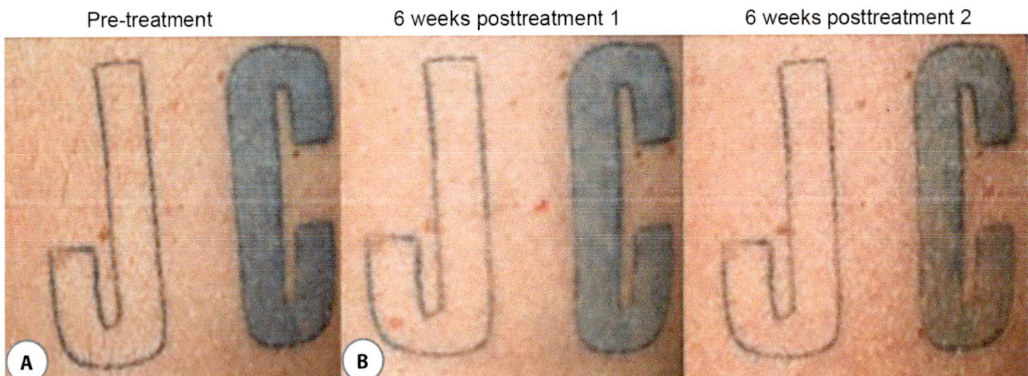

FIG. 4: Multipass treatments with the R20 method. (A) Upper half of images represent treatment of the tattoo with the standard method of a single picosecond laser treatment. (B) Lower half of images represent treatment of the tattoo with a multipass treatment technique (R20). Two passes were done at the same treatment session with 20 minutes between treatments to allow for the immediate whitening response to resolve.

tissue by minimizing scatter. This allows laser to reach ink particles residing further down in the dermis. This may be beneficial for tattoos on thicker skin locations, like hands and feet, and treatment resistant tattoos where ink particles may lie deeper out of the reach of laser energy. Silicone can also reduce the reflection of laser energy from the surface and protect the skin by absorbing heat.

Acoustic shockwave devices can also be used to enable rapid multipass treatments of tattoos. These devices apply a mechanically generated external sound wave into the body. The technology is best known for treatment of nephrolithiasis and muscle recovery in the context of physical therapy, but it is Food and Drug Administration (FDA) approved to treat cellulite and is also used to assist noninvasive fat removal. Shock waves have been shown to increase microcirculation, clear edema, stimulate angiogenesis, and remodel collagen fibers.[25] In the setting of tattoo removal, shockwave devices disrupt dermal cavitation vacuoles seen after laser treatment of tattoos, resolving the clinical whitening and allowing more efficient multipass treatments. In addition, shockwave devices may increase tattoo clearance by increasing lymphatic drainage and metabolic activity. In a study treating 34 black tattoos, 94% of patients who were treated with multiple passes assisted by shockwave therapy, had greater fading when compared to conventional treatment. 31% of patients in this study treated with multiple passes assisted by shockwave therapy achieved 75% or greater clearance and 6% achieved 90% clearance after a single session. The average clearance with the multipass treatment assisted by shockwave therapy was 45%, while the average clearance after conventional therapy was 15%.[26] Another case report showed superior tattoo clearance in one patient's black tattoo treated with multiple passes assisted by shockwave therapy when compared to multiple passes assisted by a PFD patch. The tattoo was split into two halves; both sides were treated with multiple passes. The side assisted by shockwave therapy showed an 80% clearance after 3 treatments, whereas the side assisted by a PFD patch showed a 60% clearance.[25]

Q-switched or picosecond lasers can also be combined with fractional resurfacing lasers to treat tattoos. This combination can enhance removal of ink and increases the tolerability of the treatment.[27] When columns of skin are ablated or coagulated, the ink is destroyed or extruded as well.[28] This can serve as a colorblind removal of tattoo ink and may be useful for resistant tattoos. Fractional resurfacing lasers have also been shown to successfully improve allergic tattoos when used as a standalone treatment. [29]

COMPLICATIONS

Laser tattoo removal is painful, and in most cases requires anesthesia. Topical anesthesia or local injection with lidocaine is the most common form of anesthesia used. Intradermal injection directly into a tattoo may change the skin thickness making laser penetration more difficult and may also allow ink to bleed beyond the tattoo border.[30] Therefore, local injection should be done in a ring block to avoid these complications. Ice, cold rollers, cold air chillers, and vibration can also help dull the pain of tattoo removal.

Tattoo removal leads to the immediate whitening of the tissue, which resolves within 5–20 minutes. Tissue splatter or obvious disruption of the epidermis indicates treatment beyond the desired endpoint and should be avoided. After treatment, purpura within the tattoo is usually evident. Blistering and crusting are common in the days following treatment, and are considered normal reactions. Patients should be instructed to keep the tattoo covered with a petrolatum-based ointment and a bandage for up to 2 weeks. Ointments or topicals with the potential for allergic contact dermatitis should be avoided as this can lead to discomfort and scarring.

Scarring and texture changes in tattoo removal have been reported to be 1–5%.[12] It is important to note that there may be pre-existing scars from the tattooing process. The tattoo should be evaluated closely for this prior to treatment. Tattoo removal can also result in hypo- or hyperpigmentation.

A rare side effect of tattoo removal is transient lymphadenopathy.[31] Lastly, it is important to inform patients that their tattoo can potentially contain carcinogenic or procarcinogenic materials.[32]

Patients should be advised that the number of treatments needed to remove a tattoo is unpredictable and that incomplete removal with a plateauing of results is possible. This may result in a “shadow” effect. White inks or inks with a component of white, as well as red, brown, beige, or white cosmetic tattoos, can turn black with laser treatments. Patients should be advised that this ink can lighten with repeated treatments, but that irreversible changes are possible. If possible darkening is anticipated, treating a small test area can be done. If darkening occurs, this area can be treated again to assess for clearance before treating a larger area. Reduction of titanium dioxide and iron oxides explain this immediate darkening.

Dark blue-black hyperpigmentation after treatment with a QS or picosecond laser can also represent laser-induced chrysiasis. This phenomenon is an immediate darkening of the skin in someone with a history of parenteral gold therapy who is treated with a QS or picosecond laser. After parenteral gold treatment (a therapy used for autoimmune diseases), gold particles remain in the dermis for decades. Great care should be taken to avoid this complication through patient screening, as it is very difficult to treat. Although largely considered permanent, laser-induced chrysiasis has been successfully lightened with long-pulsed (millisecond domain) ruby and alexandrite lasers in conjunction with fractional resurfacing lasers.[33] In addition to long-pulsed ruby and alexandrite lasers, pulsed dye lasers may also be effective in lightening laser-induced chrysiasis.[34]

Treatment of explosive foreign body material, like gunpowder, results in another avoidable adverse effect. In a case report of three patients with traumatic tattoos of gunpowder, treatment with QS laser resulted in microexplosions that healed with pox like scarring. The origin of traumatic tattoos should be clearly elicited before treatment.[35]

Immediate and delayed hypersensitivity reactions, both local and systemic, have been reported with tattoo removal.[36-41] Laser tattoo removal of allergic tattoos with QS or picosecond lasers is avoided to prevent systemic hypersensitivity reactions. Fractional resurfacing lasers may be useful in treating allergic tattoos, but a widespread eczematous reaction has been reported with this modality as well.[42] Fully ablative lasers with transepidermal removal of ink works best and can be very helpful at alleviating severe pruritus that these patients often experience.

CONCLUSION

After several decades of stagnation, advances in tattoo removal are increasing. New devices with shorter pulse durations and a wider range of wavelengths are now in use, better optimizing tattoo removal. In addition, combination and multipass treatments are regularly being employed. Even so, tattoo removal can still be a difficult and unpredictable task. With a staggering 40% of young Americans between the ages of 18 and 29 owning a tattoo, the demand for tattoo removal will be even greater potentially driving further innovation.[43] Future directions in tattoo removal may include creams that alter phagocytosis of ink particles in combination with laser or alone.

REFERENCES

1. Goldman L, Blaney DJ, Kindel DJ Jr, Franke EK. Effect of the laser beam on the skin. Preliminary report. J Invest Dermatol. 1963;40:121-2.
2. Goldman L, Blaney DJ, Kindel DJ Jr, Richfield D, Franke EK. Pathology of the effect of the laser beam on the skin. Nature. 1963;197:912-4.
3. Goldman L, Wilson RG, Hornby P, Meyer RG. Radiation from a Q-switched ruby laser. Effect of repeated impacts of power output of 10 megawatts on a tattoo of man. J Invest Dermatol. 1965;44:69-71.
4. Goldman L, Rockwell RJ, Meyer R, Otten R, Wilson RG, Kitzmiller KW. Laser treatment of tattoos. A preliminary survey of three year's clinical experience. JAMA. 1967;201(11):841-4.
5. Anderson RR, Parrish JA. Selective photothermolysis: precise microsurgery by selective absorption of pulsed radiation. Science. 1983;220(4596):524-7.
6. Taylor CR, Anderson RR, Gange RW, Michaud NA, Flotte TJ. Light and electron microscopic analysis of tattoos treated by Q-switched ruby laser. J Invest Dermatol. 1991;97(1):131-6.
7. Mankowska A, Kasprzak W, Adamski Z. Long-term evaluation of ink clearance in tattoos with different color intensity using the 1064-nm Q-switched Nd:YAG laser. J Cosmet Dermatol. 2015;14(4):302-9.
8. Anderson RR, Geronemus R, Kilmer SL, Farinelli W, Fitzpatrick RE. Cosmetic tattoo ink darkening. A complication of Q-switched and pulsed-laser treatment. Arch Dermatol. 1993;129(8):1010-4.
9. Jimenez G, Weiss E, Spencer JM. Multiple color changes following laser therapy of cosmetic tattoos. Dermatol Surg. 2002;28(2):177-9.
10. Taylor CR. Laser ignition of traumatically embedded firework debris. Lasers Surg Med. 1998;22(3):157-8.
11. Jow T, Brown A, Goldberg DJ. Patient compliance as a major determinant of laser tattoo removal success rates: a 10-year retrospective study. J Cosmet Laser Ther. 2010;12(4):166-9.
12. Bencini PL, Cazzaniga S, Tourlaki A, Galimberti MG, Naldi L. Removal of tattoos by Q-switched laser: variables influencing outcome and sequelae in a large cohort of treated patients. Arch Dermatol. 2012;148(12):1364-9.
13. Bernstein EF. Laser tattoo removal. Semin Plast Surg. 2007;21(3):175-92.
14. Izikson L, Farinelli W, Sakamoto F, Tannous Z, Anderson RR. Safety and effectiveness of black tattoo clearance in a pig model after a single treatment with a novel 758 nm 500 picosecond laser: a pilot study. Lasers Surg Med. 2010;42(7):640-6.
15. Ho DD, London R, Zimmerman GB, Young DA. Laser-tattoo removal—a study of the mechanism and the optimal treatment strategy via computer simulations. Lasers Surg Med. 2002;30(5):389-97.
16. Jang WH, Yoon Y, Kim W, Kwon S, Lee S, Song D, et al. Visualization of laser tattoo removal treatment effects in a mouse model by two-photon microscopy. Biomed Opt Express. 2017;8(8):3735-48.

17. Herd RM, Alora MB, Smoller B, Arndt KA, Dover JS. A clinical and histologic prospective controlled comparative study of the picosecond titanium:sapphire (795 nm) laser versus the Q-switched alexandrite (752 nm) laser for removing tattoo pigment. J Am Acad Dermatol. 1999; 40(4):603-6.
18. Ross V, Naseef G, Lin G, Kelly M, Michaud N, Flotte TJ, et al. Comparison of responses of tattoos to picosecond and nanosecond Q-switched neodymium: YAG lasers. Arch Dermatol. 1998;134(2):167-71.
19. Pinto F, Große-Büning S, Karsai S, Weiß C, Bäumler W, Hammes S, et al. Neodymium-doped yttrium aluminium garnet (Nd:YAG) 1064-nm picosecond laser vs. Nd:YAG 1064-nm nanosecond laser in tattoo removal: a randomized controlled single-blind clinical trial. Br J Dermatol. 2017;176(2):457-64.
20. Beute TC, Miller CH, Timko AL, Ross EV. In vitro spectral analysis of tattoo pigments. Dermatol Surg. 2008;34(4):508-15.
21. Kossida T, Rigopoulos D, Katsambas A, Anderson RR. Optimal tattoo removal in a single laser session based on the method of repeated exposures. J Am Acad Dermatol. 2012;66(2):271-7.
22. Biesman BS, Costner C. Evaluation of a transparent perfluorodecalin-infused patch as an adjunct to laser-assisted tattoo removal: A pivotal trial. Lasers Surg Med. 2017;49(4):335-40.
23. Reddy KK, Brauer JA, Anolik R, Bernstein L, Brightman L, Hale E, et al. Topical perfluorodecalin resolves immediate whitening reactions and allows rapid effective multiple pass treatment of tattoos. Lasers Surg Med. 2013;45(2):76-80.
24. Vangipuram R, Hamill SS, Friedman PM. Perfluorodecalin-infused patch in picosecond and Q-switched laser-assisted tattoo removal: Safety in Fitzpatrick IV-VI skin types. Lasers Surg Med. 2019;51(1):23-6.
25. Vangipuram R, Hamill SS, Friedman PM. Accelerated tattoo removal with acoustic shock wave therapy in conjunction with a picosecond laser. Lasers Surg Med. 2018;50(9):890-2.
26. Ibrahim O, Kaminer M. Accelerated tattoo removal facilitated with acoustic wave device: Delivering up to 90% fading in a single office visit. American Society for Laser and Medicine and Surgery Annual Conference Late-Breaking Abstracts #LB18. Lasers Surg Med. 2017;49:411.
27. Weiss ET, Geronemus RG. Combining fractional resurfacing and Q-switched ruby laser for tattoo removal. Dermatol Surg. 2011;37(1):97-9.
28. Wang CC, Huang CL, Sue YM, Lee SC, Leu FJ. Treatment of cosmetic tattoos using carbon dioxide ablative fractional resurfacing in an animal model: a novel method confirmed histopathologically. Dermatol Surg. 2013;39(4):571-7.
29. Ibrahimi OA, Syed Z, Sakamoto FH, Avram MM, Anderson RR. Treatment of tattoo allergy with ablative fractional resurfacing: a novel paradigm for tattoo removal. J Am Acad Dermatol. 2011;64(6):1111-4.
30. Ortiz AE, Avram MM. Redistribution of ink after laser tattoo removal. Dermatol Surg. 2012;38(10):1730-1.
31. Izikson L, Avram M, Anderson RR. Transient immunoreactivity after laser tattoo removal: report of two cases. Lasers Surg Med. 2008;40(4):231-2.
32. Kluger N, Koljonen V. Tattoos, inks and cancer. Lancet Oncol. 2012;13(4):e161-8.
33. Cohen PR, Ross EV. Q-Switched Alexandrite Laser-induced Chrysiasis. J Clin Aesthet Dermatol. 2015;8(9):48-53.
34. Yun PL, Arndt KA, Anderson RR. Q-switched laser-induced chrysiasis treated with long-pulsed laser. Arch Dermatol. 2002;138(8):1012-4.
35. Fusade T, Toubel G, Grognard C, Mazer JM. Treatment of gunpowder traumatic tattoo by Q-switched Nd:YAG laser: an unusual adverse effect. Dermatol Surg. 2000;26(11):1057-9.
36. Bernstein EF. A widespread allergic reaction to black tattoo ink caused by laser treatment. Lasers Surg Med. 2015;47(2):180-2.
37. Ashinoff R, Levine VJ, Soter NA. Allergic reactions to tattoo pigment after laser treatment. Dermatol Surg. 1995;21(4):291-4.
38. England RW, Vogel P, Hagan L. Immediate cutaneous hypersensitivity after treatment of tattoo with Nd:YAG laser: a case report and review of the literature. Ann Allergy Asthma Immunol. 2002;89(2):215-7.
39. Yorulmaz A, Onan DT, Artuz F, Gunes R. A case of generalized allergic contact dermatitis after laser tattoo removal. Cutan Ocul Toxicol. 2015;34(3):234-6.
40. Wilken R, Ho D, Petukhova T, Jagdeo J. Intraoperative localized urticarial reaction during Q-switched Nd:YAG laser tattoo removal. J Drugs Dermatol. 2015;14(3): 303-6.
41. Willardson HB, Kobayashi TT, Arnold JG, Hivnor CM, Bowen CD. Diffuse Urticarial Reaction Associated with Titanium Dioxide Following Laser Tattoo Removal Treatments. Photomed Laser Surg. 2017;35(3):176-80.
42. Meesters AA, De Rie MA, Wolkerstorfer A. Generalized eczematous reaction after fractional carbon dioxide laser therapy for tattoo allergy. J Cosmet Laser Ther. 2016;18(8):456-8.
43. Laumann AE, Derick AJ. Tattoos and body piercings in the United States: a national data set. J Am Acad Dermatol. 2006;55(3):413-21.

5 SECTION

REJUVENATION, SCAR REMODELING AND BODY CONTOURING

15

CHAPTER

Laser Resurfacing

Jill Katherine Cotseones, Lindsay Rachel Sklar, Omar A Ibrahimi, Suzanne Linsmeier Kilmer

INTRODUCTION

Resurfacing of the skin is one of the most commonly performed procedures in cosmetic dermatology and aesthetic medicine to help eliminate or soften the signs of photoaging. Initial approaches to skin resurfacing focused on fully ablative carbon dioxide (CO_2) and erbium lasers. However, the theory of selective photothermolysis proposed by Anderson and Parrish in 1983 changed the field of laser surgery; allowing us to selectively treat specific targets in the skin, such as hemoglobin, water, and melanin.[1] Advancements in laser surgery continued with further breakthroughs like the theory of fractional photothermolysis, by Anderson and Manstein in 2004.[2] As a result, these advancements have allowed us to expand our cosmetic treatment armamentarium to include a wide-array of laser resurfacing devices.

Patient Selection and Preoperative Considerations

Patient selection and screening is very important in order to achieve optimal results and safety with laser resurfacing. A thorough preoperative evaluation should be conducted in the office to gather more information about the patient's medical and surgical history prior to performing the laser procedure.

Patients that have a history of autoimmune disorders, immunodeficiencies, or who are chronically immunosuppressed are at higher risk for impaired wound healing postprocedure and may not be ideal candidates for fully ablative laser resurfacing. Also, patients should be at least 6 months out from isotretinoin use to be considered safe for most nonablative laser resurfacing procedures and around 1 year out for ablative laser resurfacing due to impaired wound healing and increased risk of scarring postprocedure [3,4] A history of keloid or hypertrophic scar formation is also important to obtain prior to laser surgery as it can lead to adverse outcomes, particularly with ablative laser resurfacing. It is important to note, that one of the authors absolute contraindications to ablative laser resurfacing is a history of vitiligo, as they are at increased risk for Koebnerization postprocedure. It is also important to be aware that this phenomenon can occur with other inflammatory conditions such as psoriasis.

Additionally, antimicrobial prophylaxis may be initiated prior to treatment in order to decrease the risk of infection. Oral antivirals are recommended when treating around the mouth for nonablative procedures and for all patients undergoing ablative laser resurfacing, regardless of a history of cold sores. The recommendations consist of starting oral acyclovir or valacyclovir one day prior and for up to seven days postablative laser resurfacing, with shorter treatment intervals for nonablative procedures.[5] Depending on the practitioner, the addition of oral antifungals or antibiotics such as oral doxycycline may be included to decrease the risk of infection or prevent flares of acne vulgaris in patients who have a prior history of acne. However, the addition of oral antibiotics prophylactically has become more controversial due to concern for opportunistic infections with gram-negative bacteria postprocedure. Some physicians may even swab the anterior nares to see if the patient is a carrier of *Staphylococcus aureus* bacteria prior to the procedure, and may pretreat the nares with topical mupirocin 2% ointment to decrease the risk of infection.[6]

Furthermore, the patient should also abstain from sun exposure 2–4 weeks both pre- and postprocedure as increased melanin can compete for absorption of the laser and increase the risk for postoperative complications such as hypo/hyperpigmentation. Patients with darker skin tones can be pretreated with topical hydroquinone prior to the procedure, although studies have shown conflicting evidence as to whether or not pretreatment results in decreased risk of postinflammatory hyperpigmentation (PIH).[7,8] Also, a prior cosmetic surgical history is important to be aware of prior to performing laser surgery as it can impact outcomes. Patients who have undergone an inferior eyelid blepharoplasty may be at higher risk for ectropion formation with fully ablative laser resurfacing. To avoid this complication, a snap test of the lower eyelid should be performed prior to the procedure. However, fractional ablative laser devices may be a safer alternative for this patient population altogether. Also, it is important to gather a prior history of a neck or face lift, where the neck skin may have been pulled onto the face. If the settings are not appropriately adjusted for the more delicate neck skin, there can be increased risk of scarring.[9]

Lastly, the practitioner should also give thoughtful consideration as to which lasers will achieve the best results for the patient. These considerations should include the patient's desired number of treatments, degree of photodamage, their skin type, the targeted chromophore (melanin, hemoglobin, and water), ability for downtime, and finally the cost of the procedure. When these factors are taken into account for a specific patient, the practitioner can then appropriately determine which type of laser resurfacing provides the safest and most effective treatment option.

Nonablative Resurfacing

Nonablative lasers were developed to reverse the signs of aging with minimal recovery time and fewer associated safety risks compared to ablative lasers. Typically, the results of nonablative lasers are much more modest, commonly requiring multiple treatments to achieve modest results. Nonetheless, nonablative laser resurfacing is a great alternative for the patient seeking a less aggressive treatment option to correct the signs of aging with minimal downtime following the procedure.

VISIBLE LIGHT LASERS

Pulsed Dye Laser

As mentioned in earlier chapters, the pulsed dye laser (PDL) emits a yellow light at a wavelength of 595 nm, which specifically targets oxyhemoglobin and selectively destroys superficial dermal blood vessels. Therefore, it is commonly used to treat telangiectasias, birthmarks, rosacea, and poikiloderma.[10] There is also some absorption of melanin at this wavelength allowing for the treatment of lentigines.[11] Additionally, Zelickson and Kilmer demonstrated that a single PDL treatment can induce collagen remodeling and improve facial rhytids for up to 12 months posttreatment. Their findings were supported histologically by an observable increase in epidermal thickness, collagen, elastin, and active fibroblasts.[12] Therefore, this may be a good treatment alternative for patients who have rosacea and telangiectasias who are looking for subtle improvements in texture and rhytids (**Figs. 1A** and **B**).

Intense Pulsed Light

Intense Pulsed Light (IPL) is a nonlaser device that emits light in a polychromatic, noncoherent, noncollimated fashion with a wide range of wavelengths ranging from 515 to 1,200 nm (**Table 1**). Cutoff filters are used to narrow the spectrum of emitted light, allowing the device to target more specific chromophores such as hemoglobin or melanin. This treatment is favored for patients who have mild photodamage, as results tend to be very gradual over a series of treatments. Caution should be used when treating darker skin types due to the risk of hyper/hypopigmentation and scarring, with longer wavelengths recommended. However, other lasers may be safer alternatives in this patient population. Many studies have shown an improvement of telangiectasias, lentigines, and texture overtime which tends to correspond histologically to an increase in collagen formation, fibroblasts and extracellular matrix proteins along with homogenization of melanin distribution.[13-16] IPL may be an excellent treatment option for patients with mild lentigines, ephelides, and telangiectasias who are looking for subtle improvements over time.

MIDINFRARED LASERS

1,320 nm Neodymium-doped Yttrium Aluminum Garnet Laser

The 1,320 nm neodymium-doped yttrium-aluminum-garnet (Nd:YAG) laser was the first laser designed for selective dermal heating.

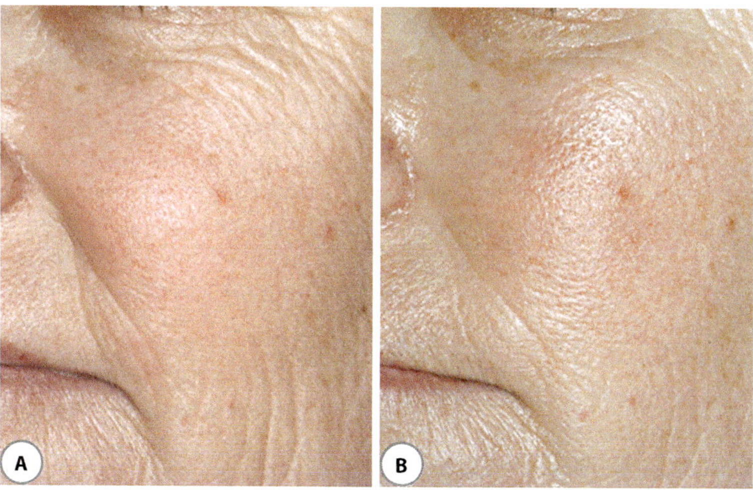

FIGS. 1A AND B: A 50-year-old Caucasian female before (A) and 2 months post two pulse dye laser treatment with settings of 10 mm spot size, 6 ms pulse width, and 7.5 J/cm^2 (B). Note improvement in wrinkles and texture as well as vasculature.

Courtesy: Suzanne Linsmeier Kilmer at the Laser and Skin Surgery Center of Northern California.

TABLE 1: Laser resurfacing types and wavelengths.

	Laser type	Wavelength (nm)
	Potassium titanyl phosphate	532
	Pulsed dye laser	595
	Picosecond	532, 585, 650, 755, and 1,064
	Diode and long pulsed	1,450
	Nd:YAG and long pulsed	1,320
	Q-switched Nd:YAG	1,064
	Fractional	1,320, 1,440, 1,470, 1,540, 1,550, 1,565, and 1,927
Nonlaser resurfacing	Intense pulse light	515–1,200
Ablative laser resurfacing	Fractional or pulsed CO_2	10,600
	Fractional or pulsed Er:YAG	2,940
	YSGG laser	2,790

(CO_2: carbon dioxide; Er: erbium; Nd:YAG: neodymium-doped yttrium aluminium garnet; YSGG: yttrium–scandium-gallium–garnet)

The dermis contains a significant amount of water which is the chromophore for this laser. When the laser heats the dermis it creates injury and stimulates extracellular matrix remodeling. The epidermis is spared due to a concomitant cryogen cooling spray. Studies with the 1,320 nm Nd:YAG laser have shown mild improvement in periocular rejuvenation as well as increased epidermal thickness. Typically, patients can start to see results after three treatments, and the results last up to 3 months posttreatment. Unfortunately, results with this laser may be limited by patient discomfort.[17,18]

1,450 nm Diode Laser

The 1,450 nm diode laser also targets dermal water as its chromophore and generates a zone of heat in the dermis up to 600 μ deep. Several authors have demonstrated the successful use of this laser in photorejuvenation. Results are seen following multiple treatments with minimal side effects consisting of erythema and edema that typically resolve within a few days posttreatment. Tanzi et al. demonstrated mild to moderate improvement of perioral and periorbital wrinkles after four treatments with this laser with an increase in collagen seen histologically for up to 6 months posttreatment.[19] No and Kilmer also found this device to be an excellent treatment option for sebaceous hyperplasia. The investigators found up to a 75% improvement after only 2–3 treatments sessions.[20] Therefore, the 1,450 nm laser may be a good treatment for patients who have mild photodamage and concomitant sebaceous hyperplasia.

Picotoning and Low-fluence Q-switched Neodymium-doped Yttrium Aluminum Garnet

Picotoning has become a popular treatment for patients looking for laser treatments with minimal downtime. This technique was originally described with the 755 nm

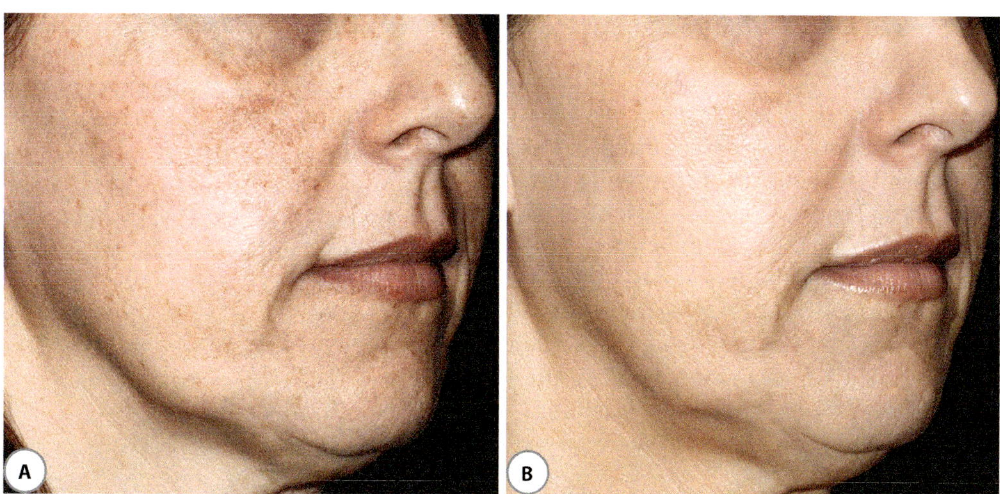

FIGS. 2A AND B: A 44-year-old Caucasian female before (A) and 3 months post five picotoning treatments with 755 nm and 750 picosecond laser using the focus lens array hand piece (B). Note improvement in wrinkles and texture as well as pigment.

Courtesy: Suzanne Linsmeier Kilmer at the Laser and Skin Surgery Center of Northern California.

wavelength picosecond laser; however, it now encompasses multiple wavelengths and lasers with a picosecond domain.[21-25] Typically, the procedure is performed using a brushstroke technique where multiple passes of the laser are administered 1–3 cm off the skin to accumulate a certain amount of energy within the treatment area. Patients often prefer this treatment because downtime is minimal, generally consisting of transient erythema that lasts for a few hours posttreatment.[26]

Studies have shown gradual improvement of rhytids and skin laxity following multiple treatments. Weiss, et al. found that after four treatments with the focus array lens, spaced one month apart, there was an overall improvement in facial rhytids by 6 months (**Figs. 2A** and **B**). This improvement corresponded to an increase in both collagen and elastin histologically.[27] Interestingly, these results may be expedited when treated at compressed treatment intervals (every 2–3 weeks) with no observable increase in side effects.[28]

Picotoning has also been shown to be safe and effective when used "off the face". A study on photorejuvenation of the chest and hands showed an improvement of rhytids, pigmentation, and texture after four treatments.[29] This is also consistent with the authors' results, which include an improvement of skin laxity and photorejuvenation of the neck and decolletage after a series of treatments.

In parallel, the Q-switched 1,064 nm Nd:YAG laser, which is often used to treat lentigines, tattoos, and nevus of Ota, can also result in a gradual improvement of photodamage, hyperpigmentation, and rhytids when used at low fluences in a similar brushstroke technique to picotoning. Likewise, there is minimal downtime following the procedure. Photorejuvenation has been shown to be secondary to increased fibrosis in the papillary dermis as early as 3 months posttreatment.[21,22] Results with this laser are gradual, and seem to be dose-dependent like with picotoning, achieving greater results with increased number of treatments.[30]

NONABLATIVE FRACTIONAL RESURFACING

Compared to nonablative resurfacing, fractional resurfacing only treats fractions of the skin while leaving the surrounding skin intact. The technology induces columns of thermal necrosis in the epidermis and dermis referred to as "microthermal zones" (MTZs). The nonablative fractional devices spare the tissue surrounding the MTZs, providing the framework necessary for healing the coagulated columns. This is an essential concept allowing for the improved safety profile of fractional lasers.[2,31]

Furthermore, immediate histology posttreatment demonstrates necrosis of the epidermis and dermis localized to the MTZs, however, there is no evidence of MTZs by 3 months posttreatment. Immunohistochemistry has also demonstrated evidence of neocollagenesis persistent for nearly 3 months posttreatment. The fractional devices do not remove epidermis and for this reason the prototype nonablative fractional laser, a 1,550 nm Erbium-fiber device, was referred to as nonablative.[2] Fractional devices offer a better safety profile for patients with quicker recovery times compared to nonfractional devices, however, this comes at the cost of more gradual results.

Dual Wavelength 1,550 nm Fractionated Erbium Glass/ 1,927 nm Thulium Fiber Laser

Aforementioned, the 1,550 nm nonablative fractional Erbium-glass laser combined with the 1,927 nm nonablative fractional thulium fiber laser on the same platform is the prototypical nonablative fractional laser. The dual wavelength allows for multiple treatment indications, and the settings can be modified to address the severity of the patient's cosmetic concerns. The pulse energy or fluence determines the depth of penetration. The treatment level determines the number of MTZs or density, and the number of passes determines the number of MTZs and kilojoules of heat laid down per pass. Treatment with one wavelength generally consists of eight passes, whereas dual wavelength treatments consist of four passes. All settings may be customized depending on the specific treatment indication, such as: Pigment, tone and texture (more superficial), versus rhytids (mid to deep range), or scars (deep range).

The 1,550 nm wavelength laser is indicated for the treatment of scars, rhytids, dyschromia, and photorejuvenation. This wavelength induces MTZs 100–200 μ wide and penetrates more deeply at 500–1,400 μ deep, with energy levels of 4–70 mJ. Treatment levels range from 5 to 48%, which corresponds to the density of the MTZs. Patients generally experience discomfort during treatment and benefit from a pretreatment topical anesthetic. Patients can expect to experience erythema and edema posttreatment which typically resolves within 3–5 days.[32]

The thulium 1,927 nm wavelength laser is indicated for the treatment of dyspigmentation, photodamage, and actinic keratoses. It is more superficial, only penetrating up to 200 μ deep and operates at fluences ranging from 5 to 20 mJ and 20 to 70% coverage. With a higher absorption coefficient for water, the 1,927 nm laser has a nonlinear depth to energy profile and therefore a greater ability to target more superficial pathology in the epidermis such as actinic keratoses, dermatoheliosis, and dyschromia (**Figs. 3A** and **B**).[32] The 1,550/ 1,927 nm lasers may be used individually or in combination with each other. The deeper wavelength should be performed first. Typically, around four passes of each laser will be performed to target both the epidermis and the dermis.

Optimal results with this nonablative fractional laser typically occur after

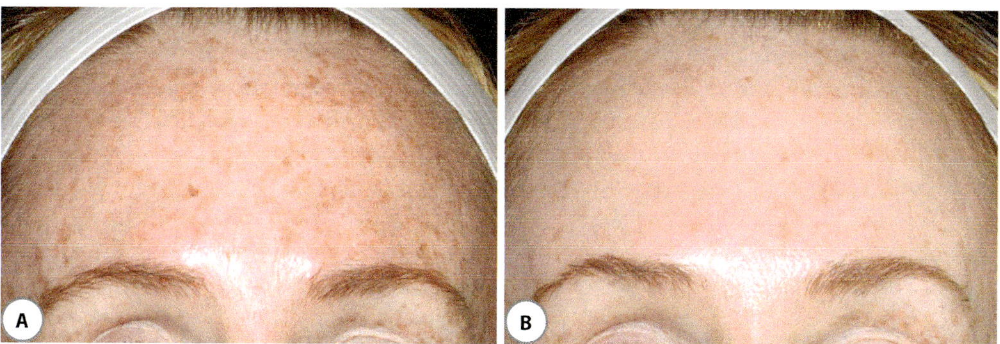

FIGS. 3A AND B: A 34-year-old Caucasian female with extensive history of sun exposure before (A) and 3 months post one fractional nonablative laser treatment with 1,927 nm wavelength (B). Note significant improvement in ephilads and lentigenes.

Courtesy: Suzanne Linsmeier Kilmer at the Laser and Skin Surgery Center of Northern California.

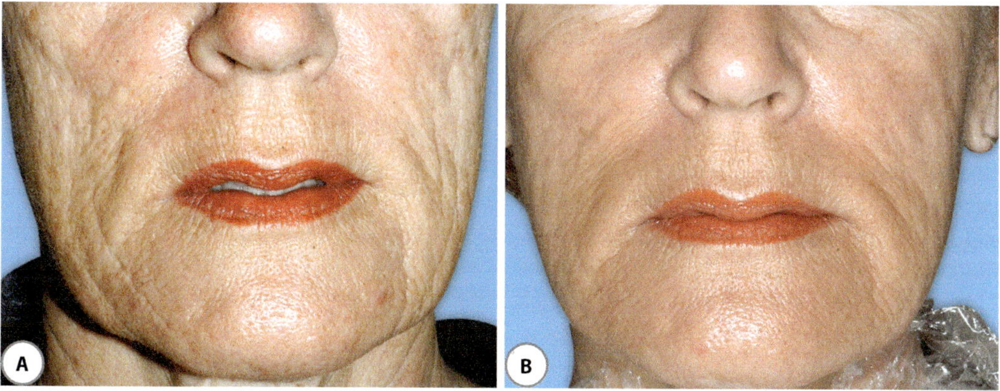

FIGS. 4A AND B: A 58-year-old Caucasian female with significant acne scarring (A) improved after a single treatment with 1,550 nm, 50 J/cm^2 and density of 29% (B).

Courtesy: Suzanne Linsmeier Kilmer at the Laser and Skin Surgery Center of Northern California.

3–4 treatments. Results with the 1,927 nm laser can be seen sooner, with over 60% of patients exhibiting significant improvement of facial photopigmentation, lentigines, and ephiledes at 1 month posttreatment.[33] In comparison, the 1,550 nm laser typically takes around 3–6 months to see improvement of fine wrinkling and tactile roughness posttreatment (**Figs. 4A** and **B**).[34] This typically corresponds to neocollagenesis histologically which takes 3–6 months to occur posttreatment. Posttreatment recovery is dependent on treatment settings, but typically includes moderate erythema and edema and mild dryness and flaking that typically resolve within 7–10 days posttreatment.[34]

Results have been shown to be more sustainable when multiple treatments are performed. Wanner, et al. found that a majority of patients treated with the 1,550 nm laser could still see observable results of up to 75% improvement in photodamage at 9 months posttreatment, when a total of three treatments were performed (spaced 3–4 weeks apart).[35]

These results were consistent with treatment on other areas of the body.[35] In summary, this laser is a great treatment option for patients who are seeking a less aggressive treatment option for hyperpigmentation, lentigines, ephelides as well as rhytids, and scarring.

1,440/1,927 nm Nonablative Fractionated Laser

The 1,440 nm diode and the diode-pumped thulium 1,927 nm lasers are low energy and low density lasers indicated for superficial skin resurfacing. This laser device is often referred to as a "lunchtime laser" as it is ideal for patients who may be looking for minimal downtime following the procedure. The settings are much more limited than the above-mentioned fractional lasers. The spot size is fixed at 140 μ and the energy level is restricted to three settings: Low (5 mJ, 5% density), medium (7 mJ, 7% density), or high (9 mJ, 9% density). Depending on the energy level, the depth of penetration ranges from 200 to 300 μ for the 1,440 nm laser and up to 170 μ for the 1,927 nm laser. The superficial penetration of the 1,927 nm laser allows for treatment of hyperpigmentation and is safer in darker Fitzpatrick skin-types due to the risk of PIH with the 1,440 nm laser.[32,36] Due to the low energy and density of the laser, multiple treatments are required, and the results are very mild. In the author's experience, patients who have epidermal melasma may exhibit improvement after a series of low energy treatments with the 1,927 nm laser in conjunction with topical therapies.

Hybrid 1,470/2,940 nm Nonablative Fractional Device

The hybrid 1,470/2,940 nm laser is unique in that it emits two different wavelengths within each laser pulse: One with nonablative coagulation at 1,470 nm, and the other with ablative vaporization at 2,940 nm.[37] The 1,470 nm laser wavelength causes MTZs up to 700 μm into the dermis whereas the 2,940 nm laser causes a much more superficial ablation of the epidermis (up to 100 μm) due to the high water absorption coefficient.[37] The ablation causes microscopic epidermal necrotic debris (MENDS) which lead to re-epithelialization within 1 week posttreatment.[38] This hybrid device has been shown to improve photodamage, rhytids as well as actinic keratoses.[38,39]

A study conducted by Waibel, et al. of 29 female patients (skin types I–IV) who underwent two treatments (4–6 weeks apart), evaluated the safety and efficacy of the hybrid laser on photodamage, dyschromia, and patient satisfaction. Up to 80% of patients showed significant skin improvement by blinded evaluators with 100% patient satisfaction. Minimal adverse effects were encountered, except for two patients who experienced PIH which resolved within 90 days posttreatment.[37] This laser is an excellent treatment option for patients who have moderate photodamage, rhytides, and scars due to the dual nonablative/ablative fractional component.

Postoperative Care

For most nonablative laser resurfacing procedures, minimal wound care is required despite avid use of mineral sunscreen. Gentle, fragrance-free cleansers, and nonocclusive emollients should be recommended for at least 3–5 days postprocedure. Patients should be advised not to rub or scrub the skin as it is healing. Certain cosmeceuticals can be applied pre- and posttreatment to enhance results and facilitate recovery of the skin, including a tripeptide and hexapeptide topical cream. Preoperative treatment with this cream has been shown to clear the extracellular matrix of debris, allowing for enhanced collagen and elastin fiber deposition posttreatment, both enhancing recovery and results.[40]

Complications of Nonablative Laser Resurfacing

A majority of the complications from nonablative laser resurfacing are self-limited. The most common side effects are acneiform eruptions and herpes simplex viral (HSV) infections, which are both reported to occur in <2% of cases following the procedure.[41] Erythema lasting >4 days after the procedure is unusual, with a reported incidence of <1.8%.[42] Also, less commonly seen in milia formation, which is attributed to the use of occlusive moisturizers posttreatment.[41]

Another potential side effect is PIH, which occurs more commonly in darker skinned patients.[41] While more aggressive treatment settings can increase the risk of PIH, this side effect has still been observed with lower treatment energy and densities.[43] Aside from decreasing treatment densities to help avoid hyper- or hypopigmentation, we recommend increasing the treatment interval between treatments and strongly encourage our patients to avoid sun exposure as mentioned earlier. Additionally, we often recommend topical lightening creams for patients of darker skin tones following the procedure to help minimize this complication. Rarely, bacterial infections with gram-negative or gram-positive bacteria can develop in the week following treatment. Close follow-up with bacterial cultures or antibiotics may be necessary if infection is suspected due to the risk of scarring or rare progression to sepsis.[44]

Lastly, to avoid ocular complications, it is very important to wear the appropriate wavelength protective eye goggles during the procedure. Intraocular eye shields should be placed when operating within the orbital rim.

ABLATIVE LASER RESURFACING

Introduction

Ablative laser skin resurfacing still remains the gold standard for patients who have a greater degree of rhytids, photodamage, skin laxity, and textural abnormalities or scarring.

The first ablative laser to truly transform the field of laser surgery was the continuous-wave (CW) CO_2 laser in the 1970s. However, bulk heating often yielded unpredictable results and led to unwanted complications such as prolonged erythema and scarring. As a result, the erbium-doped yttrium aluminum garnet laser (Er:YAG) laser as well as newer, higher powered, shorter pulsed CO_2 devices were developed. The Er:YAG laser has a much higher affinity for water than the CO_2 leading to less residual thermal damage; therefore this device may be a safer alternative for darker Fitzpatrick skin-types especially at lower densities.

As technology advanced, the concept of fractional ablative laser resurfacing was established. This led to devices that were able to approach results similar to fully ablative laser resurfacing devices, however, with a safer side effect profile and quicker recovery times. These devices may be preferable in patients of darker skin types. Although fully ablative laser resurfacing is still performed today, it is often used in combination with fractional ablative lasers.

Finally, patient selection and thorough discussion of the procedure is very important. The preoperative consult is the optimal time to properly assess the patient for the procedure, set expectations, and discuss the patient's ability for downtime and willingness to participate in postoperative wound care.

Fully Ablative Carbon Dioxide Laser

The CO_2 laser produces an infrared light at a 10,600-nm wavelength with a strong absorption coefficient for water (**Table 1**). The CO_2 was originally used in the CW mode in the 1980s, which resulted in large amounts of nonspecific thermal damage and increased risk of scarring. As a result, the CW CO_2 was quickly replaced by higher peak power, short-pulsed, and rapidly scanned CO_2 lasers. These lasers allow for >20–30 μm of ablation per pass with considerably smaller residual zones of thermal damage (only 150 μm vs. the prior 600 μm of earlier devices) (**Table 1**).[45]

The depth of ablation increases with higher fluences (in millijoules) and each subsequent pass of the CO_2. The first pass is typically confined to the epidermal layer, the second to the papillary dermis, and if a third is performed, to the superficial reticular dermis.[46,47] Typically, the papillary dermis is the goal endpoint to avoid scarring. Other ways to avoid scarring are with avoidance of pulse stacking and removal of partially desiccated tissue with a moist gauze in between passes.[48,49]

The fluence should be adjusted depending on the treatment area. For areas with thinner skin, such as the inferior eyelid or neck, lower treatment energies should be utilized to decrease the risk of ectropion and scarring. Alternatively, fractional ablative laser resurfacing may be a safer option in these high-risk areas, where lower treatment densities can be applied. Another technique to prevent bulk heating recommended by Kilmer et al., is to pretreat the skin with a hydrating topical anesthetic such as EMLA (eutectic mixture of lidocaine 2.5% and prilocaine 2.5%) in addition to other topical anesthetics [Eutectic mixture of local anesthetics (lidocaine and prilocaine), Astra, Westborough, MA].

Fully ablative CO_2 is the gold standard for the treatment of deep rhytids and severe photodamage.[50,51] On average, there is a 50% improvement in rhytids with a single treatment, although areas with high dynamic motion such as the perioral or glabella area tend to be less responsive.[52] Therefore, botulinum toxin prior to the procedure can help maximize outcomes by prolonging the correction of movement associated rhytids.[53] Improvements in infraorbital hyperpigmentation as well as atrophic scars can also be seen with fully ablative laser resurfacing in patients of both lighter and darker skin types. These results typically peak 1 year posttreatment.[54]

Additionally, ablative laser resurfacing can be used to tighten the skin, particularly in patients who want to avoid plastic surgery. Maximal skin tightening was observed initially with the fully ablative CO_2 in comparison to other lasers; however, newer Er:YAG lasers with tunable coagulation have yielded similar results.[55] The degree of skin contraction with the fully ablative CO_2 is directly proportional to the energy of the laser. Studies have found an improvement of both dermatochalasis and periorbital rhytids, with greater degrees of improvement seen in patients who have more severe rhytids and skin laxity at baseline.[56]

The benefits seen with CO_2 resurfacing are centered around wound healing and collagen remodeling which can be seen up to 6–12 months posttreatment. Immediately following the laser procedure, there is induction of the inflammatory cascade and increased expression of matrix metalloproteinases (MMPs).[57] Consequently, collagen and elastin are broken down to form new fibers that are more organized and evenly distributed within the papillary dermis.[58] Neocollagenesis and formation of new elastic fibers have been visualized on histologic biopsies as soon as 30–90 days posttreatment.[59]

Furthermore, the CO_2 laser is also an excellent treatment option for actinic damage and actinic cheilitis. Histologic examination postprocedure has shown improvement of solar elastosis, epidermal atypia, and melanocyte hyperplasia as well as decreased p53 expression that lasts for at least 6 months postprocedure.[60-62]

Moreover, the unwanted side effects of the fully ablative CO_2 laser, such as prolonged erythema, hypopigmentation, and scarring

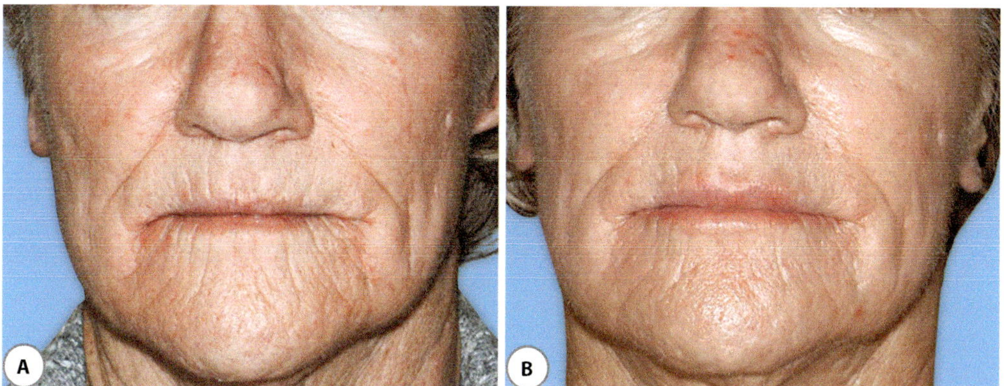

FIGS. 5A AND B: A 49-year-old Caucasian woman with history of tanning bed use and significant sun exposure before (A) and 3 months after (B) treatment with a combination fully ablative CO_2 10,600 nm and erbium 2,940 nm laser treatment. Note improvement in wrinkles as well as acne scarring.
Courtesy: Suzanne Linsmeier Kilmer at the Laser and Skin Surgery Center of Northern California.

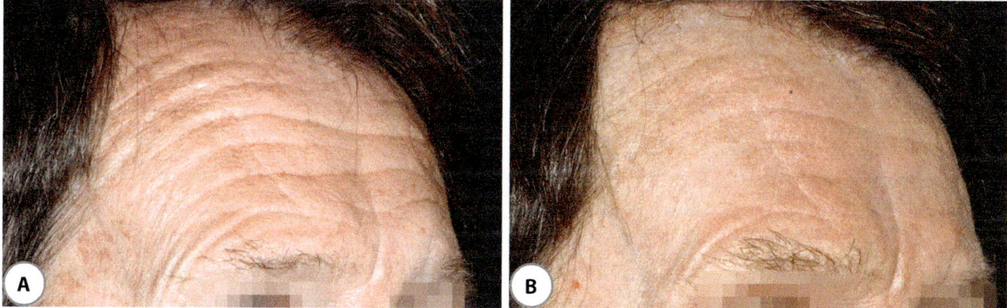

FIGS. 6A AND B: A 56-year-old Caucasian man with long history of precancers and actinic damage before (A) and after (B) a single fully ablative with two passes CO_2 laser treatment. Note improvement in rhytids as well as actinic damage.
Courtesy: Suzanne Linsmeier Kilmer at the Laser and Skin Surgery Center of Northern California.

as well as excessive downtime often limit its use in modern day medicine, as newer fractional ablative lasers have been developed. Additionally, combination treatments have become more mainstream, with fully ablative lasers concentrated around more stubborn areas such as perioral rhytids following treatment with fractional ablative resurfacing. Furthermore, combining devices can also enhance healing postprocedure and mitigate the duration of crusting, swelling, and itching postoperatively (**Figs. 5** and **6**).[63]

Ablative Erbium:Yttrium-scandium-gallium-garnet Laser

The erbium:yttrium-scandium-gallium-garnet (Er:YSGG) laser emits a wavelength at 2,790 nm and has an absorption coefficient of water somewhere in between that of the CO_2 and the Er:YAG lasers (**Table 1**). This laser was created to have the benefits of the CO_2 without the side effects of excess thermal damage.[64] The fully ablative Er:YSGG laser has been shown to improve photodamage, rhytids,

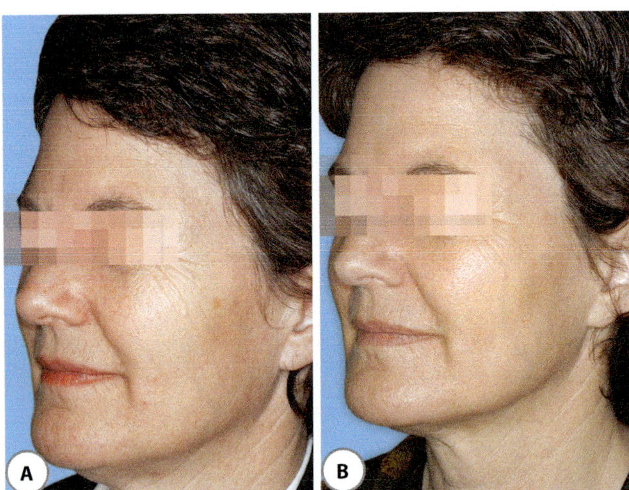

FIGS. 7A AND B: A 52-year-old Caucasian woman before (A) and after (B) a single treatment with the Erbium:Yttrium-scandium-gallium-garnet (Er:YSGG) at standard settings. Note improvement in skin texture, wrinkles, and pigmentation.

Courtesy: Suzanne Linsmeier Kilmer at the Laser and Skin Surgery Center of Northern California.

and acne scarring with 1–2 treatments spaced 4–6 weeks apart (**Figs. 7A** and **B**).[65,66] The recovery seems to be quicker (around 4 days) than other fully ablative laser resurfacing devices, with mild transient erythema noted in the week following treatment.[65-67] Higher fluences and densities may be more beneficial with this device, although more studies are needed.[67]

Fully Ablative Erbium-doped:Yttrium Aluminum Garnet Laser

The 2,940-nm Er:YAG laser operates near infrared light and has >16 times the coefficient for water absorption than the CO_2.[68] Because of the high affinity for water, the Er:YAG generates significantly less residual thermal damage (15 μm) with a more superficial ablation of 5–15 μm with each pass.[69] On average, the first pass of the short pulsed Er:YAG typically extends down to the granular layer of the epidermis, the second pass to the basal epidermal layer, the third to the papillary dermis, and passes 5–6 to the superficial reticular dermis.[70]

The characteristic "popping" sound is secondary to the explosive ejection of ablated material. There is very little scattering of the laser beam and less desiccation of the tissue which unlike the CO_2 does not prevent the Er:YAG from reaching an ablative plateau. Although there is less desiccated tissue to interfere with the depth of ablation, the Er:YAG causes vasodilation of dermal blood vessels and bleeding which can also lead to more superficial treatments.[71] For deeper treatments, the modulated Er:YAG can be used due to tunable coagulation; however, the practitioner should be cautious as the clinical endpoint of pinpoint bleeding is often absent.

Generally, there is decreased erythema and edema as well as faster re-epithelialization with the Er:YAG laser in comparison to the CO_2.[72] However, a greater number of passes are required with the short-pulsed Er:YAG laser to approach similar results as the CO_2. Patients with a greater degree of photodamage and acne scarring should be treated with the modulated Er:YAG due to the ability to penetrate more deeply.[73,74] Unfortunately, because the Er:YAG generates less heat in the tissue, there is often a lesser degree of tissue contraction/ tightening.[75] However, less heat generation may be advantageous in patients with darker skin, due to decreased risk for PIH.[76] Similarly, the Er:YAG may be a better option for patients when resurfacing areas off-the face, due to the higher risk of scarring in those areas.[77] The Er:YAG has also been reported to successfully treat many benign epidermal conditions such as: Syringomas, seborrheic keratoses, and sebaceous hyperplasia.[78] Similar to the CO_2, this laser has also been shown to be highly effective for the treatment of actinic cheilitis.[79]

Finally, for more aggressive treatments, the Er:YAG can be combined with CO_2 particularly in the perioral or periocular area without an increased risk of side effects. Goldman, et al. attributed these findings to the Er:YAG removing the thermal debris left behind from the CO_2. This allows the heat to escape from the tissue, leading to quicker re-epithelialization postprocedure and lower risk for postoperative erythema and scarring.[72]

Fractional Ablative Resurfacing

Fractional ablative laser resurfacing is similar to nonablative fractional resurfacing, as mentioned earlier in the chapter; however, instead of microthermal zones, there are columns of tissue being removed or vaporized with each pass.[80] The depth of the ablation depends on multiple variables such as the energy, wavelength, and spot size of the beam.[80] Furthermore, the density and size of the ablative columns can be adjusted depending on the intensity of treatment. Water is still the main chromophore of these devices. The ideal amount of ablation to coagulation depends on the overall treatment goal. In theory, greater amounts of coagulation should lead to greater collagen production.

Fractional ablative resurfacing works similarly to fully ablative laser resurfacing with the induction of the inflammatory cascade; however, the process may result in less collagen production.[81] This may explain why there are often inferior results for tissue tightening and deep rhytids in comparison to fully ablative modalities. Directly after treatment there is induction of heat shock proteins which is thought to act as a procollagen chaperone toward neocollagenesis.[82] Similar to fully ablative laser resurfacing, there is elevation of MMPs that breakdown damaged collagen and elastin to form newly organized fibers starting around 3 months posttreatment.[83]

Aforementioned, fractional ablative laser resurfacing may be a safer alternative for higher risk areas such as the neck or the lower eyelid where there is a greater risk of scarring or ectropion of the lower eyelid. It is also an effective treatment for photorejuvenation with considerably less down time and adverse reactions. Patients typically heal within 5–7 days with less risk of postoperative erythema or hypopigmentation. Fractional ablative resurfacing has been shown to be an effective treatment for striae, acne scarring, burn scars, surgical or traumatic scars, and can be used for topical drug-delivery (**Figs. 8** and **9**).[84,85]

Fractional Carbon Dioxide

As mentioned earlier, the fractional ablative CO_2 device has become more mainstream than fully ablative laser resurfacing due to faster wound healing and improved safety profile. This device has been shown to be effective for the treatment of photodamage, rhytids, scars, and dyschromia similar to the fully ablative CO_2; however, to a lesser degree with around 50% of the collagen induction and remodeling seen postprocedure.[81]

There are several different types of fractional ablative CO_2 devices available. One commonly used device has a microbeam with a rolling tip that allows for a certain amount

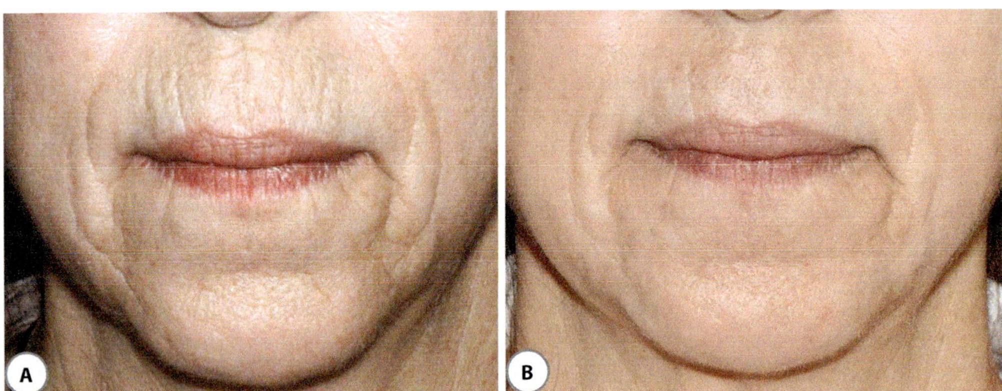

FIGS. 8A AND B: A 39–year-old Caucasian woman with history of smoking and significant upper lip lines. Botulinum toxin was utilized to two weeks prior to treatment (A). Significant improvement is noted 13 months after her fractional ablative CO_2 laser treatment and continued use of botulinum toxin to the upper lip lines (B).
Courtesy: Suzanne Linsmeier Kilmer at the Laser and Skin Surgery Center of Northern California.

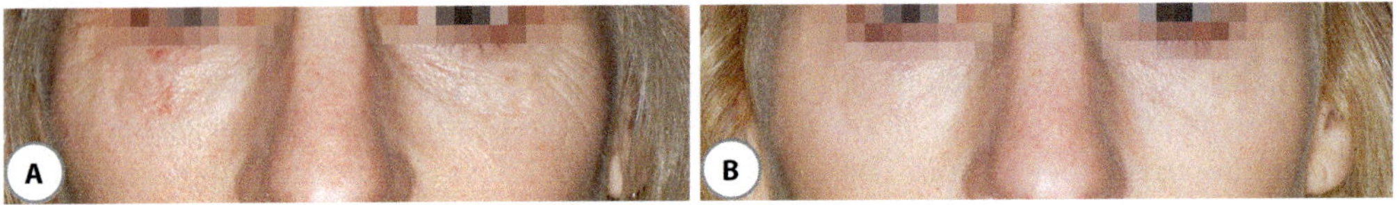

FIGS. 9A AND B: A 38-year-old woman pre (A) and post (B) a single fractional ablative CO_2 laser treatment at 20 mJ and 20% density.
Courtesy: Suzanne Linsmeier Kilmer at the Laser and Skin Surgery Center of Northern California.

of coverage per pass based upon the density. This device has a random distribution of microbeams in order to prevent bulk heating. The random distribution of the beams also allows for a more naturally blended or feathered margin of treatment. This device can go up to a peak fluence of 70 mJ/cm^2.

Another frequently used fractional ablative CO_2 device consists of two different laser handpieces on the same platform that offer dual depth ablation. It is important to note that the settings on these devices are not interchangeable. One handpiece has a 1.3-mm spot size that delivers heat in a nonsequential array with energies ranging from 2 to 225 mJ. A computer pattern generator allows you to change the size and shape of the pattern as well as the density. A density of 3 is around 82% ablation and anything above 4–9 is around 100% ablation.[81] 1–2 passes with this handpiece is typically performed with penetration up to the papillary dermis.[86]

For deeper rhytids and scars, there is an alternate handpiece that has a spot size of 0.12 mm and produces a narrower beam with energies ranging from 2.5 to 50 mJ. The depth of ablation varies from around 76 μ at the lowest energy setting of 2.5 mJ to up to 3,500 μ at the highest setting. Densities can range from 5 to 25% (**Figs. 10A** and **B**).[87]

Fractional ablative CO_2 laser resurfacing has been shown to be an effective treatment for moderate to severe acne scarring. Studies have shown after 2–3 treatments there can be up to a 66% improvement of the depths of scars with no long-term side effects from

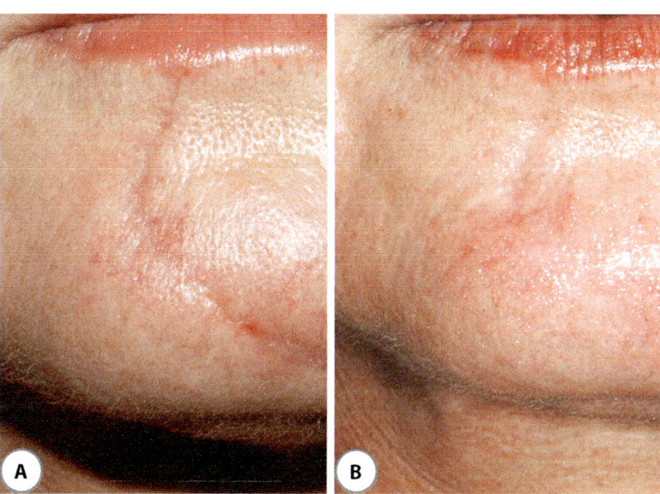

FIGS. 10A AND B: A 28-year-old woman with traumatic scar on her chin before (A) and after (B) two fractional ablative CO_2 laser treatments at 50 mJ and 25% density.

Courtesy: Suzanne Linsmeier Kilmer at the Laser and Skin Surgery Center of Northern California.

the laser.[88,89] It has also been shown to be a safe and effective treatment option for skin textural abnormalities, rhytids, and skin laxity, with a 65% improvement seen after 2–3 treatments.[87,90] Side effects include minor crusting and oozing for up to 72 hours with mild erythema resolving within 1 week posttreatment.[90]

Neocollagenesis and the formation of new elastic fibers can be seen histologically as early as 3 months posttreatment.[91] This may correspond with a peak clinical improvement seen around 3–6 months posttreatment. However, Ortiz found that up to 74% of patients maintained their results for up to 2 years posttreatment, which is similar to the authors experience.[92]

Fractional Erbium-doped:Yttrium Aluminum Garnet

Similar to fractional ablative CO_2 devices, there are also fractional ablative Er:YAG devices. Fractional ablative treatments may be a superior option for patients who have a greater degree of scarring, rhytids, or textural changes who are looking for decreased recovery time. The vaporization of skin tissue initiates the wound healing cascade, dermal remodeling, and neocollagenesis that typically occurs over the next 12 months following the procedure.

There is a profractional device that has a 20 × 20 mm scanner with a 250-μm spot size and an energy of up to 400 J/cm^2. As mentioned earlier in the nonablative section, there is also a hybrid fractional laser that delivers both nonablative and ablative wavelengths within the same pulse. This device has a 1,470 nm nonablative fractional laser that can penetrate up to 700 μ deep, as well as a 2,940 nm fractional ablative wavelength that can reach up to 100 μ in depth. The hybrid laser allows for both superficial improvements of pigmentation and dyschromia as well as improvement of deeper textural abnormalities. It is important to note, that the ablative component allows the heat to escape through the epidermis which also increases the healing time by 1–2 days.[93]

The fractional ablative Er:YAG laser has been shown to treat a wide array of conditions such as photodamage, rhytids, dyschromia, and scarring.[94,95] Typically 2–3 treatments are recommended for optimal results.[95] A split-scar study comparing the fractional ablative Er:YAG laser to the fully ablative Er:YAG laser found the fractional Er:YAG to have a 32% superior outcome as well as increased patient satisfaction (up to 94%) posttreatment.[96] Newer studies have also shown similar results, with an improvement of scar thickness observed after a series of treatments.[97] Additionally, combination treatments have become increasingly common due to excellent results and quicker recovery times.[98]

The histologic effects of the fractional ablative Er:YAG laser are similar to other laser devices. Histology has confirmed an increase in fibroblast activity leading to increased collagen deposition of type I and type III collagen fibers around 3 months posttreatment.[99] Results of the laser have been shown to be maintained for at least 9 months posttreatment.[100]

POSTOPERATIVE CARE

Wound care following the procedure is very important and careful instructions should be given prior to the patient leaving the office. Emollients are recommended immediately postprocedure to provide a protective barrier and inhibit crust formation by keeping the wound moist. Dilute white vinegar soaks are recommended to protect against microbes, as well to enhance removal of necrotic debris. The length and timing of vinegar soaks is practitioner dependent, but we generally recommend a soak every 2–3 hours for around 15–20 minutes. In between the soaks, an occlusive petrolatum is recommended. Some physicians prefer to use occlusive dressings for their postoperative wound care. Occlusive dressings have been proven to accelerate wound healing with quicker re-epithelialization occurring in up to 45% of patients.[101,102] If using occlusive dressings, it is recommended to apply the dressing within 2 hours of treatment and for it to be left in place for at least 1–2 days.[103] However, the risk of infection is often higher with occlusive dressings, so practitioners should consider broadening antibiotic coverage to include gram-negative bacteria.[103]

Postoperative swelling typically peaks on day 2–3, fully resolving by about 1 week. If the patient experiences significant swelling, topical, or oral corticosteroids can be considered; otherwise edema may be controlled with icepacks or head elevation. The combination of edema with an absent epidermal barrier creates an environment productive of a serous exudate. During postoperative days 3–5, it is recommended to avoid the use of topicals due to the increased incidence of potential contact dermatitis while the epidermal barrier is not intact. The frequency of the dilute vinegar soaks and petrolatum application may be weaned as re-epithelialization progresses.

Re-epithelialization is typically completed by days 7–10, but may be as soon as days 3–5 if fractional devices are used. At this time, a less occlusive gentle and fragrance-free moisturizer may be applied instead of petrolatum. The application of certain topicals such as vitamin C or a tripeptide/hexapeptide cream may be beneficial.[104] For darker Fitzpatrick skin types, posttreatment skin lighteners, zinc oxide sunscreen, sun avoidance, as well as mild corticosteroids are recommended to decrease the risk of PIH.

COMPLICATIONS

One of the most common complications postablative laser resurfacing is milia formation and acneiform eruptions, occurring in up to 10–15% of patients (**Table 2**).[105] It is helpful to identify this susceptible patient

TABLE 2: Complications.

• Milia	• Erythema (prolonged erythema >1 month)
• Acneiform eruptions	• Hypopigmentation
• Infections (*Pseudomonas aeruginosa* 41%, *Staphylococcus aureus* 35%, *Staphylococcus epidermidis* 35%, and *Candida* 24%)	• Postinflammatory hyperpigmentation
• Scarring	• Ectropion
• Dermatitis: Irritant/allergic contact	• Demarcation areas from missed spots/lack of feathering
Source: Alster 1999, Waldorf 1995.[45,46]	

population prior to the procedure so that less occlusive emollients can be used as well as possible antibiotic prophylaxis with oral doxycycline. As discussed earlier in the postoperative wound care section, edema is expected postprocedure and is generally no more than moderate; however, if the patient experiences significant swelling, topical or oral corticosteroids may be used.

Some degree of postoperative erythema is expected in all patients and is proportional to the depth of resurfacing. Postoperative erythema can last for an average of 4.5 weeks postprocedure, but rarely can persist.[106] For prolonged erythema following resurfacing, follow-up treatment with the PDL or application of topical brimonidine tartrate 0.33% gel has been shown to be effective.[107]

Pruritus is also a frequent complaint during postoperative week 2 that often responds to oral antihistamines; however, if the pruritus seems to be persistent or worsening, an infection or contact dermatitis must be ruled out. Symptoms of a skin infection may appear atypical due to the absent epidermis and not only present as pruritus, but as pain. Rates of infection are documented to be as high as 8.4%, with the most common microorganisms being *Staphylococcus* and *Pseudomonas*, similar to those found in burn injuries.[108] If the infection does not seem to be responding to typical antibiotics, it is important to broaden the coverage to include antifungals. Postoperative infection with HSV has also been reported to occur in 7.4% of patients, despite no prior history of the virus.[105] Therefore, we pretreat all patients with oral antivirals prior to the procedure to help prevent this complication. Nevertheless, infections still occur and should be treated according to the culture and sensitivity results. Often aerobic and anaerobic cultures are performed and a smear or tissue culture may be necessary if an atypical mycobacterial or fungal infection is suspected.

As mentioned earlier, patients with Fitzpatrick IV–VI skin types are at increased risk of PIH postprocedure.[109] Treatment of hyperpigmentation includes strict sun avoidance for 1 month following treatment as well as zinc oxide sunscreen and topical skin lighteners. We generally recommend lower density fractional ablative laser treatments spaced across greater treatment intervals for this patient population.[110]

Hypopigmentation is a complication that typically appears 6–12 months after treatment. The risk of hypopigmentation typically correlates with the treatment depth and degree of thermal injury which is more common with fully ablative laser resurfacing. The incidence of hypopigmentation is unclear, with a majority of cases suspected to be pseudohypopigmentation (where the new skin of the treated area appears lighter than the surrounding sun damaged skin).[111] Less commonly encountered, but one of the most feared complications is scarring. Scarring is more frequently seen with fully ablative laser resurfacing or with aggressive treatment settings. The neck is the highest risk area for scarring due to decreased pilosebaceous units, a thinner dermis, and increased traction which is why fractional ablative laser treatments are typically preferred in this area. Lower treatment fluences and densities should be used, however, scarring has still been reported.[112,113]

Finally, several ocular complications have been reported to occur postresurfacing with a majority of them seen with fully ablative laser resurfacing. Precaution has to be taken when working within the orbital rim or eyelid area, with moist gauze and intraocular eye shields in place to help prevent some of these complications.[114,115]

COMBINATION TREATMENTS AND LASER-ASSISTED DRUG DELIVERY

As technology continues to advance, the landscape of laser surgery is constantly evolving. Typically patients do not come in for just one cosmetic concern and often have multiple concerns that can be addressed with multiple different lasers, often on the same day.[116,117] There have also been studies that suggest combination laser treatments may lead to superior results and is theorized to be due to greater fibroblast activation and collagen production. Typically, erythema and telangiectasias should be addressed first, followed by the treatment of lentigines or dyschromia, and finally textural abnormalities or rhytids.[118,119] When treatments are individualized to specifically address a patient's cosmetic concerns, there is also a greater degree patient satisfaction.[118,119]

Finally, laser assisted drug-delivery can enhance treatment results of rhytids (with topical poly-L-lactic acid), melasma, actinic keratoses (when used in combination with PDT), and photodamage (with topical platelet rich plasma) when applied post-procedure.[84,120,121]

REFERENCES

1. Anderson RR, Parrish JA. Selective photothermolysis: precise microsurgery by selective absorption of pulsed radiation. Science. 1983;220(4596):524-7.
2. Manstein D, Herron GS, Sink RK, Tanner H, Anderson RR. Fractional photothermolysis: a new concept for cutaneous remodeling using microscopic patterns of thermal injury. Lasers Surg Med. 2004;34(5):426-38.
3. Waldman A, Bolotin D, Arndt KA, Dover JS, Geronemus RG, Chapas A, et al. ASDS Guidelines Task Force: Consensus Recommendations Regarding the Safety of Lasers, Dermabrasion, Chemical Peels, Energy Devices, and Skin Surgery During and After Isotretinoin Use. Dermatol Surg. 2017;43(10):1249-62.
4. Spring LK, Krakowski AC, Alam M, Bhatia A, Brauer J, Cohen J, et al. Isotretinoin and Timing of Procedural Interventions: A Systematic Review with Consensus Recommendations. JAMA Dermatol. 2017;153(8):802-9.
5. Lowe NJ, Lask G, Griffin ME. Laser skin resurfacing. Pre- and posttreatment guidelines. Dermatol Surg. 1995;21(12):1017-9.
6. Bellman B, Brandt FS, Holtmann M, Bebell WR. Infection with methicillin-resistant Staphylococcus aureus after carbon dioxide resurfacing of the face. Sucessful treatment with minocycline, rifampin, and mupiricin ointment. Dermatol Surg. 1998;24(2):279-82.
7. Ho C, Nguyen Q, Lowe NJ, Griffin ME, Lask G. Laser resurfacing in pigmented skin. Dermatol Surg. 1995;21(12):1035-7.
8. West TB, Alster TS. Effect of pretreatment on the incidence of hyperpigmentation following cutaneous CO_2 laser resurfacing. Dermatol Surg. 1999;25(1):15-7.
9. Kilmer SL, Chotzen VA, Silva SK, McClaren ML. Safe and effective carbon dioxide laser skin resurfacing of the neck. Lasers Surg Med. 2006;38(7):653-7.
10. Clark SM, Lanigan SW, Marks R. Laser treatment of erythema and telangiectasia associated with rosacea. Lasers Med Sci. 2002;17(1):26-33.
11. Kono T, Chan HH, Groff WF, Sakurai H, Takeuchi M, Yamaki T, et al. Long-pulse pulsed dye laser delivered with compression for treatment of facial lentigines. Dermatol Surg. 2007;33(8):945-50.
12. Zelickson BD, Kilmer SL, Bernstein E, Chotzen VA, Dock J, Mehregan D, et al. Pulsed dye laser therapy for sun damaged skin. Lasers Surg Med. 1999;25(3):229-36.
13. Goldberg DJ. New collagen formation after dermal remodeling with an intense pulsed light source. J Cutan Laser Ther. 2000;2(2):59-61.
14. Cao Y, Huo R, Feng Y, Li Q, Wang F. Effects of intense pulsed light on the biological properties and ultrastructure of skin dermal fibroblasts: potential roles in photoaging. Photomed Laser Surg. 29(5):327-32.

15. Wong WR, Shyu WL, Tsai JW, Hsu KH, Pang JH. Intense pulsed light effects on the expression of extracellular matrix proteins and transforming growth factor beta-1 in skin dermal fibroblasts cultured within contracted collagen lattices. Dermatol Surg. 2009;35(5):816-25.
16. Scattone L, de Avelar Alchorne MM, Michalany N, Miot HA, Higashi VS. Histopathologic changes induced by intense pulsed light in the treatment of poikiloderma of Civatte. Dermatol Surg. 2012;38(7 Pt 1):1010-6.
17. El-Domyati M, El-Ammawi TS, Medhat W, Moawad O, Mahoney MG, Uitto J. Effects of the Nd:YAG 1320-nm laser on skin rejuvenation: clinical and histological correlations. J Cosmet Laser Ther. 13(3):98-106.
18. Chan HHL, Lam LK, Wong DS, Kono T, Trendell-Smith N. Use of 1,320 nm Nd:YAG laser for wrinkle reduction and the treatment of atrophic acne scarring in Asians. Lasers Surg Med 2004;34(2):98-103.
19. Tanzi EL, Williams CM, Alster TS. Treatment of facial rhytides with a nonablative 1,450-nm diode laser: a controlled clinical and histologic study. Dermatol Surg. 2003;29(2):124-8.
20. No D, McClaren M, Chotzen V, Kilmer SL. Sebaceous hyperplasia treated with a 1450-nm diode laser. Dermatol Surg. 2004;30(3):382-4.
21. Tanghetti Md E, Jennings J. A comparative Study with the 755 nm picosecond Alexandrite laser with a diffractive lens array and a 532 nm/1,064 nm Nd:YAG with a holographic optic. Lasers Surg Med. 2018;50(1):37-44.
22. Tanghetti EA. The histology of skin treated with a picosecond alexandrite laser and a fractional lens array. Lasers Surg Med. 2016;48(7):646-52.
23. Gold MH. Dual wavelength treatment protocol with a picosecond laser for the reduction of facial wrinkles. J Cosmet Laser Ther. 2019;21(3):147-51.
24. Lin ET, Chiang HM, Lin BS, Huang YH, Chang CC. Photoaging Reversibility in Asian Patients With Melasma Treated Using Picosecond Lasers With Diffractive Lens Array: A 1-Year Prospective Observational Cohort Study. Dermatol Surg. 2021;47(1):e10-4.
25. Wu DC, Jones IT, Boen M, Al-Haddad M, Goldman MP. A Randomized, Split-Face, Double-Blind Comparison Trial Between Fractionated Frequency-Doubled 1064/532 nm Picosecond Nd:YAG Laser and Fractionated 1927 nm Thulium Fiber Laser for Facial Photorejuvenation. Lasers Surg Med. 2021;53(2):204-11.
26. Torbeck RL, Schilling L, Khorasani H, Dover JS, Arndt KA, Saedi N. Evolution of the Picosecond Laser: A Review of Literature. Dermatol Surg. 2019;45(2):183-94.
27. Weiss RA, McDaniel DH, Weiss MA, Mahoney AM, Beasley KL, Halvorson CR. Safety and efficacy of a novel diffractive lens array using a picosecond 755 nm alexandrite laser for treatment of wrinkles. Lasers Surg Med. 2017;49(1):40-4.
28. Khetarpal S, Desai S, Kruter L, Prather H, Petrell K, Depina J, et al. Picosecond laser with specialized optic for facial rejuvenation using a compressed treatment interval. Lasers Surg Med. 2016;48(8):723-6.
29. Saluja R. Evaluation of the Safety and Efficacy of a Low Fluence, Picopulsed, Alexandrite Laser in a Pico-Toning Technique With a Diffractive Lens Optic for the Treatment of Photodamage and Textural Improvement in "Off the Face" Applications. J Drugs Dermatol. 2016;15(11):1398-1401.
30. Huo MH, Wang YQ, Yang X. Split-face comparison of intense pulsed light and nonablative 1,064-nm Q-switched laser in skin rejuvenation. Dermatol Surg. 2011;37(1):52-7.
31. Alster TS, Lupton JR. Prevention and treatment of side effects and complications of cutaneous laser resurfacing. Plast Reconstr Surg. 2002;109(1):308-16.
32. Goldman MP, Fitzpatrick RE, Ross EV, Kilmer SL, Weiss RA. Lasers and Energy Devices for the Skin. CRC Press. 2013:178-85.
33. Brauer JA, McDaniel DH, Bloom BS, Reddy KK, Bernstein LJ, Geronemus RG. Nonablative 1927 nm fractional resurfacing for the treatment of facial photopigmentation. J Drugs Dermatol. 2014;13(11):1317-22.
34. Narurkar VA, Alster TS, Bernstein EF, Lin TJ, Loncaric A. Safety and Efficacy of a 1550nm/1927nm Dual Wavelength Laser for the Treatment of Photodamaged Skin. J Drugs Dermatol. 2018;17(1):41-6.
35. Wanner M, Tanzi EL, Alster TS. Fractional photothermolysis: treatment of facial and nonfacial cutaneous photodamage with a 1,550-nm erbium-doped fiber laser. Dermatol Surg. 2007;33(1):23-8.
36. Bae YSC, Rettig S, Weiss E, Bernstein L, Geronemus R. Treatment of Post-Inflammatory Hyperpigmentation in Patients with Darker Skin Types Using a Low Energy 1,927 nm Non-Ablative Fractional Laser: A Retrospective Photographic Review Analysis. Lasers Surg Med. 2020;52(1):7-12.
37. Waibel S, Pozner J, Robb C, Tanzi E. Hybrid Fractional Laser: A Multi-Center Trial on the Safety and Efficacy for Photorejuvenation. J Drugs Dermatol. 2018;17(11):1164-8.
38. Cohen JL, Ross EV. Combined fractional ablative and nonablative laser resurfacing treatment: a split-face comparative study. J Drugs Dermatol. 2013;12(2):175-8.
39. Brown MM, Ortiz A. Hybrid Fractional Ablative and Nonablative Laser Resurfacing of Actinic Keratoses. Dermatol Surg. 2019;45(3):468-70.
40. Robinson DM, Frulla AP. Randomized, Split-Face/Decollete Comparative Trial of Procedure Enhancement System for Fractional non-Ablative Laser Resurfacing Treatment. J Drugs Dermatol. 2017;16(7):707-10.

41. Graber EM, Tanzi EL, Alster TS. Side effects and complications of fractional laser photothermolysis: experience with 961 treatments. Dermatol Surg. 2008;34(3):301-5.
42. Lee SM, Kim MS, Kim YJ, Won CH, Lee MW, Choi JH, et al. Adverse events of non-ablative fractional laser photothermolysis: a retrospective study of 856 treatments in 362 patients. J Dermatolog Treat. 2014;25(4):304-7.
43. Chan HH, Manstein D, Yu CS, Shek S, Kono T, Wei WI. The prevalence and risk factors of post-inflammatory hyperpigmentation after fractional resurfacing in Asians. Lasers Surg Med. 2007;39(5):381-5.
44. Xu LY, Kilmer SL, Ross EV, Avram MM. Bacterial infections following non-ablative fractional laser treatment: a case series and discussion. Lasers Surg Med. 2015;47(2): 128-32.
45. Alster TS. Cutaneous resurfacing with CO_2 and erbium: YAG lasers: preoperative, intraoperative, and postoperative considerations. Plast Reconstr Surg. 1999;103(2): 619-32.
46. Waldorf HA, Kauvar AN, Geronemus RG. Skin resurfacing of fine to deep rhytides using a char-free carbon dioxide laser in 47 patients. Dermatol Surg. 1995;21(11): 940-6.
47. Trelles MA, David LM, Rigau J. Penetration depth of Ultrapulse carbon dioxide laser in human skin. Dermatol Surg. 1996;22(10):863-5.
48. Fitzpatrick RE, Smith SR, Sriprachya-anunt S. Depth of vaporization and the effect of pulse stacking with a high-energy, pulsed carbon dioxide laser." J Am Acad Dermatol. 1999;40(4):615-22.
49. Ross EV, Mowlavi A, Barnette D, Glatter RD, Grevelink JM. The effect of wiping on skin resurfacing in a pig model using a high energy pulsed CO_2 laser system. Dermatol Surg. 25(2):81-8.
50. Bernstein LJ, Kauvar AN, Grossman MC, Geronemus RG. The short- and long-term side effects of carbon dioxide laser resurfacing. Dermatol Surg. 1997;23(7):519-25.
51. Rosenberg GJ. Full face and neck laser skin resurfacing. Plast Reconstr Surg. 1997;100(7):1846-54.
52. Alster TS, Garg S. Treatment of facial rhytides with a high-energy pulsed carbon dioxide laser. Plast Reconstr Surg. 1996;98(5):791-4.
53. West TB, Alster TS. Effect of botulinum toxin type A on movement-associated rhytides following CO_2 laser resurfacing. Dermatol Surg. 1999;25(4):259-61.
54. Alster T, Hirsch R. Single-pass CO_2 laser skin resurfacing of light and dark skin: extended experience with 52 patients. J Cosmet Laser Ther. 2003;5(1):39-42.
55. Fitzpatrick RE, Rostan EF, Marchell N. Collagen tightening induced by carbon dioxide laser versus erbium: YAG laser. Lasers Surg Med. 2000;27(5):395-403.
56. Alster TS, Bellew SG. Improvement of dermatochalasis and periorbital rhytides with a high-energy pulsed CO_2 laser: a retrospective study. Dermatol Surg. 2004;30 (4 Pt 1):483-7.
57. Orringer JS, Kang S, Johnson TM, Karimipour DJ, Hamilton T, Hammerberg C, et al. Connective tissue remodeling induced by carbon dioxide laser resurfacing of photodamaged human skin. Arch Dermatol. 2004;140(11):1326-32.
58. Stuzin JM, Baker TJ, Baker TM, Kligman AM. Histologic effects of the high-energy pulsed CO_2 laser on photoaged facial skin. Plast Reconstr Surg. 1997;99(7):2036-50.
59. Ratner D, Viron A, Puvion-Dutilleul F, Puvion E. Pilot ultrastructural evaluation of human preauricular skin before and after high-energy pulsed carbon dioxide laser treatment. Arch Dermatol. 1998;134(5):582-7.
60. Orringer JS, Johnson TM, Kang S, Karimipour DJ, Hammerberg C, Hamilton T, et al. Effect of carbon dioxide laser resurfacing on epidermal p53 immunostaining in photodamaged skin. Arch Dermatol. 140(9):1073-7.
61. Trimas SJ, Ellis DA, Metz RD. The carbon dioxide laser. An alternative for the treatment of actinically damaged skin. Dermatol Surg. 1997;23(10):885-9.
62. Ross EV, Grossman MC, Duke D, Grevelink JM. Long-term results after CO_2 laser skin resurfacing: a comparison of scanned and pulsed systems. J Am Acad Dermatol. 1997;37(5 Pt 1):709-18.
63. McDaniel DH, Lord J, Ash K, Newman J. Combined CO_2/ erbium:YAG laser resurfacing of peri-oral rhytides and side-by-side comparison with carbon dioxide laser alone. Dermatol Surg. 1999;25(4):285-93.
64. Rhie JW, Shim JS, Choi WS. A Pilot Study of Skin Resurfacing Using the 2,790-nm Erbium:YSGG Laser System. Arch Plast Surg. 42(1):52-8.
65. Ross EV, Swann M, Soon S, Izadpanah A, Barnette D, Davenport S. Full-face treatments with the 2790-nm erbium:YSGG laser system. J Drugs Dermatol. 2009;8(3):248-52.
66. Kim S. Treatment of acne scars in Asian patients using a 2,790-nm fractional yttrium scandium gallium garnet laser. Dermatol Surg. 2011;37(10):1464-9.
67. Ciocon DH, Hussain M, Goldberg DJ. High-fluence and high-density treatment of perioral rhytides using a new, fractionated 2,790-nm ablative erbium-doped Yttrium Scandium Gallium Garnet Laser. Dermatol Surg. 2011;37(6):776-81.
68. Walsh JT Jr, Flotte TJ, Deutsch TF. Er:YAG laser ablation of tissue: effect of pulse duration and tissue type on thermal damage. Lasers Surg Med. 1989;9(4):314-26.
69. Alster TS. Clinical and histologic evaluation of six erbium:YAG lasers for cutaneous resurfacing. Lasers Surg Med. 1999;24(2):87-92.

70. Kauvar AN, Geronemus RG. Histology of laser resurfacing. Dermatol Clin. 1997;15(3):459-67.
71. Weinstein C. Erbium laser resurfacing: current concepts. Plast Reconstr Surg. 1999;103(2):602-16.
72. Rostan EF, Fitzpatrick RE, Goldman MP. Laser resurfacing with a long pulse erbium:YAG laser compared to the 950 ms pulsed CO(2) laser. Lasers Surg Med. 2001; 29(2):136-41.
73. Weinstein C. Computerized scanning erbium:YAG laser for skin resurfacing. Dermatol Surg. 1998;24(1):83-9.
74. Goldberg DJ, Cutler KB. The use of the erbium:YAG laser for the treatment of class III rhytids. Dermatol Surg. 1999;25(9):713-5.
75. Ross EV, Anderson RR. The erbium laser in skin resurfacing. In Alster TS Apfelberg DB, eds. Cosmetic Laser Surgery: 2nd ed. John Wiley, New York. 1999:57-84.
76. Alster TS, Lupton JR. Erbium:YAG cutaneous laser resurfacing. Dermatol Clin. 2001;19(3):453-66.
77. Jimenez G, Spencer JM. Erbium:YAG laser resurfacing of the hands, arms, and neck. Dermatol Surg. 1999;25(11):831-4.
78. Khatri KA. Ablation of cutaneous lesions using an erbium:YAG laser. J Cosmet Laser Ther. 2003;5 (3-4):150-3.
79. Cohen JL. Erbium laser resurfacing for actinic cheilitis. J Drugs Dermatol. 2013;12(11):1290-2.
80. Venugopalan V, Nishioka NS, Mikić BB. The effect of laser parameters on the zone of thermal injury produced by laser ablation of biological tissue. J Biomech Eng. 1994;116(1):62-70.
81. Orringer JS, Sachs DL, Shao Y, Hammerberg C, Cui Y, Voorhees JJ, et al. Direct quantitative comparison of molecular responses in photodamaged human skin to fractionated and fully ablative carbon dioxide laser resurfacing. Dermatol Surg. 38(10):1668-77.
82. Xu XG, Luo YJ, Wu Y, Chen JZ, Xu TH, Gao XH, et al. Immunohistological evaluation of skin responses after treatment using a fractional ultrapulse carbon dioxide laser on back skin. Dermatol Surg. 2011;37(8):1141-9.
83. Reilly MJ, Cohen M, Hokugo A, Keller GS. Molecular effects of fractional carbon dioxide laser resurfacing on photodamaged human skin. Arch Facial Plast Surg. 2010;12(5):321-5.
84. Sklar LR, Burnett CT, Waibel JS, Moy RL, Ozog DM. Laser assisted drug delivery: a review of an evolving technology. Lasers Surg Med. 2014;46(4):249-62.
85. Lee SE, Kim JH, Lee SJ, Lee JE, Kang JM, Kim YK, et al. Treatment of striae distensae using an ablative 10,600-nm carbon dioxide fractional laser: a retrospective review of 27 participants. Dermatol Surg. 2010;36(11): 1683-90.
86. Ramsdell WM. Fractional carbon dioxide laser resurfacing. Semin Plast Surg. 2012;26(3):125-30.
87. Rahman Z, MacFalls H, Jiang K, Chan KF, Kelly K, Tournas J, et al. Fractional deep dermal ablation induces tissue tightening. Lasers Surg Med. 2009;41(2):78-86.
88. Chapas AM, Brightman L, Sukal S, Hale E, Daniel D, Bernstein LJ, et al. Successful treatment of acneiform scarring with CO_2 ablative fractional resurfacing. Lasers Surg Med. 2008;40(6):381-6.
89. Elcin G, Yalici-Armagan B. Fractional carbon dioxide laser for the treatment of facial atrophic acne scars: prospective clinical trial with short and long-term evaluation. Lasers Med Sci. 2017;32(9):2047-54.
90. Tierney EP, Hanke CW, Watkins L. Treatment of lower eyelid rhytids and laxity with ablative fractionated carbon-dioxide laser resurfacing: Case series and review of the literature. J Am Acad Dermatol. 2011;64(4):730-40.
91. Shah S, Alam M. Laser resurfacing pearls. Semin Plast Surg. 26(3):131-6.
92. Ortiz AE, Tremaine AM, Zachary CB. Long-term efficacy of a fractional resurfacing device. Lasers Surg Med. 2010;42(2):168-70.
93. Orringer JS, Rittié L, Hamilton T, Karimipour DJ, Voorhees JJ, Fisher GJ. Intraepidermal erbium:YAG laser resurfacing: impact on the dermal matrix. J Am Acad Dermatol. 2011;64(1):119-28.
94. Dadkhahfar S, Fadakar K, Robati RM. Efficacy and safety of long pulse Nd:YAG laser versus fractional erbium:YAG laser in the treatment of facial skin wrinkles. Lasers Med Sci. 2019;34(3):457-64.
95. Moon HR, Yun WJ, Lee YJ, Lee MW, Chang S. A prospective, randomized, double-blind comparison of an ablative fractional 2940-nm erbium-doped yttrium aluminum garnet laser with a nonablative fractional 1550-nm erbium-doped glass laser for the treatment of photoaged Asian skin. J Dermatolog Treat. 2015;26(6):551-7.
96. Tidwell WJ, Owen CE, Kulp-Shorten C, Maity A, McCall M, Brown TS. Fractionated Er:YAG laser versus fully ablative Er:YAG laser for scar revision: Results of a split scar, double blinded, prospective trial. Lasers Surg Med. 2016;48(9):837-43.
97. Wulkan AJ, Rudnick A, Badiavas E, Waibel JS. Treatment of Hypertrophic Burn and Traumatic Scars With a 2,940-nm Fractional Ablative Erbium-doped Yttrium Aluminium Garnet Laser: A Pilot Study. Dermatol Surg. 2020;46(6):789-93.
98. Mani N, Pajk F, Vizintin Z. Full-face skin resurfacing using a combination of fractional and full spot ablative 2940 nm erbium laser. J Cosmet Dermatol. 2021;20(1):110-5.
99. Borges J, Araújo L, Cuzzi T, Martinez L, Gonzales Y, Manela-Azulay M. Fractional Laser Resurfacing Treats Photoaging by Promoting Neocollegenesis and Cutaneous Edema. J Clin Aesthet Dermatol. 2020;13(1):22-7.

100. Lapidoth M, Yagima Odo ME, Odo LM. Novel use of erbium:YAG (2,940-nm) laser for fractional ablative photothermolysis in the treatment of photodamaged facial skin: a pilot study. Dermatol Surg. 2008;34(8):1048-53.
101. Bolton LL, Johnson CL, Rijswijk LV. Occlusive Dressings: therapeutic agents and effects on drug delivery. Clin Dermatol. 1991;9(4):573-83.
102. Kannon GA, Garrett AB. Moist wound healing with occlusive dressings. A clinical review. Dermatol Surg. 1995;21(7):583-90.
103. Eaglstein WH, Davis SC, Mehle AL, Mertz PM. Optimal use of an occlusive dressing to enhance healing. Effect of delayed application and early removal on wound healing. Arch Dermatol. 1988;124(3):392-5.
104. Waibel JS, Mi QS, Ozog D, Qu L, Zhou L, Rudnick A, et al. Laser-assisted delivery of vitamin C, vitamin E, and ferulic acid formula serum decreases fractional laser postoperative recovery by increased beta fibroblast growth factor expression. Lasers Surg Med. 2016;48(3): 238-44.
105. Nanni CA, Alster TS. Complications of carbon dioxide laser resurfacing. An evaluation of 500 patients. Dermatol Surg. 1998;24(3):315-20.
106. Tanzi EL, Alster TS. Single-pass carbon dioxide versus multiple-pass Er:YAG laser skin resurfacing: a comparison of postoperative wound healing and side-effect rates. Dermatol Surg. 2003;29(1):80-4.
107. Braun SA, Artzi O, Gerber PA. Brimonidine tartrate 0.33% gel for the management of posttreatment erythema induced by laser skin resurfacing. J Am Acad Dermatol. 2017;76(2):e53-5.
108. Husain MT, Karim QN, Tajuri S. Analysis of infection in a burn ward. Burns. 1989;15(5):299-302.
109. Alster TS. Comparison of two high-energy pulsed CO_2 lasers in the treatment of periorbital rhytides. Dermatol Surg. 1996;22(6):541-5.
110. Wat H, Wu DC, Chan HHL. Fractional resurfacing in the Asian patient: Current state of the art. Lasers Surg Med. 2017;49(1):45-59.
111. Hunzeker CM, Weiss ET, Geronemus RG. Fractionated CO_2 laser resurfacing: our experience with more than 2000 treatments. Aesthet Surg J. 2009;29(4):317-22.
112. Duplechain JK. Severe neck scarring: A consequence of fractional CO_2 laser resurfacing. J Cosmet Laser Ther. 2016;18(6):352-4.
113. Avram MM, Tope WD, Yu T, Szachowicz E, Nelson SJ. Hypertrophic Scarring of the Neck Following Ablative Fractional Carbon Dioxide Laser Resurfacing. Lasers Surg Med. 2009;41(3):185-8.
114. Widder RA, Severin M, Kirchhof B, Krieglstein GK. Corneal injury after carbon dioxide laser skin resurfacing. Am J Ophthalmol. 1998;125(3)392-4.
115. Roberts TL, Lettieri JT, Elllis LB. CO_2 laser resurfacing: recognizing and minimizing complications. Aesth Surg J. 1996;16(2):142-8.
116. Mervak JE, Gan SD, Smith EH, Wang F. Facial Erosive Pustular Dermatosis After Cosmetic Resurfacing. JAMA Dermatol. 2017;153(10):1021-5.
117. Shah GM, Kilmer SL. Combined nonablative rejuvenation techniques. Dermatol Surg. 2005;31(9 Pt 2):1206-10.
118. Wu DC, Fitzpatrick RE. Facial rejuvenation via the sequential combined use of multiple laser modalities: Safety and efficacy. Lasers Surg Med. 2016;48(6):577-83.
119. Manuskiatti W, Fitzpatrick RE, Goldman MP. Treatment of facial skin using combinations of CO_2, Q-switched alexandrite, flashlamp-pumped pulsed dye, and Er:YAG lasers in the same treatment session. Dermatol Surg. 2000;26(2):114-20.
120. Ibrahim O, Ionta S, Depina J, Petrell K, Arndt KA, Dover JS. Safety of Laser-Assisted Delivery of Topical Poly-L-Lactic Acid in the Treatment of Upper Lip Rhytides: A Prospective, Rater-Blinded Study. Dermatol Surg. 2019;45(7):968-74.
121. El-Taieb MA, Ibrahim HM, Hegazy EM, Ibrahim AK, Gamal AM, Nada EA. Fractional Erbium-YAG Laser and Platelet-Rich Plasma as Single or Combined Treatment for Atrophic Acne Scars: A Randomized Clinical Trial. Dermatol Ther (Heidelb). 2019;9(4):707-17.

16

CHAPTER

Skin Tightening

Macrene Renee Alexiades

INTRODUCTION

- Skin tightening is a non-surgical approach to treating rhytids and skin laxity that is in high demand.
- The main nonsurgical skin tightening technologies include radiofrequency (RF), infrared light, and ultrasound technologies.
- Treatment protocols employ reduced energy settings or mobile delivery techniques, improving safety and comfort; needle-delivery improves efficacy.
- Skin-tightening technologies work by delivering energy into the dermis or subcutis, generating heat which results dermal and subdermal tissue remodeling.
- Patient consultation, selection, and modulating expectations are important.
- Skin tightening treatments reduce skin laxity and improve contour definition of the lower face, jawline and neck, and periorbital and brow regions.
- Combination of skin tightening devices with dermal fillers and neurotoxins serve to achieve better global improvement.
- Adverse events such as burns, indentations, scars, or changes in pigmentation are rare with these technologies.

The clinical signs of skin aging have been classified into rhytides, laxity, and the categories of photoaging, including dyspigmentation, erythema/telangiectasia, solar elastosis, keratosis, and textural changes, though skin tightening is a term ascribed to the treatment of skin laxity (**Table 1**).[1-3] Over the past several decades, lasers, light, and energy-based technologies have been developed to treat individual or grouped categories of skin aging.[1] With increasing specialization, some devices target rhytids or dyspigmentation or vascularity, while others have evolved to preferentially treat skin laxity. Among the devices targeting skin laxity and resulting in skin tightening, RF, broadband light, and ultrasound are the best known.

In the 1990s, ablative resurfacing lasers had been used for facial skin tightening.[4] Despite high efficacy for rhytid-reduction and to an extent skin tightening, ablative devices required significant recovery time, prolonged wound healing, and an increased risk of side effects and complications. Nonablative and minimally-invasive technologies with little to no recovery time and a more favorable risk-reward profile without epidermal vaporization

TABLE 1: Quantitative comprehensive grading scale of laxity. This four point grading scale has been extensively tested and employed for evaluating laser and energy-based cosmetic treatments.[1-3]

Alexiades grading scale of skin laxity		
Grading Scale	Descriptive Parameter	Laxity
0	None	None
1	Mild	Localized to nasolabial (NL) folds
1.5	Mild	Localized, NL, and early melolabial (ML) folds
2	Moderate	Localized, NL/ML folds, early jowls, and early submental/submandibular (SM)
2.5	Moderate	Localized, prominent NL/ML folds, jowls, and SM
3	Advanced	Prominent NL/ML folds, jowls, and SM, early neck strands
3.5	Advanced	Deep NL/ML folds, prominent jowls and SM, and prominent neck strands
4	Severe	Marked NL/ML folds, jowls and SM, neck redundancy, and strands

have been developed. Today, the gold standard of skin tightening remains surgical face and neck lifting, termed rhytidectomy or surgical redraping, but engenders fear in patients due to the morbidity and significant cosmetic alteration that surgery incurs. The demand for nonsurgical alternatives has resulted in the burgeoning of skin tightening technologies, which are not yet a replacement for those with advanced to severe skin laxity (see **Table 1**), but permit an alternative for mild-to-moderate skin laxity candidates willing to accept less efficacy for the promise of easy recovery and rare side effects or complications.

Pearl: It is strongly urged that standardized photographs, front and side views, before and at each follow up interval following skin-tightening procedures. Pretreatment and posttreatment photographs may need to be compared since changes with skin-tightening procedures may be subtle to the patient, especially after several months have passed.

SKIN TIGHTENING TECHNOLOGIES: SCIENTIFIC BASIS

Radiofrequency, infrared light, and ultrasound technologies work by delivering energy to the skin or underlying structures. This creates thermal, mechanical, and biochemical effects that lead to collagen denaturation and dermal remodeling that increases volume and improves the elastic properties of the skin.[5] Starting in the third decade of life, collagen and elastin synthesis decrease, and elastin fibers are degraded due to sun exposure. Collagen fibers are composed of a triple helix of protein chains linked with interchain bonds into a crystalline structure. When collagen fibers are heated to specific temperatures, they contract due to breakage of intramolecular hydrogen bonds. It had been thought that contraction causes the crystalline triple helix structure to fold, creating thicker and shorter collagen fibers resulting in tissue tightening.

However, recent findings have demonstrated that partially denatured collagen is superior to fully denatured collagen in inducing histologic dermal remodeling and clinical laxity reduction.[6] Fully denatured collagen >70°C resulted in charring of collagen and lower clinical efficacy; maximal volumes of partial collagen denaturation and optimal clinical efficacy was found at intradermal temperatures of 62–67°C. The current author theorized that exposure of RGD sequences on partially heat-denatured collagen are required for induction of neocollagenesis and neoelastinogenesis.[6] The process of neocollagenesis has been demonstrated to take up to 12 months following treatment to complete and this correlates with continued clinical improvement.

RADIOFREQUENCY

Mechanism of Action

More than any other technology, RF is known for skin tightening of the lower face and neck. Volumetric heating is delivered to dermis and this controlled thermal injury induces neocollagenesis and neoelastogenesis. These histologic changes correlate clinically with rhytid and laxity reduction. RF is in the 3 kHz–24 GHz frequency range. RF for medical use employs an oscillating electrical current which induces collisions between charged atoms and molecules in tissue generating heat. Penetration depth inversely proportional to frequency with lower RF frequencies penetrating more deeply when applied to skin surface. Heat is generated from the resistance of tissue components to the movement of electrons within the oscillating RF field as governed by Ohm's law. This resistance, called impedance, generates heat relative to the amount of current and time, converting electrical current to thermal energy.

BOX 1: Radiofrequency classification.

- Noninvasive = Skin surface
  - Monopolar
  - Unipolar
  - Bipolar: Nonablative and ablative
  - Tripolar
- Minimally-invasive = Inserted
  - Needle-based bipolar: Dermal/subdermal
  - Probe-based monopolar: Subdermal

Subtypes

Radiofrequency devices may be classified as noninvasive or skin surface applied and minimally-invasive or needle- and probe-delivered (**Box 1**). They may also be classified according to the electrode configuration. Monopolar RF contains a single electrode in the handpiece tip with a grounding pad attached to the patient, wherein the current passes from the electrode through the patient and exits via the grounding pad. Unipolar RF employs a single electrode in the handpiece; however, rather than an oscillating current, this delivers RF via antenna transmission. Bipolar and tripolar RF employs multiple electrodes in the handpiece tip such that the current passes through the skin and exits to the skin surface via a closed circuit. While the latter types of electrode configuration have a more controlled current distribution, the depth of penetration is limited to approximately one-half the distance between the electrodes.

With RF, the penetration depth depends upon mode of delivery (i.e., skin surface, needle-based or probe-based), the configuration of the electrodes (i.e., monopolar or multipolar), the tissue type (i.e., skin, fat, and other), and the frequency of the electrical current (**Table 2**). Structures with higher conductivity and impedance generate more heat. Fat, bone, and dry skin have low conductivities and

TABLE 2: Skin tightening devices.

Skin-tightening technology	Device
Monopolar radiofrequency (RF)	Thermage® (Solta)
	Exilis® (BTL)
	Trusculpt® (Cutera)
	Pelleve® (Cynosure)
Monopolar RF probe-delivery	ThermiTight® (Thermi)
Bipolar RF	Vela III, Elos Plus, Galaxy®, Aurora®, Polaris®, ReFirme® (Syneron-Candela)
	Sublime® (Syneron-Candela)
	Evoke (InMode)
	Accent/VShape® (Alma)
	Reaction, V Touch (Viora)
	EndyMed PRO (EndyMed)
	TiteFx (Invasix)
Bipolar RF + vacuum	Aluma® (Lumenis)
Bipolar RF needle-delivery	Profound® (Syneron-Candela)
	Infini/Genius
	Intensif (Endymed)
	Morpheus8 (InMode)
	Fractora (Invasix)
Bipolar RF probe	Bodytite/Facetite(R) (InMode)
Tripolar RF	Tri-Active® (DEKA)
	Pollogen (Apollo)
Broadband infrared light	Titan® (Cutera)
	NIR® (Alma)
	Icon® (Palomar)
	SkinTyte® (Sciton)
Unipolar and bipolar radiofrequency	Accent® (Alma)
Ultrasound technology	Ulthera® (Merz)

current flows around rather than through these structures; in contrast, hydrated skin possesses higher electrical conductivity allowing greater penetration of current. Improved results may be observed with coupling fluid and increased hydration.

MONOPOLAR RADIOFREQUENCY

Skin Surface Monopolar Radiofrequency

The first monopolar tissue-tightening device was Food and Drug Administration

(FDA)-cleared in 2001 (Thermage®, Solta Medical, Hayward, CA) (**Table 2**). A disposable membrane tip with a capacitive-coupled electrode is applied at a single contact point with a frequency of 6 MHz and an adhesive grounding pad to complete the circuit. Since its introduction, the protocol has been altered to a low energy multipass method which reduced the discomfort and risk of atrophic scarring, while increasing response rate. Vibration [comfort pulse technology (CPT)] has been added to the system to reduce pain sensation. Monopolar RF is used for skin tightening to the face, neck, eyelids, abdomen, and extremities.

The clinical results of monopolar RF skin tightening were first reported in 2003 by the author and colleagues for the jowls and neck, and by Fitzpatrick and colleagues for the periorbital area.[7,8] In 2007, Dover et al. compared the original single-pass, high-energy method with the low-energy, multiple-pass technique with efficacy of skin tightening of 54% and 92%, respectively, at 6 months. With the updated protocol, anesthesia is not required and the incidence of adverse events was also reduced to <0.05%.[9] The device does not provide real-time temperature feedback, so relying on patient verbal feedback regarding heat pain is still required.

Another skin surface applied monopolar RF device used for skin tightening is Trusculpt® by Cutera (**Fig. 1**). This device operates at a frequency of 1–2 MHz; electrode sizes of 16, 25, and 40 cm^2, and provides the significant advantage of real-time temperature feedback. This allows for a quantitative delivery of energy until a specified target skin surface temperature is attained and better control over outcomes. Temperatures of 42–46°C are necessary to attain tissue tightening. While the 1 MHz and 16 cm^2 tip is used for skin tightening, the recent Trusculpt 3D at 2 MHz and large handpieces targets skin tightening and fat reduction, with approximately 25% circumferential reduction in over 90% of patients.[10]

A skin surface applied monopolar RF device (Pelleve, Elliman) operates at 4 MHz and offers a range of handpiece tip sizes from 7.5 to 20 mm^2. A 50% improvement in skin laxity, rhytids, and texture were reported 1 year following six treatments.[11]

The NuEra, Lumenis platform provides three alternative frequencies of RF (470 kHz, 1 MHz, 2 MHz). Currently completing a clinical trial, the author presents the outcomes on abdomen here (**Fig. 2**, Alexiades, manuscript in preparation).

Probe-delivered Monopolar Radiofrequency

A monopolar RF device delivered via a probe to the subdermal plane has been employed for skin tightening of the jawline and neck (ThermiTight, ThermiAesthetics, Irving, TX). A blunt 10 cm long, 18-gauge percutaneous treatment probe is inserted and the distal end administers the RF. A temperature sensor is located in the probe tip that initiates an automatic feedback loop to maintain subdermal tissue temperature. The device is set to maintain a 50–60°C temperature in the subdermal plane. Subdermal temperatures of 65°C and 50°C correlated with skin surface temperatures of 41.6°C and 41.1°C, respectively.[12]

BIPOLAR RADIOFREQUENCY

Skin Surface Bipolar Radiofrequency

Skin surface applied bipolar RF skin-tightening devices combining RF energy with optical energy from laser or light sources include the Galaxy®, Aurora®, Polaris®, ReFirme®, Sublime, and Vela III systems (Syneron-Candela, Massachusetts). The hypothetical advantage to these devices is that the two

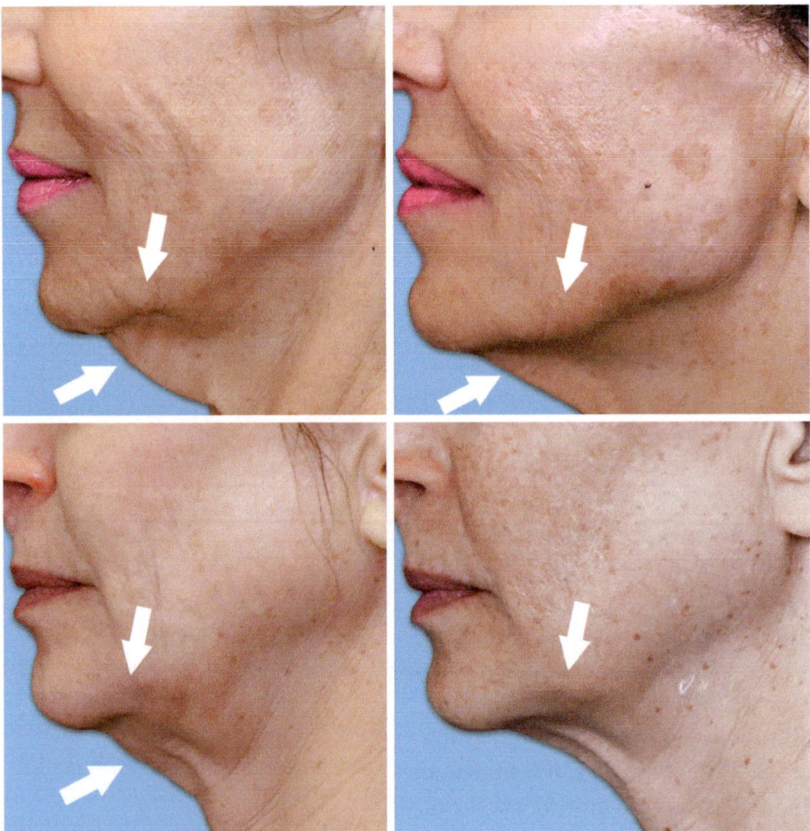

FIG. 1: Before and after photographs following a single radiofrequency microneedle (Profound, Candela Lasers) improved mandibular definition and reduced jowling.
Courtesy: Macrene Renee Alexiades.

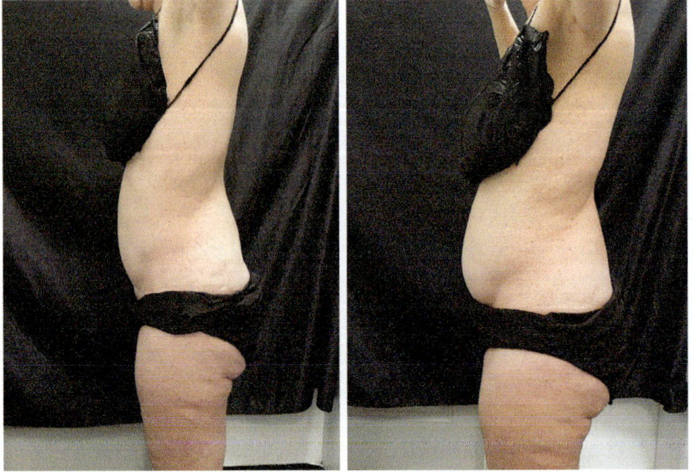

FIG. 2: Before and after monopolar radiofrequency skin tightening treatment (NuEra, Lumenis).
Courtesy: Macrene Renee Alexiades.

forms of energy may act synergistically to generate heat. The current flows between the electrodes in the handpiece tip rather than throughout the remainder of the body as with monopolar systems. One important adverse event with these devices is arcing, which occurs when inadequate coupling gel is applied and when the handpiece is not in full contact with the skin. Arcing may cause tissue burns and possible scar formation.

In 2005, Doshi and Alster reported treatment of 20 subjects with bipolar RF and diode with a (RF: 50–85 J/cm^2, optical energy: 32–40 J/cm^2). Modest improvement was reported at 3 months; with slightly less efficacy at 6 months. Sadick et al. conducted a two-center study using combination intense pulsed light and bipolar RF (RF: up to 20 J/cm^2, optical energy: 30–45 J/cm^2) over five treatments for facial rhytides and skin laxity. Modest improvements were reported with some instances of scarring and crusting. In 2006, the current author reported approximately 10% reduction in skin laxity per treatment with bipolar RF combined with diode laser and infrared light.[2] In 2007, Yu and colleagues employed combination bipolar RF and infrared energy to study skin tightening in a series of three treatments on 19 female Asian patients (RF: 70–120 J/cm^2, optical energy: 10 J/cm^2). Objective assessment showed mild to moderate improvement in 26–47% of areas treated.

Probe-delivered Bipolar Radiofrequency

A probe-based RF system was developed with energy delivered between two electrodes: One applied externally to the skin surface and an internal probe situation beneath it within the subcutaneous fat layer [BodyTite/SkinTite, InMode Corporation (R)]. Several studies have shown internal temperatures reaching 70°C with external skin surface temperatures of approximately 40°C. This device is often paired with liposuction to provide a skin tightening effect in concert.

Vacuum-assisted Bipolar Radiofrequency

Bipolar RF combined with vacuum (Aluma®, Lumenis, Santa Clara, CA) used FACES (functional aspiration controlled electro-thermal stimulation) technology. The vacuum apparatus suctions a fold of skin in alignment between two electrodes in an effort to overcome the depth limitations inherent in bipolar RF by bringing the target tissue closer to the electrodes. Vacuum technology has the added benefit of helping to reduce procedure discomfort.

Gold reported significant improvement in skin texture and a skin tightening effect in 46 adults undergoing eight facial treatments with vacuum-assisted bipolar RF. The authors noted a short-term tightening effect due to collagen contraction followed by a gradual, long-term improvement due to the wound-healing response and neocollagenesis.

Needle-delivered Bipolar Radiofrequency

The prototype device using needle-delivered bipolar RF is the Profound® (Candela-Syneron, Wayland, MA). The Profound® device pioneered a microneedle electrode array to deliver bipolar RF into the reticular dermis while bypassing the epidermis and papillary dermis and provided for the first time real-time temperature feedback using temperature thermistors in the electrode tips. Single-use treatment cartridges are utilized that contain five independently controlled, 32-gauge, bipolar microneedle pairs. The 250 μm needles are spaced 1.25 mm apart and each needle pair is independently powered by the generator. The needles are 6 mm long, with the top 3 mm insulated to protect the superficial portion of the skin during treatment, and the bottom 3 mm exposed to allow electrical current flow. The needles are inserted at a 25° angle to the epidermis so that the tip of the needle is 2 mm from the epidermis. Insertion is done by spring-loaded injection. Because current flows between the two needles in each pair, the RF energy creates fractionated zones (one between each pair) of thermal injury situated in the deep dermis 1–2 mm from the surface of the skin. Epidermal cooling is achieved via an integrated thermokinetic cooling bar on the applicator. This approach creates zones of thermal injury with real-time temperature monitoring, with temperature sensors in each electrode tip to help maintain a preselected target temperature regardless of varying skin conditions and improving consistency between patients.

The current author and colleagues compared baseline and 3–6-month follow-up photographs of 15 patients who underwent skin tightening using a microneedle RF device with those of six patients who had undergone rhytidectomy. The RF device patients were judged to have a 16% improvement from baseline and the surgical patients were judged to have a 49% improvement from baseline laxity grades, or a 0.46 versus 1.20 laxity grade reduction, respectively. The laxity grade reduction result from a single microneedle RF treatment was 37% that of a surgical facelift. In the subsequent multicenter, clinical trial and multi-arm studies of target dermal temperatures ranging from 52°C to 78°C, the current author and colleagues discovered that temperatures 67°C cohort resulted in maximal neocollagenesis, neoelastogenesis, and hyaluronic acid production and correlated clinically with maximal rhytid and laxity reduction, and a 100% response rate. Higher and lower target temperatures demonstrated less efficacy. The findings made possible by needle-delivered RF support the theory that partially denatured collagen is more effective at triggering a strong wound healing response.

Additional needle-delivered bipolar RF devices have since been developed. The Infini® (Lutronic) provides the feature of adjustable needle depths to 0.5, 1.0, 1.5, 2.0, and 3.5 mm. The device offers a 49 needle tip (10 × 10 mm, 7 × 7 needles) and a 16 needle tip (5 × 5 mm, 4 × 4 needles). The microneedles are made from surgical stainless steel, coated with gold for conductivity and then double coated with an insulating silicon compound, except for the first 300 μm of the tip. The needles have a diameter of 200 μm and a point diameter of 20 μm. The insulation of the needle shaft means that the active area of the microneedle electrodes is restricted to the tip, and there is no electrothermal damage delivered to the epidermis. Clinical trials have demonstrated wrinkle reduction following treatment with this device, with clinician-assessed overall efficacy and patient satisfaction index similar at from 80.7 to 88.9% and 81.3 to 85.9%.

The Intensif® (EndyMed Medical, Caesarea, Israel) employs 25 noninsulated gold plated microneedle electrodes with a maximum diameter of 300 μm at their base gradually tapered to a sharp edge. Penetration depth is up to 3.5 mm with digitally controlled increments of 0.1 mm. Maximal power is 25 Watts with a maximal pulse duration is 200 ms. When the needles reach the predefined insertion depth, the RF is emitted selectively heating the dermis while sparing the epidermis. The difference in electrical impedance between the epidermis (high impedance) and the dermis (low impedance) ensures RF flow through the dermis. The RF emission delivered over the whole dermal portion of the needle allows effective coagulation resulting in minimal or no bleeding, combined with deep dermal heating.

Another needle-based bipolar RF device is the Fractora® (Invasix), which employs 24 RF conducting needles, alternating current with two long side electrodes. Each needle is 2,500 μm long and 200 × 300 μm wide at the base. The coated needles are insulated along 2,000 μm, leaving the distal 500 μm uncoated. The hand piece was loaded to the Fractora™ platform (also applicable to InMode™ or BodyTite™ platforms, Invasix Ltd./InMode MD Ltd., Israel). The device has been reported to result in significant improvement in acne and acne scars.

The Morpheus[8] platform (InMode) provides a variable depth penetration from 1 to 7 mm with 24 or 12 pins. It developed the additional feature of so-called "burst mode" which delivers pulses to multiple, successive pre-selected depths in one insertion (Alexiades, manuscript in preparation). The potential advantage of this feature is the ability to target different levels pathology when the exact depth is either unknown or when the target spans a broad band of tissue.

UNIPOLAR RADIOFREQUENCY

The first system to combine unipolar and bipolar RF in one device was the Accent® (Accent/V Shape, Alma Lasers, Buffalo Grove, IL). The bipolar electrode handpiece allows for more superficial, localized (nonvolumetric) heating based on tissue resistance to the RF conductive current. The unipolar electrode handpiece targets deeper, volumetric heating via the rotational movement of water molecules in the alternating current of the electromagnetic field. The monopolar handpiece delivers a higher amount of energy since it theoretically is heating a greater tissue volume than the bipolar handpiece. Typically the monopolar handpiece is used to treat the forehead, cheeks, jawline, and neck. The bipolar handpiece is used to treat the glabella, lateral periorbital area, upper lip and chin, and leg. Despite the use of monopolar RF, this particular system uses a closed system where no grounding plate is required.

In 2007, Friedman treated 16 patients with a hybrid monopolar and bipolar RF device; 56% of participants had at least some degree of improvement in the appearance of rhytides and skin laxity. 12 patients had cheek treatments, with five achieving 51–75% improvement and two achieving >75% improvement. Nine had jowl treatments, with four achieving 51–75% improvement and one achieving >75% improvement.[18] Younger patients (25–45 years of age) were found to have a higher satisfaction rate than older patients.[18]

In 2008, the author invented the mobile delivery method using this combined unipolar/bipolar RF device. Mobile delivery was used to increase fluence delivery to the larger collagen fibrils in the dermis, while allowing the epidermis and superficial structures in the skin to cool, obviating pain sensation and improving safety.[19,20] Mild efficacy in skin tightening was observed in this split-face controlled trial comparing the unipolar to the bipolar RF handpiece. However, the current author reported that the skin surface temperature profiles of 40–43°C were required to prevent pain and assure efficacy. The same authors reported efficacy in skin tightening on the body using a similar mobile protocol.[19,20]

Infrared Light Devices

Broadband infrared light devices emitting wavelengths ranging from 800 to 1,800 nm have been utilized for nonablative skin tightening. The infrared rays are filtered to achieve dermal heating, with pre, peri, and post-cooling for epidermal protection. The first such light-based system on the market was the Titan® (Cutera, Brisbane, CAemitting 1,100–1,800 nm to target tissue water as a chromophore, causing collagen denaturation and ultimately collagen and elastin remodeling.

In 2006, Ruiz-Esparza reported treatment of 25 subjects broadband infrared light from 1,100 to 1,800 nm.[21] Following 1–3 treatments, most subjects showed minimal to excellent improvement with immediate skin tightening visible in 22 of the 25 patients. The best results were achieved when using a combination of lower fluences and a high number of pulses. Patients treated at 30 J/cm^2 expressed no pain during the procedure and had a high degree of satisfaction immediately post-procedure. The same year, Zelickson and colleagues looked at ultrastructural changes in cadaver and human skin posttreatment.[22] Collagen fibril alteration was found to be highest with greater fluences and depths of 1-2 mm. Marginal results were observed at shallower depths and lower fluences, which were possibly due to the effect of contact cooling. Comparison of the two studies emphasizes that clinical skin tightening does not always correlate with immediate positive histological findings. This is explained by the fact that full clinical effect may take weeks or months to be demonstrated owing to a secondary wound healing response.

In 2007, Taub et al. reported longer-term (12–18-month) results using the 1,100–1,800 nm infrared device at 34–36 J/cm^2. Results were both immediate and delayed up to 6 months. Clinical outcomes ranged from mild to moderate in most patients. The authors concluded that using a lower fluence range of 30–40 J/cm^2, 2–3 treatments, 1-2 passes, and extra passes on areas that need immediate contraction or along vector lines yielded best results.[23]

In 2009, the author demonstrated that mobile delivery of broad-band infrared light (1,100–1,800 nm, Titan®, Cutera) allowed for delivery of 30% higher fluences of 44–46 J/cm^2.[24] Improvement in skin laxity was demonstrated following two monthly treatments consisting of 300–450 pulses per treatment. Skin surface temperatures of 41–42°C are attained rapidly and maintained throughout the treatment with the mobile technique.[24]

Additional infrared broadband light devices have emerged. The Icon® (Cynosure, Westford, MA) delivers energy through the handpiece of the device at a wavelength range of 850 –1,350 nm, which also targets water as the principal chromophore. Multiple treatments are required for optimal results. The SkinTyte® device (Sciton, Palo Alto, CA) utilizes light at a wavelength range of 800–1400 nm. The NIR® (Alma Lasers) emits 800–1,600 nm at 50 W with a large 18 cm^2 sapphire tip that allows for shorter treatment times and faster energy delivery. The current author has reported on mobile delivery using this technology with reproducible skin tightening of approximately 10.5% reduction in laxity grade.

ULTRASOUND

High-intensity focused ultrasound (HIFU) has become a popular skin tightening treatment in recent years. The primary mechanism of action is tissue necrosis at the site of focused ultrasound secondary to heating of the tissue due to the absorption of acoustic energy. This is thought to lead to immediate tissue contraction and delayed collagen remodeling with the coagulative change limited to the focal region of the ultrasound field. However, the range of cellular changes depends on the rise in temperature and the exposure duration and can range from total necrosis to subtler ultrastructural cell damage.

Intense focused ultrasound for skin-tightening applications uses millisecond pulses and a frequency in the megahertz (MHz) domain—as opposed to the kilohertz (kHz) domain as in traditional HIFU to avoid cavitational processes. Intense focused ultrasound also uses lower energies than traditional HIFU, 0.5–10 J versus 100 J, which allows thermal tissue changes without gross necrosis. The main advantage is the potential for greater penetration depth and precisely controlled, focal tissue injury without secondary scatter, and absorption in the dermis and epidermis. Human cadaveric tissue research showed intense ultrasound energy was able to target the facial superficial musculoaponeurotic system (SMAS), producing discrete zones of thermal injury and sparing nontargeted adjacent structures.

The first intense focused ultrasound device on the market is Ulthera® (Merz Aesthetics, Raleigh, NC), which incorporates ultrasound imaging to visualize the tissue and a therapeutic ultrasound module that creates 1 mm^3, wedge-shaped zones of thermal coagulation. The thermally induced zones result from selective absorption of ultrasound energy in the area of geometric focus of the beam. The depth and volume of the thermal lesions are determined by the preset focus depth and frequency of the probe in combination with the intrinsic characteristics of the tissue being treated. The source energy is an adjustable parameter. Higher-frequency probes are associated with more superficial tissue effect whereas lower-frequency probes are associated with a deeper tissue effect. Current protocols aim for a geometric focal depth of therapy in the superficial to deep dermis. Typically, higher-frequency probes are used to treat areas of thinner skin such as that of the neck, whereas the lower-frequency probes are used to treat areas of thicker skin such as that of the cheeks.

Alam et al. (2010) assessed the safety and efficacy of intense focused ultrasound to achieve skin tightening in the brow.[25] An average brow elevation of 1.7–1.9 mm was observed in >83% of treated patients over a 90-day follow-up period sustained to 10 months. The authors found lower face tightening more difficult to assess due to a lack of fixed anatomical landmarks. In 2011, Suh and colleagues treated 22 Asian patients with facial skin laxity with intense focused ultrasound; 77% of patients reported much improvement in the nasolabial (NL) folds and 73% reported much improvement in the jaw line. Histological evaluation of skin samples showed greater dermal collagen with thickening of the dermis and straightening of elastic fibers in the reticular dermis after treatment.[25]

CONCLUSION

The demand for nonsurgical skin tightening has led to the development of an entire genre of devices targeting skin laxity. RF, infrared, and ultrasound devices may be used to treat skin laxity of the face, neck, and other body sites with mild-to-moderate improvements due to dermal remodeling. These technologies are designed for patients who have ruled out surgical face-lifting and proper management of patient expectations are required. Combining these techniques with dermal fillers and neuromodulators are recommended to achieve global improvements that will improve patient satisfaction.

REFERENCES

1. Alexiades-Armenakas MR, Dover JS, Arndt KA. The spectrum of laser skin resurfacing: nonablative, fractional and ablative laser resurfacing. J Am Acad Dermatol. 2008;58(5):719-37.
2. Alexiades-Armenakas M. Rhytides, laxity, and photoaging treated with a combination of radiofrequency, diode laser, and pulsed light and assessed with a comprehensive grading scale. J Drugs Dermatol. 2006;5(8):731-8.
3. Alexiades-Armenakas M. A quantitative and comprehensive grading scale for rhytides, laxity, and photoaging. J Drugs Dermatol. 2006;5(8):808-9.
4. Seckel BR, Younai S, Wang KK. Skin tightening effects of the ultrapulse CO_2 laser. Plast Reconstr Surg. 1998;102(3):872-7.
5. Alexiades-Armenakas M. Aging facial skin: Infrared broad band light technologies. Facial Plast Surg Clin N Am. 2011;19(2):361-37.
6. Alexiades M, Berube D. Randomized, blinded, 3-arm clinical trial assessing optimal temperature and duration for treatment with minimally invasive fractional radiofrequency. Dermatol Surg. 2015;41(5):623-32.
7. Jacobson LGS, Alexiades-Armenakas M, Bernstein L, Geronemus RG. Treatment of nasolabial folds and jowls with a noninvasive radiofrequency device. Arch Dermatol. 2003;139(10):1371-2.

8. Fitzpatrick R, Geronemus R, Goldberg D, Kaminer M, Kilmer S, Ruiz-Esparza J. Multicenter study of noninvasive radiofrequency for periorbital tissue tightening. Lasers Surg Med. 2003;33(4):232-42.
9. Dover JS, Zelickson B, 14-Physician multispecialty consensus panel. Results of a survey of 5,700 patient monopolar radiofrequency facial skin tightening treatments: assessment of a low-energy multiple-pass technique leading to a clinical end point algorithm. Dermatol Surg. 2007;33(8):900-7.
10. Sugawara J, Kou S, Kokubo K, Kuroda A, Hashizume Y, Kobayashi S, et al. Application for lower facial fat reduction and tightening by static type monopolar 1-MHz radio frequency for body contouring. Lasers Surg Med. 2017;49(8):750-5.
11. Taub AF, Tucker RD, Palange A. Facial tightening with an advanced 4-MHz monopolar radiofrequency device. J Drugs Dermatol. 2012;11(11):1288-94.
12. Key DJ. Integration of thermal imaging with subsurface radiofrequency thermistor heating for the purpose of skin tightening and contour improvement: a retrospective review of clinical efficacy. J Drugs Dermatol. 2014;13(12):1485-9.
13. Doshi SN, Alster TS. Combination radiofrequency and diode laser for treatment of facial rhytides and skin laxity. J Cosmet Laser Ther. 2005;7:11-5.
14. Sadick NS, Alexiades-Armenakas M, Bitter P Jr, Hruza G, Mulholland RS. Enhanced full-face skin rejuvenation using synchronous intense pulsed optical and conducted bipolar Radiofrequency energy (ELOS): Introducing selective radiophotothermolysis. JDrugs Dermatol. 2005;4(2):181-6.
15. Gold MH, Goldman MP, Rao J, Carcamo AS, Ehrlich M. Treatment of wrinkles and elastosis using vacuum-assisted bipolar radiofrequency heating of the dermis. Dermatol Surg. 2007;33(3):300-9.
16. Alexiades-Armenakas M, Rosenberg D, Renton B, Dover J, Arndt K. Blinded, randomized, quantitative grading comparison of minimally invasive, fractional radiofrequency and surgical face-lift to treat skin laxity. Arch Dermatol. 2010;146(4):396-405.
17. Alexiades-Armenakas M, Newman J, Willey A, Kilmer S, Goldberg D, Garden J, et al. Prospective Multicenter Clinical Trial of a Minimally-Invasive Temperature-Controlled Bipolar Fractional Radiofrequency System for Rhytid and Laxity Treatment. Dermatol Surg. 2013;39(2):263-73.
18. Friedman DJ, Gilead LT. The use of hybrid radiofrequency device for the treatment of rhytides and lax skin. Dermatol Surg. 2007;33:543-55.
19. Alexiades-Armenakas M, Dover JS, Arndt KA. Unipolar versus bipolar radiofrequency treatment of rhytides and laxity using a mobile painless delivery method. Lasers Surg Med. 2008;40(7):446-53.
20. Alexiades-Armenakas M, Dover JS, Arndt KA. Unipolar radiofrequency treatment to improve the appearance of cellulite. J Cosmet Laser Ther. 2008;10(3):148-53.
21. Ruiz-Esparza J. Painless, nonablative, immediate skin contraction induced by low-fluence irradiation with new infrared device: A report of 25 patients. Dermatol Surg. 2006;32(5):601-10.
22. Zelickson B, Ross V, Kist D, Counters J, Davenport S, Spooner G. Ultrastructural effects of an infrared handpiece on forehead and abdominal skin. Dermatol Surg. 2006;32(7):897-901.
23. Taub AF, Battle EF Jr, Nikolaidis G. Multicenter clinical perspectives on a broadband infrared light device for skin tightening. J Drugs Dermatol. 2006;5(8):771-8.
24. Alexiades-Armenakas M. Assessment of the mobile delivery of infrared light (1100-1800 nm) for the treatment of facial and neck skin laxity. J Drugs Dermatol. 2009;8(3):221-6.
25. Alam M, White LE, Martin N, Witherspoon J, Yoo S, West DP. Ultrasound tightening of facial and neck skin: A rater-blinded prospective cohort study. J Am Acad Dermatol. 2010;62(2):262-9.

17

CHAPTER

Chemical Peels

Kachiu C Lee, Gary D Monheit

INTRODUCTION

Recent developments in the field of cosmetics, including injectables and light-based technologies, have overshadowed chemical peels' popularity in treatment of cosmetic conditions. Results produced by laser technology may be more reproducible, since settings such as spot size, fluence, density, and cooling parameters, can be standardized across cosmetic providers. Results produced by chemical peels depend on the skill and artistry of the provider, relying more heavily on technique, mixture of peeling agents, and layers of peeling agents applied. Thus, the use of chemical peels is akin to other forms of art. Like any other medium of art, it is not easy to exactly reproduce the brush-strokes or heaviness of the paint to recreate a masterpiece. The peel is thus easier to individualize to the patient and not necessarily "cookbook".

A BRIEF HISTORY OF CHEMICAL PEELS

The art of chemical peeling dates back to the Ancient Egyptians, who used oils, salts, and sour milk to improve the appearance and texture of the skin. To this day, we still use the ingredients of sour milk—lactic acid—in our peel regimens. The use of chemical peels persisted beyond the Ancient Egyptians, and has been continually modified over time. The Greeks and Romans used ingredients including mustard, sulfur, and limestone to enhance their art.[1]

In modern history, dermatologists in the late 1800s started experimenting with using phenol, croton oil, salicylic acid, resorcinol, and trichloroacetic acid (TCA) for treatment of lentigines, melasma, and photorejuvenation. In the early to mid 1900s, popularity of chemical peels rose, and they were largely used to treat scarring and wrinkles. During this period, nonphysician lay peelers achieved large a celebrity following due to their ability to produce dramatic resurfacing results with deep phenol-croton oil peels. Having obtained and modified this formula from lay peelers, Baker and Gordon published their own formula for a phenol-croton peel.[2,3] The ingredients in their formula still forms the backbone of deep chemical peels used today, with the concentration of croton oil reduced.[4] After nearly half a century after the publication of this deep peel formula, Dr Gregory Hetter definitively demonstrated that croton oil, and not phenol, acted as the active ingredient in deep peels.[5,6] As such, peel depth is proportionate to concentrations of croton oil.[5]

INDICATION AND PATIENT SELECTION

Chemical peels can treat a variety of conditions, ranging from those affecting the superficial epidermis to full epidermis to the deep dermis. Peels are effective at treating actinic damage, thin seborrheic keratosis, acne, melasma and other pigmentary concerns, shallow or deep rhytides, sallowness of the skin, and other signs of photodamage. Deep peels are particularly effective at producing a resurfacing effect characterized by a reduction in deep rhytides and an improvement in skin texture and tone.[6] Medium depth chemical peels can reduce photoaging with less morbidity and downtime.

The choice of chemical peel determines the depth of the peel, as well as the results of the peel (**Table 1**). Some peeling agents, such as TCA, interact with the skin through pure chemical coagulation and have no additional biologic effect. Other chemical agents can have biochemical interactions beyond pure coagulation. Salicylic acid and pyruvic acid have anti-inflammatory actions, which can be harnessed when treating acne or other inflammatory conditions.[7-12] Retinoic acid acts directly on nuclear receptors, causing increased epidermal thickness with increased basal layer cells and nuclei.[13,14] Phenol acts as a solvent for other chemicals in solution, particularly for croton oil in deep peel formulations.

Pretreatment Considerations (Box 1)

The choice of chemical agent depends upon the patient's chief complaint, degree of photodamage, and skin type. A consultation should always start with understanding the condition being treated. For example, a patient may present with acne as his chief complaint. However, is the patient most bothered by

TABLE 1: Depth of chemical peel agents.

Depth of peel	Level of injury	Chemical peel agent
Superficial	Epidermis	TCA 10–25% (solo agent)
		Salicylic acid
		Retinoic acid
		Jessner's solution (salicylic acid, lactic acid, resorcinol, and ethanol)
		Glycolic acid 20–70% (solo agent)
		Resorcinol 20–30%
		Solid CO_2 slush
Medium	Papillary dermis	TCA 30–40%
		Glycolic acid 70% + TCA 35%
		JS + TCA 35%
		88% Phenol
Deep	Reticular dermis	Phenol-croton oil
		TCA > 50% (unstable so rarely used)

(JS: Jessner's solution; TCA: trichloroacetic acid)

BOX 1: Pretreatment considerations.

- Condition being treated
- Skin type of patient
- Degree of photodamage
- History of previous cosmetic procedures
- History of skin infections (herpes and others)
- History of cosmetic surgery
- Active infections
- Patient expectations
- Poor physician-patient relationship
- Recent or current isotretinoin usage
- Absence of pilosebaceous units on the face

the active, inflammatory acne lesions, the postinflammatory hyperpigmentation, or the pitted icepick scars? On one end of the spectrum, active acne might be best treated with a salicylic, glycolic, or retinol acid formulation. On the other end of the spectrum, ice pick scarring responds best to chemical reconstruction of skin scars (CROSS) with TCA and medium depth peel resurfacing.[15-18]

In addition, assessment of the patient's skin type is essential. Hyperpigmentation is common among skin types III, IV, V, and VI. While superficial peels are generally safe in these patients, some medium depth peels may also be used. Understanding the risks of hyperpigmentation, and discussing it with the patient in depth, will greatly influence the type of peel used. In patients with severe photodamage, higher strength or deeper peels may be necessary. The deeper peels have a higher risk of postinflammatory hypo- or hyperpigmentation. These patients often have a more resilient stratum corneum and epidermis, allowing them to better withstand UV-induced injury as well as chemical coagulation with peels.

An assessment of the patient's medical history, including history of skin infections such as herpes labialis is essential. In patients with herpes labialis, appropriate antiviral prophylaxis is necessary for perioral or deep peeling procedures to suppress any flares during the postoperative periods. Antiviral agents should be continued in the patient through the entire postoperative period, until the skin has re-epithelialized. Common prophylaxis regimens include acyclovir 400 mg three times daily, valacyclovir 500 mg twice daily, or famciclovir 250 mg twice daily. For medium or deep peels, this medication should be started on the day of the procedure, and continued for approximately 10–14 days.

Patients with active infections are contraindicated from receiving chemical peels, as are patients with unrealistic expectations. Appropriate postoperative instructions assists with patient satisfaction during the recovery period. These instructions need to clearly state what to expect and how to care for the skin.

Special Considerations in Skin Color

Due to the high risks of postinflammatory hyperpigmentation, patients with darker skin types are often pretreated with a bleaching agent such as hydroquinone 4% or higher. This can be combined with tretinoin to improve the penetration of the bleaching agent. Pretreatment with these products should begin at least 1–2 weeks prior to superficial and medium chemical peel procedures. These topical medications, especially hydroquinone, should be considered in the postoperative period to inhibit tyrosinase, thereby reducing the production of epidermal melanin and reducing the risk of postinflammatory hyperpigmentation.

Anatomic Considerations

Although chemical peels are most commonly performed on the face, they can also be used on nonfacial locations. On the chest and hands, chemical peels are particularly effective at reducing lentigines and actinic damage.[19] Nonfacial skin is less sebaceous than facial skin, so deep peels are less commonly used in these areas due to risk of scarring and poor re-epithelialization. Typically, superficial peels or superficial-medium depth peels are used in nonfacial areas.

MANAGEMENT

Superficial, medium, deep, and combination peels all have their own benefits. The depth of the peel refers to the depth of injury obtained (**Table 2**). Usually, the deeper the level of injury, the better the results that can be obtained. However, it is very important to emphasize that the risks of side effects also increases with deeper peels. Superficial peels are generally safe for all skin types, including skin types V–VI. Medium depth peels are safe for most skin types, usually up through skin types III. Deep peels should be used with caution, and are safest for skin types I–II and with caution skin type III. There are always exceptions, as medium or deep peels can be used in small, isolated areas in dark skin types.

Pre-peel Preparation

The necessity and importance of preparing the skin on the day of the procedure cannot be overstated. The skin needs to be thoroughly cleansed and degreased of residual oils, lotions, sunscreen, makeup, and other materials. This will create an even peel solution penetration and a more homogeneous result. Degreasing also helps to remove excess stratum corneum or scaling. After cleansing and degreasing, the skin is ready to serve as a canvas for the chemical peel procedure.

Superficial Chemical Peels

Superficial peels penetrate only into the epidermis, sloughing off the stratum corneum, and possibly reaching the stratum granulosum. Some agents, such as retinoic acid, help to biologically thicken the epidermal layer.[14,15] These peels are best for treatment of acne, faint lentigines, mild photoaging, mild melasma, and other superficial dyschromias. Often, multiple peels are required to achieve satisfactory results. These peels are combined with the use of topical cosmeceuticals, prescription tretinoin, or bleaching agents. The peel enhances the result of the topical agents. The benefits of these peels are the minimal downtime needed for complete recovery, making them colloquially known as the peels are further subdivided into "very light" and "light" peels. Very light peels cause only injury to the stratum corneum, creating a light exfoliation often described as a light "sloughing". Injury may extend into the stratum granulosum. Light peels penetrate through the epidermis and can biologically enhance the skin. Salicylic acid acts as a keratolytic and comedolytic, whereas retinoic acid can enhance the thickness of the epidermis.[12,14,20] Salicylic acid is a lipophilic, allowing it to

TABLE 2: Level of trichloroacetic acid frosting (ideal place for photos).

Level	Clinical observation	Depth of injury	Depth of peel
1	Irregular, patchy, and light frosting in a scattered distribution. Some erythema is also present on areas that do not show frosting	Superficial epidermis	Superficial
2	Light white frost with some erythematous background	Full thickness epidermis	Superficial
3	Solid and uniform white frost, evenly distributed	Papillary dermis	Medium

penetrate and concentrate within the pilosebaceous unit. Further, because it is produces minimal inflammation, it is ideal for treatment of postinflammatory erythema or hyperpigmentation in skin color.[12,21,22]

Very light and light peels are ideal for the treatment of acne, and in some cases, mild melasma or other pigmentary concerns. Several case series have evaluated the use of superficial peels, including salicylic acid, glycolic acid, and Jessner's solution, for acne.[9,23,24] There are a limited number of clinical trials; however, of the roughly one dozen clinical trials on the management of acne with superficial peels, the evidence is supportive of their efficacy.[25-28] Superficial peels can also induce a lightening effect, making it useful for treatment of mild melasma, pigmented lesions, and postinflammatory hyperpigmentation.[19,27,29,30] For pigmentary conditions, a series of several peels is necessary to achieve the required effect.

For photoaging, superficial peels may produce transient results, likely secondary to reduction of the stratum corneum and slight thickening of the epidermal layer. However, it is unlikely to produce long-lasting results since it has no dermal effects. Thus, any treatment related to photoaging produces very subtle, if any, results. These peels will have little effect on fine lines or other textural skin changes.

Medium Depth Peels

Medium depth peeling creates injury to papillary dermis. Depending on the peel used, damage to the upper reticular dermis can also be obtained. These peels cause epidermal necrosis, homogenization of the papillary dermis, dermal edema, and a sparse lymphocytic infiltrate initially. After the immediate postoperative period, collagen production increases with a resultant mid-dermal band of new collagen fibers. Clinically, this histologic change corresponds to improvement in skin texture, tone, and fine lines.[31]

Due to the level of injury, medium depth peels can be used to successfully treat a variety of skin conditions. Notably, these peels can be used to treat actinic keratosis, a precursor to cutaneous squamous cell carcinoma.[32-35] Using a combination of Jessner's solution and 35% TCA, the sustained reduction in number of actinic keratosis can last up to 1.5 years, and is comparable to a treatment with topical 5-fluorouracil.[36] Medium depth peels are also effective at treatment of fine wrinkles, ultraviolet-induced photoaging, pigmentary concerns, mild acne scarring, and to complement facial texture changes in patients treated with laser resurfacing procedures.

One of the most popular uses of the medium depth peel is for photorejuvenation, to remove pigmentary dyschromia and to even out the texture of the skin. It is particularly effective at refreshing the sallow, atrophic appearance of aged skin, through softening fine wrinkles and enhancing underlying collagen deposition.[37,38] Improvement can be seen after a single peel (**Figs. 1A** and **B**). A series of medium depth peels can be pursued to accomplish even better results. These should be spaced out over 3 months intervals.

In the past, 40–50% TCA was used as the prototypical peeling agent. However, TCA in strengths of ≥50% can be unstable, causing uneven penetration and resultant scarring or other negative side effects. Thus, 50% TCA is now rarely used in clinical practice. Instead, peeling agents are used in combination to produce the desired depth, with an initial agent applied to allow enhanced skin penetration of the second peeling agent, typically 35% TCA. This method allows for a controlled level of damage to achieve the desired cosmetic effects, without the volatility and risk of using 50% TCA. Current practices commonly use one of three peeling combinations to perform

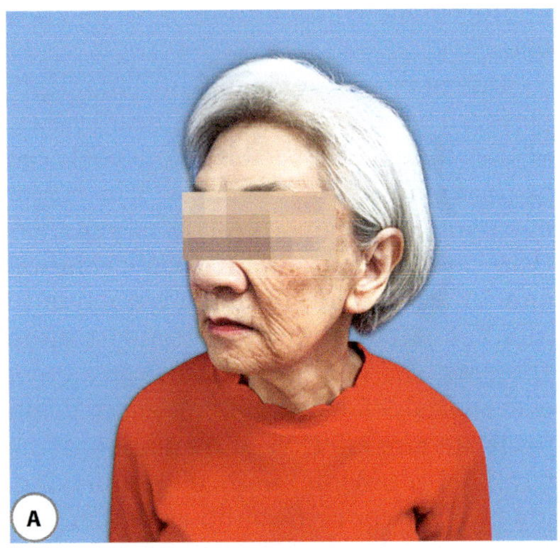

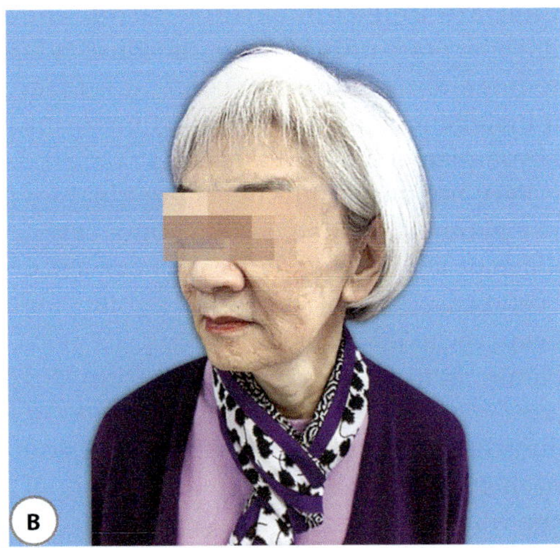

(JS: Jessner's solution; TCA: trichloroacetic acid)

FIGS. 1A AND B: (A) Baseline images of L lateral face of woman with rhytides and photodamage on the cheeks and perioral areas; (B) 1 week after JS + TCA 35% peel. Note improvement in perioral and medial cheek rhytides, as well as decreased skin lentigines. Her overall skin texture and sallowness also show improvement.

a medium depth peel: Solid CO_2, Jessner's solution, or glycolic acid 70%.

Brody and Hailey pioneered the use of solid CO_2 prior to the application of 35% TCA for use as a medium depth peel.[39,40] The CO_2 intentionally "freezes" the skin, causing epidermal sloughing and necrosis, and thus allowing for improved evenness in penetration of the subsequent 35% TCA.

Monheit used a combination of Jessner's solution and 35% TCA to achieve an enhanced medium depth peeling and allowing for evenness of penetration of 35% TCA.[41,42] Jessner's solution is initially applied to the skin, and works through destroying the epidermal barrier. Next, 35% TCA is applied to achieve destruction and inflammation of the papillary dermis.

Similarly, Coleman and Futrell developed the use of 70% glycolic acid prior to applying 35% TCA to achieve a similar effect.[43] They demonstrated clinical improvement in pigmentary dyschromia, as well as photodamage.

The technique for applying medium depth peels is similar to that of superficial peels. The first step is to completely cleanse and degrease the skin. Next, the first peeling agent, usually glycolic acid or Jessner's solution is applied using cotton tipped applicators or gauze pads. In the case of CO_2, the ice is applied in one smooth and even motion. An even coat of the solution sets the stage for even penetration of the TCA peel. In contrast to the CO_2 + 35% TCA or Jessner's + 35% TCA peels which do not need to be neutralized, glycolic acid needs to be first neutralized before a subsequent layer of 35% TCA can be applied. Thus, the 70% glycolic acid is left on the face for 2 minutes, after which it is diluted using gauze impregnated saline or another source of water. Next, 35% TCA is applied to complete the medium depth peel.[43]

Next, TCA is applied to the skin surface. Typically, anatomic areas of the face are divided into symmetric compartments: Forehead, eyelids, cheeks, nose, and perioral/chin areas. Using a systematic approach helps to ensure that all areas of the face receive an even layer of the peeling agent, and minimizes the risk of "skip" areas. The amount of TCA applied is dependent on several factors: The number of passes applied, the degree of saturation of the applicator, and amount of pressure used by the physician when applying the peel, and the duration of contact of the applicator. For larger areas, such as the cheeks, four cotton tipped applicators are commonly used. In contrast, smaller areas such as the eyelids only require one cotton tipped applicator. It is important to stretch the skin in areas with deep rhytides, so as to prevent pooling of the TCA material within these rhytides. For deep perioral furrows, the wooden tip of the cotton tipped application is used to apply TCA directly into the furrow and onto the superior edge of the vermilion border. For eyelid skin, it is best to elevate the head of the table. Immediately after applying the TCA solution to the eyelid skin, a dry cotton tipped application is rolled superior to the lid margin to catch any excess solution.

All three combination of peeling agents are effective and safe for producing a medium depth peel. The endpoints to watch for are referred to as "frosting", which appears as a white film over the skin. Areas with increased photodamage can appear to have a deeper frosting, and this effect can appear on the treated area anywhere from 30 seconds to 2 minutes after application of the peel product. Even application can prevent "skip areas". If this occurs, peel solution may need to be applied to areas with no or minimal frosting a second or third time. It is prudent to wait at least 3–4 minutes between applications of the peel solution, to allow the frosting reaction to reach its peak level. The levels of frosting, ranging from Level 1 to 3, are presented in (**Figs. 2A** to **C**).[44,45] Thicker epidermal lesions tend not to frost as evenly, due to the decreased penetration of TCA. Some physicians may decide to first debride these lesions mechanically with a curette or with light liquid nitrogen cryotherapy prior to the start of the chemical peel procedure.

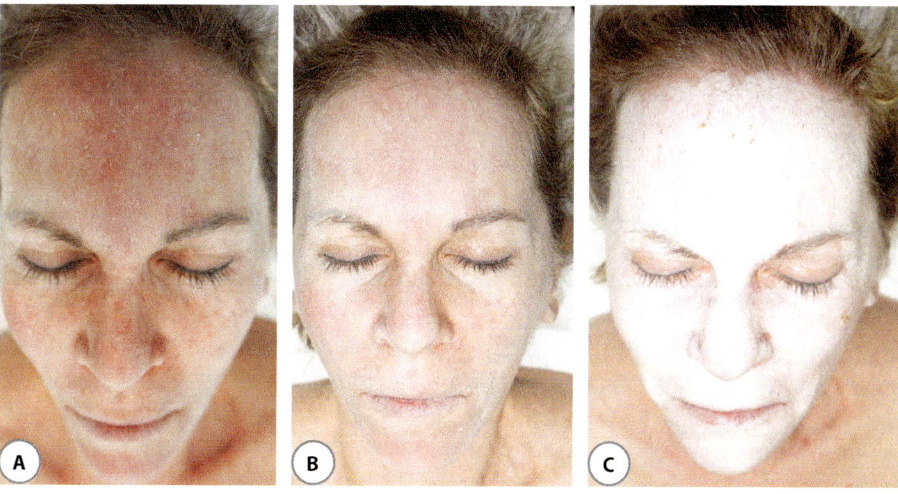

(TCA: trichloroacetic acid)

FIGS. 2A TO C: (A) Level 1 TCA frosting: Light white frosting with background of erythema; (B) Level 2 TCA frosting: Moderate white frosting with some erythema visible in the background; (C) Level 3 TCA frosting: Solid white frosting with no background erythema.

Courtesy: Dr. Marina Landau.

Although there is a burning and tingling discomfort during the TCA peel session, this sensation starts to subside as soon as the frosting reaction is complete. This discomfort is often minimal by the end of the peeling session. Cool saline compresses can provide relief after the peel, and are often welcomed by the patient.

Trichloroacetic Acid–Chemical Reconstruction of Skin Scars Technique

The TCA-CROSS technique is an effective method using high-strength TCA for treatment of atopic acne scars. After cleansing the skin, the CROSS method is performed by breaking a cotton-tipped applicator to create a fine point at one end. This point is dipped into 65% TCA or 100% TCA and focally applied to the areas of atrophic scarring. The peel solution should be firmly applied to the scars. Each of the acne scars should appear to have a Level 3 frosting. This method is repeated every 4 weeks for optimal results. Antiviral prophylaxis is not required unless a significant number of lesions are treated in the perioral area. To date, there are no case reports of herpes labialis outbreaks after performing the TCA-CROSS method. Because TCA is applied only to focal areas with clinically apparent acne scarring, it is safe for all skin colors. This technique minimizes the risk of scarring, hyper or hypopigmentation, and erosions. Several studies evaluating this technique have shown significant improvement, with high patient satisfaction rates.[17,18,46-49] CROSS can also be used concurrent with other techniques such as subcision, fillers, and dermal grafts on adjacent scars.[50,51]

Deep Chemical Peels

It is commonly accepted that the active ingredient in a deep chemical peel is croton oil.[6] Croton oil is naturally found within the seed of the plant *Croton tiglium*, and causes skin erythema and vesiculation even in low doses. Phenol is a carbolic acid which is often combined with croton oil in the preparation of a deep peel. Formulas for preparation of a phenol-croton oil peel have been previously published.[6,52] Because of the risk of cardiac toxicity when using phenol, electrocardiogram and/or other cardiac monitoring is required when performing these peels.

The technique for performing deep peels is similar to those of other peels, but the aftercare is more intensive after a deep peel. Immediately after cleansing the face thoroughly, cotton tipped applicators are used to apply the peeling solution in an even manner. All cosmetic units are generally covered, with feathering at the edges toward the hair line. The frosted skin will appear ivory white to gray white, which serves as the treatment endpoint. There are two methods of postoperative treatment; occluded and nonoccluded technique. With the occluded technique, zinc oxide nonpermeable tape is applied in strips to the skin. Each strip should be applied in an overlapping manner with the previous strips, accommodating for facial movement and swelling of the skin. The mask is removed in 24 hours and the discharge is cleansed with sterile saline. This is typically done in the physician's office. Afterwards, dry bismuth subgallate antiseptic powder is applied. It is left on for approximately 1 week, acting to absorb residual exudate and creating a firm and rigid mask. After 1 week, a gentle water rinse is used to remove the mask. This is easily accomplished through taking a lukewarm shower. The open or nonoccluded technique, as developed by McCollough, uses saline soaks followed by an occlusive ointment such as Aquaphor® or Eucerin®. The soaking and ointments are reapplied 3–4 times a day. The open technique heals faster with less risk of postoperative hypopigmentation.

Nonsteroidal anti-inflammatory drugs (NSAIDs) can be taken for pain control and swelling is to be expected. Residual erythema lasts approximately 2–3 months after the procedure. The patient must use strict sun protection, and can use nonirritating facial moisturizers. Patients with darker skin types (Fitzpatrick III or above) can use a bleaching mixture of hydroquinone, tretinoin, and hydrocortisone to prevent hyperpigmentation.

Complications

The most notable complication of deep chemical peels are risk of cardiac arrhythmia, as phenol is toxic to myocardial tissue. In one study of 181 patients underlying a deep chemical peel, 6.6% developed a cardiac arrhythmia during the procedure. Those with a history of diabetes, hypertension, and depression were more likely to develop arrhythmias. Four patients did not require treatment of their arrhythmia, which self-resolved. The remaining eight patients required 100 mg of IV lidocaine to control the arrhythmia.[53] To minimize this risk, the deep peel should be applied slowly, waiting several minutes between each cosmetic unit. The peel should be performed over >30 minutes, as the risk of arrhythmia increase when it is performed in <30 minutes. Antiarrhythmic medications are needed in the room or in an easily accessible location for possible cardiac complications during the peel.[54] Other complications of chemical peels are presented in **Table 3**.

TABLE 3: Complications of chemical peels.

Depth of peel	Complications
Superficial	• Allergic reaction • Irritant reaction • Erosions, and ulcerations (glycolic acid peels that are improperly neutralized) • Hypopigmentation • Hyperpigmentation • Stinging, irritation, and erythema (resolves after completion of peel)
Medium	• Allergic reaction • Irritant reaction • Erosions, and ulcerations • Hypopigmentation • Hyperpigmentation • Scarring • Stinging, irritation, and erythema (resolves after completion of peel)
Deep	• Cardiac arrhythmia • Scarring • Hypopigmentation • Hyperpigmentation • Delayed hypopigmentation • Delayed healing • Persistent erythema (suggestive of scarring)

CONCLUSION

Chemical peels are an effective treatment for numerous indications, ranging from acne to deep rhytides. Careful patient and peel selection will ensure operative success with satisfactory results. Superficial peels are generally safe to use in almost all skin types, while full-face medium depth and deep peels are generally contraindicated in darker skin types.

REFERENCES

1. Brody HJ, Monheit GD, Resnik SS, Alt TH. A history of chemical peeling. Dermatol Surg. 2000;26(5):405-9.
2. Baker TJ, Gordon HL. Chemical face peeling: an adjunct to surgical facelifting. South Med J. 1963;56:412-4.
3. Baker TJ. Chemical face peeling and rhytidectomy. A combined approach for facial rejuvenation. Plast Reconstr Surg Transplant Bull. 1962;29:199-207.
4. Hetter GP. An examination of the phenol-croton oil peel: Part III. The plastic surgeons' role. Plast Reconstr Surg. 2000;105(2):752-63.

5. Larson DL, Karmo F, Hetter GP. Phenol-croton oil peel: establishing an animal model for scientific investigation. Aesthet Surg J. 2009;29(1):47-53.
6. Hetter GP. An examination of the phenol-croton oil peel: part IV. Face peel results with different concentrations of phenol and croton oil. Plast Reconstr Surg. 2000;105(3):1061-83.
7. Jaffary F, Faghihi G, Saraeian S, Hosseini SM. Comparison the effectiveness of pyruvic acid 50% and salicylic acid 30% in the treatment of acne. J Res Med Sci. 2016;21:31.
8. Marczyk B, Mucha P, Budzisz E, Rotsztejn H. Comparative study of the effect of 50% pyruvic and 30% salicylic peels on the skin lipid film in patients with acne vulgaris. J Cosmet Dermatol. 2014;13(1):15-21.
9. Bae BG, Park CO, Shin H, Lee SH, Lee YS, Lee SJ, et al. Salicylic acid peels versus Jessner's solution for acne vulgaris: a comparative study. Dermatol Surg. 2013;39(2):248-53.
10. Dainichi T, Ueda S, Imayama S, Furue M. Excellent clinical results with a new preparation for chemical peeling in acne: 30% salicylic acid in polyethylene glycol vehicle. Dermatol Surg. 2008;34(7):891-9.
11. Cotellessa C, Manunta T, Ghersetich I, Brazzini B, Peris K. The use of pyruvic acid in the treatment of acne. J Eur Acad Dermatol Venereol. 2004;18(3):275-8.
12. Imayama S, Ueda S, Isoda M. Histologic changes in the skin of hairless mice following peeling with salicylic acid. Arch Dermatol. 2000;136(11):1390-5.
13. Huang P, Chandra V, Rastinejad F. Retinoic acid actions through mammalian nuclear receptors. Chem Rev. 2014;114(1):233-54.
14. Kang S, Duell EA, Fisher GJ, Datta SC, Wang ZQ, Reddy AP, et al. Application of retinol to human skin in vivo induces epidermal hyperplasia and cellular retinoid binding proteins characteristic of retinoic acid but without measurable retinoic acid levels or irritation. J Invest Dermatol. 1995;105(4):549-56.
15. Agarwal N, Gupta LK, Khare AK, Kuldeep CM, Mittal A. Therapeutic response of 70% trichloroacetic acid CROSS in atrophic acne scars. Dermatol Surg. 2015;41(5): 597-604.
16. Nofal E, Helmy A, Nofal A, Alakad R, Nasr M. Platelet-rich plasma versus CROSS technique with 100% trichloroacetic acid versus combined skin needling and platelet rich plasma in the treatment of atrophic acne scars: a comparative study. Dermatol Surg. 2014;40(8):864-73.
17. Khunger N, Bhardwaj D, Khunger M. Evaluation of CROSS technique with 100% TCA in the management of ice pick acne scars in darker skin types. J Cosmet Dermatol. 2011;10(1):51-7.
18. Bhardwaj D, Khunger N. An Assessment of the Efficacy and Safety of CROSS Technique with 100% TCA in the Management of Ice Pick Acne Scars. J Cutan Aesthet Surg. 2010;3(2):93-6.
19. Swinehart JM. Salicylic acid ointment peeling of the hands and forearms. Effective nonsurgical removal of pigmented lesions and actinic damage. J Dermatol Surg Oncol. 1992;18(6):495-8.
20. Waller JM, Dreher F, Behnam S, Ford C, Lee C, Tiet T, et al. 'Keratolytic' properties of benzoyl peroxide and retinoic acid resemble salicylic acid in man. Skin Pharmacol Physiol. 2006;19(5):283-9.
21. Lee HS, Kim IH. Salicylic acid peels for the treatment of acne vulgaris in Asian patients. Dermatol Surg. 2003;29(12):1196-9.
22. Grimes PE. The safety and efficacy of salicylic acid chemical peels in darker racial-ethnic groups. Dermatol Surg. 1999;25(1):18-22.
23. Kim SW, Moon SE, Kim JA, Eun HC. Glycolic acid versus Jessner's solution: which is better for facial acne patients? A randomized prospective clinical trial of split-face model therapy. Dermatol Surg. 1999;25(4):270-3.
24. Atzori L, Brundu MA, Orru A, Biggio P. Glycolic acid peeling in the treatment of acne. J Eur Acad Dermatol Venereol. 1999;12(2):119-22.
25. Dreno B, Fischer TC, Perosino E, Poli F, Viera MS, Rendon MI, et al. Expert opinion: efficacy of superficial chemical peels in active acne management--what can we learn from the literature today? Evidence-based recommendations. J Eur Acad Dermatol Venereol. 2011;25(6):695-704.
26. Levesque A, Hamzavi I, Seite S, Rougier A, Bissonnette R. Randomized trial comparing a chemical peel containing a lipophilic hydroxy acid derivative of salicylic acid with a salicylic acid peel in subjects with comedonal acne. J Cosmet Dermatol. 2011;10(3):174-8.
27. Garg VK, Sinha S, Sarkar R. Glycolic acid peels versus salicylic-mandelic acid peels in active acne vulgaris and post-acne scarring and hyperpigmentation: a comparative study. Dermatol Surg. 2009;35(1):59-65.
28. Kessler E, Flanagan K, Chia C, Rogers C, Glaser DA. Comparison of alpha- and beta-hydroxy acid chemical peels in the treatment of mild to moderately severe facial acne vulgaris. Dermatol Surg. 2008;34(1):45-50.
29. Joshi SS, Boone SL, Alam M, Yoo S, White L, Rademaker A, et al. Effectiveness, safety, and effect on quality of life of topical salicylic acid peels for treatment of postinflammatory hyperpigmentation in dark skin. Dermatol Surg. 2009;35(4):638-44.
30. Ahn HH, Kim IH. Whitening effect of salicylic acid peels in Asian patients. Dermatol Surg. 2006;32(3): 372-5.

31. Lawrence N, Cox SE, Cockerell CJ, Freeman RG, Cruz PD Jr. A comparison of the efficacy and safety of Jessner's solution and 35% trichloroacetic acid vs 5% fluorouracil in the treatment of widespread facial actinic keratoses. Arch Dermatol. 1995;131(2):176-81.
32. El Samahy MH, Ghoz MM, Ramzy N. Morphological investigation of chemical peel on photodamaged facial skin. Int J Cosmet Sci. 1998;20(5):269-82.
33. Humphreys TR, Werth V, Dzubow L, Kligman A. Treatment of photodamaged skin with trichloroacetic acid and topical tretinoin. J Am Acad Dermatol. 1996;34(4):638-44.
34. Nelson BR, Fader DJ, Gillard M, Majmudar G, Johnson TM. Pilot histologic and ultrastructural study of the effects of medium-depth chemical facial peels on dermal collagen in patients with actinically damaged skin. J Am Acad Dermatol. 1995;32(3):472-8.
35. Brodland DG, Roenigk RK. Trichloroacetic acid chemexfoliation (chemical peel) for extensive premalignant actinic damage of the face and scalp. Mayo Clin Proc. 1988;63(9):887-96.
36. Witheiler DD, Lawrence N, Cox SE, Cruz C, Cockerell CJ, Freemen RG. Long-term efficacy and safety of Jessner's solution and 35% trichloroacetic acid vs 5% fluorouracil in the treatment of widespread facial actinic keratoses. Dermatol Surg. 1997;23(3):191-6.
37. Chiarello SE, Resnik BI, Resnik SS. The TCA Masque. A new cream formulation used alone and in combination with Jessner's solution. Dermatol Surg. 1996;22(8): 687-90.
38. Spira M, Freeman R, Arfai P, Gero FJ, Hardy SB. Clinical comparison of chemical peeling dermabrasion, and 5-fu for senile keratoses. Plast Reconstr Surg. 1970;46(1): 61-6.
39. Brody HJ, Hailey CW. Medium-depth chemical peeling of the skin: a variation of superficial chemosurgery. J Dermatol Surg Oncol. 1986;12(12):1268-75.
40. Brody HJ. Medium-depth chemical peeling of the skin: a variation of superficial chemosurgery. Adv Dermatol. 1988;3:205-19.
41. Monheit GD. The Jessner's-trichloroacetic acid peel. An enhanced medium-depth chemical peel. Dermatol Clin. 1995;13(2):277-83.
42. Monheit GD. The Jessner's + TCA peel: a medium-depth chemical peel. J Dermatol Surg Oncol. 1989;15(9): 945-50.
43. Coleman WP 3rd, Futrell JM. The glycolic acid trichloroacetic acid peel. J Dermatol Surg Oncol. 1994;20(1):76-80.
44. Gladstone HB. The art but not the science. Dermatol Surg. 2000;26(2):173.
45. Obagi ZE, Obagi S, Alaiti S, Stevens MB. TCA-based blue peel: a standardized procedure with depth control. Dermatol Surg. 1999;25(10):773-80.
46. Dalpizzol M, Weber MB, Mattiazzi APF, Manzoni APD. Comparative Study of the Use of Trichloroacetic Acid and Phenolic Acid in the Treatment of Atrophic-Type Acne Scars. Dermatol Surg. 2016;42(3):377-83.
47. Sachdeva S. CROSS Technique with Full Strength TCA in the Management of Ice Pick Acne Scars. J Cutan Aesthet Surg. 2011;4(2):160.
48. Fabbrocini G, Cacciapuoti S, Fardella N, Pastore F, Monfrecola G. CROSS technique: chemical reconstruction of skin scars method. Dermatol Ther. 2008;21 Suppl 3:S29-32.
49. Lee JB, Chung WG, Kwahck H, Lee KH. Focal treatment of acne scars with trichloroacetic acid: chemical reconstruction of skin scars method. Dermatol Surg. 2002;28(11):1017-21.
50. Bartesaghi L, Arnaud Gouttenoire E, Prunotto A, Medard JJ, Bergmann S, Chrast R. Sox4 participates in the modulation of Schwann cell myelination. Eur J Neurosci. 2015;42(2):1788-96.
51. Ramadan SAR, El-Komy MHM, Bassiouny DA, El-Tobshy SA. Subcision versus 100% trichloroacetic acid in the treatment of rolling acne scars. Dermatol Surg. 2011;37(5):626-33.
52. Hetter GP. An examination of the phenol-croton oil peel: Part I. Dissecting the formula. Plast Reconstr Surg. 2000;105(1):227-39.
53. Landau M. Cardiac complications in deep chemical peels. Dermatol Surg. 2007;33(2):190-3.
54. Landau M. Advances in deep chemical peels. Dermatol Nurs. 2005;17(6):438-41.

18

CHAPTER

Topical Treatments

Zoe Diana Draelos

INTRODUCTION

Topical treatments can augment the final result of any facial rejuvenation procedure. These topical treatments can enhance healing, improve skin barrier function, minimize postinflammatory erythema, assist in the treatment of dyspigmentation, and improve the skin surface characteristics. These surface characteristics can be characterized as texture, radiance, and luminosity. These products are loosely termed cosmeceuticals, however this is not a recognized regulatory category, thus these topicals are simply cosmetics. Most have a moisturizer base with an added active ingredient intended to provide some skin benefits beyond simple skin hydration, although the moisturizing benefits are an important part of the formulation. This chapter examines topical treatments such as skin lightening cosmeceuticals, peptide cosmeceuticals, vitamin cosmeceuticals, botanical cosmeceuticals, and exfoliant cosmeceuticals.

SKIN LIGHTENING COSMECEUTICALS

Skin lightening cosmeceuticals may be used for the prevention and treatment of postinflammatory hyperpigmentation alone or in combination with prescription products. The most common active ingredient employed for pigment lightening is licorice extract, known as liquiritin and isoliquiritin, which are glycosides-containing flavonoids.[1] Liquiritin *in vitro* induces skin lightening by dispersing melanin. The second most common cosmeceutical skin lightening agent is kojic acid, chemically known as 5-hydroxymethyl-4H-pyran-4-one. It is a hydrophilic fungal derivative obtained from *Aspergillus* and *Penicillium* species.[2] The activity of kojic acid is attributed to its ability to prevent tyrosinase activity by binding to copper. However, kojic acid has been removed from products intended for worldwide distribution and this ingredient is no longer allowed in Japan due to the possible topic effects of kojic acid on melanocytes.[3]

Two other pigment lightening cosmeceutical ingredients are aloesin and arbutin. Aloesin is a low-molecular-weight glyco protein obtained from the *aloe vera* plant. It is a natural hydroxymethylchromone functioning to inhibit tyrosinase by competitive inhibition at the dihydroxyphenylalanine (DOPA) oxidation site.[4,5] It is sometimes mixed with arbutin, obtained from the leaves of the *Vaccinium vitis-idaea* plant, which is a naturally occurring glucopyranoside that causes decreased tyrosinase activity without affecting messenger ribonucleic acid (RNA) expression and inhibits melanosome maturation in vitro.[6]

Finally, vitamin C is used in some cosmeceutical formulations as a pigment lightening active for its ability to interrupt melanin production by interacting with copper ions to reduce dopaquinone and blocking dihydrochinindol-2-carboxylic acid oxidation.[7] The concentration of vitamin C must be relatively low; however, as it can easily lower pH and cause cutaneous irritation.[8]

PEPTIDE COSMECEUTICALS

Peptides, composed of amino acids, are the building blocks for proteins and are used in many cosmeceutical moisturizers. They have a variety of purported activities, which include functioning as cellular messengers allowing receptor modulation, activating enzyme release, and regulating the production of proteins. Peptides are safe cosmeceutical actives belonging to the following functional families: Carrier peptides, signal peptides, and neurotransmitter peptides.[9]

Carrier Peptides

The first commercialized peptides were carrier peptides designed to hook to another ingredient and facilitate transportation of the agent to the active site.[10] The first carrier peptide GHK-Cu was designed to deliver copper, a trace element necessary for wound healing.[11] GHK, composed of glycine, histidyl, and lysine, was originally isolated from human plasma and then synthetically engineered. GHK-Cu was commercialized into a line of skin care products to minimize the appearance of fine lines and wrinkles based on the in vitro observation of dermal keratinocytes proliferation induction and this carrier peptide is sometimes used post laser resurfacing.

Signal Peptides

Signal peptides are the most commonly used peptide family in cosmeceuticals. Signal peptides are designed in vitro to increase collagen, elastin, fibronectin, proteoglycan, and glycosaminoglycan production.[12] The most popular signal peptide is palmitoyl pentapeptide, abbreviated as Pal-KTTKS, and is composed of the amino acids lysine, threonine, threonine, lysine, and serine. It is a procollagen I fragment demonstrated to stimulate the production of collagen I, III, and IV *in vitro*.[13] It is used in a low concentration of four parts per million, since it theoretically acts as a "signal" whereby one molecule has a cascading effect. The idea is to present the body with procollagen fragments that will downregulate the production of collagenase, thereby increasing dermal collagen.

Neurotransmitter Peptides

Neurotransmitter peptides are purported to function by inhibiting the release of acetylcholine at the neuromuscular junction. They are similar to botulinum toxin in that both selectively modulate synaptosome-associated protein of 25,000 Daltons, more commonly known as SNAP-25. Botulinum toxin A proteolytically degrades SNAP-25 while acetyl hexapeptide-3, a neurotransmitter peptide, mimics the N-terminal end of the SNAP-25 protein that inhibits the SNARE (soluble N-ethylmaleimide-sensitive factor attachment protein receptor) complex formation.[14] Acetyl hexapeptide-3, the most widely commercialized neurotransmitter peptide, *in vitro* inhibits vesicle docking through prevention of the SNARE complex formation inducing muscle relaxation.

VITAMIN COSMECEUTICALS

Vitamins are commonly used active ingredients in cosmeceutical moisturizers.[15] They are safe for topical application as they can be consumed and are considered foods. The most common topical vitamins are discussed.

Retinoids

Topical cosmeceutical retinoids are synthetic vitamin A derivatives, which include retinol (vitamin A alcohol), retinyl esters, retinoic acid (tretinoin), and retinyl palmitate. Retinoids are biologic modifiers producing receptor-specific effects including regulating growth of epidermal cells and promoting differentiation of cell lines.[16,17] They are difficult to topically formulate due to their inherent photo instability and degradation upon exposure to oxygen.

Retinyl palmitate is the most stable form of vitamin A esters and can be easily incorporated into the oil phase of creams and lotions, due to its lipophilic nature, however it is not very biologically active.[18] Topical activity of retinyl palmitate is thought to occur following cutaneous enzymatic cleavage of the ester bond and subsequent conversion of retinol to retinoic acid. It is this cutaneous conversion of retinol to retinoic acid that is responsible for the biologic activity of some of the new stabilized over-the-counter (OTC) retinol preparations. Unfortunately, only small amounts of retinol can be converted by the skin, accounting for the increased efficacy seen with prescription preparations containing retinoic acid.[19]

Vitamin C

The active form of vitamin C is L-ascorbic acid, which is also light and oxygen sensitive, functioning as an antioxidant by scavenging and quenching free radicals and by regenerating vitamin E from its radical form.[20,21] Some investigators have demonstrated enhanced cutaneous vitamin C levels following topical application of 10% L-ascorbic acid, however this work was performed on a porcine model.[22] Other human studies have demonstrated a decrease in the minimal erythema dose and less erythema following ultraviolet B (UVB) exposure in subjects treated with topical 10% L-ascorbic acid.[23] Vitamin C has also been purported to produce lightening of skin dyspigmentation in the form of magnesium L-ascorbyl-2-phosphate.[24]

Vitamin E

Vitamin E is a lipid soluble antioxidant with alpha tocopherol possessing greater biologic activity than gamma-tocopherol. Vitamin E is naturally found in the membranes of cells and organelles preventing oxidation of the polyunsaturated fatty acids of the phospholipids in the membranes by capturing singlet oxygen species.[25] A variety of claims have been made regarding the topical cosmeceutical effects of vitamin E on the skin to include: Improved moisturization, increased softness, and better smoothness. Topically applied alpha-tocopherol has been shown to inhibit UVB-induced edema and erythema, conferring a sun protection factor (SPF) of 3, after multiple applications.[18] This is thought to be due to its ability to marginally absorb light and function as a free radical quenching, lipid-soluble antioxidant.[26] Vitamin E is lipophilic and can be incorporated into cosmeceuticals in the form of vitamin E acetate, the stable esterified form of vitamin E, and vitamin E linoleate.

Niacin

Niacin is one component of the B vitamin complex, known as vitamin B3. It is an important part of two coenzymes of intermediate metabolism: Nicotinamide adenine dinucleotide (NAD) and nicotinamide adenine dinucleotide phosphate (NADP). It is found in moisturizers as niacinamide with a variety of purported cosmeceutical effects: sebum inhibition, increased epidermal lipids, reduced inflammation, increased collagen production, increased dermal elasticity, and UV protection.[27-29]

Panthenol

Panthenol is the biologically active alcohol form of pantothenic acid, also known as vitamin B5, and is enzymatically converted to pantothenic acid in the skin. It is widely used topically as a cosmeceutical skin conditioning agent. Its function is best characterized as a humectant, since it can both hold and attract water.[30]

Four forms of cosmeceutical panthenol are available: D-panthenol, the dextrorotatory isomer, and dl-panthenol, the racemic form, d-calcium pantothenate, and ethyl panthenol. The physiologic activity of the racemic form is 50% less than the dextrorotatory isomer.[18] D-Panthenol is a colorless liquid and DL-Panthenol is white crystalline powder, but both are oil insoluble. Panthenol can be used to control viscosity, maintain water content in formulation, increase spreadability, act as a plasticizer, impart better glide, and improve the clarity of gel formulations. In skin preparations, it is usually found at a concentration of 5%.

Essential Fatty Acids

Essential fatty acids (EFAs), sometimes referred to as vitamin F, are composed of unsaturated linoleic, linolenic, and arachidonic acid. These fatty acids are termed essential since they cannot be synthesized by the body, requiring oral ingestion. EFAs are very important in maintenance of the barrier function of the stratum corneum. Linoleic acid is found in high concentration in ceramides, which are a major component of the intercellular lipids filling the spaces between the corneocytes. Topical application of pure linoleic acid is not desirable, since it is a strong cutaneous irritant and unstable. Vitamin E linoleate is a better choice for topical cosmeceutical supplementation of EFAs.

COSMECEUTICAL BOTANICALS

Botanicals are frequent cosmeceutical moisturizer additives.[31] They are generally recognized as safe (GRAS) ingredients not requiring food and drug administration (FDA) approval since they are not consumed as foods. Thus, plant derivatives comprise the most commonly used active ingredient category due to their diversity, formulation ease, and presumed safety. Since plants live in a UV-rich outdoor environment, they must all contain antioxidants for survival that can be adapted to provide increased oxidative protection when applied topically on humans.[32] Botanicals are used to support cosmetic appearance claims purporting the related benefits listed in **Box 1**.

The list of possible botanicals for inclusion in cosmeceuticals is endless, limited by only the imagination of the cosmetic chemist. **Table 1** lists some of the more popular extracts in current use and the chemical class that accounts for their activity.

This section will discuss some of the more interesting botanicals with current dermatologic relevance to include: Soy, curcumin, silymarin, pycnogenol, and gingko.

- *Soy*: Fermented soy, found in tofu and roasted soy nuts, contains two primary isoflavones: genistein and daidzein. These isoflavones function as phytoestrogens, which are plant-derived estrogens with

BOX 1: Purported botanical cosmeceutical benefits.

- Photoprotection against ultraviolet B
- Quenching of reactive oxygen species
- Metal chelation
- Inhibition of targeted enzymes
- Hormonal modulation
- Anti-inflammatory activity
- Microorganism growth inhibition
- Antioxidant effect of multiple organ systems

TABLE 1: Novel botanical antioxidants.[33]

Common botanical name	Chemical class
Rutin (apples, blueberries)	Flavone
Quercetin (apples, blueberries)	Flavone
Hesperidin (lemons, oranges)	Flavone
Diosmin (lemons, oranges)	Flavone
Mangiferin (mango plant)	Xanthone
Mangostin (bilberry plant)	Xanthone
Astaxanthin (tomatoes)	Carotenoid
Lutein (tomatoes)	Carotenoid
Lycopene (tomatoes)	Carotenoid
Rosmarinic acid (rosemary)	Polyphenol
Hypericin (St. John's wort)	Polyphenol
Ellagic acid (pomegranate fruit)	Polyphenol
Chlorogenic acid (blueberry leaf)	Polyphenol
Oleuropein (olive leaf)	Polyphenol

structural homology to human estrogens. It is theorized that plants generate estrogens to reduce male mammal fertility preventing extinction from overgrazing. Orally consumed soy has been associated with the decrease in cardiovascular disease and breast cancer seen in Asian women.[34,35] Topical genistein may function as an antioxidant scavenging peroxyl radicals and protecting against lipid peroxidation in vivo.[36] A study on mice documented the ability of soy to protect against UVB-induced skin damage where a topical application of nondenatured soy extracts reduced UVB-induced cyclooxygenase-2 expression, prostaglandin-E2 secretion, and inhibited p38 mitogen-activated protein (MAP) kinase activation.[37] It is unknown whether this rodent data translates into UVB photoprotection in humans.

- *Curcumin*: Curcumin is a botanical utilized as a spice and rediscovered as a topical antioxidant. It is used in cosmetics as a natural yellow coloring derived from the rhizome of the turmeric plant. Tetrahydrocurcumin, a hydrogenated form of curcumin, is off-white in color and can be added to skin care products as a natural preservative to prevent moisturizer lipid rancidity. The antioxidant effect of tetrahydrocurcumin is said to be greater than vitamin E. The skin benefits accrue when curcumin quenches oxygen radicals and inhibits nuclear factor-κB.[38]
- *Silymarin*: Another family of flavonoids comes from the milk thistle plant (*Silybum marianum*), which belongs to the *aster* family of plants including daisies, thistles, and artichokes. The cosmeceutical extract is termed silymarin and contains three flavonoids derived from the fruit, seeds, and leaves of the plant. These flavonoids are silybin, silydianin, and silychristine, which possess antioxidant effects demonstrated topically in hairless mice by the 92% reduction of skin tumors following UVB exposure.[39] The mechanism for this decrease in tumor production is unknown, but topical silymarin has been shown to decrease the formation of pyrimidine dimers in a mouse model and improve healing of burn wound in albino rats.[40,41] A double-blind placebo-controlled study in 46 subjects with rosacea found improvement in skin redness, papules, itching, hydration, and skin color, which was postulated to be due to direct activity on cytokine and angiokine activity.[42]
- *Pycnogenol*: Pycnogenol is an extract of French marine pine bark (*Pinus pinaster*), which grows only on the southwest coast of France in Les Landes de Gascogne. The extract is a water-soluble liquid containing several phenolic constituents, including taxifolin, catechin, and procyanidins. It also contains several phenolic acids, including p-hydroxybenzoic, protocatechuic, gallic,

vanillic, p-couric, caffeic, and ferulic.[43] It is a potent-free radical scavenger that can reduce vitamin C radicals, returning the vitamin C to its active form.[44] The active vitamin C in turn regenerates vitamin E to its active form maintaining the natural oxygen scavenging mechanisms of the skin.[44]

- Ginkgo: *Ginkgo biloba*, also named the maidenhair tree, is the last member of the Ginkgoaceae family, which developed some 200–250 million years ago. For this reason, ginkgo contains flavonoids not found in other botanicals. It possesses bilobalide (a sequiterpene), ginkgolides (diterpenes with 20 carbon atoms), and other aromatic substances such as ginkgol, bilobdol, and ginkgolic acid. The plant leaves are said to contain unique polyphenols such as terpenoids (ginkgolides and bilobalides), flavonoids, and flavonol glycosides that have anti-inflammatory effects. These anti-inflammatory effects have been linked to antiradical and antilipoperoxidant effects in experimental fibroblast models.[45] Ginkgo flavonoid fractions containing quercetin, kaempferol, sciadopitysin, ginkgetin, and isoginkgetin have been demonstrated to induce human skin fibroblast proliferation in vitro. Increased collagen and extracellular fibronectin were also demonstrated by radioisotope assay.[46]

COSMECEUTICAL EXFOLIANTS

Exfoliation of the skin is a cosmeceutical benefit achieved by encouraging the desquamation of corneocytes to create a smoother skin surface with enhanced light reflection. Cosmetic terminology that is used to describe well-exfoliated skin includes enhanced luminosity, radiance, glow, and shine. While some exfoliation can improve skin appearance, too much exfoliation can create sensitive skin and even dermatitis. The two exfoliant substances, most commonly used in cosmeceuticals, are glycolic and salicylic acid.

1. *Alpha hydroxy acid (AHA): Glycolic acid*: AHAs are a group of organic carboxylic acids distinguished by a substituted hydroxy group covalently bonded to the α-carbon of a carboxylic acid.[47] They are linear, aliphatic water-soluble substances that can be added to cosmeceutical moisturizer bases.[48] Glycolic acid is the most popular AHA in cosmeceutical moisturizers, inducing exfoliation through corneocyte disadhesion, which is thought to require disruption of ionic bonding.[49,50] The corneocyte disadhesion occurs at the level of the stratum granulosum followed by dermal penetration.[51,52] The epidermal effects of AHAs are a thinned stratum corneum with epidermal acanthosis and decreased melanogenesis while the dermal effects of AHAs are increased synthesis of glycosaminoglycans and increased dermal thickness, possibly due to enhanced collagen production via fibroblast proliferation.[53,54] Glycolic acid has been purported to function as an anti-inflammatory agent and antioxidant by alleviating erythema associated with UV exposure conferring an SPF of 2.4.[55]
2. *Beta hydroxy acid (BHA): Salicylic acid*: Salicylic acid (ortho-hydroxybenzoic acid), the only so-called BHA, is a lipophilic aromatic carboxylic acid with a hydroxy group in the beta position. It is a phenolic white crystalline powder with the ability to enter the milieu of the sebaceous unit, inducing exfoliation in the oily areas of the face.[56] For this reason, it has been used for years by dermatologists as a monographed comedolytic in OTC acne preparations, but it is also an excellent keratolytic-inducing facial exfoliation in cosmeceutical moisturizers.[57,58]

Salicylic acid is thought to function through solubilization of intercellular cement, thereby reducing corneocyte adhesion. It appears to eliminate the stratum corneum layer by layer from the outermost level downward.[59] This is in contrast to AHAs, which appear to diminish cellular cohesion between the corneocytes at the lowest levels of the stratum corneum.[60] This difference is probably due in part to the water-soluble characteristics of the AHAs, which readily penetrate into the stratum corneum, and the oil-soluble characteristics of salicylic acid, which remains on the stratum corneum.

CONCLUSION

This chapter has examined some of the relevant categories of cosmeceuticals for topical treatment of aging and postprocedure use. All of these products possess a moisturizer vehicle with an added ingredient suitable for OTC sale. These products can be incorporated in the dermatologists' treatment armamentarium as needed.

REFERENCES

1. Amer M, Metwalli M. Topical Liquiritin improves melasma. Int J Dermatol. 2000;39(4):299-301.
2. Lim JT. Treatment of melasma using kojic acid in a gel containing hydroquinone and glycolic acid. Dermatol Surg. 1999;25(4):282-4.
3. Garcia A, Fulton JE Jr. The combination of glycolic acid and hydroquinone or kojic acid for the treatment of melasma and related conditions. Dermatol Surg. 1996;22(5):443-7.
4. Choi S, Lee SK, Kim JE, Chung MH, Park YI. Aloesin inhibits hyperpigmentation induced by UV radiation. Clin Exp Dermatol. 2002;27(6):513-5.
5. Jones K, Hughes J, Hong M, Jia Q, Orndorff S. Modulation of melanogenesis by aloesin: a competitive inhibitor of tyrosinase. Pigment Cell Res. 2002;15(5):335-40.
6. Hori I, Nihei K, Kubo I. Structural criteria for depigmenting mechanism of arbutin. Phytother Res. 2004;18(6):475-9.
7. Espinal-Perez LE, Moncada B, Castanedo-Cazares JP. A double blind randomized trial of 5% ascorbic acid vs. 4% hydroquinone in melasma. Int J Dermatol. 2004;43(8):604-7.
8. Herndon JH, Jiang LI, Kononov T, Fox T. An open label clinical trial to evaluate the efficacy and tolerance of a retinol and vitamin C facial regimen in women with mild-to-moderate hyperpigmentation and photodamaged facial skin. J Drugs Dermatol. 2016;15(4):476-82.
9. Litner K. Peptides, amino acids and proteins in skin care? Cosmet Toilet. 2007;122:26-34.
10. Gruchlik A, Jurzak M, Chodurek E, Dzierzewicz Z. Effect of gly-gly-his, gly-his-lys and their copper complexes on TNF-alpha-dependent IL-6 secretion in normal human dermal fibroblasts. Acta Pol Pharm. 2012;69(6):1303-6.
11. Maquart FX, Pickart L, Laurent M, Gillery P, Monboisse JC, Borel JP. Stimulation of collagen synthesis in fibroblast cultures by the tripepetide-copper complex glycyl-L-histidyl-L-lysine-Cu^{2+}. FEBS Lett. 1988;238(2):343-6.
12. Zhang L, Falla TJ. Cosmeceuticals and peptides. Clin Dermatol. 2009;27(5):485-94.
13. Katayama K, Armendariz-Borunda J, Raghow R, Kang AH, Seyer JM. A pentapeptide from type I procollagen promotes extracellular matrix production. J Biol Chem. 1993;268(14):9941-4.
14. Blanes-Mira C, Clemente J, Jodas G, Gil A, Fernández-Ballester G, Ponsati B, et al. A synthetic hexapeptide (Argireline) with antiwrinkle activity. Int J Cosmet Sci. 2002;24(5):303-10.
15. Manela-Azulay M, Bagatin E. Cosmeceuticals vitamins. Clin Dermatol. 2009;27(5):469-74.
16. Goodman DS. Vitamin A and retinoids in health and disease. N Eng J Med. 1984;310(16):1023-31.
17. Noy N. Interactions of retinoids with lipid bilayers and with membranes. In: MA Livrea, L Packer (Eds). Retinoids. New York: Marcel Dekker; 1993. pp. 17-27
18. Idson B. Vitamins and the skin. Cosmet Toilet. 1993;108:79-94.
19. Babamiri K, Nassab R. Cosmeceuticals: The evidence behind the retinoids. Aesthetic Surg J. 2010;30(1):74-7.
20. Chan AC. Partners in defense, vitamin E and vitamin C. Can J Physiol Pharmacol. 1993;71:725-31.
21. Beyer RE. The role of ascorbate in antioxidant protection of biomembranes: interaction with vitamin E and coenzyme Q. J Bioenerg Biomembr. 1994;26(4):349-58.
22. Darr D, Combs S, Dunston S, Manning T, Pinnell S. Topical vitamin C protects porcine skin from ultraviolet radiation-induced damage. Br J Dermatol. 1992;127(3):247-53.
23. Murray J, Darr D, Reich J, Pinnell S. Topical vitamin C treatment reduces ultraviolet B radiation-induced erythema in human skin (abstract). J Invest Dermatol. 1991;96:587.
24. Kameyama K, Sakai C, Kondoh S, Yonemoto K, Nishiyama S, Iagawa M, et al. Inhibitory effect of magnesium L-ascorbyl-2-phosphate (VC-PMG) on melanogenesis in vitro and in vivo. J Am Acad Dermatol. 1996;34(1):29-33.

25. Burton GW, Joyce A, Ingold KU. Is vitamin E the only lipid-soluble, chain-breaking antioxidant in human blood plasma and erythrocyte membranes? Arch Biochem Biophys. 1983;221(1):281-90.
26. Mayer P, Pittermann W, Wallat S. The effects of vitamin E on the skin. Cosmet Toilet. 1993;108:99-109.
27. Bissett DL, Miyamoto K, Sun P, Li J, Berge CA. Topical niacinamide reduces yellowing, wrinkling, red blotchiness, and hyperpigmented spots in aging facial skin. Int J Cosmet Sci. 2004;26(5):231-8.
28. Bissett DL, Oblong J, Saud A. Topical niacinamide provides skin aging appearance benefits while enhancing barrier function. J Clin Dermatol. 2003;32S:9-18.
29. Farris P, Zeichner J, Berson D. Efficacy and tolerability of a skin brightening/anti-aging cosmeceutical containing retinol 0.5%, niacinamide, hexylresorcinol, and resveratrol. J Drugs Dermatol. 2016;15(7):863-8.
30. Camargo FB Jr, Gaspar LR, Maia Campos PM. Skin moisturizing effects of panthenol-based formulations. J Cosmet Sci. 2011;62(4):361-70.
31. Draelos ZD. A pilot study investigating the efficacy of botanical anti-inflammatory agents in an OTC eczema therapy. J Cosmet Dermatol. 2016;15(2):117-9.
32. Epstein H. Cosmeceuticals and polyphenols. Clin Dermatol. 2009;27(5):475-8.
33. Arct J, Pytkowska K. Flavonoids as components of biologically active cosmeceuticals. Clin Dermatol. 2008;26(4):347-57.
34. Glazier MG, Bowman MA. A review of the evidence for the use of phytoestrogens as a replacement for traditional estrogen replacement therapy. Arch Intern Med. 2001;161(9):1161-72.
35. Friedman M, Brandon DL. Nutritional and health benefits of soy proteins. J Agric Food Chem. 2001;49(3):1069-86.
36. Wiseman H, O'Reilly JD, Adlercreutz H, Mallet AI, Bowey EA, Rowland IR, et al. Isoflavone phytoestrogens consumed in soy decrease F(2)-isoprostane concentrations and increase resistance of low-density lipoprotein to oxidation in humans. Am J Clin Nutr. 2000;72(2):395-400.
37. Chen N, Scarpa R, Zhang L, Seiberg M, Lin CB. Nondenatured soy extracts reduce UVB-induced skin damage via multiple mechanisms. Photochem Photobiol. 2008;84(6):1551-9.
38. Hatcher H, Planalp R, Cho J, Torti FM, Torti SV. Curcumin: from ancient medicine to current clinical trials. Cell Mol Life Sci. 2008;65(11):1631-52.
39. Katiyar SK, Korman NJ, Mukhtar H, Agarwal R. Protective effects of silymarin against photocarcinogenesis in a mouse skin model. J Natl Cancer Inst. 1997;89(8):556-66.
40. Chatterjee ML, Agarwal R, Mukhtar H. Ultraviolet B radiation-induced DNA lesions in mouse epidermis: an assessment using a novel 32P-postlabelling technique. Biochem Biophys Res Commun. 1996;229(2):590-5.
41. Toklu HZ, Tunali-Akbay T, Erkanli G, Yüksel M, Ercan F, Sener G. Silymarin, the antioxidant component of Silybum marianum, protects against burn-induced oxidative skin injury. Burns. 2007;33(7):908-16.
42. Berardesca E, Cameli N, Cavallotti C, Levy JL, Piérard GE, de Paoli Ambrosi G. Combined effects of silymarin and methylsulfonylmethane in the management of rosacea: clinical and instrumental evaluation. J Cosmet Dermatol. 2008;7(1):8-14.
43. Rohdewald P. A review of the French maritime pine bark extract (Pycnogenol), a herbal medication with a diverse clinical pharmacology. Int J Clin Pharmacol Ther. 2002;40(4):158-68.
44. Cossins E, Lee R, Packer L. ESR studies of vitamin C regeneration, order of reactivity of natural source phytochemical preparations. Biochem Mol Biol Int. 1998;45(3):583-97.
45. Schönlau F. The cosmeceutical Pycnogenol. J Appl Cosmetol. 2002;20:241-46.
46. Joyeux M, Lobstein A, Anton R, Mortier F. Comparative antilipoperoxidant, antinecrotic and scavenging properties of terpenes and biflavones from Ginkgo and some flavonoids. Planta Med. 1995;61(2):126-9.
47. Kim SJ, Lim MH, Chun IK, Won YH. Effects of flavonoids of Ginkgo biloba on proliferation of human skin fibroblast. Skin Pharmacol. 1997;10(4):200-5.
48. Green BA, Yu RJ, Van Scott EJ. Clinical and cosmeceutical uses of hydroxyacids. Clin Dermatol. 2009;27(5):495-501.
49. Stiller MJ, Bartolone J, Stern R, Smith S, Kollias N, Gillies R, et al. Topical 8% glycolic acid and 8% L-lactic acid creams for the treatment of photodamaged skin. A double-blind vehicle-controlled trial. Arch Dermatol. 1996;132(6):631-6.
50. Ditre CM, Griffin TD, Murphy GF, Sueki H, Telegan B, Johnson WC, et al. Effects of alpha-hydroxy acids on photoaged skin. J Am Acad Dermatol. 1996;34(2 Pt 1):187-95.
51. Berardesca E, Maibach H. AHA mechanism of action. Cosmet Toilet. 1995;110:30-1.
52. Van Scott EJ, Yu RJ. Hyperkeratinization, corneocyte cohesion, and alpha hydroxy acids. J Am Acad Dermatol. 1984;11(5 Pt 1):867-79.
53. Bernstein EF, Uitto J. Connective tissue alterations in photoaged skin and the effects of alpha hydroxy acids. J Geriatr Derm. 1995;3(suppl):7A-18A.

54. Lavker RM, Kaidbey K, Leyden JJ. Effects of topical ammonium lactate on cutaneous atrophy from a potent topical corticosteroid. J Am Acad Dermatol. 1992;26(4):535-44.
55. Perricone NV, DiNardo JC. Photoprotective and antiinflammatory effects of topical glycolic acid. Dermatol Surg. 1996;22(5):435-7.
56. Davies M, Marks R. Studies on the effect of salicylic acid on the normal stratum corneum. Br J Dermatol. 1980;103:191-6.
57. Kligman A, Kligman AM. Salicylic acid as a peeling agent for the treatment of acne. Cosmet Dermatol. 1997;10: 44-7.
58. Draelos ZD. Salicylic acid in the dermatologic armamentarium. Cosmet Derm. 1997;10(suppl 4):7-8.
59. Roberts DL, Marshall R, Marks R. Detection of the action of salicylic acid on the normal stratum corneum. Br J Dermatol. 1980;103(2):191-6.
60. Huber C, Christophers E. Keratolytic effect of salicylic acid. Arch Dermatol Res. 1977;257:293-7.

19

CHAPTER

Scars: Burn, Traumatic, and Surgical

John P Tsatalis, Ali Rajabi-Estarabadi, Caiwei Zheng, Keyvan Nouri

INTRODUCTION

Scars resultant from burns, traumatic injury, and surgical procedures are a significant cause of morbidity for millions of people, negatively impacting functional and psychosocial domains. Scarring can produce contractures, pruritus, and pain, in addition to significant visual disfigurement that diminishes quality of life and can lead to decreased self-esteem, depression, social avoidance, and anxiety.[1-5]

There are a variety of nonlaser interventions available for the management of scars. These include nonsurgical therapies like silicone sheeting, compression garments, corticosteroid therapy, massage therapy, and physical therapy.[6] None of these management options provides a definitive treatment and as such are often combined in a treatment protocol. Surgical management with skin grafting, stepwise resection, or release of contractures can also be combined with the aforementioned therapies, although surgical intervention is, itself, associated with additional morbidity.[7]

Laser scar revision represents a safe, effective modality for improvement of scar symptoms and appearance. Lasers utilize photothermal energy to remodel tissue,[8] resulting in functional (range of motion, pain, and pruritus) and cosmetic improvements with generally high patient satisfaction. Currently, there are a variety of lasers available for scar revision that represent a relatively noninvasive technique to reduce the need for surgical scar revision. Like the aforementioned interventions, laser scar revision should be a portion of a multimodal therapy approach tailored to a patient's specific indications.

PRETREATMENT CONSIDERATIONS

During consultation, it should be explained to patients that laser scar treatment is a multimodal approach that often requires multiple sessions over a long period of time. Patients should also understand that cosmetic outcomes typically improve with more sessions; achieving outcomes satisfactory to the patient may require multiple costly treatments. Finally, effectively communicating the potential for natural scar improvement with time, risk of common adverse events, and realistic expectations in relation to the patient's desired outcome is crucial prior to commencing treatment (**Box 1**).

BOX 1: Pretreatment considerations.

- Obtain a detailed history and examination of the patient's scars with special considerations to determine anesthesia plan, indications for prophylactic treatment, and preventative measures in skin of color
- Proper, evidence-based laser settings should be determined according to scar characteristics and patient characteristics, including Fitzpatrick skin type
- Scars should be assessed according to the Vancouver Scar Scale (VSS) or Patient and Observer Scar Assessment Scale (POSAS) and photographs and measurements should be taken to document scar improvement
- Topical anesthetic should be applied at least an hour prior to and removed immediately preceding treatment

Laser scar revision requires careful management as procedures are typically performed in the outpatient setting. Application of anesthetic, prophylactic treatment of viral infections, and preventative measures in skin of color are important preprocedural considerations that are further discussed in the "complications" section. Additionally, photographs and measurements of the scar should be taken to document and monitor treatment response.[8]

KEY CONSULTATION QUESTIONS

A detailed history and examination of the patient's scars as well as a complete patient history is required for appropriate management. A scar history as well as information about previous scar treatments help inform appropriate laser selection and determine the correct time to commence therapy.[8,9] Determining the extent of injury, patient's age, and pain sensitivity guides the development of a plan for anesthesia.

It is also important to be aware of contraindications to laser therapy and to elucidate this information from patients.[8] Some common contraindications include:

- Pregnancy or breastfeeding
- Immunosuppression
- Connective tissue disorders
- Concomitant skin disease at the site of treatment

Although an expert task force concluded that laser scar treatment does not need to be delayed in patients taking isotretinoin, full-field ablative laser resurfacing is an indication to delay treatment until 6 months after isotretinoin cessation.[10]

Fractional laser treatment is contraindicated during an active infection, in the presence of cultured epithelial autografts, and in unstable epithelium in the initial weeks following injury.[7] Although not a contraindication, patients with a history of herpes simplex virus require prophylactic antiviral therapy.[8]

DIAGNOSTIC TOOLS

Choosing proper, evidence-based laser settings is contingent upon thorough assessment of scar characteristics. Scar presentation is heterogeneous, with characteristics that vary by pigmentation, degree of erythema, regularity of texture, thickness, tension, anatomic location, and pathology. Although there is not an established consensus method for scar assessment, a clinical assessment of scar and patient characteristics is utilized to guide therapy.[8,11] A review of published articles found the Patient and Observer Scar Assessment Scale (POSAS) and Vancouver Scar Scale (VSS) are most often used for scar assessment.[12] The VSS reflects an aggregate score taking into account categories of vascularity, pigmentation, pliability, and scar height, while the POSAS is a composite of observer and patient scar assessment scales. The observer component of the POSAS quantifies vascularity, pigmentation, thickness, relief, and pliability; the patient component quantifies subjective symptoms of pain, itching, color, stiffness, thickness, and relief.[13]

A promising technology for the objective diagnosis and assessment of scars is optical coherence tomography, which may be applied to determine scar collagen thickness and optimize determination of laser settings.[14]

ANATOMIC CONSIDERATIONS AND DIAGRAMS

Anatomic considerations are informative in the development of a treatment plan. Generally, surgical scars resultant from closure following large skin excision or scars located on the chest, back, or extensor surfaces are susceptible to and should be suspected for high-tension forces.[9]

Adnexal-rich skin (head and neck) can re-epithelialize more rapidly than adnexal-poor areas (trunk and extremities), permitting more aggressive energy and density settings.[9] Conversely, more conservative energy and density settings are recommended when treating dependent areas in patients with venous insufficiency, photo-damaged areas on the neck,[15] areas with skin graft,[9] and sensitive areas such as the eyelids, upper neck, lower neck, and chest.[16]

It is also important to classify the patient's skin type with the conventionally used Fitzpatrick scale as this consideration affects prognosis and warrants distinct modification of laser settings.[17] Patients with higher Fitzpatrick skin types are at a particularly increased risk for postinflammatory pigmentation changes, further addressed in the "complications" section.

MANAGEMENT

Evidence- and consensus-based guidelines for laser scar revision provide useful algorithms and insight that should be referred to for comprehensive guidance of burn scars and traumatic and surgical scars (addressed together to reflect current literature) treatment.[7,9,18,19]

Most scars require the use of multimodal laser therapy or combination with medical, surgical, or other traditional approaches. Different laser modalities are indicated in different patients and scars to maximize improvement and minimize risk profile. Laser modality can be selected by accounting for presence of dyschromia, scar type (hypertrophic, atrophic, and flat), scar location, patient's skin type, and comorbid conditions.[7,19] This strategy holds for burn, traumatic, and surgical scars (**Table 1**).

Treatment Options and Efficacy

Vascular Lasers

The millisecond duration pulsed dye laser (PDL) (585 and 595 nm) and potassium titanyl phosphate (KTP) laser (532 nm) emit wavelengths of radiation selectively absorbed by oxyhemoglobin chromophores, causing selective photothermolysis of microvessels.[20] These lasers, commonly referred to as vascular lasers, are clinically applied to reduce inflammation and edema in erythematous scars.[19,21] Guidelines also recommend PDL for severe pruritus associated with scarring.[22]

Pulsed dye lasers are considered safe and have a low risk of adverse effects in the treatment of scars. Postoperative blisters, rash, and purpura persisting for 7–10 days are the most common complications and are mild.[17,23] Hypopigmentation is a more serious adverse effect in patients with higher Fitzpatrick skin types.[17]

Accounting for its good safety profile, PDL treatment of erythematous scars can commence within 3–6 weeks following injury, with early intervention for prevention of scars improving responses.[9,23] Large spot size and low-fluence settings are recommended, with

TABLE 1: Laser treatment options for burn, traumatic, and surgical scars.

Laser type	Use
Ablative lasers:	
10,600 nm carbon dioxide (CO_2) laser	• Hypertrophic burn scars • Assist topical steroid delivery
2,940 nm erbium-doped yttrium-aluminum-garnet (Er:YAG) laser	• Hypertrophic burn scars • Assist topical steroid delivery
Nonablative fractional lasers:	
1,540 nm erbium-doped phosphate glass laser	Normotrophic and atrophic scars > hypertrophic scars
Vascular lasers and pigment lasers:	
1,064 nm Q-switched neodymium-doped yttrium aluminum garnet (Nd:YAG) laser	Dyschromic scars
585 nm and 595 nm flash lamp-pumped pulsed dye laser (PDL)	• Erythematous scars • Prevention of surgical scar formation

treatment occurring between 1 and 2 month intervals.[9,17,21]

The efficacy of PDL is limited by penetration depth and in thicker hypertrophic scars PDL is combined with other therapies (**Box 2**). This principle further enforces the benefits of early intervention with PDL when scars are still thin.[23]

Burn and trauma injury can produce complex scars with areas of hypertrophy and atrophy. Early intervention in flat or atrophic scars or areas should include PDL, which is effective in these thin scars (**Figs. 1A** and **B**).

Pulse dye laser is also an option for treatment of mildly hypertrophic (<3 mm) erythematous scars under low tension (**Figs. 2A** and **B**).[9] PDL combined with adjunctive intralesional triamcinolone (TAC) and intralesional 5-fluorouracil (5-FU) is recommended (**Figs. 3A** and **B**), having demonstrated greater improvements in size, erythema, pliability, and pruritus as compared to intralesional TAC alone.[24] Comparison between monotherapy with intralesional TAC, intralesional 5-FU, and PDL saw equivalent improvements.[25]

Pulse dye laser also plays a role in the treatment of hypertrophic scars (>3 mm) under high tension. Scars under 60 days old are initially treated with a combination of PDL, intralesional TAC, and intralesional 5-FU.[7,9,21] After 60 days, as the scar matures and growth

BOX 2: Tips for efficacy and safety.

- Appropriately calibrate and set laser parameters according to the patient's skin type and scar characteristics
- Burn patients treated with the ablative fractional laser may require greater doses of anesthesia
- Start with a test spot to predict the efficacy and any potential side effects
- Use a lower energy setting in skin of color to reduce risk of complications
- Ablative fractional lasers can penetrate up to 4 mm. Depth penetration should be proportional to and not exceed scar thickness. Selecting a density setting <15% can help prevent excess thermal injury
- Instruct the patient to avoid the sun and keep the treatment area clean and protected postoperation
- Following ablative laser therapy, appropriate postoperative analgesia, and dressing should be applied, along with antibiotic coverage

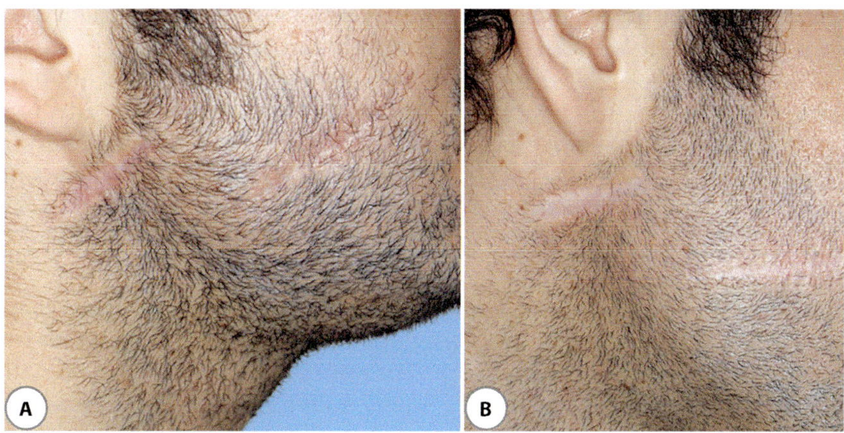

FIGS. 1A AND B: Baseline and after 1 pulsed dye laser (PDL) treatment. Atrophic scar of the face with demonstrable improvement in erythematous and hypotrophic areas.
Courtesy: Dr. Zeina Tannous.

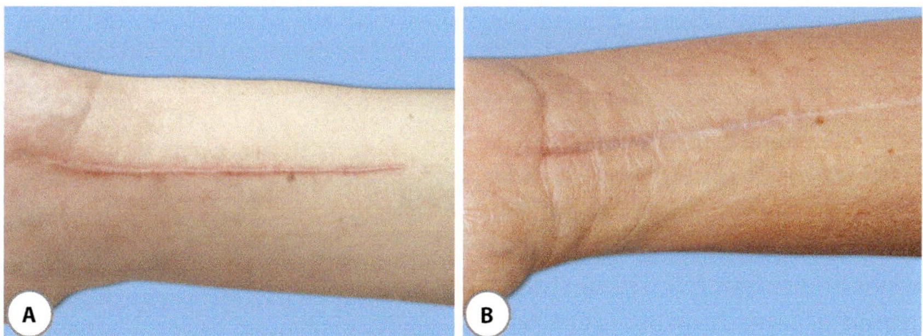

FIGS. 2A AND B: Baseline and after 1 pulsed dye laser (PDL) treatment. Hypertrophic scar of the wrist and forearm exhibiting improved thickness and coloration.
Courtesy: Dr. Zeina Tannous.

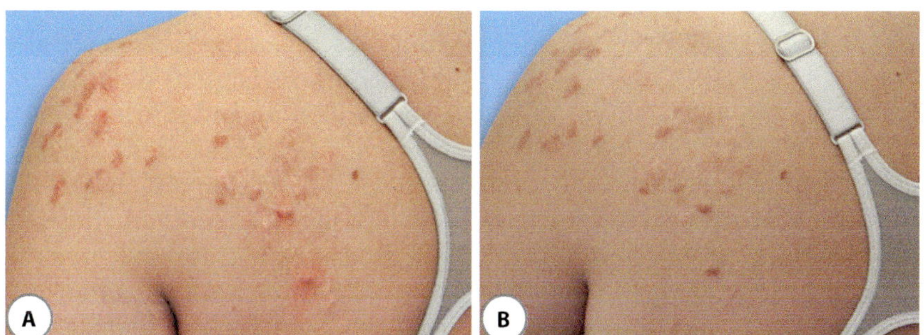

FIGS. 3A AND B: Baseline and 1.5 months after 1 session pulsed dye laser (PDL) + intralesional steroid injection. Hypertrophic scars of the upper back with improvements in thickness, size, and color.
Courtesy: Dr. Zeina Tannous.

stabilizes, nonablative fractional laser (NAFL) therapy can be added in addition to this regimen. As the scars are still relatively young at this point, low-energy and low-density settings (15–20%) are recommended;[26] same session treatment can be repeated at intervals of 4–6 weeks.[9]

Literature also suggests PDL holds potential in prevention of scar formation and adverse outcomes following burn, traumatic, and surgical injury.[27,28] Nouri et al. conducted a randomized, controlled clinical trial to determine the optimal time period for PDL in prevention of surgical scars.[29] Therapy with the 585 nm PDL (10 mm, 3.5 J/cm^2) commenced upon suture removal, with three total treatments at 4–10 week intervals. Compared to untreated controls, the study found early PDL treatment safe and effective for improving scar quality and cosmetic outcomes according to VSS score, visual analog scale, and histologic examination.[29] Further studies comparing the effects of wavelength and pulse duration in the treatment of postoperative scars beginning on the day of suture removal reported similar improvement and safety.[30,31] These studies demonstrated greater improvement with 585 nm than 595 nm wavelength, and similar effectiveness and safety with short-pulse (450-μs) and long-pulse (1.5-ms) 585-nm PDL.[30,31] The investigators advocated for future research to further refine laser settings for prophylactic PDL treatment of scars.

Fractional Lasers

Fractional lasers have revolutionized laser scar revision by delivering nonselective thermal energy through evenly spaced microscopic columns that penetrate into the dermis. These columns selectively cause thermal injury while sparing surrounding skin. After fractional laser revision, improvement in pigmentation can occur rapidly in weeks, with improvements in texture following.[7]

Laser density is an important variable that reflects the concentration of thermal columns in a given treatment area. Adopting lower treatment density settings advantageously reduces adverse effects resultant from excessive thermal damage but may also require additional treatment sessions to achieve equivalent improvement.[7] Energy or fluence (energy per unit area) setting is another variable that must be correctly selected for safe, effective fractional laser treatment. An appropriate energy setting allows for penetration that matches but does not exceed the scar tissue thickness.[9] In the clinical setting, scar depth can be sufficiently approximated by palpation for scar pliability and thickness in both ablative fractional laser (AFL) and NAFL.[7] In AFL, increasing laser energy setting to the point of pinpoint bleeding signifies complete penetration.[32] Ultrasonography can also be utilized to better clarify scar depth.[7] Conversely, mild erythema and edema are clinical indications of appropriate energy setting in NAFL treatment.

Although NAFLs generate less tissue regeneration than AFL, they are generally safer and less likely to cause adverse effects, and can improve scar appearance, texture, and color.[33] Low-density (10–20%) settings have been demonstrated to reduce the risk of adverse events while maintaining similar effectiveness as higher density settings in NAFL revision of surgical scars.[34] Hypertrophic surgical scars under tension are also treated with NAFL revision as ablative lasers may cause widening and further hypertrophy of the scar.[9] NAFL treatment sessions should occur at 4–6 week intervals.[9] NAFLs (1,400, 1,540, 1,550, 1,565 nm) are preferred for the initial treatment of atrophic or normotrophic burn scars, because penetration depth is sufficient for these scars and the safety profile is favorable in comparison to AFL (**Figs. 4A and B**).[19] The relative safety of NAFL makes them a preferred modality to AFL when treating

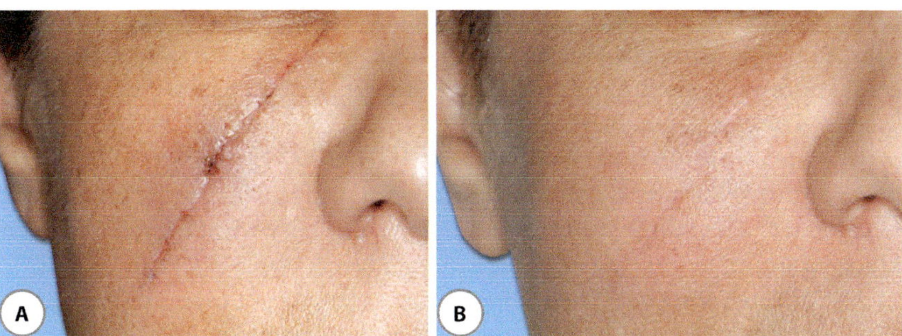

FIGS. 4A AND B: Baseline at suture removal and after 2 pulsed dye lasers (PDLs) + 2 fraxel laser treatments. Surgical scar of the face with improved texture and erythematous features.
Courtesy: Dr. Zeina Tannous.

immature scars, or skin of color [less likely to induce postinflammatory hyperpigmentation (PIH) in these patients].[9,35]

Conversely, AFLs [erbium-doped yttrium aluminum garnet (Er:YAG) 2,940 nm and CO_2 10,600 nm] are capable of greater depth penetration as compared to NAFLs, generating a more robust improvement that makes these lasers the preferred modality for treatment of mature, thick hypertrophic, and contracture scars.[7,9] AFL revision carries a relatively greater risk for adverse events, which can be mitigated by using low-density settings (5–10%) when appropriate.[9] Mature hypertrophic scars are safely permissive of high-energy AFL revision, which demonstrates superior improvements to NAFL.[36] Combination therapy of AFL, intralesional TAC, and intralesional 5-FU represents first-line therapy for mature burn scars and has been shown to improve contractures.[37] AFL is also useful for improving complex burn or trauma scars, demonstrating beneficial improvement in both hypertrophic and atrophic areas.[36,38] Extra care is warranted to avoid high-density AFL in atrophic areas of scar tissue that are particularly susceptible to injury.[9] Although mature scars are more tolerant of high-energy settings, Kauver et al. recommends waiting at least 3 months postinjury or until the scar fully matures and growth stops to commence high-energy AFL.[9]

High-energy AFL sessions should occur at 8–12 week intervals, while low-energy AFL permits more frequent intervals of 4–6 weeks.[9]

While mature scars respond well to high-density and high-energy AFL, it is less clear how aggressively immature scars can be treated.[9] Immature scars can be destabilized by aggressive laser treatment leading to potentially permanent complications.[7] Although Kauvar et al. found low-fluence vascular lasers valuable early in scar formation, the authors recommend avoiding high-fluence PDL, high-density NAFL, and high-density or high-energy AFL which may destabilize immature scars.[9] Anderson et al., however, suggest that AFL and NAFL, at conservative density and energy settings, may be beneficial within the first 3 months after a traumatic injury or burn.[7] AFL-assisted drug delivery offers a combination approach to scar revision that demonstrates improved outcomes, reduced side effects, and permits superior drug distribution penetration as compared to intralesional delivery.[36,39-41] Low-energy, low-density AFL has also been safely utilized to enhance topical delivery of drugs like TAC or 5-FU in immature burn and trauma scars.[42,43]

Finally, although future study is warranted, expert clinical consensus suggests AFLs may also be combined prior to, concurrently with, or after surgery to improve outcomes in scars complicated by contracture.[7]

Per treatment, fractional lasers generate greater improvement in burn scars than PDLs or Q-switched neodymium-doped YAG (QS Nd:YAG) lasers.[7] NAFL has been demonstrated to improve the appearance, texture, thickness, and pliability of burn scars as compared to untreated scars.[44,45] The same studies also found NAFL scar improvement was reduced in hypertrophic scars as compared to thinner scars. Several studies utilizing the VSS and POSAS scores have demonstrated statistically significant improvement of AFL-treated burn scars as compared to baseline,[46-49] and Willows et al. summarize reports supporting AFL revision to improve thickness, texture, and color of burn scars.[19] AFL revision is preferred for hypertrophic or contracture burn scars, while NAFL can be used in normotrophic or atrophic burn scars. Comparing fractional lasers demonstrates AFL generates a greater response and is more effective than NAFL in burn scars.[7,50] For this reason, NAFL may require additional treatments to achieve results comparable to AFL.[7]

Atrophic scars may result from burn or other traumatic injuries and require careful treatment. The dermis is thinned in atrophic scars and more susceptible to tissue necrosis.[9] To avoid excess thermal injury, NAFL revision should be considered first even though AFL has been shown to improve burn and traumatic atrophic scars.[51] High-density and high-fluence energy settings should be avoided with either laser type. Laser-assisted delivery of topical poly-L-lactic acid following low-energy, low-density AFL treatment is an interesting combination technique reported to synergistically affect collagen synthesis.[52] AFL has also been successfully utilized to re-epithelialize chronic, ulcerated scars of traumatic, burn, and surgical origin.[53]

Mature surgical scars or lacerations scars located in adnexal-rich areas (such as the face) are better able to re-epithelialize and can therefore tolerate fractional or full-field ablative laser revision.[9] Large, uncomplicated surgical or laceration scars located in adnexal-poor areas may be treated with AFL or NAFL.[9]

Intense Pulsed Light and Pigment Lasers

A pilot study investigating intense pulsed light for treatment of dyschromic burn scars found high levels of patient satisfaction.[51] Authors, however, did not recommend intense pulsed light due to minimal observed improvement and risk of complications.[9,35,54]

Nanosecond domain lasers, most prominently including the QS Nd:YAG; 1,064 nm, cause selective thermal injury to small blood vessels and pigmented cells.[19,55] The QS Nd:YAG also produces less hypopigmentation as compared to other nanosecond domain lasers (QS ruby, alexandrite).[56] These lasers can be used to treat hyperpigmented and dyschromic scars. QS Nd:YAG may be considered for hyperpigmented scars that are unresponsive to other therapies and NAFLs can also be considered for hyperpigmentation.[36]

Conversely, hypopigmentation may occur in burn, trauma, and surgical scars and can be improved with both AFL and NAFL. Treatment response may be enhanced by combining laser therapy with topical prostaglandin analogs.[57,58] Safely administered AFL is more effective than NAFL.[9]

COMPLICATIONS

Procedural pain is common and most associated with AFL. Epidermal cooling or application of a topical anesthetic like lidocaine 4% cream (allowed to occlude for an hour prior to treatment) is suitable for NAFL and low-energy, low-density AFL. Chuang et al. report cases of ulceration in chronic stable surgical scars following NAFL with pretreatment intralesional injection of 1% lidocaine with epinephrine. Instead of intralesional anesthesia, authors recommended preferential treatment with topical anesthetic or deeper dermal injection for ring block.[59] Intralesional anesthesia may be considered for high-energy AFL procedures.[9] PDL is not typically associated with pain requiring anesthesia. It is important to exercise caution when using lidocaine due to the difficult-to-predict nature of lidocaine toxicity and the potential relationship with occlusive dressings.[60] Although treatments do not generally require sedation and postprocedure discomfort is minimal, sensitivity, age, and extent of injury are considerations for general anesthesia or conscious sedation.[61] Burn patients treated with AFL traditionally report lower pain tolerance and often require procedural intralesional anesthesia and postprocedural intravenous opioids. One cohort study found adoption of multimodal anesthesia including a topical anesthetic reduced pain and the need for postprocedural intravenous opioids.[62]

Avoiding lidocaine toxicity is also a serious consideration, which potentially occurs due to increased percutaneous absorption following fractional therapy. Removal of the topical anesthetic prior to laser treatment can easily minimize this risk.[63]

Postoperative complications associated with laser treatment of scars are typically minor and transient, although more serious adverse events can more rarely occur. While comprehensive safety data for fractional laser therapy is lacking, review articles are available to reflect the published literature. Metelitsa and Alster provide a literature review of complications arising from fractional laser therapy,[64] Willows et al. summarize the literature on adverse effects of laser treatment for burn scars,[19] and a retrospective review of adverse events following laser treatment of hypertrophic burn scars reports recommendations to avoid and manage complications.[17]

Ablative fractional laser and NAFL are well tolerated and risk of complications is low, especially when considered in comparison to full-field ablative therapy.[7] Immediately following fractional laser therapy, local edema and erythema are common transient symptoms expected to resolve within days. Persistent erythema is a rare outcome. Infection, ecchymoses, and blistering are other minor effects.[65] Ablative therapy with the Er:YAG laser is more likely to cause pinpoint bleeding than with the CO_2 laser.[9] AFL therapy may also be followed by mild serous discharge that persists for 1–2 days, warranting nonstick dressings.[7] Postprocedure pain is typically minimal, with pain to a degree requiring medical treatment being rare.[7] New or worsening scarring is a rare adverse effect that can be avoided by utilizing low-density settings and selecting an appropriate penetration depth (energy setting).[7]

Dyschromia (changes in pigmentation) is a moderate complication[65] significantly associated with higher Fitzpatrick skin type.[17,65] Melanin absorbs radiation of wavelengths between 550 and 1,100 nm, with hypopigmentation more clinically noticeable in skin of color.[9] PIH is similarly a concern in skin of color, and it is critical that preventative measures be taken to reduce this risk. Chaowattanapanit et al. reviewed options for preventing PIH, recommending low-density NAFL or picosecond laser for flat or atrophic scars.[35] AFL is more effective than NAFL for revision of mature hypertrophic scars in skin of color but also carries a higher risk of PIH; for both AFL and NAFL revision, it is recommended that low-density settings be used to reduce risk of PIH.[35,36] Combination of low-density AFL with TAC and 5-FU can also safely improve outcomes.[35] Other strategies to prevent PIH include: Pre- and postoperative photoprotection, procedural epidermal cooling to minimize epidermal injury, and postoperative continuation of topical corticosteroid (several days).[35] Early initiation of treatment and photoprotection prevent worsening of PIH. Hydroquinone, along with other topical bleaching agents, is widely used in the management of PIH.[35] Additional treatment options are chemexfoliation and laser therapy.[66]

CONCLUSION

Lasers are a safe, effective treatment modality that should be considered part of a multimodal first-line therapy for scar improvement alongside traditional options. Surgical and traumatic scars are addressed as a single category as scar characteristics (e.g., tension, location, age, and thickness) are considered more important than wound origin in selecting appropriate laser treatment. Effectively treating burn scars also involves recognizing scar characteristics (dyschromia, erythema, thickness, and scar type) that provide indications for selecting the proper treatment modality. Expert consensus and reviews provide useful algorithms for safe treatment of burn, traumatic, and surgical scars to guide treatment,[7,9,18,19,35] and research into prophylactic implementation of PDL is changing the perception of when safe, effective laser therapy may commence. While new literature continues to refine implementation of this technology, laser therapy currently stands as an important component of scar treatment offering significant esthetic, functional, and symptomatic improvements with minimal risk.

REFERENCES

1. Monstrey S, Middelkoop E, Vranckx JJ, Bassetto F, Ziegler UE, Meaume S, et al. Updated scar management practical guidelines: non-invasive and invasive measures. J Plast Reconstr Aesthet Surg. 2014;67(8):1017-25.
2. Gladstone HB, Berg D, McDonald M. Scar revision. Dermatol Res Pract. 2010;2010:545796.
3. Namazi MR, Fallahzadeh MK, Schwartz RA. Strategies for prevention of scars: what can we learn from fetal skin? Int J Dermatol. 2011;50(1):85-93.
4. Smith OJ, McGrouther DA. The natural history and spontaneous resolution of keloid scars. J Plast Reconstr Aesthet Surg. 2014;67(1):87-92.
5. Walliczek U, Engel S, Weiss C, Aderhold C, Lippert C, Wenzel A, et al. Clinical Outcome and Quality of Life After a Multimodal Therapy Approach to Ear Keloids. JAMA Facial Plast Surg. 2015;17(5):333-9.
6. Gauglitz GG, Korting HC, Pavicic T, Ruzicka T, Jeschke MG. Hypertrophic scarring and keloids: pathomechanisms and current and emerging treatment strategies. Mol Med. 2011;17(1-2):113-125.
7. Anderson RR, Donelan MB, Hivnor C, Greeson E, Ross EV, Shumaker PR, et al. Laser treatment of traumatic scars with an emphasis on ablative fractional laser resurfacing: consensus report. JAMA Dermatol. 2014;150(2):187-93.
8. Xiao A, Ettefagh L. Laser Revision Of Scars. In: StatPearls. Treasure Island (FL). StatPearls Publishing; 2019.
9. Kauvar ANB, Kubicki SL, Suggs AK, Friedman PM. Laser Therapy of Traumatic and Surgical Scars and an Algorithm for Their Treatment. Lasers Surg Med. 2020;52(2):125-36.
10. Waldman A, Bolotin D, Arndt KA, Dover JS, Geronemus RG, Chapas A, et al. ASDS Guidelines Task Force: Consensus Recommendations Regarding the Safety of Lasers, Dermabrasion, Chemical Peels, Energy Devices, and Skin Surgery During and After Isotretinoin Use. Dermatol Surg. 2017;43(10):1249-62.
11. van Zuijlen PP, Angeles AP, Kreis RW, Bos KE, Middelkoop E. Scar assessment tools: implications for current research. Plast Reconstr Surg. 2002;109(3):1108-22.
12. Bae SH, Bae YC. Analysis of frequency of use of different scar assessment scales based on the scar condition and treatment method. Arch Plast Surg. 2014;41(2):111-5.
13. Draaijers LJ, Tempelman FR, Botman YA, Tuinebreijer WE, Middelkoop E, Kreis RW, et al. The patient and observer scar assessment scale: a reliable and feasible tool for scar evaluation. Plast Reconstr Surg. 2004;113(7):1960-5.
14. Waibel JS, Rudnick AC, Wulkan AJ, Holmes JD. The Diagnostic Role of Optical Coherence Tomography (OCT) in Measuring the Depth of Burn and Traumatic Scars for More Accurate Laser Dosimetry: Pilot Study. J Drugs Dermatol. 2016;15(11):1375-80.
15. Avram MM, Tope WD, Yu T, Szachowicz E, Nelson JS. Hypertrophic scarring of the neck following ablative fractional carbon dioxide laser resurfacing. Lasers Surg Med. 2009;41(3):185-8.
16. Fife DJ, Fitzpatrick RE, Zachary CB. Complications of fractional CO_2 laser resurfacing: four cases. Lasers Surg Med. 2009;41(3):179-84.
17. Clayton JL, Edkins R, Cairns BA, Hultman CS. Incidence and management of adverse events after the use of laser therapies for the treatment of hypertrophic burn scars. Ann Plast Surg. 2013;70(5):500-5.
18. Mustoe TA, Cooter RD, Gold MH, Hobbs FD, Ramelet AA, Shakespeare PG, et al. International clinical recommendations on scar management. Plast Reconstr Surg. 2002;110(2):560-71.

19. Willows BM, Ilyas M, Sharma A. Laser in the management of burn scars. Burns. 2017;43(7):1379-1389.
20. Keaney TC, Tanzi E, Alster T. Comparison of 532 nm Potassium Titanyl Phosphate Laser and 595 nm Pulsed Dye Laser in the Treatment of Erythematous Surgical Scars: A Randomized, Controlled, Open-Label Study. Dermatol Surg. 2016;42(1):70-6.
21. Anderson RR, Parrish JA. Selective photothermolysis: precise microsurgery by selective absorption of pulsed radiation. Science. 1983;220(4596):524-7.
22. Nast A, Eming S, Fluhr J, Fritz K, Gauglitz G, Hohenleutner S, et al. German S2k guidelines for the therapy of pathological scars (hypertrophic scars and keloids). J Dtsch Dermatol Ges. 2012;10(10):747-62.
23. Brewin MP, Lister TS. Prevention or treatment of hypertrophic burn scarring: a review of when and how to treat with the pulsed dye laser. Burns. 2014;40(5):797-804.
24. Asilian A, Darougheh A, Shariati F. New combination of triamcinolone, 5-Fluorouracil, and pulsed-dye laser for treatment of keloid and hypertrophic scars. Dermatol Surg. 2006;32(7):907-15.
25. Manuskiatti W, Fitzpatrick RE. Treatment response of keloidal and hypertrophic sternotomy scars: comparison among intralesional corticosteroid, 5-fluorouracil, and 585-nm flashlamp-pumped pulsed-dye laser treatments. Arch Dermatol. 2002;138(9):1149-55.
26. Karmisholt KE, Wenande E, Thaysen-Petersen D, Philipsen PA, Paasch U, Haedersdal M. Early intervention with non-ablative fractional laser to improve cutaneous scarring-A randomized controlled trial on the impact of intervention time and fluence levels. Lasers Surg Med. 2018;50(1):28-36.
27. Gaston P, Humzah MD, Quaba AA. The pulsed tuneable dye laser as an aid in the management of postburn scarring. Burns. 1996;22(3):203-5.
28. McCraw JB, McCraw JA, McMellin A, Bettencourt N. Prevention of unfavorable scars using early pulse dye laser treatments: a preliminary report. Ann Plast Surg. 1999;42(1):7-14.
29. Nouri K, Jimenez GP, Harrison-Balestra C, Elgart GW. 585-nm pulsed dye laser in the treatment of surgical scars starting on the suture removal day. Dermatol Surg. 2003;29(1):65-73; discussion 73.
30. Nouri K, Rivas MP, Stevens M, Ballard CJ, Singer L, Ma F, et al. Comparison of the effectiveness of the pulsed dye laser 585 nm versus 595 nm in the treatment of new surgical scars. Lasers Med Sci. 2009;24(5):801-10.
31. Nouri K, Elsaie ML, Vejjabhinanta V, Stevens M, Patel SS, Caperton C, et al. Comparison of the effects of short- and long-pulse durations when using a 585-nm pulsed dye laser in the treatment of new surgical scars. Lasers Med Sci. 2010;25(1):121-6.
32. Bowen RE. A novel approach to ablative fractional treatment of mature thermal burn scars. J Drugs Dermatol. 2010;9(4):389-92.
33. Waibel J, Wulkan AJ, Lupo M, Beer K, Anderson RR. Treatment of burn scars with the 1,550 nm nonablative fractional Erbium Laser. Lasers Surg Med. 2012;44(6):441-6.
34. Lin JY, Warger WC, Izikson L, Anderson RR, Tannous Z. A prospective, randomized controlled trial on the efficacy of fractional photothermolysis on scar remodeling. Lasers Surg Med. 2011;43(4):265-72.
35. Chaowattanapanit S, Silpa-Archa N, Kohli I, Lim HW, Hamzavi I. Postinflammatory hyperpigmentation: A comprehensive overview: Treatment options and prevention. J Am Acad Dermatol. 2017;77(4):607-21.
36. Issler-Fisher AC, Waibel JS, Donelan MB. Laser Modulation of Hypertrophic Scars: Technique and Practice. Clin Plast Surg. 2017;44(4):757-66.
37. Shumaker PR, Kwan JM, Landers JT, Uebelhoer NS. Functional improvements in traumatic scars and scar contractures using an ablative fractional laser protocol. J Trauma Acute Care Surg. 2012;73(2 Suppl 1):S116-21.
38. Sklar LR, Burnett CT, Waibel JS, Moy RL, Ozog DM. Laser assisted drug delivery: a review of an evolving technology. Lasers Surg Med. 2014;46(4):249-62.
39. Waibel JS, Rudnick A. Laser-Assisted Delivery to Treat Facial Scars. Facial Plast Surg Clin North Am. 2017;25(1):105-17.
40. Waibel JS, Wulkan AJ, Shumaker PR. Treatment of hypertrophic scars using laser and laser assisted corticosteroid delivery. Lasers Surg Med. 2013;45(3):135-40.
41. Waibel JS, Wulkan AJ, Rudnick A, Daoud A. Treatment of Hypertrophic Scars Using Laser-Assisted Corticosteroid Versus Laser-Assisted 5-Fluorouracil Delivery. Dermatol Surg. 2019;45(3):423-30.
42. Zhang Y, Liu Y, Cai B, Luo C, Li D, Wang S, et al. Improvement of Surgical Scars by Early Intervention With Carbon Dioxide Fractional Laser. Lasers Surg Med. 2020;52(2):137-48.
43. Clayton NA, Haertsch PA, Maitz PK, Issler-Fisher AC. Ablative Fractional Resurfacing in Acute Care Management of Facial Burns: A New Approach to Minimize the Need for Acute Surgical Reconstruction. J Burn Care Res. 2019;40(3):368-72.
44. Taudorf EH, Danielsen PL, Paulsen IF, Togsverd-Bo K, Dierickx C, Paasch U, et al. Non-ablative fractional laser provides long-term improvement of mature burn scars--a randomized controlled trial with histological assessment. Lasers Surg Med. 2015;47(2):141-7.
45. Haedersdal M, Moreau KE, Beyer DM, Nymann P, Alsbj ørn B. Fractional nonablative 1540 nm laser resurfacing for thermal burn scars: a randomized controlled trial. Lasers Surg Med. 2009;41(3):189-95.

46. Ozog DM, Liu A, Chaffins ML, Ormsby AH, Fincher EF, Chipps LK, et al. Evaluation of clinical results, histological architecture, and collagen expression following treatment of mature burn scars with a fractional carbon dioxide laser. JAMA Dermatol. 2013;149(1):50-7.
47. Qu L, Liu A, Zhou L, He C, Grossman PH, Moy RL, et al. Clinical and molecular effects on mature burn scars after treatment with a fractional $CO_{(2)}$ laser. Lasers Surg Med. 2012;44(7):517-24.
48. Kawecki M, Bernad-Wisniewska T, Sakiel S, Nowak M, Andriessen A. Laser in the treatment of hypertrophic burn scars. Int Wound J. 2008;5(1):87-97.
49. Khandelwal A, Yelvington M, Tang X, Brown S. Ablative fractional photothermolysis for the treatment of hypertrophic burn scars in adult and pediatric patients: a single surgeon's experience. J Burn Care Res. 2014;35(5):455-63.
50. Kim HS, Lee JH, Park YM, Lee JY. Comparison of the effectiveness of nonablative fractional laser versus ablative fractional laser in thyroidectomy scar prevention: A pilot study. J Cosmet Laser Ther. 2012;14(2):89-93.
51. Keen A, Sheikh G, Hassan I, Jabeen Y, Rather S, Mubashir S, et al. Treatment of post-burn and post-traumatic atrophic scars with fractional CO_2 laser: experience at a tertiary care centre. Lasers Med Sci. 2018;33(5):1039-46.
52. Rkein A, Ozog D, Waibel JS. Treatment of atrophic scars with fractionated CO_2 laser facilitating delivery of topically applied poly-L-lactic acid. Dermatol Surg. 2014;40(6):624-31.
53. Shumaker PR, Kwan JM, Badiavas EV, Waibel J, Davis S, Uebelhoer NS. Rapid healing of scar-associated chronic wounds after ablative fractional resurfacing. Arch Dermatol. 2012;148(11):1289-93.
54. Hultman CS, Friedstat JS, Edkins RE. Efficacy of intense pulsed light for the treatment of burn scar dyschromias: a pilot study to assess patient satisfaction, safety, and willingness to pay. Ann Plast Surg. 2015;74 Suppl 4:S204-8.
55. Friedman PM, Jih MH, Skover GR, Payonk GS, Kimyai-Asadi A, Geronemus RG. Treatment of atrophic facial acne scars with the 1064-nm Q-switched Nd:YAG laser: six-month follow-up study. Arch Dermatol. 2004;140(11):1337-41.
56. Gorouhi F, Davari P, Kashani MN, Firooz A. Treatment of traumatic tattoo with the Q-switched Nd:YAG laser. J Cosmet Laser Ther. 2007;9(4):253-5.
57. Siadat AH, Rezaei R, Asilian A, Abtahi-Naeini B, Rakhshanpour M, Raei M, et al. Repigmentation of Hypopigmented Scars Using Combination of Fractionated Carbon Dioxide Laser with Topical Latanoprost Vs. Fractionated Carbon Dioxide Laser Alone. Indian J Dermatol. 2015;60(4):364-8.
58. Massaki AB, Fabi SG, Fitzpatrick R. Repigmentation of hypopigmented scars using an erbium-doped 1,550-nm fractionated laser and topical bimatoprost. Dermatol Surg. 2012;38(7 Pt 1):995-1001.
59. Chuang GS, Manstein D, Tannous Z, Avram MM. Ulceration of mature surgical scars following nonablative fractional photothermolysis associated with intralesional lidocaine injections. Dermatol Surg. 2012;38(11):1879-81.
60. Oni G, Brown S, Burrus C, Grant L, Watkins J, Kenkel M, et al. Effect of 4% topical lidocaine applied to the face on the serum levels of lidocaine and its metabolite, monoethylglycinexylidide. Aesthet Surg J. 2010;30(6):853-8.
61. Griffin AC. Laser resurfacing procedures in dark-skinned patients. Aesthet Surg J. 2005;25(6):625-7.
62. Edkins RE, Hultman CS, Collins P, Cairns B, Hanson M, Carman M. Improving Comfort and Throughput for Patients Undergoing Fractionated Laser Ablation of Symptomatic Burn Scars. Ann Plast Surg. 2015;74(3):293-9.
63. Marra DE, Yip D, Fincher EF, Moy RL. Systemic toxicity from topically applied lidocaine in conjunction with fractional photothermolysis. Arch Dermatol. 2006;142(8):1024-6.
64. Metelitsa AI, Alster TS. Fractionated laser skin resurfacing treatment complications: a review. Dermatol Surg. 2010;36(3):299-306.
65. Alam M, Warycha M. Complications of lasers and light treatments. Dermatol Ther. 2011;24(6):571-80.
66. Davis EC, Callender VD. Postinflammatory hyperpigmentation: a review of the epidemiology, clinical features, and treatment options in skin of color. J Clin Aesthet Dermatol. 2010;3(7):20-31

20

CHAPTER

Laser Treatment of Acne Scars

Oge C Onwudiwe, Elizabeth L Tanzi

INTRODUCTION

Millions of Americans have suffered from acne at some point in their lives. Unfortunately for some, disfiguring acne scars are left behind. In the USA, this disease has a high cost burden with respect to treatment and loss of productivity.[1] Although without cure, many treatments, including lasers, are used to help improve the appearance. With respect to lasers in the treatment of acne scars, pulse dye and neodymium-doped yttrium aluminum garnet (Nd:YAG) lasers have been used to treat hypertrophic/keloid scars as well as prolonged erythema within scars. Both ablative and nonablative fractional laser devices are typically employed for atrophic scars. Radiofrequency (RF)-based devices have also shown promise in the treatment of atrophic acne scars and have an added benefit of being "color blind" which allows their use in skin of color.

Acne is a disorder of the pilosebaceous unit caused by several factors including hormonal factors, increased sebum production, follicular debris, the bacterium *Propionibacterium acnes*, and an inflammatory response.[2] Clinically, one typically presents with comedones, papules, pustules, and/or a nodulocystic eruption, which can subsequently lead to varying degrees of scarring.

Residual scarring on the face is often more worrisome to the patients than the original insult. Patients tend to seek treatment for resultant scarring because of the appearance as well as the psychosocial impact, which places limitations on self-esteem and interpersonal relationships.[3] It has been associated with depression and suicidal ideation.[4]

Acne scarring can be generally classified into categories: Atrophic and hypertrophic. The former is more common and is broadly defined as a localized loss of collagen secondary to abnormal wound healing. Based on factors such as size, depth, and shape, atrophic scars can be further divided: icepick, rolling, and boxcar.

Icepick scars are narrow, typically <2 mm wide, deep, and sharply demarcated scars that extend vertically to the deep dermis or subcutaneous tissue. The surface opening is usually wider as the scar tapers from the surface to its base.

Rolling scars are usually wider than 4–5 mm and have smoother and more rounded edges. They possess fibrotic bands extending from the dermis to the subcutaneous tissue.

Boxcar scars are usually 1.5–4.0 mm in diameter with varying depths: Superficial (0.1–0.5 mm) and deep (≥0.5 mm). They possess well-demarcated vertical edges. They are clinically wider at the surface than icepick scars and do not taper to a point at the base.

Sinus tracts, hypertrophic scars, and keloidal scars may also occur after acne.[5] Hypertrophic scars have an abundance of collagen deposition confined to the borders of the original injury. In contrast, keloidal scars proliferate and extend beyond these borders.

Current treatment modalities for acne scars include, but are not limited to, punch excision, dermal filler, autologous fat transfer, chemical peels, intralesional injections of kenalog and fluorouracil, subcision, microneedling, dermabrasion, RF, and laser treatments such as pulsed dye laser (PDL) and skin resurfacing devices.[6] Recent pilot studies have also suggested a possible role for injectable autologous bone marrow stem cells (BMSCs) and a topical synthetic epidermal growth factor (EGF) serum in the treatment of atrophic scars.[7,8] Of note, some of these modalities can be combined for better outcomes. The focus herein will be the application of lasers in the treatment of acne scars.

Pretreatment considerations: Previous treatments, type and depth of the scar, skin phototype, and the patient's medical history are important things to consider (**Box 1**). For example, does the patient have a history of herpes simplex virus (HSV) or methicillin-resistant *Staphylococcus aureus* (MRSA)? Is there a recent history of isotretinoin use?

BOX 1: Considerations prior to treatment.

- Scar characteristics
- Skin phototype
- Past medical history: HSV, MRSA, current acne, and isotretinoin use
- Pain control
- Pretreating with doxycycline for acneiform eruptions

(HSV: herpes simplex virus; MRSA: methicillin-resistant *Staphylococcus aureus*)

There are key considerations that should be tackled during the initial consultation such as patient's expectations, use of diagnostic tools, and the anatomic location being treated. First, obtaining an accurate picture of patient's expectations and then setting realistic expectations with respect to outcomes is paramount. In addition, implementing good standardized photography is a key diagnostic tool that can be used to assess the patient, develop a treatment plan, and compare results with baseline. Scar scales and other scar measuring devices can be used, but are not necessary in the day-to-day clinical setting. With respect to anatomic considerations, the practitioner should bear in mind that the energy settings on most laser devices used to treat acne scars are commonly lower when treating off the face.

MANAGEMENT

Treatment of acne scars must be individually customized for each patient depending on the type of scars present, recent treatment history, skin phototype, downtime, and cost. Acne scar treatments within 6 months of isotretinoin were reported to have a high risk of hypertrophic scarring.[9-13] On this premise, surgical and laser intervention has typically been delayed for 6–12 months post isotretinoin. A recent consensus document reviewed 32 relevant publications, which reported 1,485 procedures. Their conclusions were that there was inadequate evidence to support delaying procedures such as manual dermabrasion, superficial chemical peels, cutaneous surgery, laser hair removal, and fractional ablative and nonablative laser procedures for patients being treated with or who have recently completed isotretinoin therapy. On the other hand, modalities such as mechanical dermabrasion and fully ablative lasers were not recommended in the setting of systemic isotretinoin treatment.[14]

Pulsed dye lasers have shown great utility when treating persistent erythematous scars as well as hypertrophic scars, and in some cases—keloids.[15-18] It has been suggested that their mechanism is through the suppression of fibroblast proliferation and induction of apoptosis.[19] They also produce an increase in collagenase-3 activity and a decrease in collagen type III deposition.[20] Improvement in characteristics such as scar thickness, erythema, and pliability has been noted.[15-18] The authors find the PDL helpful in the treatment of early scar formation with active acne. These so-called "prescars" respond well to PDL treatments and can be effectively delivered during topical and/or oral acne treatment (**Figs. 1A** and **B**). Of note, the 532 nm potassium titanyl phosphate (KTP) laser has been shown to be comparable in efficacy and safety in the treatment of erythematous surgical scars when compared to PDL, and would be expected to improve acne prescars similarly to the PDL.[21]

Success with the use of Nd:YAG in the treatment of hypertrophic/keloid scars has been shown in the literature.[22-24] Its mechanism, in part, may be due to selective suppression of collagen production.[25] One comparison study between PDL and long-pulsed Nd:YAG lasers in the treatment of hypertrophic and keloid scars showed improvement in scar characteristics, but no statistically significant difference between the two modes.[26]

Ablative skin resurfacing (ASR) with carbon dioxide (CO_2) and erbium-doped yttrium aluminum garnet (Er:YAG) lasers was once considered the gold standard with respect to outcome in the treatment of atrophic acne scars.[27-32] The mechanism of action was essentially via vaporization of a layer of skin and thermal coagulation necrosis of cells with a subsequent residual zone of thermal injury at a precisely defined depth.

While highly effective in improving scar appearance, patients typically experienced significant side effects such as edema, oozing, crusting, burning, prolonged erythema, infection, scarring, and delayed onset hypopigmentation.[33,34] In light of these potential risks, nonablative dermal remodeling (NDR) using long-pulsed infrared 1,450-nm diode and 1,320-nm Nd:YAG subsequently emerged. Their mechanism of action was through selective heating/stimulation of dermal tissue

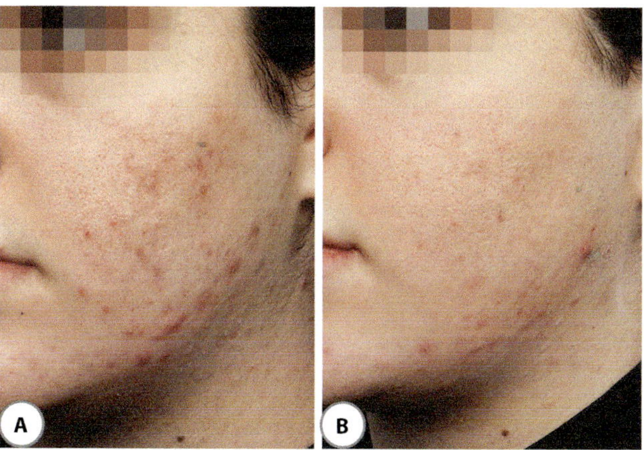

FIGS. 1A AND B: Before and after topical therapy and pulsed dye laser × 2 sessions for prescars.

to induce a wound response, while sparing damage to the epidermis.[35-38] The clinical outcomes of these devices lacked comparable clinical efficacy seen with the aforementioned ablative devices.

Fractional photothermolysis (FP) was introduced in an attempt to overcome the limitations associated with ASR and NDR procedures. This system involves the use of mid-infrared light emitted by a 1,550-nm erbium-doped laser to create microscopic spatially arranged columns of thermal injury in the dermis [microscopic thermal zones (MTZ)] surrounded by regions of unaffected tissue. The microscopic zones of thermal injury produce localized epidermal necrosis and denatured collagen. The reservoir of unaffected cells surrounding each MTZ contributed to more rapid wound healing allowing for complete re-epithelialization is as little as one day.[39] In addition, preservation of the stratum corneum allows for continued epidermal barrier function including helping to minimize infection risks. Side effects include transient erythema and edema, postinflammatory hyperpigmentation, HSV outbreaks, and an acneiform eruption.[40] Oozing, crusting, and scarring are typically not seen in nonaggressive settings (**Figs. 2A** and **B**).

Although not a laser device, RF microneedling is an energy-based device used in the treatment of various skin conditions including acne scars (**Figs. 3A** and **B**). It has been shown to stimulate new collagen and elastin formation through electrical currents that heat dermal tissue. It utilizes the resistance of dermal tissue or other layers of the skin to transform the RF energy into thermal energy. The creation of RF thermal injury is not dependent on a specific chromophore and does not adhere to the theory of selective photothermolysis. Three main types exist: (1) Monopolar, (2) Bipolar, and (3) Unipolar devices. Fractional RF is a subset of bipolar RF. There are multiple devices in the market for RF for acne scars; however, no comparative studies have been performed. Side effects such as mild erythema, postinflammatory hyperpigmentation, and track marks from the device have been reported.[41-43]

Of the modalities mentioned, Nd:YAG, nonablative fractional technologies as well as RF when proper settings are utilized can be safe in skin of color. Fractional ablative

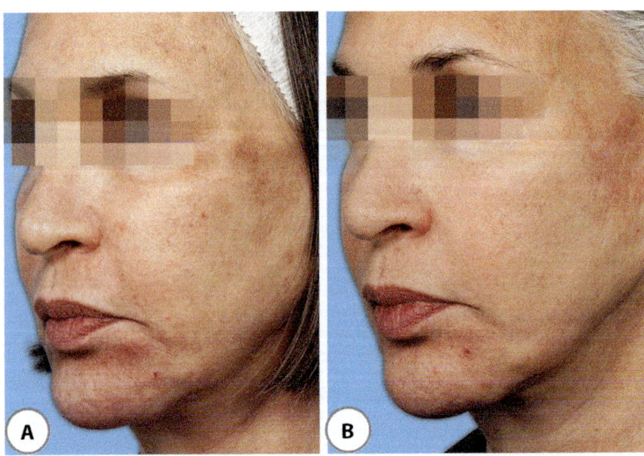

FIGS. 2A AND B: Baseline after 1,550 nm nonablative fractional resurfacing with postinflammatory hyperpigmentation (PIH) and then 3 months after with resolution of PIH and improvement of atrophic scars.

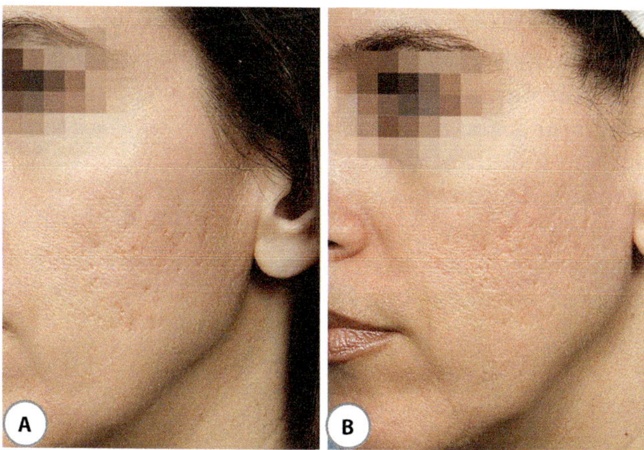

FIGS. 3A AND B: Before and 3 months after a series of three radiofrequency microneedling treatments for acne scars.

treatments can be used, but with caution as permanent pigmentary changes and scarring may occur. PDL and fully ablative resurfacing should be avoided, if possible, in the darkest of phototypes.

Treatment Options

Treatments must be tailored to each patient. The scar type, its depth, the patient's phototype, downtime, and financial restrictions will all be important factors to consider. All else being equal, the scar type and its depth are the main factors to consider when choosing a laser device (**Table 1**).

Treatment Efficacy

Treatment efficacy is dependent on a number of factors including but not limited to: The type of scar and its depth, the laser employed, and the number of treatments delivered in the series. Icepick scars, as previously mentioned, are typically narrow and deep. Its depth can sometimes be deeper than the depth of penetration of some skin resurfacing lasers, thus making it a bit more challenging. Rolling scars are usually wider than deep, which is advantageous when using resurfacing lasers.

TABLE 1: Treatment options for different types of scars.

Type of scar	Laser devices of choice
Hypertrophic scars	PDL, Nd:YAG, ablative fractional
Icepick scars	Radiofrequency-fractional ablative type, ablative fractional CO_2/Er:YAG fully ablative resurfacing
Boxcar scars	Radiofrequency, fully ablative resurfacing, ablative fractional CO_2/Er:YAG, and nonablative fractional resurfacing
Rolling scars	Radiofrequency, fully ablative resurfacing, ablative fractional CO_2/Er:YAG, and nonablative fractional resurfacing

(Er:YAG: erbium-doped yttrium aluminum garnet; Nd:YAG: neodymium-doped yttrium aluminum garnet; PDL: pulsed dye laser)

One must bear in mind that there can be fibrous tethering of the dermis, which must be addressed for treatment success.

Boxcar scars can be shallow or deep. The deeper variants tend to be less responsive to laser resurfacing treatments as a single modality.

Significant improvement in the appearance of scars is typically seen after 4–6 treatments. The treatments are usually performed on a monthly basis. Recalcitrant scars, at times, tend to be responsive to a multimodality approach. This typically includes combination treatments with laser resurfacing and punch excision, subcision, etc. Lastly, skin phototype, patient history, and downtime are also key considerations.

COMPLICATIONS

Potential complications will vary based on the laser device used. It is of paramount importance to review potential complications and expected side effects in detail during the initial consultation and obtain informed consent prior to the procedure (**Box 2**). The patient should be aware of the "expected" side effects during the healing phase, but cautioned to monitor for the onset of certain symptoms that could indicate a potential infection. Lastly, the patient should be informed of which side effects are temporary in nature, delayed in onset, prolonged, and potentially permanent. In general, all lasers can potentially cause erythema, edema, pain, and dyschromia. However, side effects such as acneiform eruptions, infection, and scarring are most likely to be seen when utilizing fractional and/or ablative energy-based devices.

BOX 2: Tips for avoiding complications.

- Avoid utilizing more aggressive settings
- Avoid bulk heating
- Respect skin phototypes and recent skin tanning/sun exposure
- Consider treatment with doxycycline prior to fractionated laser treatments to prevent acneiform eruptions
- Prophylactically treat patients with history of HSV with appropriate antivirals
- Stress sun avoidance, sunscreen, and other sun protective factors posttreatment

(HSV: herpes simplex virus)

CONCLUSION

Acne scarring can cause a tremendous loss of self-esteem and can be burdensome for affected patients. Key aspects when evaluating the patient during the initial consultation include setting realistic expectations, discussing side effects, treatment options, number of treatments, cost, and downtime. It should be stressed to the patient that the various modalities can significantly improve the appearance of scars, but will not eradicate them. Treatments can continue as long as improvement does not plateau. A tailored treatment based on the scar type is needed for optimal treatment outcomes. Treatment recommendations will vary because of scar type and severity, length of recovery, affordability, and practitioner comfort level. Good clinical photography is the key in tracking improvement. The practitioner should anticipate side effects such as acneiform eruptions and postinflammatory hyperpigmentation and be prepared to treat these relatively common side effects when they arise. Lastly, these modalities as well as other nonlaser treatments can potentially be combined for better outcomes, but caution should be employed as this carries greater risks of adverse events and prolonged recovery periods.

REFERENCES

1. Bhate K, Williams HC. Epidemiology of acne vulgaris. Br J Derm. 2013;168(3):474-85.
2. Kurokawa I, Danby FW, Ju Q, Wang X, Xiang LF, Xia L, et al. New developments in our understanding of acne pathogenesis and treatment. Exp Dermatol. 2009;18(10):821-32.
3. Lasek RJ, Chren MM. Acne vulgaris and the quality of life of adult dermatology patients. Arch Dermatol. 1998;134(4):454-8.

4. Picardi A, Mazzotti E, Pasquini P. Prevalence and correlates of suicidal ideation among patients with skin disease. J Am Acad Dermatol. 2006;54(3):420-6.
5. Jacob CI, Dover JS, Kaminer MS. Acne scarring: a classification system and review of treatment options. J Am Acad Dermatol. 2001;45(1):109-17.
6. Rivera AE. Acne scarring: a review and current treatment modalities. J Am Acad Dermatol. 2008;59(4):659-76.
7. Ibrahim ZA, Eltatawy RA, Ghaly NR, Abd El-Naby NM, Abou El Fetouh HM, Abd Elateef AE, et al. Autologous bone marrow stem cells in atrophic acne scars: A pilot study. J Dermatolog Treat. 2015;26(3):260-5.
8. Seidel R, Moy RL. Improvement in atrophic acne scars using topical synthetic epidermal growth factor (EGF) serum: a pilot study. J Drugs Dermatol. 2015;14(9):1005-10.
9. Rubenstein R, Roenigk HH Jr, Stegman SJ, Hanke CW. Atypical keloids after dermabrasion of patients taking isotretinoin. J Am Acad Dermatol. 1986;15(2 Pt 1):280-5.
10. Zachariae H. Delayed wound healing and keloid formation following argon laser treatment or dermabrasion during isotretinoin treatment. Br J Dermatol. 1988;118(5):703-6.
11. Katz BE, Mac Farlane DF. Atypical facial scarring after isotretinoin therapy in a patient with previous dermabrasion. J Am Acad Dermatol. 1994;30(5 Pt 2):852-3.
12. Roenigk HH Jr., Pinski JB, Robinson JK, Hanke CW. Acne, retinoids, and dermabrasion. J Dermatol Surg Oncol. 1985;11:4:396-8.
13. Roenigk HH Jr. Dermabrasion: state of the art. J Dermatol Surg Oncol. 1985;11(3):306-14.
14. Spring LK, Krakowski AC, Alam M, Bhatia A, Brauer J, Cohen J, et al. Isotretinoin and Timing of Procedural Interventions: A Systematic Review With Consensus Recommendations. JAMA Dermatol. 2017;153(8):802-9.
15. Alster TS, Handrick C. Laser treatment of hypertrophic scars, keloids, and striae. Semin Cutan Med Surg. 2000;19(4):287-92.
16. Alster TS, McMeekin TO. Improvement of facial acne scars by the 585nm flashlamp-pumped pulsed-dye laser. J Am Acad Dermatol. 1996;35(1):79-81.
17. Alster TS, Nanni CA. Pulsed dye laser treatment of hypertrophic burn scars. Plast Reconstr Surg. 1998;102(6):2190-5.
18. Manuskiatti W, Fitzpatrick RE. Treatment response of keloidal and hypertrophic sternotomy scars: comparison among intralesional corticosteroid, 5-fluorouracil, and 585-nm flashlamp-pumped pulsed-dye laser treatments. Arch. Dermatol. 2002;138(9):1149-55.
19. Zhu R, Yue B, Yang Q,, Ma Y, Huang G, Guan M, et al. The effect of 595 nm pulsed dye laser on connective tissue growth factor (CTGF) expression in cultured keloid fibroblasts. Lasers Surg Med. 2015;47(2):203-9.
20. Kuo YR, Wu WS, Jeng SF, Wang FS, Huang HC, Lin CZ, et al. Suppressed TGF-beta1 expression is correlated with up-regulation of matrix metalloproteinase-13 in keloid regression after flashlamp pulsed-dye laser treatment. Lasers Surg Med. 2005;36(1):38-42.
21. Keaney TC, Tanzi E, Alster T. Comparison of 532 nm Potassium Titanyl Phosphate Laser and 595 nm Pulsed Dye Laser in the Treatment of Erythematous Surgical Scars: A Randomized, Controlled, Open-Label Study. Dermatol Surg. 2016;42(1):70-6.
22. Rossi A, Lu R, Frey MK, Kubota T, Smith LA, Perez M. The use of the 300 microsecond 1064 nm Nd:YAG laser in the treatment of keloids. J Drugs Dermatol. 2013;12(11):1256-62.
23. Sherman R, Rosenfeld H. Experience with the Nd:YAG laser in the treatment of keloid scars. Ann Plast Surg. 1988;21(3):231-5.
24. Abergel RP, Dwyer RM, Meeker CA, Lask G, Kelly AP, Uitto J. Laser treatment of keloids: a clinical trial and an in vitro study with Nd:YAG laser. Lasers Surg Med. 1984;4(3):291-5.
25. DJ Castro, RP Abergel, C Meeker, RM Dwyer, MA Lesavoy, Uitto J. Effects of the Nd:YAG laser on DNA synthesis and collagen production in human skin fibroblast cultures. Ann Plast Surg. 1983;11(3):214-22.
26. Al-Mohamady Ael-S, Ibrahim SM, Muhammad MM. Pulsed dye laser versus long-pulsed Nd:YAG laser in the treatment of hypertrophic scars and keloid: A comparative randomized split-scar trial. J Cosmet Laser Ther. 2016;18(4):208-12.
27. Hruza GJ, Dover JS. Laser skin resurfacing. Arch Dermatol. 1996;132(4):451-5.
28. Kaufmann R, Hibst R. Pulsed Erbium:YAG laser ablation in cutaneous surgery. Lasers Surg Med. 1996;19(3):324-30.
29. Tanzi EL, Alster TS. Treatment of atrophic acne scars with a dual-mode Er:YAG laser. Dermatol Surg. 2002;28(7):551-5.
30. Alster TS. Cutaneous resurfacing with CO2 and erbium: YAG lasers: preoperative, intraoperative, and postoperative considerations. Plast Reconstr Surg. 1999;103(2):619-32.
31. Alster TS, West TB. Resurfacing of atrophic facial acne scars with a high-energy, pulsed carbon dioxide laser. Dermatol Surg. 1996;22(2):151-4.
32. Walia S, Alster TS. Prolonged clinical and histologic effects from CO2 laser resurfacing of atrophic acne scars. Dermatol Surg. 1999;25(12):926-30.

33. Nanni CA, Alster TS. Complications of carbon dioxide laser resurfacing. An evaluation of 500 patients. Dermatol Surg. 1998;24(3):315-20.
34. Tanzi EL, Alster TS. Side effects and complications of variable-pulsed erbium:yttrium-aluminum-garnet laser skin resurfacing: extended experience with 50 patients. Plast Reconstr Surg. 2003;111(4):1524-9.
35. Tanzi EL, Alster TS. Comparison of a 1450-nm diode laser and a 1320-nm Nd: YAG laser in the treatment of atrophic facial scars: a prospective clinical and histologic study. Dermatol Surg. 2004;30(2 Pt 1):152-7.
36. Chua SH, Ang P, Khoo LS, Goh CL. Nonablative 1450-nm diode laser in the treatment of facial atrophic acne scars in type IV to V Asian skin: a prospective clinical study. Dermatol Surg. 2004;30(10):1287-91.
37. Keller R, Júnior WB, Valente NY, Rodrigues CJ. Nonablative 1,064-nm Nd:YAG laser for treating atrophic facial acne scars: histologic and clinical analysis. Dermatol Surg. 2007;33(12):1470-6.
38. Min SU, Choi YS, Lee DH, Yoon MY, Suh DH. Comparison of a long-pulse Nd:YAG laser and a combined 585/1,064-nm laser for the treatment of acne scars: a randomized split-face clinical study. Dermatol Surg. 2009;35(11):1720-7.
39. Manstein D, Herron GS, Sink RK, Tanner H, Anderson RR. Fractional photothermolysis: a new concept for cutaneous remodeling using microscopic patterns of thermal injury. Lasers Surg Med. 2004;34(5):426-38.
40. Graber EM, Tanzi EL, Alster TS. Side effects and complications of fractional laser photothermolysis: experience with 961 treatments. Dermatol Surg. 2008;34(3):301-5.
41. Cho SI, Chung BY, Choi MG, Baek JH, Cho HJ, Park CW, et al. Evaluation of the clinical efficacy of fractional radiofrequency microneedle treatment in acne scars and large facial pores. Dermatol Surg. 2012;38(7 Pt 1):1017-24.
42. Gold MH, Biron JA. Treatment of acne scars by fractional bipolar radiofrequency energy. J Cosmet Laser Ther. 2012;14(4):172-8.
43. Forbat E, Al-Niaimi F. Fractional radiofrequency treatment in acne scars: Systematic review of current evidence. J Cosmet Laser Ther. 2016;18(8):442-7.

21

CHAPTER

Fat and Cellulite

Catherine DiGiorgio, Mathew M Avram

INTRODUCTION

Given the risks associated with general anesthesia required for invasive surgical procedures to remove unwanted adipose tissue, noninvasive procedures have become the focus of lower risk cosmetic procedures. There are many noninvasive therapeutic options for the removal of unwanted subcutaneous adipose tissue. Additionally, mostly for women, cellulite is an undesirable appearance for which patients seek treatment. It is important to remember the treatments described in this chapter should be considered body-sculpting procedures as they may be less effective than conventional surgical procedures. This chapter will review laser- and energy-based modalities for the removal of unwanted fat including: cryolipolysis, radiofrequency (RF), ultrasound, and low-level light therapy (**Table 1**). We will also discuss laser- and energy-based modalities used to improve the appearance of cellulite (**Table 2**).

DESTRUCTION OF UNWANTED FAT

Cryolipolysis

Manstein et al. first demonstrated in a pig model that human adipose tissue can be selectively damaged by cold exposure.[1] Based on the well-defined but rare clinical conditions of "popsicle panniculitis" and "equestrian panniculitis" in which prolonged exposure to cold results in fat necrosis, their study demonstrated that prolonged cold exposure resulted in selective necrosis of fat with sparing of epidermal and dermal structures.[1-3] "Popsicle panniculitis" and "equestrian panniculitis" are types of cold panniculitides that occur due to the physical properties of lipids compared to water. Other components of skin and subcutaneous tissue are composed mostly of water and freezing of lipids occurs at a higher temperature than that of water.[1] Therefore, when controlled cooling is applied to areas containing unwanted adipose tissue, cold panniculitis of fat occurs with resultant selective necrosis of fat without permanent damage to skin or other subcutaneous tissues. The necrotic fat undergoes apoptosis and is eliminated. This results in contoured body areas after several months.

To date, studies in both human and animal models show that cryolipolysis does not cause alterations in liver function tests or serum lipid levels. Common complications after treatment with cryolipolysis include pain, edema, purpura, edema, and numbness.[4-6] Less common complications include intense

TABLE 1: Destruction of unwanted fat.

Technology	Mechanism of action	Commercial name(s)
Cryolipolysis	Selective destruction of adipocytes by cold panniculitis resulting in necrosis	Coolsculpting (Allergan. Dublin, IE)
High-intensity focused ultrasound (HIFU)	Delivery of energy (2 MHz, >1,000 W/cm^2) via acoustic waves resulting in coagulative necrosis and mechanical destruction of adipocytes	Liposonix (Solta. Pleasanton, CA)
Low-frequency focused ultrasound	Delivery of lower intensity energy (200 kHz, 17.5 W/cm^2) via acoustic waves causing mechanical destruction via cavitation of adipocytes	Ultrashape (Candela. Wayland, MA)
Radiofrequency	Rapidly alternating direct electrical causes oscillation of cellular structures and heating of fat based on properties of low thermal conductivity and high electrical resistance	**Unipolar** Monopolar: • Exilis (BTL. Marlborough, MA) monopolar radiofrequency (RF) and nonfocused ultrasound • truSculpt iD (Cutera. Brisbane, CA) monopolar RF Bipolar: • Velashape (Candela. Wayland, MA) bipolar RF and infrared light Multipolar: • Vanquish (BTL. Marlborough, MA)
Infrared lasers	Molecular vibration resulting in collisions and adipocyte injury (1060 nm)	Sculpsure (Cynosure. Westford, MA)
Low-level laser therapy (LLLT)	Mechanism is controversial and not well defined	Zerona (Erchonia Corporation. Melbourne, FL)

neuropathic pain and paradoxical adipose tissue hyperplasia.[5,7,8]

High-intensity Focused Ultrasound

The application of high-intensity focused ultrasound (HIFU) delivers energy to the subcutaneous fat in the form of acoustic waves to selectively destroy adipose tissue by coagulative necrosis and mechanical destruction.[5,9,10] Properties of adipose tissue that allow its selective destruction by HIFU waves include a lower heat conductivity, lower specific heat capacity, and lower perfusion in comparison to the surrounding epidermal and subcutaneous tissues.[10] High-frequency ultrasound waves can be focused due to the short wavelengths used in these devices (1-mm wavelengths).[11] These focused ultrasound waves penetrate through the skin and subcutaneous tissues to reach the desired focal zone. The temperature at the focus of the ultrasound waves is rapidly increased beyond 55°C, resulting in coagulative necrosis of the cells and mechanical destruction of collagen. The high-intensity ultrasonic energy

TABLE 2: Treatment of cellulite.

Technology	Commercial Name(s)	
Extracorporeal shock wave therapy (acoustic wave therapy)	D-Actor®200 (Storz Medical AG, Tagerwilen, Switzerland)	
Low level laser	Zerona (Erchonia, McKinney, TX)	
Laser assisted subcision (1440 nm)	Cellulaze (Cynosure, Inc, Westford, MA)	
Radiofrequency (RF)	**Unipolar RF**	**Thermage (Solta Medical, Hayward, CA)**
	Unipolar RF + Bipolar RF	• Accent (Alma Lasers Ltd, Caesarea, Israel)
	Monopolar RF + Ultrasonic energy	• Exilis (BTL Industries, Inc, Prague, Czech Republic)
	Electromagnetic energy + Infrared light + RF + mechanical manipulation	• VelaSmooth (Syneron Medical Ltd, Yokneam Illit, Israel)
	RF + IR + vacuum + mechanical manipulation	• VelaShape (Syneron Medical Ltd, Yokneam Illit, Israel)

(2 MHz, >1000 W/cm^2) enables adequate heat production to induce this destruction in the focal zone at a depth of 1.3 cm.[5,10,12]

Studies have demonstrated the effectiveness of HIFU technology to reduce waist circumference, with the initial clinical response evident as early as 2 weeks and complete clinical response at 3 months.[11] However, there has been slight variation in the reported amount of waist circumference reduction. Two retrospective chart reviews performed by Fatemi et al. reviewed 367 patients after a single HIFU treatment to the abdomen and flanks and demonstrated a mean waist circumference reduction measured at 12 weeks ranging from 4.2 to 4.7 cm.[11-13] A randomized study of 188 subjects performed by Robinson et al. found a mean waist circumference reduction at 12 weeks of 2.3 ± 2.9 cm.[14] Results have also demonstrated that reduction of waist circumference correlates with the total fluence delivered, not the total number of passes performed.[5]

Adverse events experienced with HIFU are mild and self-limited and include pain during treatment, tenderness (which can be prolonged), edema, and ecchymosis.[5,11] Destruction of adipose tissue by HIFU has not been shown to affect serum lipid levels or other serum laboratory values and has not resulted in dystrophic calcification.[11]

Low-frequency (Nonthermal) Focused Ultrasound

Low-frequency focused ultrasound delivers energy in the form of acoustic waves at a lower intensity compared to HIFU. The low-intensity focused ultrasound energy (200 kHz, 17.5 W/cm^2) destroys adipocytes at the focal point depth of 1.5 cm through mechanical damage resulting in cavitation without damage to skin and surrounding subcutaneous tissue (**Figs. 1A** to **C**).[15-17]

A study by Teitelbaum et al. in which 137 subjects were treated with a single treatment of low-frequency focused ultrasound demons-

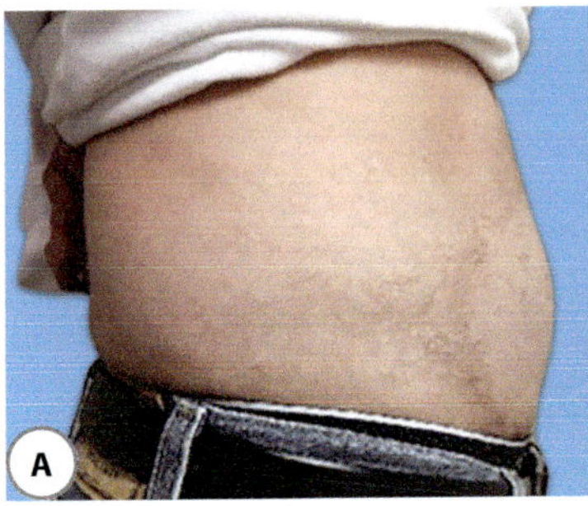

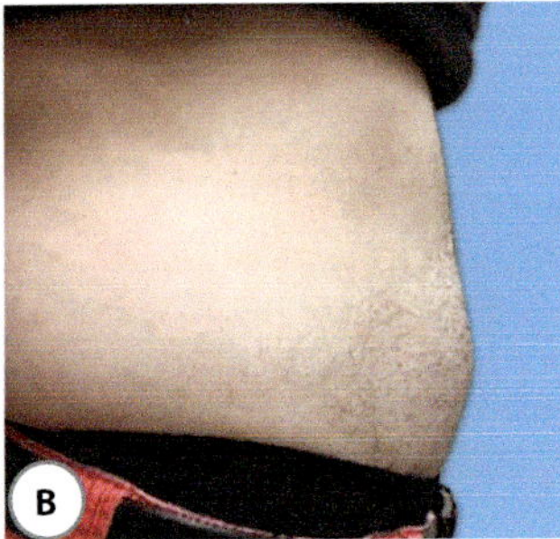

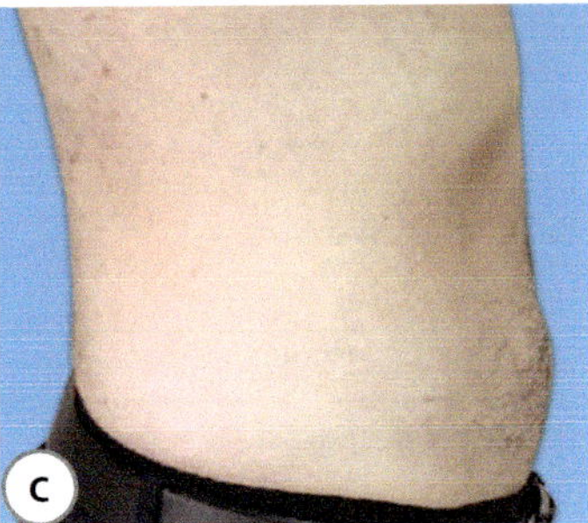

FIGS. 1A TO C: Treatment with low-frequency (nonthermal) focused ultrasound at baseline, 2 weeks posttreatment, and 6 weeks posttreatment.
Courtesy: Dana Marshall, MD.

trated approximately 2 cm of fat reduction in the treated areas of the abdomen, flanks, and thighs.[18] A more recent multicenter, randomized, control study by Coleman et al. evaluated the effects of multiple treatments with low-frequency focused ultrasound at 2-week intervals in two groups of subjects. They demonstrated a reduction in abdominal circumference of 2.5–3.5 cm after three consecutive treatments. This study also showed that multiple treatments resulted in a greater reduction in abdominal circumference.[19]

Adverse events experienced with low-frequency focused ultrasound are mild and self-limited and include pain, erythema, ecchymosis, and blistering.[5,19]

Radiofrequency

Radiofrequency devices deliver a rapidly alternating direct electric current to tissue causing oscillation of cellular structures and, with continued delivery of current, molecular collisions that create energy in the form of heat. Although RF is nonselective, physical properties of adipose tissue, such as low thermal conductivity and high electrical resistance, allow selective destruction of fat while sparing surrounding dermal and epidermal structures.[20] In addition to destruction of adipose tissue, RF also heats collagen type I resulting in denaturation, remodeling, and repair, theoretically also tightening the tissue to improve laxity.[21]

Radiofrequency devices can be monopolar, unipolar, bipolar, or multipolar. Monopolar RF devices use one electrode and a grounding pad to deliver the electrical current into the skin resulting in heating. These devices have had success for tissue tightening but studies demonstrating reduction of adipose tissue are lacking. Unipolar RF devices use one electrode to deliver electromagnetic radiation, not electrical current, to produce heat. Limited data is available for unipolar RF and adipose tissue destruction; however, one study showed a decrease in thigh circumference after sequential repeated sessions. Unipolar RF has been shown to improve the appearance of cellulite, which will be further discussed in this chapter. Bipolar RF devices use two electrodes, between which the electrical current flows. Some bipolar RF devices combine use of a light source such as infrared light (**Figs. 2A** and **B**), or [intense pulsed light (IPL)], or diode, while others use a vacuum system to increase the depth of penetration and effectiveness. Multipolar RF devices utilize three or more electrodes to deliver electrical current that can reach a depth of 20 mm allowing volumetric heating of deeper subcutaneous tissues. Reduction of abdominal circumference has

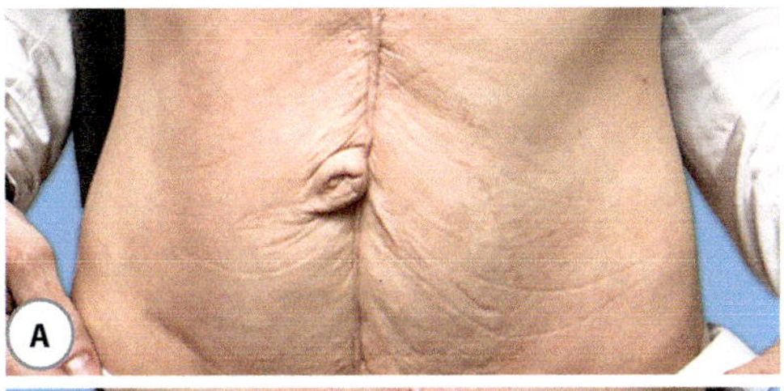

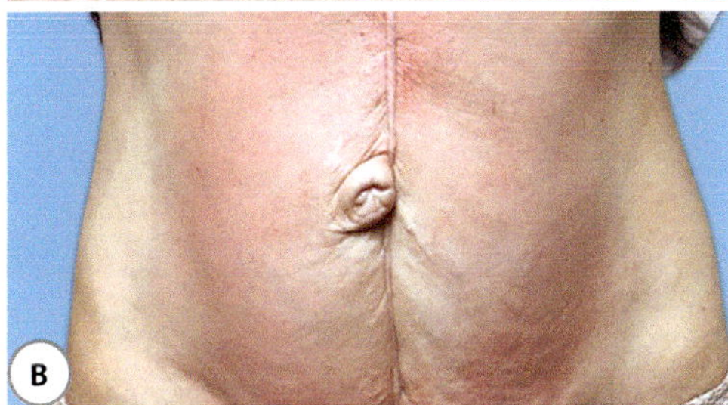

FIGS. 2A AND B: Before and immediately after treatment with bipolar radiofrequency and infrared light device—Velashape (Candela. Wayland, MA).
Courtesy: Dana Marshall, MD.

been demonstrated in several trials using the bipolar and multipolar RF devices indicating these may be an effective treatment option for destruction of unwanted subcutaneous adipose tissue.[5,20]

Adverse events reported with RF devices are mostly transient and include pain, erythema, edema, purpura, postinflammatory pigmentary alteration, and, rarely, blisters and burns.[5,20]

Infrared Lasers

Based on the theory of selective photothermolysis, near-infrared lasers operating at wavelengths of 1,210 nm and 1,720 nm have been used to selectively target and destroy lipid molecules based on molecular vibration.[22-24] A 1,060-nm diode laser is cleared by the Food and Drug Administration (FDA) for selective destruction of adipose tissue. This laser delivers energy in the form of heat that is selectively absorbed by subcutaneous adipose tissue resulting in molecular collisions and adipocyte injury (**Figs. 3A** to **D**). The device utilizes a sapphire window to protect overlying epidermis from injury.[25,26] Temperature of adipocytes must be maintained at 42–47°C to achieve adipocyte injury by delayed cell death.[25,26] Side effects are minimal and include mild discomfort during the procedure, and mild to moderate tenderness postprocedure. There have been no reports of prolonged pain postprocedure.[25]

Although there are no long-term studies demonstrating sustained improvement with use of the 1,060-nm diode infrared laser for fat reduction, several studies show patient satisfaction at 90%.[25] In one two-center prospective controlled study of treatment of the abdomen with evaluations performed at 6 weeks and 12 weeks posttreatment, blinded evaluators were able to differentiate pretreatment photos from posttreatment photos on an average of 95% of the time. Ultrasound analysis revealed decreased fat layer from baseline both at 6 weeks (1.5 ± 1.23 mm) and 12 weeks (2.65 ± 1.41 mm).[27] Another two-center prospective study analyzing treatment of the flanks also showed improvement at 12 weeks, with blinded evaluators able to differentiate pre- and posttreatment photos 90% of the time on average.[28] Ultrasound analysis showed fat reduction from baseline was approximately 9% ± 5% at 6 weeks and 13% ± 6% at 12 weeks. Control site fat reduction was 1% ± 5% at both 6 weeks and 12 weeks.[28] Although these short-term studies show mild improvement with a decrease in fat layer in the treated areas, long-term studies demonstrating the efficacy of this device are not available.[28]

Low-level Laser Therapy

Low-level laser therapy (LLLT) involves the application of laser light at a low irradiance. Initial studies performed by Niera et al. used a 635-nm light source operating at 10 mW for pulse durations ranging from 0 to 6 minutes,[29] while others have attempted lipolysis with

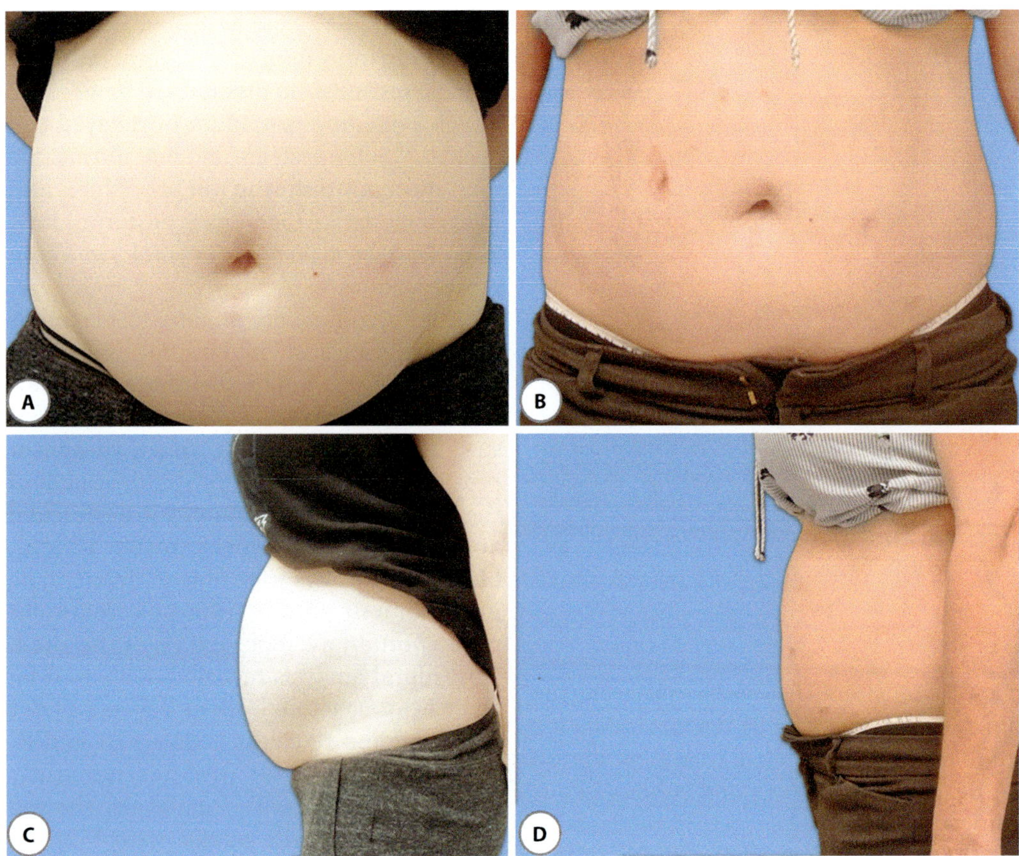

FIGS. 3A TO D: Treatment with a 1060-nm diode laser. This patient received two treatments. Photos are at baseline and 3 months from initial treatment.

Courtesy: Nazanein Saedi, MD.

other wavelengths such as 850 nm, 650 nm and irradiances ranging from 1 mW to 5 W/cm^2.[30] The mechanism of action for destruction of adipose tissue by LLLT is controversial and not well defined.[5,30] Niera et al. proposed that LLLT created a transient pore within the wall of adipocytes allowing leakage of lipid from the intracellular space to the extracellular space.[29] Other studies have suggested that LLLT induces mobilization of triglycerides out of cells without damage to the cell membrane.[31] Furthermore, some studies have suggested that LLLT indirectly modulates autocrine or paracrine processes within the adipocyte to alter lipid metabolism without cell lysis.[30] Additional studies have also suggested that destruction of adipocytes by LLLT occurs through complement activation or mitochondrial releases of cytochrome c oxidase.[32] None of these proposed mechanisms have been validated, therefore, the exact mechanism of action for destruction of adipose tissue by LLLT is not understood.[5]

Some studies have demonstrated a reduction in abdominal circumference after treatment with LLLT. However, the results are confounded by subjects undergoing rigorous exercise programs and subjects using dietary weight loss supplements. In addition, the studies themselves lack appropriate clinical control sites.[30] One split abdomen study showed no clinically significant difference in fat thickness on the treatment site compared to control site, and 8 of 17 patients in this study had an increase in fat thickness on the treatment site.[30] Given the controversial and contradictory evidence surrounding LLLT for reduction of adipose tissue, further studies must be performed in order to elucidate the mechanism of action, safety, and efficacy for this modality.

CELLULITE

Cellulite is a medically normal, cosmetically unfavorable appearance of the skin mostly on the posterior thighs, lateral thighs, and buttocks affecting up to 90% of postpubertal women.[33-35] The appearance of cellulite has been described as "cottage cheese" or "orange peel."[35] The exact etiology of cellulite is still being defined in the literature and several factors have been suggested to be associated with the appearance of cellulite including postpubertal age, female gender, decreased dermal collagen, hormonal imbalance, genetics, and thickened fibrous septae.[32,34] Although not identified as medical causes of cellulite, diet, obesity, weight gain, and lack of exercise do contribute to a worsening clinical appearance of cellulite.[33]

Studies using magnetic resonance imaging have described the anatomy of cellulite as thickened fibrous septae tethering the dermis to the underlying fascia and running in a perpendicular angle to skin.[31-34] This tension allows fat lobules to extend upward and protrude into the dermal fat layer.[34,36]

While the exact etiology of cellulite has yet to be proven, there are numerous theories in the literature, particularly focusing on the reasoning behind cellulite being more common in women. The first theory for the cause of the appearance of cellulite being more common in women than men was first described by Nürnberger and Muller in 1978.[37,38] Their studies demonstrated structural variations of dermal and subcutaneous tissue in men versus women and the body's response to estrogen (**Figs. 4A** and **B**). In women, collagen fibers are rectangular and organized perpendicular to the skin surface with lobules of adipocytes between these fibers. In men, collagen fibers are randomly organized around adipose tissue creating unorganized polygonal adipose lobules. This description of the structural variations in cellulite for men and women is widely accepted. Additionally, they hypo-

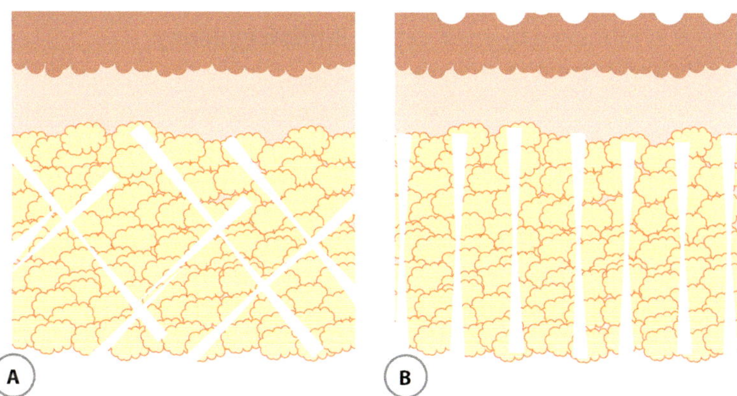

FIGS. 4A AND B: Schematic demonstrating the anatomy of cellulite in men in which fibrous septae are arranged haphazardly (A) versus women in which thickened fibrous septae run perpendicular to the skin and tether the dermis to the underlying fascia (B).

thesized that estrogen causes thickening of collagen fibers, and in women, this results in compression of mature adipose lobules by thickened organized collagen fibers, which leads to the appearance of cellulite.[37,39]

A second theory, hypothesized by Merlin and Curri in the 1980s, suggested differing lymphatic draining patterns and vascular circulation leading to fibrosis visualized on skin biopsies and suggested as the cause of cellulite.[38,40,41] Others have expanded on this vascular theory and have suggested that disruption of capillary vasculature networks results in accumulation of fluid within adipocyte lobules that then clump together and inhibit venous return resulting in impaired tissue repair and deposition of protein around adipocyte lobules leading to the clinical appearance of cellulite.[42]

A third theory is based on dermal collagen destruction mediated by hormones released in women during menstruation. Collagenase [matrix metalloproteinase-1 (MMP-1)] and gelatinase (MMP-2) are metalloproteases that break down the fibrillar collagen lattices in the endometrium resulting in menstruation, and as suggested by this theory, in the dermis as well. During the late proliferative phase and postovulation phase of the menstrual cycle, gelatinase B is produced by mast cells and stromal cells and results in release of inflammatory mediators. Synthesis of glycosaminoglycans (GAGs) in the dermis may be a component of this inflammatory cascade. GAGs deposited in the dermal-subcutaneous junction enhance water binding resulting in edema, which may contribute to the appearance of cellulite. Repeated cycles of menstruation result in cyclical production of collagenases and cyclical deposition of GAGs in the dermis, which theoretically contributes to worsened appearance of cellulite in women that increases with age.[38,42]

Given the social distress patients experience due to the presence of cellulite, several treatments have been developed, however, lack of long-term improvement, unpredictable efficacy, and cost are likely reasons; such treatments have not become more common.[33] This chapter will focus on treatment of cellulite via the following laser- and energy-based modalities: Extracorporeal shock wave therapy (acoustic wave therapy), RF, and laser lipolysis. Other modalities that do not use laser- and energy-based technology (including topical therapy, injectables, and subcision) will not be discussed.

Treatment of Cellulite

Extracorporeal Shock Wave Therapy (Acoustic Wave Therapy)

Extracorporeal shock wave therapy or acoustic wave therapy utilizes low-energy, non-focused sound waves to nonselectively destroy target tissue and may improve the appearance of cellulite through neocollagenesis and improvement in microcirculation and lymphatic drainage.[43] Limited studies have shown improvement in cellulite using acoustic wave therapy, therefore further studies are needed to demonstrate the effectiveness of this modality.[43,44]

Radiofrequency

Radiofrequency, as described earlier in this chapter, delivers energy by electrical current and can be monopolar, unipolar, bipolar, or multipolar. One device used primarily for tissue tightening utilizes transcutaneous monopolar RF delivery and can temporarily improve the appearance of cellulite in some patients (**Figs. 5A** and **B**). However, studies investigating improvement of cellulite with this device are limited and results are variable.[33] Several devices combining RF with other modalities are currently being used to treat cellulite in combination with treatment of

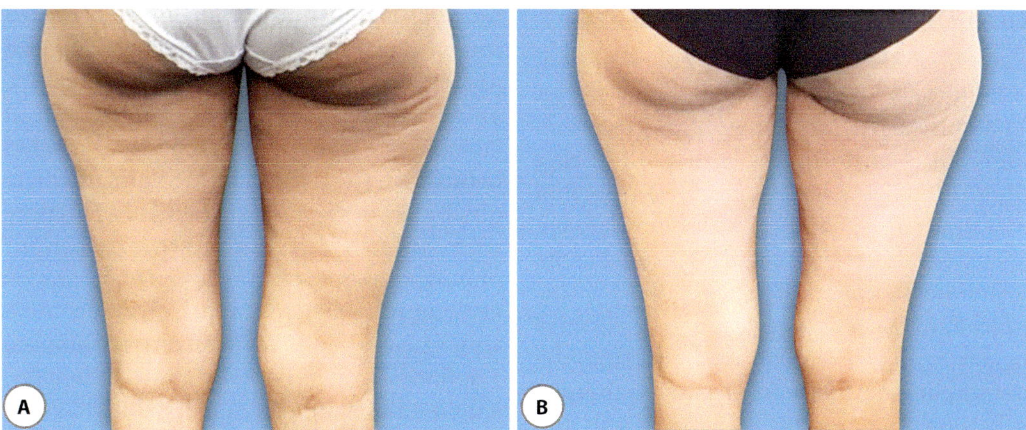

FIGS. 5A AND B: Before and 3 months after treatment with monopolar radiofrequency (Thermage. Solta, Pleasanton, CA) to improve the appearance of cellulite.

unwanted adipose accumulation and to achieve tissue tightening.[33] Since bipolar RF only reaches a superficial depth, it is usually combined with other modalities in the treatment of cellulite.[33] One device combines bipolar RF with mechanical massage and controlled infrared light energy (700–2000 nm) that manipulates the tissue via vacuum suction. Treatments can be refined based on the patient by adjusting settings on any of the three modalities.[35]

Unipolar RF devices can deliver energy deeper and, therefore, have been studied for the treatment of cellulite. Off-label treatment of cellulite with a device (traditionally used for treatment of rhytides) that combines monopolar RF with ultrasound has been anecdotally reported to improve the appearance of cellulite. Since these devices are also used for destruction of unwanted adipose tissue, treatment of cellulite is similar and has the same side effect profile.[35]

Laser

A combination device with a triple treatment approach was developed and uses laser, massage, and contact cooling to improve the appearance of cellulite. Laser energy is delivered via six 808-nm diode lasers. Delivery of laser energy is thought to promote neovascularization and enhance vascular flow of the arterial, venous, and lymphatic systems. The massage component of the device is rhythmic and can be adjusted for depth and intensity based on the patient. Depth is adjusted based on frequency of aspirations; higher frequencies target superficial tissue while lower frequencies target deeper tissue. Intensity is tunable by changing the duration of active aspirations. Increasing the duration of each aspiration increases the intensity of the treatment while decreasing the duration of each aspiration decreases the intensity of treatment. The massage component of the device stretches and smoothes tissue between the dermis and epidermis while also stimulating vascular flow and lymphatic drainage. The contact cooling system also increases mobilization of vascular fluid resulting in decreased edema.[35] Studies have shown improvement in the appearance of cellulite after treatment with these devices, but results have not been permanent.[33,45]

Laser Lipolysis

Laser lipolysis to improve the appearance of cellulite was first demonstrated in 2008.[46] A 1440-nm Nd:YAG (neodymium-doped yttrium aluminum garnet) laser with a side-firing fiber tip delivers laser energy via insertion of a thermal-sensing cannula into the skin such that laser energy can be delivered at the anatomical location of the cellulite.[33,36] This procedure has been suggested to be effective by destroying fat lobules protruding into the dermis, destroy thickened septae via thermal subcision, and promote neocollagenesis and tissue tightening by delivering energy to the dermis. It is usually combined with manual subcision to achieve optimal results.[33,36] The procedure requires tumescent anesthesia. Common side effects are transient and include bruising, pain, edema, and numbness.[33,36]

Studies demonstrating the effectiveness of the 1440 nm laser for the treatment of cellulite are sparse. The device does not appear to substantially destroy the fibrous bands that theoretically cause the appearance of cellulite nor does the device result in significant adipolysis.[47]

One multicenter study enrolled 57 female subjects in total that received one single treatment with the 1440 nm laser for cellulite. 47 subjects (82%) returned for 6 month follow-up evaluation and 30 subjects (53%) returned for the 12 month follow-up evaluation. Blinded evaluators were asked to view two treatment sites per patient and identify pretreatment photographs from posttreatment photographs (at 6 months and 12 months), evaluate contour and dimpling, and an assessment of physician and subject satisfaction was performed. At the 6-month follow-up visit, a total of 94 photographs were available for blinded evaluation; however, 32 photographs were determined to be inadequate in quality and were removed from evaluation. A total of 62 photographs from various sites were included and blinded investigators were able to differentiate pretreatment from posttreatment in 97% on average. At the 12-month follow-up of 30 subjects, only 52 photographs were included because 8 were determined to be of inadequate quality. On average 91% of blinded evaluators were able to differentiate pretreatment photographs from posttreatment photographs at 12 months. Dimples were also graded on a scale of 0–4, where 0 was defined as no dimples, 1 defined as 1 dimple, 2 defined as 2 dimples, 3 defined as 3 dimples, and 4 defined as 4 or more dimples. Similarly, a contour score ranged in severity from 0 (no contour irregularities) to 4 (severe contour irregularities). The authors report an average of 1 score of improvement for both contour and dimpling and an average physician satisfaction score at 6 months of 5.4 on a 6-point scale (6 being extremely satisfied) and subject satisfaction score of 5.0 (45 subjects completed questionnaire). At 12 months, average physician satisfaction score was 5.6 and average subject satisfaction score 5.3 (11 subjects completed questionnaire).[36] A similar study was performed by the same authors in 2013 and had similar methodology, photography, evaluations, and results.[48] Another study by Katz et al. utilized two-dimensional (2D) surface imaging and results showed that blinded investigators were able to differentiate between pretreatment and posttreatment photos on an average of 90%, and with 3D imaging found improvement of dimpling in 49% at 6 months.[49] In summary, the efficacy of the 1440 nm laser in the treatment of cellulite is unclear given the paucity of scientific evidence.

CONCLUSION

Noninvasive and minimally invasive body contouring procedures for the treatment of fat and cellulite have increased since the innovation in this field began about 10 years ago. Patients continue to seek procedures to improve the appearance of their body and prefer to avoid large surgical procedures with longer recovery times. As physicians continue to try to meet the needs and desires of their patients, innovation will continue to grow. We are certainly on the forefront of the development of additional laser- and energy-based modalities to treat unwanted fat and improve the appearance of cellulite in a safe, noninvasive manner. The future is bright for more effective noninvasive and minimally invasive treatments to improve the appearance of fat and cellulite.

REFERENCES

1. Manstein D, Laubach H, Watanabe K, Farinelli W, Zurakowski D, Anderson RR. Selective cryolysis: a novel method of non-invasive fat removal. Lasers Surg Med. 2008;40(9):595-604.
2. Beacham BE, Cooper PH, Buchanan CS, Weary PE. Equestrian cold panniculitis in women. Arch Dermatol. 1980;116(9):1025-7.
3. Epstein EH, Oren ME. Popsicle panniculitis. N Engl J Med. 1970;282(17):966-7.
4. Coleman SR, Sachdeva K, Egbert BM, Preciado J, Allison J. Clinical efficacy of noninvasive cryolipolysis and its effects on peripheral nerves. Aesthetic Plast Surg. 2009;33(4):482-8.
5. Friedmann DP. A review of the aesthetic treatment of abdominal subcutaneous adipose tissue: background, implications, and therapeutic options. Dermatol Surg. 2015;41(1):18-34.
6. Keaney TC, Gudas AT, Alster TS. Delayed Onset Pain Associated With Cryolipolysis Treatment: A Retrospective Study With Treatment Recommendations. Dermatol Surg. 2015;41(11):1296-9.
7. Jalian HR, Avram MM, Garibyan L, Mihm MC, Anderson RR. Paradoxical adipose hyperplasia after cryolipolysis. JAMA Dermatol. 2014;150(3):317-9.
8. Singh SM, Geddes ERC, Boutrous SG, Galiano RD, Friedman PM. Paradoxical adipose hyperplasia secondary to cryolipolysis: An underreported entity? Lasers Surg Med. 2015;47(6):476-8.
9. Lee HJ, Lee M-H, Lee SG, Yeo U-C, Chang SE. Evaluation of a novel device, high-intensity focused ultrasound with a contact cooling for subcutaneous fat reduction. Lasers Surg Med. 2016;48(9):878-86.
10. Winter PM, Lanier M, Partanen A, Dumoulin C. Initial investigation of a novel noninvasive weight loss therapy using MRI-Guided high intensity focused ultrasound (MR-HIFU) of visceral fat. Magn Reson Med. 2016;76(1):282-9.
11. Jewell ML, Solish NJ, Desilets CS. Noninvasive body sculpting technologies with an emphasis on high-intensity focused ultrasound. Aesthetic Plast Surg. 2011;35(5):901-12.
12. Fatemi A, Kane MAC. High-intensity focused ultrasound effectively reduces waist circumference by ablating adipose tissue from the abdomen and flanks: a retrospective case series. Aesthetic Plast Surg. 2010;34(5):577-82.
13. Fatemi A. High-intensity focused ultrasound effectively reduces adipose tissue. Semin Cutan Med Surg. 2009;28(4):257-62.
14. Robinson DM, Kaminer MS, Baumann L, Burns AJ, Brauer JA, Jewell M, et al. High-intensity focused ultrasound for the reduction of subcutaneous adipose tissue using multiple treatment techniques. Dermatol Surg. 2014;40(6):641-51.
15. Shek SYN, Yeung CK, Chan JCY, Chan HHL. The efficacy of a combination non-thermal focused ultrasound and radiofrequency device for noninvasive body contouring in Asians. Lasers Surg Med. 2016;48(2):203-7.
16. Zhou B, Leung BYK, Sun L. The Effects of Low-Intensity Ultrasound on Fat Reduction of Rat Model. Biomed Res Int. 2017;2017:4701481.
17. Brown SA, Greenbaum L, Shtukmaster S, Zadok Y, Ben-Ezra S, Kushkuley L. Characterization of nonthermal focused ultrasound for noninvasive selective fat cell disruption (lysis): technical and preclinical assessment. Plast Reconstr Surg. 2009;124(1):92-101.
18. Teitelbaum SA, Burns JL, Kubota J, Matsuda H, Otto MJ, Shirakabe Y, et al. Noninvasive body contouring by focused ultrasound: safety and efficacy of the Contour I device in a multicenter, controlled, clinical study. Plast Reconstr Surg. 2007;120(3):779-89.
19. Coleman WP, Coleman W, Weiss RA, Kenkel JM, Ad-El DD, Amir R. A Multicenter Controlled Study to Evaluate Multiple Treatments With Nonthermal Focused Ultrasound for Noninvasive Fat Reduction. Dermatol Surg. 2017;43(1):50-7.
20. Boisnic S, Divaris M, Nelson AA, Gharavi NM, Lask GP. A clinical and biological evaluation of a novel, noninvasive radiofrequency device for the long-term reduction of adipose tissue. Lasers Surg Med. 2014;46(2):94-103.
21. Hruza GJ, Tanzi EL (Eds). Lasers and Lights. Elsevier: 2018.
22. Anderson RR, Farinelli W, Laubach H, Manstein D, Yaroslavsky AN, Gubeli J 3rd, et al. Selective photothermolysis of lipid-rich tissues: a free electron laser study. Lasers Surg Med. 2006;38(10):913-9.

23. Anderson RR, Parrish JA. Selective photothermolysis: precise microsurgery by selective absorption of pulsed radiation. Science. 1983;220(4596):524-7.
24. Sakamoto FH, Doukas AG, Farinelli WA, Tannous Z, Shinn M, Benson S, et al. Selective photothermolysis to target sebaceous glands: theoretical estimation of parameters and preliminary results using a free electron laser. Lasers Surg Med. 2012;44(2):175-83.
25. Schilling L, Saedi N, Weiss R. 1060 nm Diode Hyperthermic Laser Lipolysis: The Latest in Non-Invasive Body Contouring. J Drugs Dermatol. 2017;16(1):48-52.
26. Decorato JW, Chen B, Sierra R. Subcutaneous adipose tissue response to a non-invasive hyperthermic treatment using a 1,060 nm laser. Lasers Surg Med. 2017;49(5):480-9.
27. Bass LS, Doherty ST. Safety and Efficacy of a Non-Invasive 1060 nm Diode Laser for Fat Reduction of the Abdomen. J Drugs Dermatol. 2018;17(1):106-12.
28. Katz B, Doherty S. Safety and Efficacy of a Noninvasive 1,060-nm Diode Laser for Fat Reduction of the Flanks. Dermatol Surg. 2018;44(3):388-96.
29. Neira R, Arroyave J, Ramirez H, Ortiz CL, Solarte E, Sequeda F, et al. Fat liquefaction: effect of low-level laser energy on adipose tissue. Plast Reconstr Surg. 2002;110(3):912-22;discussion 923-5.
30. Jankowski M, Gawrych M, Adamska U, Ciescinski J, Serafin Z, Czajkowski R. Low-level laser therapy (LLLT) does not reduce subcutaneous adipose tissue by local adipocyte injury but rather by modulation of systemic lipid metabolism. Lasers Med Sci. 2017;32(2): 475-9..
31. Caruso-Davis MK, Guillot TS, Podichetty VK, Mashtalir N, Dhurandhar NV, Dubuisson O, et al. Efficacy of low-level laser therapy for body contouring and spot fat reduction. Obes Surg. 2011;21(6):722-9.
32. Avci P, Nyame TT, Gupta GK, Sadasivam M, Hamblin MR. Low-level laser therapy for fat layer reduction: a comprehensive review. Lasers Surg Med. 2013;45(6): 349-57.
33. Friedmann DP, Vick GL, Mishra V. Cellulite: a review with a focus on subcision. Clin Cosmet Investig Dermatol. 2017;10:17-23.
34. Kaminer MS, Coleman WP, Weiss RA, Robinson DM, Grossman J. A Multicenter Pivotal Study to Evaluate Tissue Stabilized-Guided Subcision Using the Cellfina Device for the Treatment of Cellulite With 3-Year Follow-Up. Dermatol Surg. 2017;43(10):1240-8.
35. Peterson JD, Goldman MP. Laser, light, and energy devices for cellulite and lipodystrophy. Clin Plast Surg. 2011;38(3):463-74;vii.
36. DiBernardo BE, Sasaki GH, Katz BE, Hunstad JP, Petti C, Burns AJ. A Multicenter Study for Cellulite Treatment Using a 1440-nm Nd:YAG Wavelength Laser with Side-Firing Fiber. Aesthet Surg J. 2016;36(3):335-43.
37. Nürnberger F, Müller G. So-called cellulite: an invented disease. J Dermatol Surg Oncol. 1978;4(3):221-9.
38. Conti G, Zingaretti N, Amuso D, Dai Prè E, Brandi J, Cecconi D, et al. Proteomic and Ultrastructural Analysis of Cellulite-New Findings on an Old Topic. Int J Mol Sci. 2020;21(6):2077.
39. Nürnberger F. [Practically important diseases of the subcutaneous fatty tissue (including so-called cellulite)]. Med Welt. 1981;32(18):682-8.
40. Merlen JF, Curri SB. [Anatomico-pathological causes of cellulite]. J Mal Vasc. 1984;9 Suppl A:53-4.
41. Curri SB, Merlen JF. [Microvascular disorders of adipose tissue]. J Mal Vasc. 1986;11(3):303-9.
42. Draelos ZD. The disease of cellulite. J Cosmet Dermatol. 2005;4(4):221-2.
43. Alizadeh Z, Halabchi F, Mazaheri R, Abolhasani M, Tabesh M. Review of the Mechanisms and Effects of Noninvasive Body Contouring Devices on Cellulite and Subcutaneous Fat. Int J Endocrinol Metab. 2016;14(4): e36727.
44. Russe-Wilflingseder K, Russe E, Vester JC, Haller G, Novak P, Krotz A, et al. Placebo controlled, prospectively randomized, double-blinded study for the investigation of the effectiveness and safety of the acoustic wave therapy (AWT(®)) for cellulite treatment. J Cosmet Laser Ther. 2013;15(3):155-62.
45. Knobloch K, Joest B, Krämer R, Vogt PM. Cellulite and focused extracorporeal shockwave therapy for non-invasive body contouring: a randomized trial. Dermatol Ther (Heidelb). 2013;3(2):143-55.
46. Goldman A, Gotkin RH, Sarnoff DS, Prati C, Rossato F. Cellulite: a new treatment approach combining subdermal Nd: YAG laser lipolysis and autologous fat transplantation. Aesthet Surg J. 2008;28(6):656-62.
47. Sadick N. Treatment for cellulite. Int J Womens Dermatol. 2018;5(1):68-72.
48. DiBernardo B, Sasaki G, Katz BE, Hunstad JP, Petti C, Burns AJ. A multicenter study for a single, three-step laser treatment for cellulite using a 1440-nm Nd:YAG laser, a novel side-firing fiber, and a temperature-sensing cannula. Aesthet Surg J. 2013;33(4):576-84.
49. Katz B. Quantitative & qualitative evaluation of the efficacy of a 1440 nm Nd:YAG laser with novel bi-directional optical fiber in the treatment of cellulite as measured by 3-dimensional surface imaging. J Drugs Dermatol. 2013;12(11):1224-30.

6 SECTION

SOFT TISSUE FILLERS AND NEUROMODULATORS

22 CHAPTER

Soft Tissue Fillers

*Lauren Meshkov Bonati, *Mona Sadeghpour, Thomas E Rohrer

INTRODUCTION

The use of soft tissue fillers for noninvasive rejuvenation continues to grow. The wide variety of products available, ease of use, enhanced safety profile, and increased patient awareness make filler procedures particularly appealing. Before treatment, a well-thought-out consultation will help establish patient goals and set realistic expectations. Treatment strategy should be guided by knowledge of each filler's unique properties and of age-related changes in anatomy, gender ideals, and desired outcome as it relates to the individual patient. Mastery of facial vasculature and competence in preventing and managing complications are absolute prerequisites for any injector.

The number of patients considering cosmetic medical procedures continues to grow. According to the American Society of Dermatologic Surgery (ASDS) Consumer Survey On Cosmetic Dermatologic Procedures, this number has steadily increased from 30% of consumers considering cosmetic medical procedures in 2014 to 70% in 2017.* This growth is due to increased supply and a demand for minimally invasive esthetic procedures, including soft tissue fillers. Unlike the high cost and prolonged downtime of conventional cosmetic surgery, such as the facelift, today's minimally invasive procedures allow patients to enjoy the benefits of esthetic rejuvenation with lower risks, shorter recoveries, and decreased costs.

These trends are reflected in the increasing popularity and utilization of soft tissue fillers. The 2017 American Society of Plastic Surgeons statistics report ranked soft tissue fillers as the second most common noninvasive cosmetic procedure, with 2.7 million treatments performed in 2017,[2] and the third most common cosmetic treatment performed by dermatologic surgeons according to the 2016 ASDS Survey on Dermatologic Procedures.[3] Recent data from the ASDS showed that dermatologic surgeons performed 1.35 million soft tissue filler procedures in 2016, which represents a 47% increase from 2012.

Since the advent of bovine collagen fillers in the 1970s, the increase in demand has translated to a booming supply market with more than 300 commercially available forms of injectable fillers world-wide. Several methods

*Authors contributed equally to chapter.

for categorization of these fillers have been proposed in the past. Reflecting the current utilization of fillers in our own practice, this chapter will discuss two general categories of filler, hyaluronic acid (HA) fillers and non-HA fillers, based on their chemical composition and reversible property, or lack thereof, with hyaluronidase.

PRETREATMENT CONSIDERATIONS

Consultation and Evaluation

Prior to filler injection, history should be obtained from the patient. More specifically, patients should be asked about prior filler injection (type, date, location, and outcome) and allergy to any prior filler or lidocaine (as many current fillers come premixed with lidocaine). Due to reports of infection and biofilm formation after dental procedures, it is advisable to ask about recent or future dental cleaning or procedures.[4] In our practice, we counsel patients to avoid any such procedures for 2–4 weeks before or after the filler injection. However, these recommendations vary, with some practices avoiding dental procedures after the procedure only. If the treatment will target the lips or perioral skin, prophylactic treatment of herpes simplex virus (HSV) with valacyclovir 500 mg twice daily for 7–10 days or famciclovir 500 mg twice daily for 7–10 days starting the day prior to the procedure should be considered in those with a positive history.[5,6]

Evaluation and management of patient goals and expectations is paramount in achieving posttreatment satisfaction. Careful listening will reveal which anatomic area is of highest treatment priority, as this may differ from the esthetic assessment of the physician. A candid discussion should be about cost, volume, and duration of the filler recommended, as well as an explanation of the temporary, permanent, or semipermanent nature of the filler to be used. Realistic expectations should be agreed upon by patient and physician, with deferral of treatment if unrealistic expectations persist.

Any baseline asymmetry of the patient's anatomy should be pointed out and captured in pretreatment photography, as patients often examine their facial structure more carefully posttreatment. In the authors' practice, 3-view photos from the front, the right and left oblique angles are obtained. Common postprocedure complications and side effects should be discussed, including immediate or delayed bruising. Treatment may be delayed if patients have important life or social events in the near future. Informed consent, detailing risk for common, temporary, and/or permanent complications, should be provided and signed by patient. A summary of pretreatment considerations is displayed in **Table 1**.

Patient Positioning and Preparation

Evaluation for soft tissue filler begins with the patient sitting comfortably in the upright position. This allows for more accurate assessment of facial contour and the effects of gravity. If concurrent botulinum toxin or laser treatments are to be performed on the same day, it is recommended to do the filler treatment first, as temporary erythema, bleeding, and edema associated with toxin or laser may obscure facial landmarks and contour.

It is imperative to maintain a clean technique prior to and during the injection of fillers to reduce the risk of biofilm or infectious nodules. This precaution includes any staff who may be assisting or adding lidocaine or saline to fillers. Care should be taken to remove all makeup, and/or topical anesthetic before injection, and the skin should be cleaned with alcohol or other topical antimicrobial. Treatment should be deferred in the case of infection in or near the treatment areas.

TABLE 1: Pretreatment evaluation/considerations.

Patient driven factors	Management of expectations and goals
History of prior procedures in the area (surgeries and related scars, radiation therapy, facial implants, and facelifts)	Listen to and understand patient's exact priority for the treatment
History of prior filler injection (location, type, complication, and patient satisfaction with results)	Set up realistic expectation for degree of correction and longevity of filler posttreatment
History of autoimmune or connective tissue disease (may increase risk for bruising or delayed immune-mediated complications)	Assess patient's tolerance of "downtime" and common complications, including immediate and delayed bruising
History of herpes simplex virus	Discuss different types, amount, and cost of available filler treatments
History of prior hypersensitivity or allergy (including to lidocaine)	Evaluate and discuss any baseline asymmetry if present and potential effect on results
Medications (medically or nonmedically indicated anticoagulants and supplements)	Discuss and obtain informed consent
Pregnancy/lactation	Obtain baseline pretreatment photos (3-views recommended)
Plans for upcoming dental procedure/dental cleaning or other surgery/trauma in the area	

TREATMENT

Injection Technique

For esthetic restoration, filler should be placed in areas of shadowing and volume loss. Knowledge of fat pad location, common areas of bony recession, and age-related anatomical change will help guide placement. Correct depth of injection will also help achieve optimal outcomes and is determined by both the depth of the deficit and the structure and thickness of individual products being used. A variety of techniques for filler injections exist and are reviewed below.

Crosshatching Technique

This technique involves using the needle to inject parallel cords of filler in one direction followed by overlap of another series of parallel cords in the perpendicular direction. This method can be associated with increased bruising, but can be used in locations where more diffuse bulk volume of filling is needed, such as cheeks, marionette lines, or jowls.

Linear Threading Technique

This involves a single insertion point (usually at the inferior end of the fold) where the needle is advanced forward to a desired end point and filler material injected in an anterograde or retrograde fashion as the needle is being advanced or removed. This method is commonly used in the filling of nasolabial folds or jawline.

Fanning Technique

This method begins similarly to the linear threading technique, but instead of the needle being withdrawn from the skin, the needle is readvanced into the skin in different directions in a fan-like fashion. This technique poses a higher risk for bruising and should be used with caution.

Depot Technique

Here, the filler product is injected through a single insertion point. Depot injections may be very superficial to fill in fine lines or deep to restore areas of bony resorption. Massage or light pressure over the treatment area will smooth out any contour irregularities following injection. Common areas for use include perioral rhytides, oral commissures, cheeks, marionette lines, and prejowl sulcus.

HYALURONIC ACID FILLERS

Soft tissue fillers may be categorized into HA fillers and non-HA fillers based on the filler's chemical composition and reversible or irreversible properties. HA fillers are the most widely used soft tissue fillers in today's esthetic market, with 2 million HA injections performed in 2017.[2] This is likely due to ease of use right off the shelf, without need for dilution, adaptability, tolerability, and reversibility through hyaluronidase.

Hyaluronic acid is a member of the glycosaminoglycan (GAG) polysaccharide family, which includes dermatan sulfate, dextran sulfate, heparan sulfate, and heparin. Structural similarity of the HA molecule to heparin is important as it has been shown to weakly interact with the coagulation cascade and possibly lead to the phenomenon of delayed bruising in some patients.[7] Structurally, HA is composed of repeating nonsulfated disaccharide units of N-acetyl-glucosamine and B-glucuronic acid forming a polymer capable of attracting a large volume of water through its negatively-charged sugar molecules. This hydrophilicity allows HA to form a fluid matrix that functions in stabilizing the intercellular components of the dermis including collagen and elastic fibers.

With age, the amount of natural HA in the dermis diminishes, predisposing the skin to wrinkle formation. The hydrophilicity of HA allows it to provide a hydrating and volumizing effect to the skin making it an ideal candidate for correction of facial wrinkles and volume loss. In addition to the volumizing nature of HA, evidence from the 2007 study by Wang et al. showed that injection of cross-linked HA can further stimulate collagen synthesis through mechanical stretching and activation of dermal fibroblasts.[5]

Unlike collagen, HA is generally considered a nonimmunogenic molecule given its lack of protein epitopes. However, this notion juxtaposes the clinical finding of inflammatory-mediated delayed onset nodules, which can form months to years after injection of HA fillers.[7-9] In fact, there has been increasing clinical and scientific evidence to support the proinflammatory role of HA,[10-12] which can predispose to susceptible individuals to immune-mediated reactions following injection. Increased incidence of these delayed inflammatory reactions has recently been reported with the use of the newer classes of HA filler products that utilize a novel and proprietary Vycross® crosslinking technology. Although investigation is currently underway, it is thought that these reactions may be the result of incorporation of both high- and low-molecular-weight HA in the crosslinking process, which can result in a differential proinflammatory response within the immune system.[8,13] Fortunately, the incidence of such reactions with HA remains very low, especially when compared to other types of fillers.

While native HA maintains a half-life of only 1–2 days, HA fillers in today's market are cross-linked through conjugation with butanediol diglycidyl ether (BDDE) to confer longevity to the products. The cross-linked HA is then processed to produce either a homogeneous gel, referred to as monophasic HA fillers (Juvederm family), or a suspension of particles in gel carriers, referred to as biphasic HA fillers (Restylane family).

The process of crosslinking varies between different HA products, as does the concentration of HA, giving each product its own unique esthetic properties and longevity. As such, injectors must be familiar with the unique property, concentration, and consistency of each filler so that proper injection technique and depth are employed. In general, the higher the concentration of HA, the more stiff the product and the longer the durability.

Hyaluronic acid fillers can be further categorized by the source of the HA molecule, either animal-derived or nonanimal-derived. The animal-derived, stabilized HA group from rooster combs, which includes the formerly used Hylaform® group of fillers, will not be discussed in this chapter. Below are the different HA fillers currently approved for use by the US Food and Drug Administration (FDA). **Table 2** includes a full summary of all FDA-approved HA fillers including current on- and off-label uses.

Nonanimal Stabilized Hyaluronic Acid Fillers

Nonanimal stabilized hyaluronic acid (NASHA) fillers are comprised of HA molecules derived from bacterial (*Streptococcus*) fermentation. Because NASHA products are not fully saturated or hydrated in the syringe, their filling effect will continue to improve 24 hours after injection. It is therefore important to not overcorrect.

Restylane® Family

The first injectable stabilized HA filler approved by the FDA was Restylane® in 2003. A randomized prospective study showed it to be safe, more effective, and more durable when compared to bovine collagen (Zyplast) for treatment of nasolabial folds (**Figs. 1A** and **B**).

Juvederm® Family

Juvederm was initially approved by the FDA in 2006 for use in the nasolabial fold. The Juvederm family of fillers are comprised of a homogeneous (monophasic) gel produced through either the Hylacross or Vycross technology. The first generation of products (Juvederm Ultra® and Juvederm Ultra Plus®) are produced through the propriety Hylacross technology, where high-molecular-weight HA is used in the cross-linking process. In contrast, the later generation of products (Juvederm Voluma®, Juvederm Vollure®, and Juvederm Volbella®) are produced through the Vycross technology, which utilizes cross-linking of both high- and low-molecular-weight HA. Vycross products are considered more efficient and durable, whereas Hylacross products are twice as hydrophilic.

Belotero Family

Belotero is formed through cross-linking with BDDE into a cohesive and polydensified matrix (CPM). It is known for ease of injection and histological studies showing excellent integration with the dermis. Currently the only FDA-approved product from the Belotero family in the US is Belotero Balance®. Belotero is best suited for injection of superficial lines, such as those found periorally.

NONHYALURONIC ACID FILLERS

Calcium Hydroxylapatite

Calcium hydroxylapatite (CaHA), or Radiesse®, is FDA approved for the correction of moderate-to-severe facial lines and folds, hand rejuvenation, and lipoatrophy associated with human immunodeficiency virus (HIV). It is composed of 25–45 mm spherical particles suspended in a 30% sodium carboxymethylcellulose gel.[14] It offers a 1:1 correction ratio of implant to tissue volume, which means overcorrection is unnecessary.[15]

Once injected, the gel vehicle is eventually phagocytized, leaving behind CaHA particles that become fixed in the tissue. This prevents

TABLE 2: Currently available hyaluronic acid fillers approved by the US Food and Drug Administration (FDA).

Filler trade name (company)	Year FDA approved	Concentration	Longevity	Contains lidocaine (yes/no)	Approved for	Other unique properties; common off-label uses
Restylane® and Restylane-L® *(Galderma Laboratories)*	• Restylane®: 2003 • Restylane-L®: 2012	20 mg/mL	6–12 months	• Restylane®: No • Restylane-L®: Yes	Injection into the mid-to-deep dermis for correction of moderate for severe facial wrinkles; Restylane-L is also indicated for lips	*Off-label use:* Versatile use: Tear-troughs, marionettes, prejowl sulcus, temples
Restylane Lyft®; previously marketed as Perlane® *(Galderma Laboratories)*	2015	20 mg/mL	6–12 months	Yes	Deep implantation for moderate-to-severe facial folds such as nasolabial folds; cheek and midface augmentation	*Off-label use:* Prejowl sulcus, jawline
Restylane Defyne® *(Galderma Laboratories)*	2016	20 mg/mL	6–12 months	No	Injection into the mid-to-deep dermis for correction of moderate for severe facial wrinkles including nasolabial folds	• Bigger gel particles and more extensive HA crosslinking making it firmer and better suited for lift and volume compared to Restylane Refyne • *Off-label use*: Smile lines, cheeks, forehead, and temples
Restylane Refyne® *(Galderma Laboratories)*	2016	20 mg/mL	6–12 months	No	Injection into the mid-to-deep dermis for correction of moderate for severe facial wrinkles including nasolabial folds	• Smaller size particles, less HA cross-linking, and a softer gel compared to Restylane Defyne • *Off-label use*: Marionette lines, oral commissures, and tear-troughs

Cont'd...

Cont'd...

Filler trade name (company)	Year FDA approved	Concentration	Longevity	Contains lidocaine (yes/no)	Approved for	Other unique properties; common off-label uses
Restylane Silk® (*Galderma Laboratories*)	2014	20 mg/mL	6–12 months	Yes	Lip augmentation and dermal implantation for correction of perioral rhytids	• Smallest gel size of the Restylane® family, faster flowing with less volumizing effect; can place injection more superficially compared to other Restylane family; associated with increased swelling (to avoid, inject slowly using small volume aliquots and do not place large total volume in one session) • *Off-label use*: Tear-troughs, glabellar lines • Smile lines
Juvederm Ultra XC® *(Allergan)*	2010* 2015 (lips)	24 mg/mL	6–9 months	Yes	• Use in mid-to-deep dermis for correction of moderate-to-severe facial wrinkles and folds (such as nasolabial folds) • Additional FDA approval in 2015 for injection into the lips and perioral areas for lip augmentation	• Hylacross technology, lower G' compared to Juvederm Ultra Plus® with 9% crosslinking of HA; best for contouring and correcting medium-depth wrinkles, can cause more gel swelling compared to Vycross products due to increased hydrophilicity (at risk for overcorrection) • *Off-label uses*: Versatile use including cheeks, marionettes, prejowl sulcus, temples

Cont'd...

Cont'd...

Filler trade name (company)	Year FDA approved	Concentration	Longevity	Contains lidocaine (yes/no)	Approved for	Other unique properties; common off-label uses
Juvederm Ultra Plus® XC *(Allergan)*	2010*	24 mg/mL	6–12 months	Yes	Use in mid-to-deep dermis for correction of moderate to severe facial wrinkles and folds (such as nasolabial folds).	• Hylacross technology; slightly higher G′ compared to Juvederm Ultra with 11% crosslinking of HA. Better for volumizing and correcting deeper folds. Can cause more gel swelling compared to Vycross products due to increased hydrophilicity (at risk for overcorrection) • *Off-label uses*: Versatile use: Cheeks, marionettes, prejowl sulcus, temples
Juvederm Voluma® *(Allergan)*	2013	20 mg/mL	12–24 months	Yes	Deep (subcutaneous and/or supraperiosteal) injection for cheek augmentation to correct age-related volume deficit in the mid-face	• Vycross technology (first one to be approved) with highest concentration, highest cohesivity, and durability of the Vycross products. Injections should be placed deep in preperiosteal plane in small boluses of 0.1–0.3 cc to avoid visibility and nodule formation; Often mixed with lidocaine to ease injection and malleability of product • *Off-label uses*: Temples, jawline

Cont'd...

Cont'd...

Filler trade name (company)	Year FDA approved	Concentration	Longevity	Contains lidocaine (yes/no)	Approved for	Other unique properties; common off-label uses
Juvederm Vollure® *(Allergan)*	2017	17.5 mg/mL	6–12 months	No	Injection into mid-to-deep dermis for correction of moderate-to-severe facial wrinkles including the nasolabial folds	• Vycross technology; falls in between Voluma and Volbella with regards to its concentration and cohesivity • *Off-label use*: Restoration of forehead, tear trough, temporal fossa, brow, nasal dorsum, and nasal tip contouring
Juvederm Volbella® *(Allergan)*	2016	15 mg/mL	6–12 months	Yes	Injection into the lips for augmentation and for correction of perioral rhytids	• Vycross technology, softest and least cohesive of the Vycross products; ideally designed for superficial plane injection of fine lines • *Off-label use:* Tear troughs, superficial lines of the glabella, forehead and cheeks
Belotero Balance® *(Merz Aesthetics)*	2011	22.5 mg/mL	6 months	No	Mid-to-deep dermis for correction of moderate-to-severe facial wrinkles such as the nasolabial fold	• Soft gel suited for superficial injection of fine lines; can be directly injected into superficial dermal wrinkles without risk of Tyndall effect • *Off-label use*: Tear troughs, superficial lines of the glabella, forehead and cheeks

*Initial form approved by FDA in 2006 without added lidocaine and marketed under Juvéderm 24HV, Juvéderm 30, and Juvéderm 30HV.
(HA: hyaluronic acid)

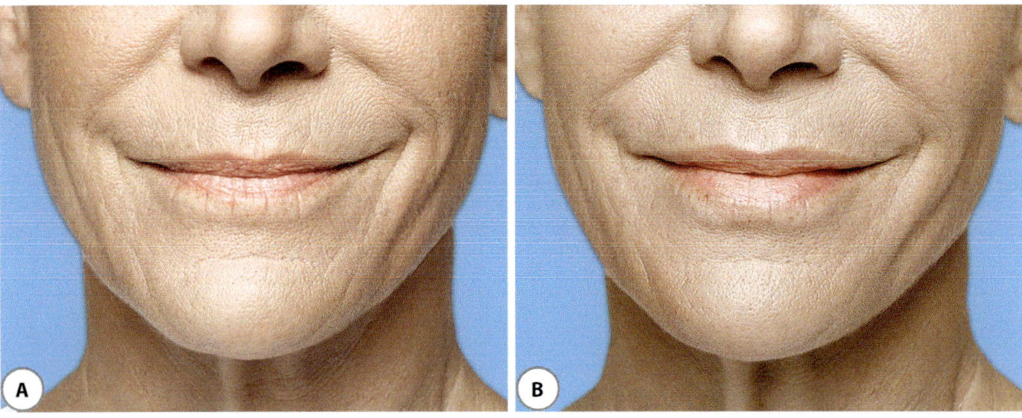

FIGS. 1A AND B: Lip augmentation and correction of perioral lines with 2.8 mL of Restylane silk. (A) Before; (B) After.
Courtesy: Galderma Laboratories, L.P.

product migration. New collagen deposition around the particles restores lost volume, with structural improvement lasting up to 2.5 years.[16] Over a 12-month period, CaHA particles break down into calcium and phosphate ions that are metabolized by the body. Results may last up to 15 months in dynamic locations and 24–30 months in more static locations.[17]

Several clinical trials have confirmed the safety of CaHA in all skin types.[18] No calcification or ossification of tissue has been known to occur[19] and the product does not interfere with radiographic imaging.[20] The most common side effects include mild and transient ecchymosis, edema, erythema, pain, and pruritus.

Lip augmentation and injection within the orbital rim with CaHA is discouraged, as nodules have been reported in up to 12.4% of patients after lip augmentation.[21] Unlike HA fillers, there is no reversal agent for CaHA. Therefore, nodules or undesirable outcomes may be treated with needle disruption, massage, or injection of normal saline plus lidocaine or 5-fluorouracil plus lidocaine with or without epinephrine.

Poly-L-lactic Acid

Poly-L-lactic acid (PLLA), or Sculptra® and Sculptra Aesthetic®, is a biostimulatory agent that is FDA approved for the treatment of HIV-associated lipoatrophy as well as facial folds and wrinkles. PLLA offers a gradual and long-lasting correction for panfacial volume loss by providing a sugar-based scaffold on which neocollagenesis may occur (**Figs. 2A** and **B**).

Evaluation of the patient's facial structure in relation to known areas of fat pad and bony volume loss is crucial for guiding placement. Key areas for injection are the lateral temporal superficial fat pads and the deep medial cheek fat pads, which increase anterior projection of the midface.[22] Deep supraperiosteal injections are ideal for the temple, zygoma, maxilla, and mandible, while subcutaneous depth is recommended for the midcheek, lateral cheek, and preauricular area to avoid the parotid gland and duct.[23]

Preparation of PLLA must be done with meticulous care. Proper reconstitution will reduce the risk of clogged needles and nodule formation. Product should be reconstituted with 8–9 mL of sterile water at least 24 hours before injection. The vial should not be shaken,

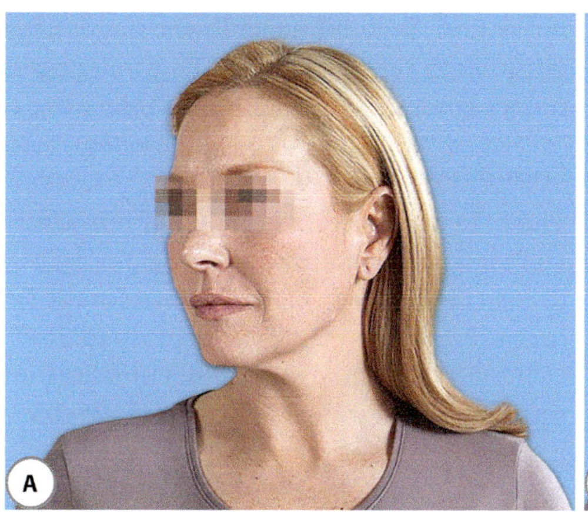

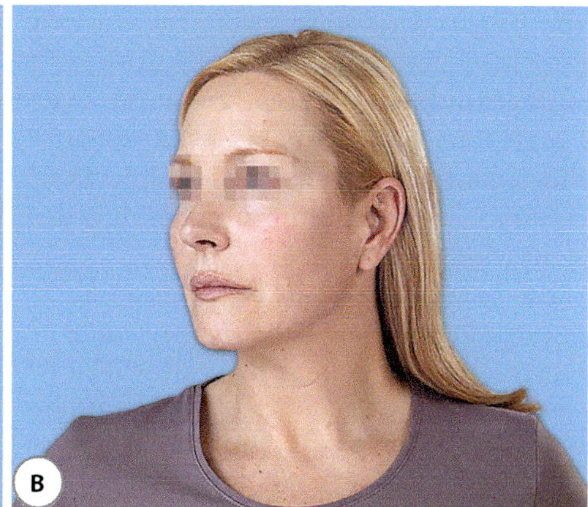

FIGS. 2A AND B: Before and 7-months after photographs of panfacial volume loss restored with 5 vials of poly-L-lactic acid (PLLA) (Sculptra®).
Courtesy: Galderma Laboratories, L.P.

as dry product deposited on the walls of the container may not hydrate appropriately. Lidocaine 1–2% with or without epinephrine may be added immediately prior to injection. Reconstituted product may be stored at room temperature for 24–48 hours before injection, but should be refrigerated if stored 3–4 weeks before injection.

Immediately before injection, the skin should be prepped with chlorhexidine 4% or isopropyl alcohol 70%. The vial should be gently rolled in the hands or mixed using a laboratory vortex to create a homogeneous suspension and to loosen microparticles from the vial base. Vigorous shaking should be avoided, as it creates unusable foam that can clog the needle during injection. Treatment is generally performed using a 25- or 26-gauge needle, or a cannula of 1 or 1.5 inch length.

Off-label use includes injection under acne scars, varicella scars, and soft tissue loss after surgery.[24] A larger volume 16 mL dilution has been described for treating the decollete[25] and a 12–14-mL dilution may be used for cellulite dimples and volume loss of the lower thighs just above the knees. Treatment of the hands and neck should be avoided due to reports of subsequent papules and nodules.

Postprocedural care includes massaging the treatment areas for 5 minutes, 5 times per day, for 5 days, commonly known as the "rule of fives." The message is an important deterrent to particle conglomeration, which may lead to nodule formation. Patients should be counseled that the immediate volumizing effect from dilutional fluid will fade over 1–4 days, and that long-term neocollagenesis will take approximately 2 months to appreciate.[26]

Poly-l-lactic acid is typically injected over several treatment sessions, at 4–6 week intervals. The number of treatment sessions will depend upon individual baseline volume loss. Results may last up to 25 months, as seen in 80% of patients in the FDA trials.[27]

The development of PLLA-related papules or nodules is often related to poor preparation of material, suboptimal injection technique, inadequate postprocedural massage, or delayed inflammation. Product placed too superficially in the dermis may lead to neocollagenesis-related lumps or bumps. Product placed in the dynamic musculature of the perioral or periocular region can clump and cause pseudogranulomas.[28] Pseudogranulomas typically resolve over 2–3 years, but may be treated with excision, needle subcision with sterile water injection, thalidomide, ciprofloxacin, or by blending the contour with HA filler.

True granulomas can be distinguished from pseudogranulomas by the presence of inflammation in all treatment sites due to an overactive host response. These nodules respond to intralesional corticosteroids and or 5-flourouracil. Delayed nodules may occur at 14–24 months after treatment.

Permanent Fillers

Nonbiodegradable fillers currently available in the United States include polymethylmethacrylate (PMMA) and liquid injectable silicone (LIS), or polymethylsiloxane. These products offer longer lasting results, but carry the risk of permanent side effects.

Polymethylmethacrylate

Bellafill®, previously known as Artefill®, is a PMMA agent with FDA approval for the correction of nasolabial folds and moderate-to-severe atrophic acne scars. It is comprised of 30–50-um microspheres that are suspended in a 3.5% bovine collagen gel and 0.3% lidocaine. An allergy test should be performed 28 days prior to use.

Once injected, PMMA microspheres are surrounded by a thin fibrous capsule and left behind permanently. The bovine collagen dissipates around 1–3 months. PMMA particles then serve as a scaffold for neocollagenesis, which occurs around 4 months. Optimal results typically require multiple treatment sessions, but persistent results have been noted at 5-year follow-up.[29]

When placed too superficially, PMMA can cause beading, scarring, and or nodule formation. Bellafill has a lower incidence of granuloma formation than its predecessors, but a higher incidence than HA fillers.[30]

Liquid Injectable Silicone

The FDA approved LIS for ocular purposes in 1959 but has been used off-label for decades to treat facial volume loss. Products in the USA include Silikon 1000® and Adatosil 5000®. Using sterile technique, product may be drawn up using a 16-gauge needle and injected with a 27-gauge needle.[31] Experts recommend the microdroplet technique, whereby small 0.005–0.01-mL aliquots are placed subcutaneously at intervals of 2–5 mm.[32] Treatment volume should not exceed 2.0-mL for larger areas and 0.5-mL for smaller areas.

Multiple small volume treatments spaced 1–2 months apart will prevent bolus-related migration that that can lead to striking facial bumps at distant sites. Intradermal injection should also be avoided, as this may cause erythema, postinflammatory hyperpigmentation, or ridging.

Permanent fillers do not have an antidote and side effects, such as silicone granulomas or product migration, may occur weeks to years after injection. Excessive collagen growth may create firm nodules or local areas of persistent swelling due to inflammation that may or may not respond to intralesional steroids or antimetabolites. Impurities and adulterants are also a concern with nonmedical, industrial grade LIS, resulting in infection, ulceration, or chronic inflammation.

ANATOMIC CONSIDERATIONS AND SAFETY

Fillers enjoy a favorable safety profile, but still run the risk of serious complications. Injecting physicians should employ preventative strategies and be prepared to manage all complications.

Periprocedural

The most common adverse events with all filler types are mild and transient, including swelling, erythema, pruritus, bruising, and procedural pain. Patients will likely experience worsened ecchymosis if taking antiplatelets, anticoagulants, nonsteroidal anti-inflammatories, or blood-thinning supplements (**Fig. 3**). Supplements should be stopped 5 days in advance, but therapeutic medications should be continued.

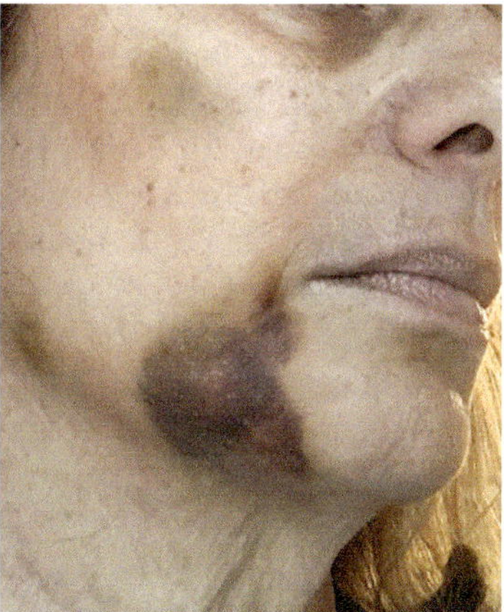

FIG. 3: Significant ecchymoses after various types of hyaluronic acid injection to the lateral cheek, jawline, and marionette lines.

Nodules

Filler placed too superficially can result in papules or nodules. Visible nodules of any type may be manually pressed, aspirated, or relieved by incision and drainage. Other treatment options include watchful waiting, hyaluronidase for HA-induced nodules, intralesional triamcinolone with or without 5-fluorouracil, oral prednisone, and manually breaking up nodules with a needle.[33]

Delayed nodules represent inflammatory host reactions that may be associated with immunologic triggers, such as infection, flu-like illness, dental procedure, or trauma. Median time of onset from injection to nodule formation is about 4 months, but may occur years later.[4] Regardless of etiology, patients are often retreated without further episodes.

Infection

Infections typically present as fluctuant, tender, erythematous nodules with or without systemic involvement (**Figs. 4A** and **B**). Infections are typically caused by *Staphylococcus* or *Streptococcus*, but empiric antibiotics should be initiated while waiting for culture or biopsy results. The authors recommend clarithromycin or minocycline. Atypical *Mycobacterium* should raise suspicion for counterfeit or adulterated product.

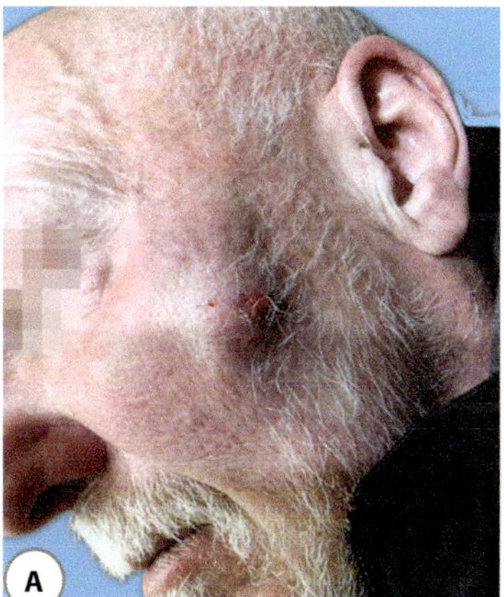

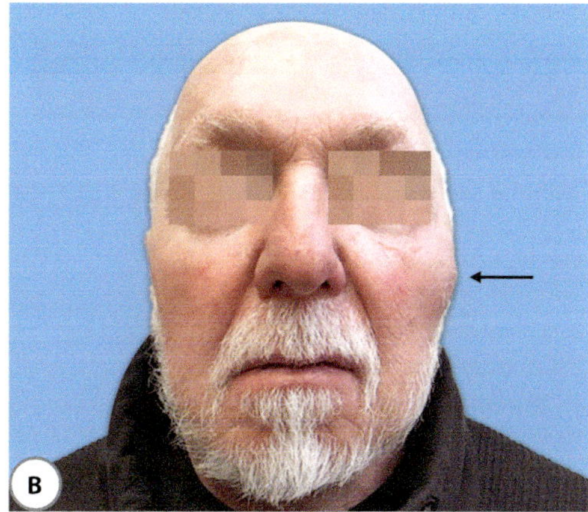

FIGS. 4A AND B: Nodule and abscess on the left cheek after injection of a large quantity of Voluma.

Biofilms

A biofilm is a highly structured group of microorganisms that adheres to the surface of injected filler. Typically comprised of *Staphylococcus aureus* or *epidermidis*, *Pseudomonas aeruginosa*, *Enterococcus* species, and *Candida*, biofilms are introduced at the time of filler injection. They are uniquely protected from host immunity and exogenous treatment by their polymeric matrix capsule. Culture of a biofilm is typically negative.

In the skin, biofilms give rise to active or chronic infections, abscesses, cellulitis, chronic inflammation, nodules, and granulomas that may occur months to years later.[34]

Often biofilms are quiescent until they are activated by trauma or subsequent injection. Biofilms are more common with permanent fillers, but can occur with any product type. The risk may be reduced with proper antiseptic technique using isopropyl alcohol or chlorhexidine.

Angry red nodules with or without pain should be treated with antibiotics, such as clarithromycin or minocycline, for 2–6 weeks.[35] Intralesional steroids and 5-fluorouracil should only be used in conjunction with oral antibiotics, as injectable monotherapy may aggravate the process. Excision should be considered for permanent filler nodules and biofilms. Treatment recommendations for nodules are listed in **Box 1**.

BOX 1: Treatment strategy for inflammatory nodules.

- Incise and drain any material
- Send for culture
- Minocycline or clarithromycin × 2–6 weeks. Consider multiple antibiotics or IV administration if severe
- Avoid intralesional steroids until patient is on established antibiotic regimen
- Hyaluronidase injection if used HA filler
- Excise or debride if persistent

(HA: hyaluronic acid; IV: intravenous)

Granulomas

Persistent nodules may be caused by a granulomatous foreign body reaction against synthetic filler or may be due to a biofilm. Reactions may be local or regional, delayed or recurrent. Granulomas have been reported after injection of all filler types.

VASCULAR COMPROMISE

The most dangerous complication of soft tissue fillers is vascular compromise due to intravascular injection. Blanching or significant pain are early warning signs, followed by a violaceous or dusky patch with mottled or reticulated pattern over the next 24–48 hours. Without intervention, necrosis, ulceration, and eventual scarring can occur.

All injectors should possess a firm knowledge of vascular anatomy, both in depth of plane and location. While this can reduce the risk of such events, the variability in anatomy makes avoiding the risk entirely impossible. Past surgical history should also be noted as it may indicate anomalous vasculature.

Injection technique and product choice may help reduce risk for vascular events. Smaller gauge needles and slow injections will prevent plunger pressure from overcoming that of arterial pressure. Injecting small volumes of 0.1 mL or less and continual movement of the needle will prevent large boluses from being deposited in one location. Choosing an HA filler product will allow for immediate reversal with hyaluronidase. Other fillers lack an antidote. The use of cannulas or mixing filler with epinephrine remains controversial. Strategies for preventing vascular events are listed in **Box 2**.

Management of Vascular Compromise

Physicians should have an established protocol and readily available supplies in the case of vascular compromise (**Box 3**). If blanching,

BOX 2: Strategies for preventing vascular compromise.

- Obtain surgical history for possible anomalous vasculature, particularly around the nose
- Master the location and depth of facial vasculature, including common variations
- Choose an HA filler for its ability to dissolve with hyaluronidase injection
- Use small diameter needles
- Use larger grade cannulas
- Use small volume syringes
- Inject small volumes of 0.1 mL or less
- Inject slowly with minimal pressure
- Continually move the needle tip to prevent large deposit in one location
- Consider mixing filler with epinephrine to reduce vessel diameter
- Consider using a cannula to reduce risk of piercing a vessel
- Consider aspirating to check needle location, though technique may not work due to pressure gradient between filler and vessel

(HA: hyaluronic acid)
Source: Adapted from Beleznay K et al.[36]

pain out of proportion, or a dusky violaceous hue develops, stop the injection immediately and administer hyaluronidase if using an HA filler.

Hyaluronidase will hydrolyze HA product and reduce edema that may be contributing to vessel occlusion.[33] Vascular compromise has been reported to reverse with doses ranging from 200 to 1500 IU, most at a dilution of 150 IU/mL.[37,38] Due to variability in dosing strategy and no known upper limit, it may be most effective to simply flood the injection point and surrounding area in urgent situations. Injections may be repeated hourly until clinical resolution. Those with bee sting allergies should not be treated with hyaluronidase and skin testing should be done if using sheep- or bovine-derived formulas. In severe situations of vascular compromise, it may be worth risking hypersensitivity.

BOX 3: Management of vascular compromise.

- Stop injection as soon as blanching or pain is noted
- Inject hyaluronidase if HA filler was used
- Warm compress every 10 minutes for the first few hours
- Vigorous massage
- Consider topical nitroglycerin paste 2% q 1–2 hours initially
- Consider aspirin 325 mg sublingual immediately, then 81 mg PO daily. May also consider Ibuprofen 400–600 mg q8h to reduce swelling
- Consider prednisone 20–40 mg PO daily × 3–5 days
- Consider hyperbaric oxygen
- Consider low-molecular-weight heparin
- Reevaluate the area frequently and see patient in follow-up as reocclusion may occur

(HA: hyaluronic acid; PO: per os)
Source: Adapted from Beleznay K.[39]

Other strategies to restore perfusion, before or after hyaluronidase, are listed in **Box 3**. Patients should be followed closely to optimize outcome. Those with necrosis will require wound care and a treatment plan for subsequent scarring.

Blindness

Retrograde embolization of product into the ocular vessels is the most dreaded of filler complications. There are currently 98 cases of filler-related blindness reported in the literature, with 48% caused by autologous fat and 24% caused by HA fillers.[36] The most high-risk location is the glabella, followed by the nasal region, nasolabial fold, and forehead, however any location is at risk due to anastomosing vessels.

BOX 4: Management of ocular compromise.

- Stop injection immediately if ocular pain, headache, nausea, or vomiting occurs
- Immediately contact and transfer to ophthalmologist or oculoplastic surgeon
- If HA filler was used, inject hyaluronidase into the treatment and surrounding areas
- If HA filler was used, consider retrobulbar injection with 300–600 U of hyaluronidase (2–4 mL)
- Consider ocular massage, anterior chamber paracentesis, IV mannitol, and acetazolamide

(HA: hyaluronic acid; IV: intravenous)
Source: Adapted from Beleznay K et al.[39]

There is an approximate window of 90 minutes or less before permanent blindness becomes irreversible. If the patient reports ocular pain, vision changes, headache, or nausea, stop the injection immediately. If an HA filler was used, inject a large volume of hyaluronidase at the filler location and surrounding areas, as the reverser will diffuse through vessel walls. Seek emergent help from an ophthalmologist or oculoplastic surgeon, with whom a relationship has already been established and a description of this situation previously discussed.

In the case of vision loss, a retrobulbar injection of 300–600 units of hyaluronidase may be attempted. The lower lateral lid should be anesthetized first. A 25-gauge needle is advanced at least 1-inch in depth into the inferolateral orbit before injecting 2–4-mL of hyaluronidase. Other strategies for reducing intraocular pressure are listed in **Box 4**.

CONCLUSION

The multitude of HA and non-HA fillers allows for individualized treatment plans that address unique esthetic goals. Despite the procedure's popularity and user-friendly products, soft tissue filler augmentation remains a complex and technically demanding procedure. Rheological understanding, meticulous technique, and the ability to prevent and treat complications will set apart the expert injector from the novice in both safety and outcome.

REFERENCES

1. ASDS. (2017). ASDS Consumer Survey on Cosmetic Dermatologic Procedures. [online] Available from https://www.asds.net/medical-professionals/practice-resources/asds-consumer-survey-on-cosmetic-dermatologic-procedures [Last accessed March, 2021].
2. American Society of Plastic Surgeons. (2016). ASPS National Clearinghouse of Plastic Surgery Procedural Statistics. [online] Available from https://www.plasticsurgery.org/documents/News/Statistics/2016/plastic-surgery-statistics-full-report-2016.pdf [Last accessed March, 2021].
3. ASDS. (2012). ASDS Survey on Dermatologic Procedures. [online] Available fom https://www.asds.net/medical-professionals/practice-resources/asds-survey-on-dermatologic-procedures [Last accessed March, 2021].
4. Beleznay K, Carruthers JD, Carruthers A, Mummert ME, Humphrey S. Delayed-onset nodules secondary to a smooth cohesive 20 mg/mL hyaluronic acid filler: cause and management. Dermatol Surg. 2015;41:929-39.
5. Onwudiwe OC, Marmur ES, Cohen JL. Are we too cavalier about antiviral prophylaxis? J Drugs Dermatol. 2013;12(2):199-205.
6. Chi CC, Wang SH, Delamere FM, Wojnarowska F, Peters MC, Kanjirath PP. Interventions for prevention of herpes simplex labialis (cold sores on the lips). Cochrane Database Syst Rev. 2015;2015(8):CD010095.
7. Sadeghpour M, Dover JS. Understanding Delayed Bruising After Hyaluronic Acid Injections: Why the Molecule and Not Just the Injection Matters. Dermatol Surg. 2019;45(3):471-3.
8. Sadeghpour M, Quatrano NA, Bonati LM, Arndt KA, Dover JS, Kaminer KS. Delayed-Onset Nodules to Differentially Crosslinked Hyaluronic Acids: Comparative Incidence and Risk Assessment. Dermatol Surg. 2019;45(8):1085-94.
9. Wang F, Garza LA, Kang S, Varani J, Orringer JS, Fisher GJ, et al. In vivo stimulation of de novo collagen production caused by cross-linked hyaluronic acid dermal filler injections in photodamaged human skin. Arch Dermatol. 2007;143:155-63.
10. Artzi O, Loizides C, Verner I, Landau M. Resistant and Recurrent Late Reaction to Hyaluronic Acid-Based Gel. Dermatol Surg. 2016;42:31-7.
11. Alijotas-Reig J, Fernández-Figueras MT, Puig L. Inflammatory, immune-mediated adverse reactions related to soft tissue dermal fillers. Semin Arthritis Rheum. 2013;43:241-58.

12. Baeva LF, Lyle DB, Rios M, Langone JJ, Lightfoote MM. Different molecular weight hyaluronic acid effects on human macrophage interleukin 1β production. J Biomed Mater Res A. 2014;102:305-14.
13. Mummert ME. Immunologic roles of hyaluronan. Immunol Res. 2005;31:189-206.
14. Ridenour B, Kontis TC. Injectable calcium hydroxylapatite microspheres (Radiesse). Facial Plast Surg. 2009;25:100-5.
15. Yutskovskaya Y, Kogan E, Leshunov E. A randomized, split-face, histomorphologic study comparing a volumetric calcium hydroxylapatite and a hyaluronic acid-based dermal filler. J Drugs Dermatol. 2014;13:1047-52.
16. Lemperle G, Morhenn V, Charrier U. Human histology and persistence of various injectable filler substances for soft tissue augmentation. Aesthetic Plast Surg. 2003;27:354-66; discussion 67.
17. Silvers SL, Eviatar JA, Echavez MI, Pappas AL. Prospective, open-label, 18-month trial of calcium hydroxylapatite (Radiesse) for facial soft-tissue augmentation in patients with human immunodeficiency virus-associated lipoatrophy: one-year durability. Plast Reconstr Surg. 2006;118:34S-45S.
18. Marmur ES, Taylor SC, Grimes PE, Boyd CM, Porter JP, Yoo JY. Six-month safety results of calcium hydroxylapatite for treatment of nasolabial folds in Fitzpatrick skin types IV to VI. Dermatol Surg. 2009;35 Suppl 2:1641-5.
19. Marmur ES, Phelps R, Goldberg DJ. Clinical, histologic and electron microscopic findings after injection of a calcium hydroxylapatite filler. J Cosmet Laser Ther. 2004;6:223-6.
20. Carruthers A, Carruthers J. Evaluation of injectable calcium hydroxylapatite for the treatment of facial lipoatrophy associated with human immunodeficiency virus. Dermatol Surg. 2008;34:1486-99.
21. Jansen DA, Graivier MH. Evaluation of a calcium hydroxylapatite-based implant (Radiesse) for facial soft-tissue augmentation. Plast Reconstr Surg. 2006;118:22S-30S, discussion 1S-3S.
22. Rohrich RJ, Pessa JE, Ristow B. The youthful cheek and the deep medial fat compartment. Plast Reconstr Surg. 2008;121:2107-12.
23. Palm MD, Woodhall KE, Butterwick KJ, Goldman MP. Cosmetic use of poly-l-lactic acid: a retrospective study of 130 patients. Dermatol Surg. 2010;36:161-70.
24. Beer K. A single-center, open-label study on the use of injectable poly-L-lactic acid for the treatment of moderate to severe scarring from acne or varicella. Dermatol Surg. 2007;33 Suppl 2:S159-67.
25. Vanaman M, Fabi SG. Decolletage: Regional Approaches with Injectable Fillers. Plast Reconstr Surg. 2015;136:276S-81S.
26. Rotunda AM, Narins RS. Poly-L-lactic acid: a new dimension in soft tissue augmentation. Dermatol Ther. 2006;19:151-8.
27. Burgess CM, Quiroga RM. Assessment of the safety and efficacy of poly-L-lactic acid for the treatment of HIV-associated facial lipoatrophy. J Am Acad Dermatol. 2005;52:233-9.
28. Fitzgerald R, Vleggaar D. Facial volume restoration of the aging face with poly-l-lactic acid. Dermatol Ther. 2011;24:2-27.
29. Mills DC, Camp S, Mosser S, Sayeg A, Hurwitz D, Ronel D. Malar augmentation with a polymethylmethacrylate-enhanced filler: assessment of a 12-month open-label pilot study. Aesthet Surg J. 2013;33:421-30.
30. Narins RS, Coleman WP 3rd, Rohrich R, Monheit G, Glogau R, Brandt F, et al. 12-Month controlled study in the United States of the safety and efficacy of a permanent 2.5% polyacrylamide hydrogel soft-tissue filler. Dermatol Surg. 2010;36 Suppl 3:1819-29.
31. Jones DH, Carruthers A, Orentreich D, Brody HJ, Lai MY, Azen S, et al. Highly purified 1000-cSt silicone oil for treatment of human immunodeficiency virus-associated facial lipoatrophy: an open pilot trial. Dermatol Surg. 2004;30:1279-86.
32. Prather CL, Jones DH. Liquid injectable silicone for soft tissue augmentation. Dermatol Ther. 2006;19:159-68.
33. Alam M, Dover JS. Management of complications and sequelae with temporary injectable fillers. Plast Reconstr Surg. 2007;120:98S-105S.
34. Dayan SH, Arkins JP, Brindise R. Soft tissue fillers and biofilms. Facial Plast Surg. 2011;27:23-8.
35. Narins RS, Jewell M, Rubin M, Cohen J, Strobos J. Clinical conference: management of rare events following dermal fillers--focal necrosis and angry red bumps. Dermatol Surg. 2006;32:426-34.
36. Beleznay K, Humphrey S, Carruthers JD, Carruthers A. Vascular compromise from soft tissue augmentation: experience with 12 cases and recommendations for optimal outcomes. J Clin Aesthet Dermatol. 2014;7:37-43.
37. Cohen JL, Biesman BS, Dayan SH, DeLorenzi C, Lambros VS, Nestor MS, et al. Treatment of hyaluronic acid filler-induced impending necrosis with hyaluronidase: consensus recommendations. Aesthet Surg J. 2015;35(7):844-9.
38. Signorini M, Liew S, Sundaram H, De Boulle KL, Goodman GJ, Monheit G, et al. Global aesthetics consensus: avoidance and management of complications from hyaluronic acid fillers-evidence- and opinion-based review and consensus recommendations. Plast Reconstr Surg. 2016;137(6):961e-71e.
39. Beleznay K, Carruthers JD, Humphrey S, Jones D. Avoiding and Treating Blindness From Fillers: A Review of the World Literature. Dermatol Surg. 2015;41:1097-117.

23

CHAPTER

Cosmetic Neuromodulators

Jean Diana Carruthers, James Alastair Carruthers

INTRODUCTION

Botulinum toxin type A (BoNTA) produces temporary muscle paralysis and is the most requested noninvasive cosmetic procedure worldwide. Increased knowledge about the pathology of aging in the face has changed the approach to facial rejuvenation; BoNTA is rarely used in isolation but is combined with soft-tissue fillers and other cosmetic procedures for optimal esthetic outcomes in the face and neck. Regular treatment over several years produces cumulative improvements in wrinkle reduction and skin quality for higher levels of patient and physician satisfaction.

Derived from the bacterium *Clostridium botulinum*, botulinum toxin produces temporary muscle weakening by binding to presynaptic cholinergic nerve terminals and blocking the release of acetylcholine from motor neurons at the neuromuscular junction.[1] Of the seven serotypes, BoNTA is the most potent and widely used across the world in multiple formulations for cosmetic and therapeutic indications. BoNTA was originally tested in primates for ophthalmologic indications[2] and has been used therapeutically for over 30 years.[3] In 1992, we published the first report of the cosmetic use of BoNTA for the treatment of glabellar frown lines.[4] After numerous open-label studies involving >800 subjects, and two large, double-blind, placebo-controlled randomized clinical trials, the Food and Drug Administration (FDA) approved BoNTA for the nonsurgical reduction of glabellar furrows in 2002.[5] Since then, BoNTA has become the most frequently performed cosmetic procedure in the world and is considered the gold standard treatment for dynamic facial wrinkles.[6] To date, the FDA has approved three distinct formulations of BoNTA for both therapeutic and cosmetic purposes, and one formulation of BoNTB for therapeutic use only. All products differ in terms of diffusion, potency, and clinical effect. Likewise, clinical doses vary according to product and are not interchangeable. All doses discussed herein refer to onabotulinumtoxinA, the most widely studied of all available formulations for cosmetic and therapeutic purposes.[7]

COSMETIC USE OF BOTULINUM TOXIN

Every face differs in terms of facial musculature, symmetry, and expressivity. An individualized assessment is the key to successful treatment with BoNTA (**Box 1**).

Full examination considers anatomy, function, qualitative, and quantitative status of hard and soft tissues, and observation of both static and dynamic rhytides. A thorough understanding of facial anatomy (**Fig. 1**) and the interplay of adjacent musculature is mandatory.

Recognition of the multifactorial nature of aging has revolutionized the approach to facial rejuvenation. Current treatment guidelines for the use of BoNTA stress the importance of an integrated, panfacial approach in which multiple areas are treated concurrently using decreased doses, the fewest number of injection points, and wider injection intervals, alone or in combination with other cosmetic procedures, particularly soft-tissue fillers, for optimal clinical outcomes (**Figs. 2A and B**) (**Table 1**).[7,8] Because aging occurs as a continuum across areas, treatment of two adjacent areas can produce the same or potentially better results with reduced doses per injection point.[7] Modulation of muscular activity, rather than paralysis, is the goal. Studies show that treatment of multiple

BOX 1: Treatment considerations.

- Use an individualized approach to assessment and treatment planning
- Observe spontaneous facial expression at rest and on animation
- Analyze the target muscles in the context of adjacent muscles and associated soft and hard tissues
- Modulation of muscular activity is the goal, rather than paresis
- Treatment of multiple areas in combination with other cosmetic procedures improves outcomes
- Regular and repeated injections overtime produce progressive wrinkle reduction and cumulative improvements in skin quality

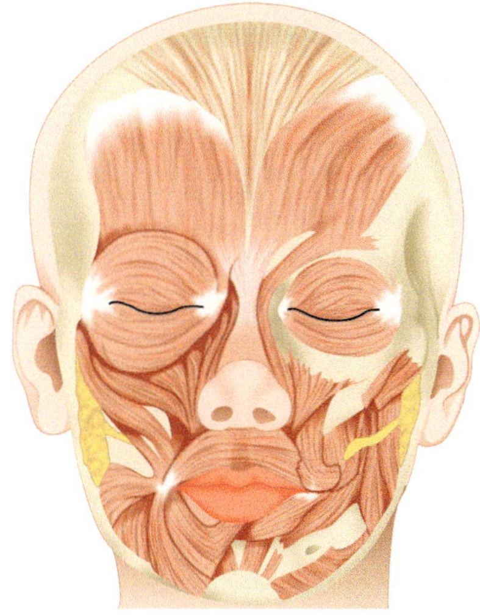

FIG. 1: A detailed knowledge of facial anatomy is essential to successful treatments with neuromodulators.

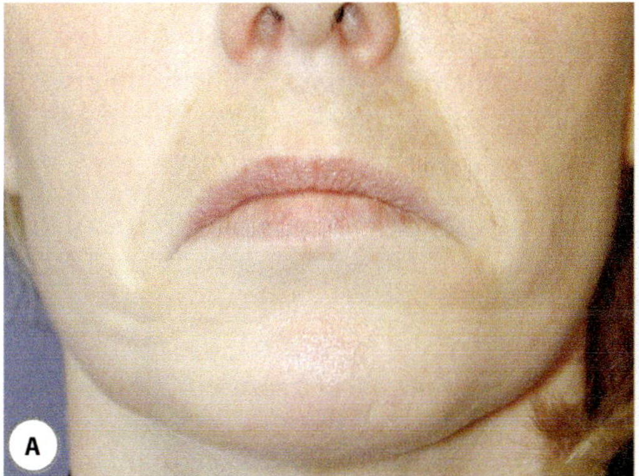

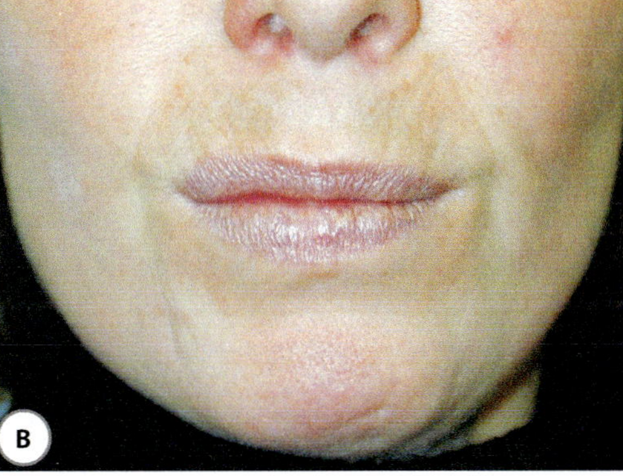

FIGS. 2A AND B: Combination therapy with neuromodulators, fillers, and noninvasive energy-based devices which tighten skin gives much greater esthetic benefit and subject satisfaction.

TABLE 1: Suggested injection parameters with onabotulinumtoxinA.

Indication	Number of injection points	Total dose
Glabellar rhytides	3–7	12–40 U
Horizontal forehead lines	4–8	8–15 U
Lateral canthal rhytides	1–5 per side	6–15 U per side
Infraorbital rhytides	1–3 per side	0.5–2 U per side
Nasal flare	2	1–4 U
Bunny lines	2–3	4–8 U
DAO overactivity	1–2 per side	2–5 U per side
Mentalis overactivity	1–4 per side	4–10 U
Masseteric hypertrophy	1–5 per side	15–40 U
Perioral rhytides	2–5	1–6 U
Platysmal bands Nefertiti Lift	3–6 per band 5–6 per side	6–12 U per band 10–30 U per side

(DAO: depressor anguli oris)

Source: Sundaram H, Signorini M, Liew S, Trindade de Almeida AR, Wu Y, Vieira Braz A, et al. Global Aesthetics Consensus: Botulinum toxin type A–Evidence-based review, emerging concepts, and consensus recommendations for esthetic use, including updates on complications. Plast Reconstr Surg. 2016;137(3):518e-29e.

facial lines with BoNTA significantly improves patient-reported outcomes,[9,10] and patients who receive regular treatment over many years experience a greater reduction in perceived age the longer the treatment continues[11] with sustained patient and physician satisfaction.[12] Moreover, several studies have demonstrated progressive wrinkle reduction and cumulative improvements in skin quality after repeated treatment.[13-16]

TREATMENT OF THE UPPER FACE

Wrinkles amenable to treatment with BoNTA in the upper face include glabellar, lateral canthal, and horizontal forehead lines, and all three regions are often treated simultaneously for optimal esthetic improvement.[7] Injection sites and doses will depend on the location, size, and use of the target muscles, all of which varies greatly between individuals.

Glabellar Rhytides

Frown lines in the glabellar region are caused by contraction of the corrugator supercilii and orbicularis oculi muscles which move the brow medially, and the procerus and depressor supercilii muscles which pull the brow inferiorly. Treatment aims to significantly weaken the corrugator and procerus muscles. We currently use five injection sites when treating glabellar frown lines and vary the dosage depending on the individual brow.

Crow's Feet

Contraction of the lateral fibers of the orbicularis oculi muscle produces lateral canthal rhytides or (crow's feet). Since, forceful closure of the eyelids requires orbicularis contraction, the goal of treatment is to produce weakening just in the lateral orbital area, rather than a complete paralysis of the muscle.

Multiple injections using small doses are required to weaken broad areas of the muscle.

Forehead Rhytides

Deep horizontal creases in the forehead are produced by the repeated contraction of the frontalis muscle, the brow elevator. Since, too much toxin in the frontalis can result in brow ptosis or complete immobility, treatment aims to soften, rather than eliminate horizontal lines, allowing for some mobility after injection. Brow depressors should always be treated at the same time as the frontalis in order avoid brow ptosis. In some subjects with pre-existing brow ptosis, the glabellar region is treated first, and the frontalis re-evaluated for subsequent treatment.

Shaping the Brow

Women prefer a higher, more arched eyebrow than men.[17] Frankel first noted subtle brow elevation after treatment of the brow depressors,[18] while central injections into the glabella alone produced a dramatic lateral eyebrow elevation followed by an entire chemical brow lift due to diffusion of the toxin into the inferomedial frontalis and compensatory increase in the resting tone of the lateral remainder of this muscle.[19] Understanding that the shape and height of the eyebrow is determined by the opposing activity of the frontalis muscle and the brow depressors allow the clinician to manipulate eyebrow position at will to improve esthetic appearance and correct asymmetry (**Figs. 3A** and **B**).

Widening the Eye

The palpebral aperture can be widened by subcutaneous injections of BoNTA into the lower lid with concomitant treatment of crow's feet.[20] Small doses placed subdermally in the lower eyelid in the midpupillary line, 3 mm below the ciliary margin, will simultaneously increase the vertical palpebral aperture by 2–3 mm at rest and full smile, respectively, lending a more rounded appearance to the lower eyelid.

MIDFACE INJECTIONS

The midface is a complex area that demands full anatomical familiarity and precise injection techniques. It is not an area for novice injectors. Muscles in this region are important in expressing emotion, elevating the upper lip, and smiling. Even minor miscalculations

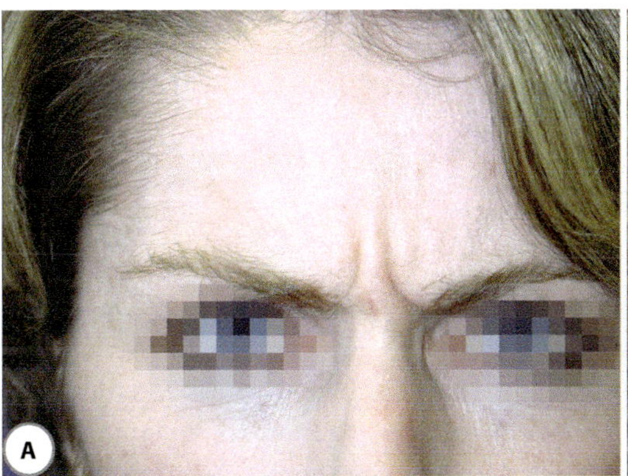

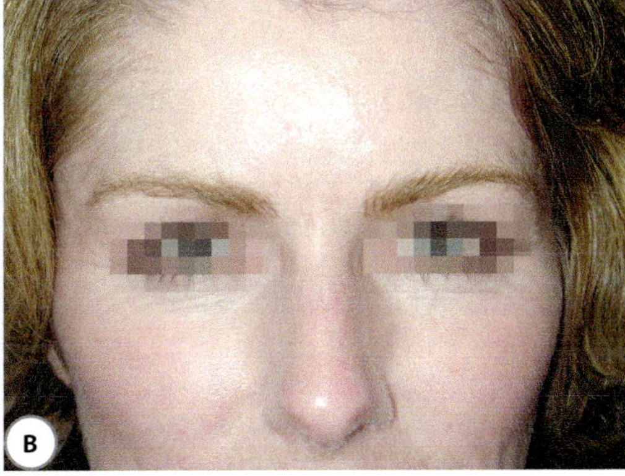

FIGS. 3A AND B: Understanding that the opposing activity of the frontalis muscle and the brow depressors allow the clinician to manipulate eyebrow position.

in dosing or placement can have dire consequences. In general, the muscles in the midface require smaller doses than the muscles in the upper face. It is critical to avoid initial overtreatment; start low and titrate as needed.

Contraction of the upper nasalis muscle causes fanning rhytides (bunny lines) at the radix (root) of the nose. BoNTA treatment weakens the upper nasalis effectively and dramatically softens these lines. Bunny lines are typically treated in conjunction with the glabellar complex. Similarly, contraction of the nasalis muscle accentuates nasal flare and the repeated dilation of nostrils. Small doses of BoNTA can produce a satisfactory decrease in involuntary nostril flare in some patients for 3–4 months. Nasal tip droop is common during aging. Contraction of the depressor septi nasi, a small muscle located at the external base of the nasal septum, pulls the tip of the nose downward. BoNTA slightly elevates the nasal tip. Caution should be taken with individuals who already have a long nonvermilion upper lip because of an associated risk of lip ptosis.

TREATMENT OF THE LOWER FACE

In the lower face, BoNTA can lift mouth corners and improve the appearance of the chin and jaw, but it is usually combined with fillers or other rejuvenating procedures to produce optimal and durable results.[7,8,21-23] In the first systematic comparison of its kind to date for the treatment of the aging lower face, combination therapy with neurotoxins, and hyaluronic acid (HA) fillers in the perioral region resulted in higher overall satisfaction scores than BoNTA alone and the greatest increase in the percentage of participants reporting their appearance to be younger than their current age.[22]

A thorough understanding of muscular anatomy in the lower face and the way in which muscles interact is necessary to maintain facial balance, especially in the perioral region. Because paralysis of the muscles in the lower face can lead to functional impairment, the goal of treatment is to soften the rhytides through muscular relaxation rather than complete paresis of the target muscle.

Radial Lip Lines

As the mouth ages, the cutaneous upper lip lengthens and dense vertical perioral rhytides appear. These vertical lines are commonly referred to as "smoker's lines" but can have other causes such as heredity, photodamage, or activities such as playing a musical instrument that require pursing of the lips. Small doses of BoNTA that produce localized microparesis of the orbicularis oris can dramatically reduce radial lip lines and improve the appearance of the lips. Conservative doses are a must to maintain competence of the mouth and superficial injections are recommended over deep injections. Even conservative dosing, however, may affect the function of the mouth. This procedure may not be desirable for musicians who play wind instruments and professional singers or speakers. Some patients have difficulty with lip proprioception after treatment, but eating, drinking, and singing are typically not affected. BoNTA injections for radial lip lines may be particularly useful in combination with perioral laser or electrosurgical resurfacing or in combination with a filling agent.

Mouth Frown

The frowning expression created when the lateral corners of the mouth are permanently angled downward can create an impression of disapproval and unpleasantness and is caused by overactivity of the depressor anguli oris (DAO) muscle which pulls down the corner of the mouth in opposition to the zygomaticus major and minor muscles. BoNTA can be used to weaken the DAO and reset muscular balance, allowing the zygomaticus to elevate the corners of the mouth and return them to a horizontal position. Contraction of the DAO also exacerbates the appearance of marionette lines which extend from the down-turned corner of the mouth to the lateral mentum. Marionette lines are traditionally treated with fillers; the addition of BoNTA as an adjunct prevents the repeated molding and contortion of the implant in this highly mobile area, thus extending the duration of the soft-tissue augmentation.

The Chin and Jaw

Contraction of the mentalis muscle can produce a deep groove or convexity (mental crease) between the lower lip and the prominence of the chin. Injection of BoNTA into the mentalis muscle gives a satisfactory softening of the crease while avoiding complications from weakening of the orbicularis oris (**Box 2**). An "orange peel" (peau d'orange) appearance of the chin results from the loss of dermal collagen and subcutaneous fat at the mentum overtime and is worsened by mastication or speech. BoNTA can be used alone or in combination with fillers to improve the appearance of the chin.

BoNTA can be used to reduce muscle bulk in patients with masseteric hypertrophy which can be due to a number of reasons; most commonly, it is a side effect of bruxism (the nonfunctional gnashing or grinding of teeth) to which adequate dosing of BoNTA to the masseter muscle overtime offers relief. Esthetic recontouring of the lower face—using BoNTA to shape the jaw—was initially attempted for East Asian patients but is now a common procedure for any individual desiring a less prominent jawline or to correct asymmetry or unwanted bulk.[24-27]

BOX 2: Avoiding complications.

- Understand the mechanism of action of BoNTA on functional anatomy and muscles of expression
- Use a conservative approach, especially when injecting near muscles that can cause functional impairment
- Avoid over-large doses and complete paresis of target muscles

(BoNTA: botulinum neurotoxin type A)

TREATMENT OF THE NECK

The aging neck presents with vertical bands, horizontal lines, and loss of lower face contour, all of which can be effectively treated with BoNTA, alone, or increasingly in combination with fillers and energy-based devices.[23,28,29] The platysma is a broad and flat muscle that covers the anterior and lateral aspects of the neck, inserting into the mentum, mandible, orbicularis oris, DAO, and risorius.[30] Platysmal bands are formed when the anterior fibers of the platysma separate into two discrete vertical bands that often tighten and become more visible on animation in older individuals. When the upper and lower portions of the platysma contract, they pull the skin to the center of the muscle, forming horizontal neck lines.[29] Most BoNTA injection techniques have targeted platysmal bands and horizontal necklace lines by way of deep intradermal injections using small doses of BoNTA at multiple sites along each band.[31-33] Alternatively, multiple microdroplets of diluted BoNTA injected as superficially as possible across the entire sweep of the platysma muscle has been demonstrated to improve skin texture, color, and smoothness, reduces the appearance of horizontal necklace lines and vertical banding, and create a lifting effect of the jowls and jawline for better cervicomental contouring.[34] Levy described the Nefertiti lift to correct loss of definition along the jaw, in which small doses of BoNTA are injected in multiple sites under the mandible and intradermally into the upper half of the actively contracting posterior platysmal band to sharpen the contours of the jaw and raise the corners of the mouth.[35] However, the Nefertiti Lift does not address the anterior fibers of the platysma which may be recruited during neck contraction, resulting in local wrinkling, worsening of bands, and loss of anterior facial contour.[29]

Typical treatment of the neck has its limitations. In individuals with extensive cutaneous laxity and large quantities of subcutaneous fat, the effect may not be noticeable. Large doses into the anterior strap muscles can not only produce weakness in the neck flexors but can diffuse deeply, causing dysphagia. Lateral injections away from the strap muscles of deglutition, however, can result in remarkable improvements in cervical contour.[29,33,35]

A new understanding of the role of the upper platysma and its impact on lower facial dynamics and contour has altered the approach to treatment in the neck. In a retrospective analysis of 161 patients, the lower face was treated as a whole unit with a standardized pattern of injection: Intramuscular injections at two sites in the mentalis muscle, followed by superficial injections along with two horizontal lines from the mandibular border, stretching from the level of the DAO to the mandibular angle, spaced 2 cm apart.[29] The injections targeted the upper platysma and produced marvellous if sometimes surprising results: Enhancement of the lower facial contour (especially during lower facial muscular contraction), and relaxation or even complete effacement of oblique and horizontal lines and wrinkles and lower vertical deep smile lines. All patients were satisfied with treatment at follow-up.

Combination Therapy

When used alone, BoNTA effectively reduces the appearance of dynamic rhytides and superficial lines and is able to alter the contours of a face but fails to address the underlying loss of volume or changes in skin texture or pigmentation that occurs overtime. As a result, neurotoxins are increasingly used in conjunction with other interventions. Combination therapy with BoNTA, soft-tissue fillers, and light or energy-based therapies often procures a kind of synergy, leading to enhanced esthetic outcomes of greater duration in the face and neck.[8,21,23,28,36]

A number of studies have shown superior efficacy and patient satisfaction in association with a combination of fillers and neuromodulators, especially in individuals with deep resting rhytides.[22,37-39] BoNTA and fillers work by the dual mechanisms of reflation and relaxation—restoring volume and decreasing activity of the muscles of expression responsible for the creation of glabellar rhytides, lateral canthal rhytides, horizontal forehead lines, melomental folds, and mouth frown, as well as lines and wrinkles around the mouth and in the neck. Traditionally, BoNTA treatment preceded fillers by a week or two in order to assess the need for the treatment of residual static lines, deep folds, and volume deficiencies. Currently, we treat with neuromodulators and three-dimensional superficial fillers at the same time. If energy-based devices are required at the same visit, we usually treat with fillers first, ask the individual to lie down for treatment with the energy-based devices, and finally treat with the neuromodulator when the subject is again vertical to prevent ptosis.

Similarly, the overall esthetic benefit of light and energy-based systems, such as intense-pulsed light, radiofrequency devices, and microfocused ultrasound which were developed to treat the envelope of the skin by tightening, lifting, improving texture, and correcting skin tone, and discoloration appears to be greater when combined with BoNTA than when used alone.[23,36,40-42]

SIDE EFFECTS AND COMPLICATIONS

Most side effects of BoNTA are injection-related and transient such as swelling, bruising, and pain. Complications occur when the toxin diffuses into nontargeted or glandular tissue surrounding the site of injection due to overenthusiastic doses, inappropriate injection sites, or poor technique.[43] Each point of injection is associated with an area of denervation of about 1–1.5 cm (2–3 cm diameter) due to the spread of toxin. Careful injection techniques targeting the appropriate muscles and using concentrated, low doses to limit its diffusion to nontargeted muscles, or glands are recommended. A higher concentration allows for more accurate placement, greater duration of effect, and fewer side effects, since, lower concentrations may encourage the spread of toxin. In the upper face, adverse events translate into a drooping eyelid or brow (ptosis), watery, dry, or crossed eyes, and eyebrows that can appear askew or asymmetrical. Lower face complications impact muscle function, resulting in a flaccid cheek, lopsided smile, incompetent mouth, the inability to whistle, dysphagia, and neck weakness. However, when used appropriately by experienced injectors, cosmetic doses of BoNTA are well tolerated and safe, and over 30 years of clinical use has demonstrated a strong record of safety.[44] Serious adverse events are rare and more likely to occur with the much higher doses used for therapeutic indications in larger muscle groups such as in cervical dystonia, particularly in individuals who may have underlying medical conditions that increase the risk of complications.[45]

CONCLUSION

Injections of BoNTA have been an integral part of cosmetic practice for over 30 years, the first-line treatment for smoothing hyperkinetic lines in the face and neck. Treatment is both an art and a science in the hands of an adept clinician who is able to use the toxin to lift the brows, widen the eyes, correct asymmetry and imbalance, and sculpt the jaw, and lift the neck. The current treatment paradigm favors a multifaceted approach to rejuvenation, targeting aging changes across all tissue levels, from the epidermis to bone. To that end, BoNTA is rarely used in isolation but is combined with fillers and other cosmetic procedures such as energy-based devices and surgery to produce optimal, natural, and durable esthetic outcomes.

REFERENCES

1. Frevert J. Pharmaceutical, biological, and clinical properties of botulinum neurotoxin type A products. Drugs R D. 2015;15(1):1-9.
2. Scott AB. Botulinum toxin injection into extraocular muscles as an alternative to strabismus surgery. Ophthalmology. 1980;87:1044-9.
3. Carruthers A, Carruthers J. Botulinum toxin type A: History and current cosmetic use in the upper face. Semin Cutan Med Surg. 2001;20:71-84.
4. Carruthers JDA, Carruthers JA. Treatment of glabellar frown lines with C. botulinum A exotoxin. J Dermatol Surg Oncol. 1992;18:17-21.
5. Carruthers A, Carruthers J. History of cosmetic botulinum toxin. In: Carruthers A, Carruthers J, Dover JS, (eds). Procedures in Cosmetic Dermatology: Botulinum Toxin. New York: Saunders Elsevier; 2013. pp. 13-7.
6. American Society of Plastic Surgeons. (2016). 2015 Plastic Surgery Statistics Report. [online] Available from: www.plasticsurgery.org (Last accessed August, 2021.
7. Sundaram H, Signorini M, Liew S, Trindade de Almeida AR, Wu Y, Vieira Braz A, et al. Global Aesthetics Consensus: Botulinum toxin type A—Evidence-based review, emerging concepts, and consensus recommendations for aesthetic use, including updates on complications. Plast Reconstr Surg. 2016;137(3):518e-29e.
8. Sundaram H, Liew S, Signorini M, Vieira Braz A, Fagien S, Swift A, et al. Global Aesthetics Consensus: Hyaluronic acid fillers and botulinum toxin type A-Recommendations for combined treatment and optimizing outcomes in diverse patient populations. Plast Reconstr Surg. 2016;137(5):1410-23.
9. Carruthers A, Carruthers J. Patient-reported outcomes with botulinum neurotoxin type A. J Cosmet Laser Ther. 2007;9(Suppl 1):32-7.

10. Moers-Carpi M, Carruthers J, Fagien S, Lupo M, Delmar H, Jones D, et al. Efficacy and safety of onabotulinumtoxinA for treating crow's feet lines alone or in combination with glabellar lines: A multicenter, randomized, controlled trial. Dermatol Surg. 2015;41(1):102-12.
11. Carruthers A, Sadick N, Brandt F, Trindade de Almeida AR, Fagien S, Goodman GJ, et al. Evolution of facial aesthetic treatment over five or more years: A retrospective cross-sectional analysis of continuous onabotulinumtoxin A treatment. Dermatol Surg. 2015;41(6):693-701.
12. Trindade de Almeida A, Carruthers J, Cox SE, Goldman MP, Wheeler S, Gallagher CJ. Patient satisfaction and safety with aesthetic onabotulinumtoxinA after at least 5 years: A retrospective cross-sectional analysis of 4,402 glabellar treatments. Dermatol Surg. 2015;41(Suppl 1):S19-28.
13. Binder WJ. Long-term effects of botulinum toxin type A (Botox) on facial lines: A comparison in identical twins. Arch Facial Plast Surg. 2006;8:426-31.
14. Dailey RA, Philip A, Tardie G. Long-term treatment of glabellar rhytides using onabotulinumtoxina. Dermatol Surg. 2011;37:918-28.
15. Bonaparte JP, Ellis D. Alterations in the elasticity, pliability, and viscoelastic properties of facial skin after injection of onabotulinum toxin A. JAMA Facial Plast Surg. 2015;17:256-63.
16. Rivkin A, Binder WJ. Long-term effects of onabotulinumtoxin A on facial lines: a 19-year experience of identical twins. Dermatol Surg. 2015;41(Suppl 1):S64-6.
17. Carruthers J, Carruthers A. Social significance of the eyebrows and periorbital complex. J Drugs Dermatol. 2014;13(1 Suppl):s7-11.
18. Frankel AS, Kamer FM. Chemical brow lift. Arch Otolaryngol Head Neck Surg. 1998;124:321-23.
19. Carruthers A, Carruthers J. Eyebrow height after botulinum toxin type A to the glabella. Dermatol Surg. 2007;33(1):S26-31.
20. Flynn TC, Carruthers JA, Carruthers JA. Botulinum-A toxin treatment of the lower eyelid improves infraorbital rhytides and widens the eye. Dermatol Surg. 2001;27:703-8.
21. Carruthers JD, Glogau RG, Blitzer A. Advances in facial rejuvenation: Botulinum toxin type a, hyaluronic acid dermal fillers, and combination therapies--consensus recommendations. Plast Reconstr Surg. 2008;121(5 Suppl):5S-30S.
22. Carruthers J, Carruthers A, Monheit GD, Davis PG. Multicenter, randomized, parallel-group study of onabotulinumtoxinA and hyaluronic acid dermal fillers (24-mg/ml smooth, cohesive gel) alone and in combination for lower facial rejuvenation: Satisfaction and patient-reported outcomes. Dermatol Surg. 2010;36(4):2135-45.
23. Carruthers J, Burgess C, Day D, Fabi SG, Goldie K, Kerscher M, et al. Consensus recommendations for combined aesthetic interventions in the face using botulinum toxin, fillers, and energy-based devices. Dermatol Surg. 2016:42:S86-97.
24. To EW, Ahuja AT, Ho WS, King WW, Wong WK, Pang PC, et al. A prospective study of the effect of botulinum toxin A on masseteric muscle hypertrophy with ultrasonographic and electromyographic measurement. Br J Plast Surg. 2001;54(3):197-200.
25. von Lindern JJ, Niederhagen B, Appel T, Bergé S, Reich RH. Type A botulinum toxin for the treatment of hypertrophy of the masseter and temporal muscle: an alternative treatment. Plast Reconstr Surg. 2001;107(2):327-32.
26. Park MY, Ahn KY, Jung DS. Application of botulinum toxin A for treatment of facial contouring in the lower face. Dermatol Surg. 2003;29:477-83.
27. Liew S, Dart A. Nonsurgical reshaping of the lower face. Aesthet Surg J. 2008;28:251-7.
28. Vanaman M, Fabi SG, Cox SE. Neck rejuvenation using a combination approach: Our experience and a review of the literature. Dermatol Surg. 2016;42(Suppl 2):S94-100.
29. de Almeida ART, Romiti A, Carruthers JDA. The facial platysma and its underappreciated role in lower face dynamics and contour. Dermatol Surg. 2017;43:1042-9.
30. Fagien S, Raspaldo H. Facial rejuvenation with botulinum neurotoxin: An anatomical and experiential perspective. J Cosm Laser Ther. 2007;9(Suppl 1):23-31.
31. Brandt FS, Bellman B. Cosmetic use of botulinum A exotoxin for the aging neck. Dermatol Surg. 1998;24:1232-4.
32. Matarasso A, Matarasso SL, Brandt FS, Bellman B. Botulinum A exotoxin for the management of platysma bands. Plast Reconstr Surg. 1999;103:645-52.
33. Carruthers J, Carruthers A. Aesthetic botulinum A toxin in the mid and lower face and neck. Dermatol Surg. 2003;29:468-76.
34. Wu WT. Microbotox of the lower face and neck: Evolution of a personal technique and its clinical effects. Plast Reconstr Surg. 2015;136(5 Suppl):92S-100S.
35. Levy PM. The 'Nefertiti lift': A new technique for specific re-contouring of the jawline. J Cosmet Laser Ther. 2007;9:249-52.
36. Fabi SG, Goldman MP, Mills DC, Werschler WP, Green JB, Kaufman J, et al. Combining microfocused ultrasound with botulinum toxin and temporary and semi-permanent dermal fillers: Safety and current use. Dermatol Surg. 2016;42(Suppl 2):S168-76.
37. Carruthers J, Carruthers A. A prospective, randomized, parallel group study analyzing the effect of BTX-A (Botox) and nonanimal sourced hyaluronic acid (NASHA, Restylane) in combination compared with NASHA (Restylane) alone in severe glabellar rhytides in adult female subjects: treatment of severe glabellar rhytides with a hyaluronic acid derivative compared with the derivative and BTX-A. Dermatol Surg. 2003;29:802-9.

38. Dubina M, Tung R, Bolotin D, Mahoney AM, Tayebi B, Sato M, et al. Treatment of forehead/glabellar rhytide complex with combination botulinum toxin a and hyaluronic acid versus botulinum toxin A injection alone: A split-face, rater-blinded, randomized control trial. J Cosmet Dermatol. 2013;12(4):261-6.
39. Beer KR, Julius H, Dunn M, Wilson F. Remodeling of periorbital, temporal, glabellar, and crow's feet areas with hyaluronic acid and botulinum toxin. J Cosmet Dermatol. 2014;13:143-50.
40. Carruthers J, Carruthers A. The effect of full-face broadband light treatments alone and in combination with bilateral crow's feet Botulinum toxin type A chemodenervation. Dermatol Surg. 2004;30:355-66.
41. Khoury JG, Saluja R, Goldman MP. The effect of botulinum toxin type A on full-face intense pulsed light treatment: a randomized, double-blind, split-face study. Dermatol Surg. 2008;34:1062-9.
42. Cuerda-Galindo E, Palomar-Gallego MA, Linares-Garcíavaldecasas R. Are combined same-day treatments the future for photorejuvenation? Review of the literature on combined treatments with lasers, intense pulsed light, radiofrequency, botulinum toxin, and fillers for rejuvenation. J Cosmet Laser Ther. 2015;17:49-54.
43. Klein AW. Complications, adverse reactions, and insights with the use of botulinum toxin. Dermatol Surg. 2003;29:549-56.
44. Carruthers J, Carruthers A. Complications of botulinum toxin A. Facial Plast Surg Clin North Am. 2007;15:51-4.
45. Coté TR, Mohan AK, Polder JA, Walton MK, Braun MM. Botulinum toxin type A injections: Adverse events reported to the US Food and Drug Administration in therapeutic and cosmetic cases. J Am Acad Dermatol. 2005;53:407-15.

7 SECTION

MEDICAL APPLICATIONS

24

CHAPTER

Laser and Light-based Therapies for Acne Vulgaris

H Ray Jalian

INTRODUCTION

Acne vulgaris is a near-ubiquitous skin disorder characterized by comedones, inflammatory papules, and nodules. While lifelong prevalence is estimated to be upward of 85%, the exact pathogenesis of the disease is poorly understood. For most, the disease is most pronounced during adolescence, but often can linger into adulthood particularly in female patients. Despite its transient nature, acne scarring and psychologic impact of the disease has appreciable morbidity well into adulthood with many seeking laser and energy-based treatments for acne scarring.

The pathogenesis of the disease is multifactorial and includes an interplay between follicular hyperkeratinization (e.g., "clogged pore"), excess sebum production, overgrowth of gram-positive anaerobe *Propionibacterium acnes*, and host immune and inflammatory response. Many of the treatments are aimed at addressing aspects of the pathogenesis and can be quite successful in the appropriate clinical settings. Topical treatments, such as antibiotics and retinoids, help with bacterial overgrowth, inflammation, and follicular keratinization and are appropriate therapies in patients with mild-to-moderate disease. Oral treatments, including systemic antibiotics and isotretinoin, are reserved for those with moderate-to-severe disease, or if significant scarring is present. While effective treatments are present, providers and patients alike are turning to alternative treatments, including laser and light-based treatments.

Many of the currently available laser and light-based treatments utilize preexisting technology, and were not developed specifically for acne. While effective, they lack selectivity and rely largely on an indirect thermal effect resulting in transient improvement. Luckily, several selective treatments for acne vulgaris with promising preclinical and early clinical data are in the pipeline ushering in a new era of treatment based on targeting species aspects of disease pathogenesis.

LASERS

Vascular Selective Lasers

Early studies using purpuric settings with pulsed dye lasers (PDLs) resulted in variable clinical efficacy for the treatment of inflammatory acne. An initial study found a statistically and clinically significant reduction in acne 12 weeks after a single PDL treatment, though a subsequent near identical study failed to reproduce the same results.[1,2] While there is weak evidence in the literature to support its efficacy, reports remain inconsistent and very few well-controlled studies comparing it to standard topical regimens have been conducted. Moreover, the wide variety of parameters utilized in these studies makes it difficult to draw a conclusive comparison.

The clinical effect of the PDL is theorized to be related to its passive photothermal effect on tissue through targeting of dilated blood vessels in hyperemic inflammatory lesions. There is no demonstrable decrease in *P. acnes* counts or sebum excretion rate following PDL treatments.[3] Other studies demonstrate altered expression of inflammatory mediators, such as transforming growth factor beta (TGF-β), following treatment with PDL suggesting the mechanism of nonselective light-based treatments is related to soluble factors that are upregulated following treatment. This may also explain the global improvement seen in split-face trials where both treatment and nontreatment side improve.[3]

Mid-infrared Lasers

The pursuit of the use of mid-infrared lasers for the treatment of acne stemmed from the histologic observation of sebaceous gland damage in both an in vivo rabbit ear model as well as ex vivo in human skin. This observation spurred clinical trials investigating the efficacy of a 1450-nm diode laser for the treatment of acne. A preliminary split-back study consisted of 27 subjects treated for four treatments separated by 3 weeks at various dosimetries. 24 weeks following the final treatment, lesion counts were improved in the 15 subjects who completed the study. One biopsy specimen demonstrated photothermal coagulation of the pilosebaceous unit, though specimens taken later, including from the same subject, showed normal sebaceous gland and skin adnexal architecture.[4] With these preliminary results, follow-up studies with the same device confirmed efficacy for the use of this device for inflammatory acne on the face.[5] Subsequent dose–response studies demonstrated longevity of clinical results as well as safety in darker skin phototypes.[6] Several flaws in study design limit the impact of these studies. None of the initial trials used standardized acne measures now required by the Food and Drug Administration (FDA) for any device seeking clearance of the treatment of acne. Moreover, one of the studies allowed subjects to continue their current topical or oral acne regimens, confounding interpretation of the efficacy of the device as a monotherapy.[5] Larger blinded studies utilizing standardized acne scales demonstrated a statistically significant reduction between treatment and control sites at 12-month follow-up after a third treatment session.[7] There was, however, an improvement in both the treatment and control sites suggesting that there may be a systemic effect of acne treatments mediated by a soluble factor. This has been suggested by others who failed to show a statistically significant difference between treated and untreated side, despite global improvement in acne severity.

The paucity of clinical evidence for the 1450-nm diode laser as a monotherapy led most to use it as an adjunctive treatment for medical therapies. Due to relatively painful nature of the treatment, topical anesthesia is highly recommended. Adverse effects of the treatment are limited to transient erythema and pigmentary alteration in darker skin phenotypes. Low fluence multiple pass techniques may improve tolerability and decrease risk postinflammatory pigment alteration in darker Fitzpatrick phototypes.[8,9] In similar studies, a 1320-nm infrared laser demonstrated transient improvement in comedone count, though failed to improve inflammatory acne lesions.[10]

Similar to the PDL, the mechanism of action of mid-infrared lasers is likely related to their photothermal effect on the sebaceous gland. Passive heating of the sebaceous gland is thought to temporary alter sebaceous gland function and architecture. Indeed, we observe transient decrease in sebum production following treatment with these devices.[6,11] Despite preliminary evidence to suggest targeting of sebaceous glands directly, no permanent effect on sebaceous glands occurs. Moreover, as these devices have narrow therapeutic windows and minimal long-term efficacy, most providers no longer use these lasers for the treatment of acne.

NONCOHERENT LIGHT SOURCES

The use of broadband light sources for the treatment of acne is not a novel practice. Historically, natural sunlight and ultraviolet light were used to treat acne but were largely replaced by medical therapies. The mechanism of action is likely related to photochemical effects by directly activating endogenous bacterial porphyrins. This results in the formation of reactive oxygen species (ROS), damage to bacterial membranes, and a decrease in bacterial load.[12]

Narrow-band Blue Light Sources

Narrow-band blue light continuous wave (CW) light sources have modest effects on acne. Most treatment protocols involve a series of treatments resulting in moderate efficacy, though long-term improvement is unknown. Because the action spectrum for killing *P. acnes* has a relative peak from 400 to 420 nm (blue light),[13] many studies have focused on this spectrum of light. Reduction in inflammatory lesions was sustained 8 weeks following twice weekly treatment with a blue light device.[14] Others have demonstrated the efficacy of blue light in comparison to 1% topical clindamycin solution.[15] While effective for inflammatory lesions, there is minimal effect on comedonal lesions and it is best combined with a topical keratolytic (such as a retinoid).[16] Additional peaks can be extrapolated from the action spectrum of protoporphyrin IX (PPIX), the main endogenous porphyrin produced by *P. acnes*, corresponding to green, yellow, and red light and others have demonstrated efficacy with these corresponding wavelengths.[16-18]

Visible light sources are uniformly safe with adverse effects related to posttreatment erythema and dryness. It is of the author's opinion that low-energy CW visible light sources can be an adjunct to topical or oral medical regimen and can be an appropriate choice for those patients who wish to take an "active" role in the management of their acne. Moreover, with the recent FDA clearance of home versions of these devices, it improves accessibility and cost effectiveness of this treatment.

Intense Pulsed Light sources

Flashlamp light sources administer broad-spectrum, noncoherent pulses of visible light. The evidence for intense pulsed light (IPL) sources as a monotherapy is weak, with most studies pairing IPL with an exogenous photosensitizer resulting in conflicting results for efficacy.[19,20] Many of these devices now are combined with gentle negative pressure, so called photopneumatic devices, with modest efficacy to treat acne.[21]

Photodynamic Therapy

Photodynamic therapy (PDT) involves the application of an exogenous photosensitizer followed by activation by a light source. For the treatment of acne, numerous studies have used various photosensitizers combined with both laser and CW light sources. The definitive study describing the utility of PDT defined a high-dose red light protocol that resulted in long-term remission of acne and demonstrable reduction in sebum production after four treatment sessions.[22] Long incubations with aminolevulinic acid allow for PPIX accumulation within the sebaceous gland. CW red light (635 nm) at dosimetry of 200 J/cm^2 results in activation of PPIX, generation of ROS, and subsequent desired clinical effect. Many iterations of PDT exist for the treatment of acne, with variability in photosensitizer, incubation time, and light source (both wavelength and CW vs. pulsed laser/light sources).[23,24] These variabilities make standardization and comparison between studies difficult.

It is the author's opinion that in order to achieve appreciable clearance and longevity in treatment response prolonged, incubation times (>90 min) are necessary to allow for accumulation of activated PPIX within the sebaceous gland. Moreover, in order to target at the depth of the sebaceous gland, CW red light is the most effective light source.

Of all the currently available laser and light-based options available for the treatment of acne, high-dose red light PDT is by far the most effective and definitive treatment. This makes it an attractive treatment option for clinicians. However, in practical terms, high-dose red light PDT is rarely performed given the adverse effects. In addition to treatment discomfort, many patients have photosensitivity for approximately 48 hours after treatment. Erythema, swelling, crusting, sterile pustulation, and desquamation are common and expected side effects following treatment. While these are all transient side effects and resolved typically within 7–10 days, the prolonged downtime discourages many providers and patients alike from having the procedure. Further discussion of PDT for acne is available in articles by Sakamoto et al.[23,24]

LIPID SELECTIVE LIGHT: TOWARD A TRUE SEBACEOUS GLAND SELECTIVE LASER

The theory of selective photothermolysis involves the selection of a wavelength and pulse duration that targets a specific chromophore while also confining the heat to the target. This thermal confinement of heat allows for the targeting of individual chromophores without disruption of adjacent tissue.[25] Selective targeting of lipid-rich tissues is possible by vibrational bands within the tissue. Anderson et al. measured the absorption spectrum of fat, identifying peaks at 1210 nm and 1720 nm where the absorption coefficient of lipid is greater than that of water.[26] Given the similarities in lipid content between adipose tissue and sebum, investigators identified absorption peaks near 1210 nm, 1728 nm, 1760 nm, 2306 nm, and 2346 nm. Histologic confirmation of selective damage to sebaceous glands was confirmed using 1700 nm at 100–135 ms pulse durations on ex vivo tissue. Further studies using a tabletop device with similar wavelengths demonstrate similar histologic outcomes.[27,28] At this present time, clinical trials are underway to explore the clinical efficacy for this device for the treatment of acne. While there is no clinical evidence that the destruction of sebaceous glands will improve acne, medical therapies which reduce sebaceous gland volume or sebum production historically result in a significant clinical improvement in acne.[28]

Selective Cryolipolysis

Cryosurgery of the skin has a variety of dermatologic uses including the nonselective destruction of epidermal lesions such as actinic keratosis or verruca vulgaris. By exploiting the different freezing points of lipid-rich versus water-rich tissues, selective damage to adipose tissue with controlled cooling, termed cryolipolysis, has evolved into an effective methodology for noninvasive body contouring. Historically speaking, the use of cryotherapy to treat acne has significant clinical support. Moreover, sebaceous gland damage in animals after localized cryoinjury was first reported decades ago.[29] With these facts in mind, investigators sought to investigate the feasibility of controlled cooling to target sebaceous glands. In animal and human models, selective destruction of sebaceous glands was seen on standard histology and various time points following treatment. In addition, suppressed sebum production up to 2 weeks following treatment was seen in a pilot human clinical trial.[30] While no clinical effects of efficacy for the treatment of acne vulgaris exist, this technology may prove to be a useful treatment for acne in the future.

Nanotechnology

Advances in nanotechnology now allow for the use of inorganic, inert nanoparticles for various medical applications. From this, the development of silica-gold nanoshells has been commercialized for the treatment of acne. These 150 nm size nanoshells are introduced into the hair follicle and subsequently the sebaceous gland, allowing the targeting of these structures with commercially available infrared lasers. The resulting thermal effect attenuates the sebaceous gland. Randomized controlled trials utilizing this technique for acne showed statistically significant improvement of inflammatory lesions as well as prolonged reduction up to 16 weeks posttreatment. This technology was recently cleared by the FDA and is currently awaiting commercialization.[31,32]

CONCLUSION

A critical appraisal of laser and light-based therapies leaves many questions unanswered. It is clear from the evidence presented that, for the most part, laser and light-based treatment should not be used as a monotherapy. In those patients who are motivated, the addition of light-based therapies as an adjunctive treatment may be a plausible option. While efficacy was not always reproducible, studies support the safety of these devices with a low incidence of adverse events.

REFERENCES

1. Seaton ED, Charakida A, Mouser PE, Grace I, Clement RM, Chu AC. Pulsed-dye laser treatment for inflammatory acne vulgaris: randomised controlled trial. Lancet. 2003;362(9393):1347-52.
2. Orringer JS, Kang S, Hamilton T, Schumacher W, Cho S, Hammerberg C, et al. Treatment of acne vulgaris with a pulsed dye laser: a randomized controlled trial. JAMA. 2004;291(23):2834-9.
3. Seaton ED, Mouser P, Charakida A, Alam S, Seldon PM, Chu AC. Investigation of the mechanism of action of nonablative pulsed-dye laser therapy in photorejuvenation and inflammatory acne vulgaris. Br J Dermatol. 2006;155(4):748-55.
4. Paithankar DY, Ross VE, Saleh BA, Blair MA, Graham BS. Acne treatment with a 1,450 nm wavelength laser and cryogen spray cooling. Lasers Surg Med. 2002;31(2):106-14.
5. Friedman PM, Jih MH, Kimyai-Asadi A, Goldberg LH. Treatment of inflammatory facial acne vulgaris with the 1450-nm diode laser: a pilot study. Dermatol Surg. 2004;30(2 Pt 1):147-51.
6. Jih MH, Friedman PM, Goldberg LH, Robles M, Glaich AS, Kimyai-Asadi A. The 1450-nm diode laser for facial inflammatory acne vulgaris: dose-response and 12-month follow-up study. J Am Acad Dermatol. 2006;55(1):80-7.
7. Darne S, Hiscutt EL, Seukeran DC. Evaluation of the clinical efficacy of the 1,450 nm laser in acne vulgaris: a randomized split-face, investigator-blinded clinical trial. Br J Dermatol. 201;165(6):1256-62.
8. Bernstein EF. A pilot investigation comparing low-energy, double pass 1,450 nm laser treatment of acne to conventional single-pass, high energy treatment. Lasers Surg Med. 2007;39(2):193-8.
9. Yeung CK, Shek SY, Yu CS, Kono T, Chan HH. Treatment of inflammatory facial acne with 1,450-nm diode laser in type IV to V Asian skin using an optimal combination of laser parameters. Dermatol Surg. 2009;35(4):593-600.
10. Orringer JS, Kang S, Maier L, Johnson TM, Sachs DL, Karimipour DJ, et al. A randomized, controlled, split-face clinical trial of 1320-nm Nd:YAG laser therapy in the treatment of acne vulgaris. J Am Acad Dermatol. 2007;56(3):432-8.

11. Perez-Maldonado A, Runger TM, Krejci-Papa N. The 1,450-nm diode laser reduces sebum production in facial skin: a possible mode of action of its effectiveness for the treatment of acne vulgaris. Lasers Surg Med. 2007;39(2):189-92.
12. Arakane K, Ryu A, Hayashi C, Masunaga T, Shinmoto K, Mashiko S, et al. Singlet oxygen (1 delta g) generation from coproporphyrin in Propionibacterium acnes on irradiation. Biochem Biophys Res Commun. 1996;223(3):578-82.
13. Kjeldstad B, Johnsson A. An action spectrum for blue and near ultraviolet inactivation of Propionibacterium acnes; with emphasis on a possible porphyrin photosensitization. Photochem Photobiol. 1986;43(1):67-70.
14. Elman M, Slatkine M, Harth Y. The effective treatment of acne vulgaris by a high-intensity, narrow band 405-420 nm light source. J Cosmet Laser Ther. 2003;5(2):111-7.
15. Gold MH, Rao J, Goldman MP, Bridges TM, Bradshaw VL, Boring MM, et al. A multicenter clinical evaluation of the treatment of mild to moderate inflammatory acne vulgaris of the face with visible blue light in comparison to topical 1% clindamycin antibiotic solution. J Drugs Dermatol. 2005;4(1):64-70.
16. Sigurdsson V, Knulst AC, van Weelden H. Phototherapy of acne vulgaris with visible light. Dermatology. 1997;194(3):256-60.
17. Papageorgiou P, Katsambas A, Chu A. Phototherapy with blue (415 nm) and red (660 nm) light in the treatment of acne vulgaris. Br J Dermatol. 2000;142(5):973-8.
18. Konig K, Teschke M, Sigusch B, Glockmann E, Eick S, Pfister W. Red light kills bacteria via photodynamic action. Cell Mol Biol (Noisy-le-grand). 2000;46(7):1297-303.
19. Rojanamatin J, Choawawanich P. Treatment of inflammatory facial acne vulgaris with intense pulsed light and short contact of topical 5-aminolevulinic acid: a pilot study. Dermatol Surg. 2006;32(8):991-6; discussion 996-7.
20. Santos MA, Belo VG, Santos G. Effectiveness of photodynamic therapy with topical 5-aminolevulinic acid and intense pulsed light versus intense pulsed light alone in the treatment of acne vulgaris: comparative study. Dermatol Surg. 2005;31(8 Pt 1):910-5.
21. Rajabi-Estarabadi A, Choragudi S, Camacho I, Moore KJ, Keri JE, Nouri K. Effectiveness of photopneumatic technology: a descriptive review of the literature. Lasers Med Sci. 2018;33(8):1631-7.
22. Hongcharu W, Taylor CR, Chang Y, Aghassi D, Suthamjariya K, Anderson RR. Topical ALA-photodynamic therapy for the treatment of acne vulgaris. J Invest Dermatol. 2000;115(2):183-92.
23. Sakamoto FH, Lopes JD, Anderson RR. Photodynamic therapy for acne vulgaris: a critical review from basics to clinical practice: part I. Acne vulgaris: when and why consider photodynamic therapy? J Am Acad Dermatol. 2010;63(2)183-93.
24. Sakamoto FH, Torezan L, Anderson RR. Photodynamic therapy for acne vulgaris: a critical review from basics to clinical practice: part II. Understanding parameters for acne treatment with photodynamic therapy. J Am Acad Dermatol. 2010;63(2):195-211.
25. Anderson RR, Parrish JA. Selective photothermolysis: precise microsurgery by selective absorption of pulsed radiation. Science. 1983;220(4596):524-7.
26. Wanner M, Avram M, Gagnon D, Mihm MC Jr, Zurakowski D, Watanabe K, et al. Effects of non-invasive, 1,210 nm laser exposure on adipose tissue: results of a human pilot study. Lasers Surg Med. 2009;41(6):401-7.
27. Sakamoto FH, Doukas AG, Farinelli WA, Tannous Z, Shinn M, Benson S, et al. Selective photothermolysis to target sebaceous glands: theoretical estimation of parameters and preliminary results using a free electron laser. Lasers Surg Med. 2012;44(2):175-83.
28. Janiczek-Dolphin N, Cook J, Thiboutot D, Harness J, Clucas A. Can sebum reduction predict acne outcome? Br J Dermatol. 2010;163(4):683-8.
29. Gage AA, Meenaghan MA, Natiella RJ, Greene GW Jr. Sensitivity of pigmented mucosa and skin to freezing injury. Cryobiology. 1979;16(4):348-61.
30. Jalian HR, Tam J, Vuong LN, Fisher J, Garibyan L, Mihm MC, et al. Selective Cryolysis of Sebaceous Glands. J Invest Dermatol. 2015;135(9):2173-80.
31. Paithankar D, Hwang BH, Munavalli G, Kauvar A, Lloyd J, Blomgren R, et al. Ultrasonic delivery of silica-gold nanoshells for photothermolysis of sebaceous glands in humans: Nanotechnology from the bench to clinic. J Control Release. 2015;28:206:30-6.
32. Paithankar DY, Sakamoto FH, Farinelli WA, Kositratna G, Blomgren RD, Meyer TJ, et al. Acne Treatment Based on Selective Photothermolysis of Sebaceous Follicles with Topically Delivered Light-Absorbing Gold Microparticles. J Invest Dermatol. 2015;135(7):1727-34.

25

CHAPTER

Hyperhidrosis

Yakir Levin, Cameron Rokhsar

INTRODUCTION

Hyperhidrosis, or excessive sweating, is usually categorized as primary or secondary. Primary hyperhidrosis is the most common type, typically affecting a focal area such as the palms, soles, axillae, and/or craniofacial region. Secondary hyperhidrosis is due to an underlying condition or medication, and may be localized or generalized. This chapter will focus on primary focal hyperhidrosis. However, a brief discussion of secondary hyperhidrosis is undertaken because of the importance of identifying this condition and its causes.

There are many causes of secondary hyperhidrosis. These include genodermatoses that affect palmoplantar skin and therefore cause palmoplantar hyperhidrosis, as well as hereditary autonomic neuropathies. Hypothalamic stimulation in response to temperature elevation can also cause hyperhidrosis. This is most commonly seen in febrile illnesses such as chronic infection or lymphoma, but can also be associated with a variety of metabolic and endocrine disorders. Many drugs can also cause hyperhidrosis, including cholinomimetic agents, cholinesterase inhibitors, adrenomimetic agents, hypoglycemic agents, CNS stimulants, antidepressants, opioids, and others. Gustatory hyperhidrosis can be a normal physiologic response to eating, and usually affects the upper cutaneous lip or cheeks. It can also occur in response to injury of any of a number of nerves associated with sweating. One such example is Frey's syndrome, characterized by gustatory flushing and sweating, which occurs after injury to the auriculotemporal nerve and is most commonly seen after parotid surgery. Hyperhidrosis in one area can also be compensatory of hypohidrosis in another. Secondary hyperhidrosis can also be nonneural in origin, through direct stimulation of the eccrine glands. This is usually a localized phenomenon and is associated with cutaneous malformations or localized stimuli.[1,2]

The distinction between primary and secondary hyperhidrosis is important in that secondary hyperhidrosis can sometimes be treated by elimination of the cause. More importantly, because secondary hyperhidrosis can be associated with systemic disease (e.g., malignancy, endocrine disorder, infection), identification of a potential cause is paramount.

As noted above, the remainder of this chapter will focus on primary hyperhidrosis.

PREVALENCE

The prevalence of primary hyperhidrosis has been the subject of a number of studies, and the results are somewhat inconsistent. In one study, US prevalence was estimated at 2.8%.[3] Hyperhidrosis prevalence was highest among those 25–64 years of age (3.5–4.5%) and lowest among those younger than 12 (0.5–0.7%). A second study estimated United States prevalence of 4.8%.[4] By comparison, prevalence of psoriasis in the United States among adults age 20 and more is estimated at 3.2%;[5] hyperhidrosis is a similarly common condition. Reports of prevalence of primary hyperhidrosis in other countries are also variable, with estimates of 4.6% in Germany,[6] 5.5% in Sweden, 12.3% in Vancouver,[7] 12.8% in Japan,[8] and 14.5% in Shanghai[7]. Despite the significant variation in prevalence estimates, it is clear that primary hyperhidrosis is of significant clinical issue.

ASSESSMENT OF HYPERHIDROSIS

Diagnostic Criteria

Proper diagnosis of primary focal hyperhidrosis is necessary before consideration of a treatment approach.

The diagnosis of primary focal hyperhidrosis is made based on the following criteria:[2]

- Focal, visible, excessive sweating
- At least 6 months' duration
- Lack of apparent secondary causes
- Presence of two or more of the following characteristics:
    - Bilateral and approximately symmetric
    - Age of onset less than 25 years
    - Frequency of episodes at least once per week
    - Positive family history
    - Cessation of excessive sweating on sleep
    - Impairment of daily activities

BOX 1: Pretreatment considerations.

- Hyperhidrosis diagnosis: Primary vs. secondary
- Severity of hyperhidrosis
- Health history including contraindications for botulinum toxin or systemic medications
- Physical examination including location of hyperhidrosis and skin type
- Prior treatment methods
- Patient desire for a permanent solution
- Insurance coverage and cost constraints

Assessment of Severity and Response to Treatment

Several measures have been used to assess the severity of hyperhidrosis and response to treatment. One is the Hyperhidrosis Disease Severity Scale (HDSS), in which patients assess sweating based on tolerability and impact on daily activities (see **Box 1**). Another is the starch iodine test, in which iodine and starch are placed on the skin; a dark blue to black color emerges when the patient's sweat comes into contact with this mixture. Although this does not quantify sweat at each location, authors have used semiquantitative scales that estimate the total area experiencing the color change. The most quantitative measurement of sweat is gravimetry, in which a piece of preweighed filter paper is placed onto the affected area and is then weighed after it has absorbed sweat for a given period of time. Other commonly used measures include use of the Dermatology Quality of Life Index (DLQI), as well as numerical scales that report subjective response.

The key pretreatment considerations are reviewed in **Box 1**, and the hyperhidrosis severity scale is reviewed in **Table 1**.

TREATMENT OF HYPERHIDROSIS

Treatment options for hyperhidrosis include topical medications, systemic medications,

TABLE 1: Hyperhidrosis Disease Severity Scale.

How would you rate the severity of your hyperhidrosis?	
Score	**Patient response**
1	My axillary sweating is never noticeable and never interfered with my daily activities
2	My axillary sweating is tolerable but sometimes interferes with my daily activities
3	My axillary sweating is barely tolerable and frequently interferes with my daily activities
4	My axillary sweating is intolerable and always interferes with my daily activities

surgery, injectable medications, iontophoresis and laser and energy based devices. These are reviewed in **Tables 2** and **3**.

TABLE 2: Management options.

Topical	• Aluminum chloride • Glycopyrronium tosylate
Systemic	• Glycopyrrolate • Beta-blocker • Alpha-adrenergic agonist
Surgical	• Sympathotomy
Injectable	• Abobotulinum toxin • Onabotulinum toxin • Incobotulinum toxin
Iontophoresis	• Tap water • Botulinum toxin • Anticholinergic • Baking soda
Laser	• Subdermal 924/975 • Subdermal Nd:YAG • 800 nm laser • 1,064 nm laser
Other energy based device	• Microwave destruction • Microfocused ultrasound • Fractional microneedle radiofrequency

Drugs

Pharmacologic treatment of hyperhidrosis has included topical, systemic, and injectable agents.

Aluminum Chloride

Aluminum salts have long been used in varying concentrations to treat localized hyperhidrosis, particularly of the axillae. Aluminum chloride is the partially neutralized form used in cosmetic antiperspirants, while aluminum chloride hexahydrate is used in prescription strength products. The mechanism of action is believed to be obstruction of the distal sweat duct. It is thought that metal ions precipitate with mucopolysaccharides, damaging epithelial cells lining the ducts and forming a plug that blocks sweat output. The efficacy is of limited duration due to epidermal turnover. However, some studies have shown long-term destruction of some secretory cells, resulting in reduced severity of hyperhidrosis over time. Holzle and Braun-Falco reported morphological changes in eccrine glands in skin biopsies from patients who had received long-term treatment with aqueous aluminum chloride solution. These included vacuolization of the secretory epithelium, dilatation of eccrine acini with atrophy of secretory cells, and accumulation of PAS-positive, diastase-resistant material in the dilated lumen of the secretory coils. The authors concluded that long-term blockage of the distal acrosyringium due to aluminum salts may lead to functional and structural degeneration of eccrine acini.[9] Other metal salts such as zirconium, vanadium, and indium are thought to work by the same mechanism as aluminum salts, though they are less commonly used.

Hyperhidrosis may respond to OTC aluminum chloride antiperspirants, but more severe cases may require the 20% aluminum chloride hexahydrate solution. In order to

TABLE 3: Energy based devices.

Author	Modality	Study method	Number of subjects	Primary outcome measure(s)	Outcome
Nestor and Park[23]	Microfocused ultrasound	RCT: Two treatments in one axilla vs. sham treatments in other axilla	*n* = 14	50% reduction in baseline spontaneous axillary sweat production measured gravimetrically on day 120	>50% of subjects achieved the primary outcome measure
Nestor and Park[23]	Microfocused ultrasound	RCT: Two treatments in both axillae versus two sham treatments in both axillae	*n* = 20 (12 received treatment and 8 received sham)	Reduction in HDSS score by 2 points on day 60	67% response in the treatment group and 0% in the sham group
LeClere et al.[24]	Minimally invasive laser (laser fiber introduced into subdermal space)	• RCT: Single treatment • Four groups: i. 975 nm alone ii. 975/924 nm iii. Curettage alone iv. 975/924 nm + curettage	*n* = 102: 25 in group 1, 26 in group 2, 26 in group 3 25 in group 4	HDSS, starch iodine test (semiquantitative 4 point scale), GAIS	Summarized in **Table 4**
Goldman and Wollina[25]	Minimally invasive laser (300 μm optic fiber inserted into subdermal space)	Single treatment in bilateral axillae	*n* = 17	Patient global assessment and physician global assessment	Patient global assessment: 12 subjects: "excellent" 3 subjects: "good" 2 subjects: "fair" Physician global assessment: 10 subjects: "excellent" 4 subjects: "good" 3 subjects: "fair"

Cont'd...

Cont'd...

Author	Modality	Study method	Number of subjects	Primary outcome measure(s)	Outcome
Bechara et al.[26]	800 nm diode laser	RCT: 5 treatments in one axilla vs. untreated contralateral control	$n = 19$	Gravimetry at 4 weeks, patient evaluation of sweat reduction at 4 weeks and 12 months (VAS), and patient satisfaction at 4 weeks and 12 months (VAS)	Gravimetry: Treated side: 89 mg/min (range 42–208) 48 mg/min (17–119) at 4 weeks Untreated side: 78 mg/min (25–220) 65 mg/min (24–399) at 4 weeks Subjective perception of reduction in hyperhidrosis: 32.4% at 4 weeks, 25% at 12 months Patient satisfaction: 5.9 at 4 weeks, 4.1 at 12 months
Letada et al.[28]	1,064 nm laser	RCT: 5–6 treatment in one axilla vs. untreated contralateral control	$n = 6$	Global assessment questionnaire (efficacy rated 0–3 for "poor", "fair", "good", and "excellent")	All patients reported some improvement after each treatment, and all reported good to excellent improvement at 1 month after final treatment
Aydin et al.[27]	1,064 nm laser	6–10 treatments in both axillae	$n = 38$	Starch iodine test and patient scoring using VAS. Measured at baseline and at 1 month and 12 months following treatment	Significant increase in sweating at 1 month and at 12 months for both starch iodine test and patient scoring

Cont'd...

Cont'd...

Author	Modality	Study method	Number of subjects	Primary outcome measure(s)	Outcome
Kim et al.[29]	Fractionated microneedle RF	Two treatments separated by 4 weeks	$n = 20$	HDSS and TEWL (transepidermal water loss) at baseline, 4 weeks after first treatment, 4 weeks after second treatment, and 8 weeks after second treatment	HDSS: 3.5 (baseline) 1.5 (4 weeks after first treatment) 1.8 (4 weeks after second treatment) 2.3 (8 weeks after second treatment) TEWL: Significant decrease at 4 weeks, but steady rise thereafter
Fatemi Naeni et al.[30]	Fractionated microneedle RF	RCT: Three treatments at 3-week intervals in one axilla vs. sham treatment in contralateral control	$n = 25$	HDSS at baseline, 3 weeks, 6 weeks, 9 weeks, 3 months. Response defined as two point reduction in HDSS	HDSS: Significant decrease in treatment vs. control starting after treatment #2
Schick et al.[32]	Fractionated microneedle RF	Three treatment sessions at 6 week intervals	$n = 30$	HDSS, DLQI, gravimetry at baseline and at 6 months following third treatment	HDSS: 3.5 (baseline) to 2.1 (6 months) DLQI: 16 to 7 Gravimetry: 221 mg/min to 33 mg/min All $p < 0.05$

(DLQI: dermatology life quality index; GAIS: global aesthetic improvement scale; HDSS: Hyperhidrosis Disease Severity Scale; RCT: randomized controlled trial; RF: radiofrequency; TEWL: transepidermal water loss; tx: treatment; VAS: visual analog scale; wk: week)

limit skin irritation, to increase efficacy, and to limit damage to clothing, the solution should be applied at night time, before bed, to dry skin. Because of lower sweat output at night, the solution remains on the skin for a longer period of time, resulting in more efficient uptake into the sweat ducts.[10]

Topical Glycopyrronium Tosylate

Topical glycopyrronium tosylate became available in the United States, in the form of a prescription topical cloth (Qbrexza™, Dermira), as of October 2018, for patients of 9 years of age or older suffering from axillary hyperhidrosis. In the Food and

Drug Administration (FDA) clinical trials, a total of 344 patients were randomized to apply single-use cloths premoistened with 2.4% glycopyrronium solution, once daily for 4 weeks. Patients were assessed to have a statistically significant improvement in sweating both according to a verified scale as well as in gravimetric measurements compared to a vehicle group. Responses were seen as early as 1 week post initiation of treatment, with further gradual improvement over the course of the next 3 weeks.

The most frequently related side effects were anticholinergic in nature, namely dry mouth and mydriasis. Blurred vision associated with mydriasis was noted to be either unilateral or bilateral. Other side effects seen, were urinary retention or hesitancy. These side effects were reported to be seen in the first week of treatment but decreased thereafter. The side effects were managed by either temporarily withholding the drug, or applying the drug every other day as opposed to daily. The presence of these side effects suggests that there can be notable systemic absorption of the drug. It is important to wash the hands after the use of the cloths, as it was postulated that the cases of unilateral mydriasis were likely related to the inadvertent transfer of the drug from the hands to one eye.

Botulinum Toxin type A

Botulinum toxin functions to decrease sweating by blocking presynaptic release of acetylcholine, the neurotransmitter involved in stimulation of the eccrine gland. Botulinum toxin injections must be administered by a physician. Many small injections are made into the subcutis of the axilla. Sweating can be typically decreased for 3–6 months, depending on the severity of the case and the anatomical location of the condition. The same medication can be used to treat craniofacial or palmoplantar hyperhidrosis, but currently, this is considered an off-label use by the United States FDA. The treatment of palmar or plantar hyperhidrosis with injected botulinum toxin may require some form of local anesthesia due to the rich nerve endings in this area. Effective regional anesthesia can be achieved using a regional block (e.g., Bier's block), but not all physicians can reliably perform this procedure. Application of ice packs for 15 minutes prior to the procedure is adequate for many patients. If needed, topical lidocaine cream and/or vibration can be added.[11] Other methods of cryoanalgesia have also been described.[12] Because botulinum toxin also weakens muscles, a side effect of treatment of the palms can be a weakened grip; patients must be cautioned about this possibility. Typically if encountered, weakness is most prominent at about 2 weeks post injection and usually improves within 4 weeks of injections. When using onabotulinum toxin for palmar hyperhidrosis, 50–100 units are injected into each palm, divided among many injections at a density of approximately 1 injection per square centimeter. A sample injection scheme is depicted in **Figure 1**. The dose for plantar hyperhidrosis is typically higher, requiring

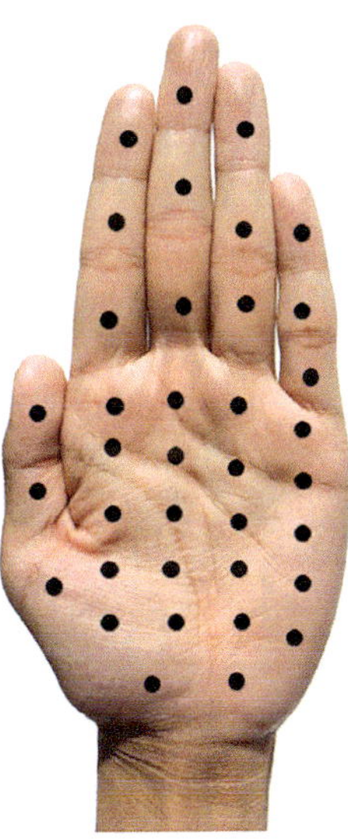

FIG. 1: Sample injection scheme.

50–150 units per sole. For axillary hyperhidrosis, 50 units per axilla are usually sufficient, but some patients may require as much as 100 units per each underarm.

Onabotulinum toxin is FDA-approved for the treatment of axillary hyperhidrosis in subjects age 18 and older. The product packaging cites two randomized, multicenter, double-blind, placebo-controlled studies as the basis for the efficacy and safety of this product. In one study, 322 subjects with axillary hyperhidrosis were randomized in a 1:1:1 ratio to receive 50 units, 75 units, or placebo in the axilla. HDSS and gravimetry were used to measure response. Responders were identified based on improvement of at least two grades in HDSS score or gravimetric reduction in sweating of at least 50% 4 weeks after treatment. 55% of those receiving 50 units and 49% of those receiving 75 units responded as measured by HDSS score. Only 6% of the placebo group responded by this criterion. 81% of the 50-unit group, 86% of the 75 unit group, and 41% of the placebo group achieved a response as measured by gravimetry. Median duration of response (defined as the number of days between injection and the date of the first visit at which patients return to 3 or 4 on the HDSS) was 201 days.[13]

In the second study,[14] 320 adults were randomized to receive 50 units of onabotulinum toxin or placebo. Treatment response was defined as reduction of at least 50% in axillary sweating as measured by gravimetry 4 weeks after injection. 91% of the treatment group and 36% of the placebo group responded ($p < 0.001$).

Many other studies have been conducted to demonstrate the efficacy of all commercially available botulinum toxin type A products, including abobotulinum toxin, onabotulinum toxin, and incobotulinum toxin, in the treatment of hyperhidrosis.

Systemic Treatments

Localized treatments are usually considered first-line therapy for primary focal hyperhidrosis. Oral medications can be beneficial when focally targeted therapies are ineffective or unavailable, or if multiple areas of the body are effective. The most common category of systemic agents used for hyperhidrosis is anticholinergics. These are useful because sweat glands are innervated by sympathetic postganglionic nerves that have acetylcholine as their primary neurotransmitter. Anticholinergic agents work by competitive inhibition of acetylcholine at the muscarinic receptor. Their use is limited by systemic side effects; muscarinic receptors are present throughout the central and autonomic nervous systems. Glycopyrrolate (glycopyrronium bromide) is favored over other anticholinergics such as atropine and scopolamine because glycopyrrolate has limited penetration of the blood brain barrier. Side effects can be additive when patients concurrently use other anticholinergic medications such as phenothiazines, TCAs, and anti-Parkinson drugs. Anticholinergic therapy may be contraindicated in patients with glaucoma, obstructive uropathy, obstructive disease of the GI tract, paralytic ileus, severe ulcerative colitis, and myasthenia gravis. Glycopyrrolate is usually started at 1 mg once to twice daily, and then increased by 1 mg/d at 2-week intervals based on therapeutic response and side effects. Oxybutynin is another common anticholinergic drug used to treat hyperhidrosis. Because it is a tertiary amine, it has greater penetration of the blood brain barrier than glycopyrrolate. Nonetheless, it has been used extensively and successfully for this condition. 5–10 mg daily is a usual dose for hyperhidrosis, but doses up to 15 or 20 mg daily may be required.[15] Anticholinergic medication side effects include, dry mouth, urinary retention, constipation, flushing, blurred vision and glaucoma.

Rarer serious side effects of these medications include hyperthermia and seizures and should be reviewed with patients when prescribing these medications.

Other systemic medications for hyperhidrosis include beta blockers and alpha adrenergic agonists. The use of beta blockers for hyperhidrosis is usually in the context of their use to improve the symptoms of phobias and performance anxiety. Commonly used doses are 10–20 mg of propranolol taken approximately 1 hour before a performance. Care must be taken in patients with low resting blood pressure, slow baseline heart rate, or low body mass index. Clonidine, a centrally active alpha-2-adrenergic agonist used to treat hypertension and some anxiety disorders, has been used to treat hyperhidrosis, usually at a dose of 0.1 mg BID. Case reports of other systemic medications for the treatment of hyperhidrosis are published, but these are beyond the scope of this chapter.[15]

Devices

Iontophoresis

Iontophoresis is the passing of an ionized substance through intact skin by the application of electrical current. For hyperhidrosis, the simplest method uses tap water, although in some situations, the addition of baking soda, anticholinergics, aluminum chloride, or botulinum toxin to the water may be performed.[16,17] Palms or soles are placed in a shallow water bath, through which the electrical current is passed. Three iontophoresis devices are available in the US and registered with the USFDA for treatment of hyperhidrosis. These are the RA Fischer (both MD-1a and MD-2 models) and the Drionic® devices.[18]

The precise mechanism of tap water iontophoresis has not been definitively identified, but hypotheses have included the development of keratinaceous plugs leading to mechanical ductal obstruction, inhibition of secretion of sweat by decoupling of the sweat stimulus from the secretion of sweat, and destruction of the secretory and ductal portions of the gland due to accumulation of hydronium ions in these portions of the eccrine apparatus.[19]

Stolman[20] conducted a study of 18 subjects in which one hand was treated by iontophoresis and the other hand served as a control. Subjects underwent tap water iontophoresis three times per week for 20 minutes each over a 3 week period. Fifteen of the 18 subjects experienced significant improvement, as measured by the subject's subjective report and by qualitative assessment using the starch iodine test.[20]

In a study by Kim et al.,[21] tap water iontophoresis was performed five times per week for 2 weeks for 20 minutes at each session. Twenty seven subjects completed the study, 14 of whom received active treatment and 13 of whom served as sham-treated controls. Starch iodine testing demonstrated improvement in 92.9% of treated subjects in comparison to 38.5% of untreated controls ($p = 0.001$). Sweat secretion rate (measured by gravimetry) was reduced by 91.8% in treated subjects and by 39.1% in untreated controls.[21]

Karakoc et al.,[22] treated 112 patients with palmar hyperhidrosis using 15-minute iontophoresis eight times over a 28 days period. Among all participants, sweat intensity at baseline was 2.98 ± 1.19 g/h for the right hand and 3.04 ± 1.32 g/h for the left. Among 91 responders, sweat intensity decreased to 0.39 ± 0.12 g/h for the right and 0.52 ± 0.15 for the left ($p < 0.0001$ for both right and left). For nonresponders, final sweat intensity was 2.82 ± 0.98 g/h for the right and 2.91 ±1.02 for the left.

Iontophoresis has been used to treat palmoplantar hyperhidrosis since at least 1952. More recently, additional devices have been studied for their potential to achieve longer lasting improvement in hyperhidrosis. These devices are discussed here.

Microwave Destruction of Sweat Glands

A microwave device has been FDA-cleared for the treatment of primary axillary hyperhidrosis since 2011, but was in use for a couple of years prior to this in Canada. After infiltration with a local anesthetic, electromagnetic energy at 5.8 GHz is delivered to the skin. Because of the different dielectric properties of the dermis and fat, much of this energy is reflected at the dermohypodermal junction. This energy in turn causes dielectric heating of the tissue, resulting in tissue destruction. The epidermis and upper dermis are relatively spared because the incident and reflected waves exhibit destructive interference in the more superficial region and because contact cooling is also used at the epidermis.[23]

In a randomized controlled study of 120 subjects by Glaser et al.,[24] bilateral axillae were treated by the active device ($n = 81$) or a sham device ($n = 39$) for a total of 1–3 treatments. Clinical efficacy was assessed using HDSS and gravimetric measurement. Total 89% of the active treatment group and 54% of the sham group achieved the endpoint of HDSS score of 1 or 2 at day 30 ($p < 0.001$). At 6 months, this endpoint was achieved by 69% of the active group and 44% of the sham group and the difference was still statistically significant ($p = 0.02$). A 50% reduction in sweat production by gravimetric measurement was achieved by 80% of the active group and 67% of the sham group ($p = 0.07$) at day 30. At 6 months this was 63% and 59%, respectively ($p = 0.69$). Side effects in the treatment group included persistent pain as well as persistent swelling, pustules or blisters; these resulted in the exclusion of 7 subjects from a second treatment. Subsequent protocol improvements by the manufacturer have decreased the incidence of these complications. As noted above, the device was initially cleared by the FDA in 2011 for treatment of primary axillary hyperhidrosis. Because destruction is nonselective, it subsequently received FDA clearance for permanent axillary hair reduction as well.

In clinical practice, a majority of patients require two treatment sessions, spaced 3 months apart for ideal long-term sweat reduction, although some individuals achieve satisfactory results only after one session. 5% of patients require three sessions. These patients typically suffer from the most severe form of sweating and have exhausted all other options. Patients typically report 50–60% improvement after one session, and 70–90% improvement after two treatment sessions. Tumescent anesthesia has enabled clinicians to use maximal energy settings improving efficacy outcomes, allowing the treatments to be administered with little to no discomfort, while almost eliminating most side effects seen in the FDA clinical trials. Most patients will develop edema; this usually resolves within a week. Hard nodules may be seen for a few weeks, sometimes lasting up to 3 months. One author (Cameron Rokhsar) has extensive experience with this device and estimates the nonresponder rate at <1%. In this author's opinion, microwave technology has revolutionized the treatment of axillary hyperhidrosis and should be considered the reference standard.

Microfocused Ultrasound

Nestor and Park[25] conducted two randomized controlled studies using microfocused ultrasound (MFU) in the treatment of focal axillary hyperhidrosis. In the first study, each subject received two MFU treatments in one axilla 30 days apart, and two sham treatments in the other axilla 30 days apart. Two passes were performed during each treatment. On the treatment side, one pass used a 7 MHz transducer (with a focal depth of 3 mm) while the other pass used a 4 MHz (with a focal depth of 4.5 mm). Each pass used the maximum allowable energy for the given transducer. On the sham side, treatment energy was set to 0 J. Positive treatment response was defined as >50% reduction in spontaneous axillary sweat production in the treated axilla on day 120 of the study (90 days following the second treatment). A total of 14 patients completed this study. The authors reported that >50% of patients achieved a positive response.

In the second study, subjects were randomized to receive two bilateral MFU ultrasound treatments or two bilateral sham treatments, 30 days apart. Efficacy assessments consisting of the HDSS, gravimetric measurements, and starch iodine tests were made on days 7, 14, 30, 37, 44, 60, 90, 120 and 365. Patient satisfaction questionnaires were also completed on days 60, 90, 120, and 365. A total of 20 subjects were enrolled in the study, 12 in the MFU treatment group and 8 in the sham treatment group. On day 60, a positive HDSS response rate of 67% was achieved in the MFU group versus 0% in the sham group. HDSS response rate was ≥50% at all-time points for the MFU group (except for day 7), and remained zero percent at all-time points in the sham group. In aggregate, baseline sweat production decreased by ≥50% at all-time points in the MFU group, but not the sham group. 10 of 12 patients in the MFU group (and none in the sham group) achieved ≥50% reduction in gravimetric measurement of sweat production. Patients also reported higher levels of satisfaction in the MFU group than in the sham group. Total 12-month follow-up was available for a subset of the subjects; 5 of 6 in the MFU group continued to report noticeable clinical improvement and remained satisfied with the treatment; five maintained a positive treatment response based on gravimetric measurement.

Laser Treatment

Minimally Invasive Laser

A minimally invasive subdermal 924/975 nm laser treatment has been evaluated for efficacy in axillary hyperhidrosis in a randomized controlled study. Leclère et al.,[26] conducted a four-arm investigation in 100 patients with axillary hyperhidrosis. Subjects were divided into one of four groups (see **Table 4**): Group 1 was treated with laser alone at 975 nm. A Toledo cannula was used without suction to create a plane in the superficial subdermis, after which the laser fiber was introduced. Group 2 was treated with laser alone at 924/975 nm simultaneously, while curettage alone (using a Toledo cannula with suction) was used for group 3. Laser at 924/975 nm followed by curettage was used for group 4. All laser treatments were performed at a treatment power of 20 W using a 1.5 mm optical fiber introduced into the subdermal space and passed back and forth beneath the skin. HDSS, starch iodine test, and global aesthetic improvement scale (GAIS) were used to assess efficacy. The authors used a semiquantitative 4-point scale to assess improvement on the starch-iodine test. Assessments were performed at 1 month and at 1 year following treatment. The authors reported minimal improvement in group 1 (975 nm laser alone), but notable improvement in groups 2 and 3. Group 4 (924/975 nm laser followed by curettage) achieved the most improvement. Quantitative scores are provided, but significance values are not.

Goldman and Wollina[27] evaluated a subdermal Nd-YAG laser for axillary hyperhidrosis in a nonrandomized study. Seventeen patients were treated with a pulsed 1,064 nm Nd:YAG system, in which energy is delivered via a 300 μm fiber optic through an 18 gauge Tuohy disposable epidural needle. Under tumescent anesthesia, bilateral axillae were

TABLE 4: Results from LeClere, et al.[24]

Group	HDSS Baseline, 1 month and 12 months Mean (standard deviation)	Starch iodine Baseline, 1 month and 12 months Mean (standard deviation)	GAIS 1 month and 12 months Mean (standard deviation)
975 nm	3.88 (0.33) 3.40 (0.50) 3.44 (0.51)	2.60 (0.48) 2.48 (0.51) 2.76 (0.44)	1.04 (0.35) 0.92 (0.28)
975 nm and 924 nm	3.84 (0.37) 1.96 (0.68) 1.96 (0.61)	2.60 (0.60) 1.36 (0.49) 1.48 (0.51)	2.36 (0.49) 2.72 (0.46)
Curettage	3.85 (0.37) 2.20 (0.41) 2.32 (0.48)	2.58 (0.48) 1.56 (0.51) 1.76 (0.60)	2.28 (0.46) 2.64 (0.49)
975 and 924 nm, Curettage	3.88 (0.33) 1.24 (0.44) 0.48 (0.51)	2.64 (0.49) 0.40 (0.50) 0.44 (0.51)	3.72 (0.54) 3.76 (0.44)

treated using 15 mJ/pulse, pulse duration of 100 µs, 40 pulses/s. Needles and fiber were moved back and forth approximately at the level of the dermal/subdermal junction. Patient global assessment (outcome assessment by patient of poor, fair, good, and excellent) and physician global assessment (classification of result by pre- and postsurgery photographs based on estimated percentage reduction in hyperhidrosis area) were used to assess efficacy. Twelve of 17 patients reported "excellent" results, while three reported "good" and two reported "fair." Physician global assessment was excellent in 10, good in four, and fair in three patients. The authors report follow-up periods of 12 to 43 months, but it is unclear to which time point(s) the results correspond.

Noninvasive Laser

Noninvasive lasers, including 800 nm and 1064 nm lasers, have been assessed in randomized and nonrandomized studies for their efficacy in treating hyperhidrosis.

Bechara et al.[28] enrolled 21 subjects (19 of whom completed the study) in a study using long pulsed 800 nm diode laser at 50 J/cm^2 and pulse duration of 30 ms. A total of five treatments were performed on one axilla while the other served as a control. Gravimetry was used to compare sweat rates before therapy and 4 weeks after the last laser treatment. Subjects estimated their decrease in sweating and reported their satisfaction using visual analog scales at 4 weeks and 12 months after the last laser treatment. Sweat rate measured by gravimetry was significantly lower after treatment on the treated side, decreasing from a median of 89 mg/min (range 42–208) to a median of 48 mg/min (range 17–119, $p < 0.001$). Sweat rate on the untreated side also decreased, however, from a median of 78 mg/min (25–220) to a median of 65 mg/min (range 24–399 mg/min, $p = 0.04$). There was no significant difference in reduction in sweat rate between the treated and nontreated sides ($p = 0.10$). Patient satisfaction with reduction in sweating was 5.9 at 4 weeks and 4.1 at

12 month follow-up. Histologic examination of skin biopsies before and after laser treatment did not demonstrate any significant changes in appearance of apocrine and eccrine glands. The authors concluded that although an overall reduction in hyperhidrosis was observed in the study population, it could not be attributed to the treatment. The study may simply not have been adequately powered to distinguish between the treatment and control groups.

Aydin et al.[29] studied 38 patients receiving axillary laser hair removal treatments with a 1,064 nm Nd:YAG laser. Both axillae were treated at fluences and pulse durations appropriate for skin type, and patients received a total of 6–10 monthly treatments until desirable hair removal results were achieved. The iodine starch test was performed in both axillae before treatment and again 1 month and 1 year after the final treatment. Computerized analysis of photos was used to determine the total area with active sweating, recorded as number of active pixels. The authors controlled for room temperature and time of day in order to make a valid comparison between measurements at different time points. In addition to the iodine starch test, patient assessment of intensity of sweat production was performed using a 10-point VAS. The authors found a significant increase in sweat area at 1 month and at 12 months in comparison to pretreatment values in both axillae. Involved area increased from 579.5 ± 1582.5 at baseline in the right axilla to 8822.5 ± 16761.8 at 1 month and 7001.961 ± 12688.3 at 12 months following final treatment. Left axilla values were 593.5 ± 1140.4, 7748.5 ± 14051.8, and 6864.7 ± 11056.9, respectively. VAS scores were also increased from 4.55 ± 1.05 to 6.15 ± 1.66 at 1 month and 5.81 ± 1.37 at 12 months.

Letada et al.,[30] investigated treatment of axillary hyperhidrosis with a 1,064 nm Nd:YAG laser using hair reduction settings in six adults with a history of intolerable hyperhidrosis refractory to standard therapies. For each subject, one side was randomized to treatment and the other side to control. Treatment parameters were spot size of 12 mm and pulse duration of 20 ms. Fluences ranged from 24 to 56 J/cm^2 and were determined by Fitzpatrick skin type. Five or six treatments were performed for each subject. Assessments of efficacy were based on a Global Assessment Questionnaire, which rates efficacy on a scale of 0 to 3 depending on level of improvement. Qualitative evaluation of improvement was also made using Minor's starch iodine test. All subjects reported subjective improvement following each treatment, and all reported good to excellent subjective improvement in sweating at 1 month follow-up after final treatment. Histologic analysis of pre- and posttreatment did not reveal any significant changes in sweat gland density or morphology.

Fractionated Microneedle Radiofrequency

Fractionated microneedle radiofrequency devices have been used in randomized as well as nonrandomized studies in the treatment of axillary hyperhidrosis.

Kim et al.,[31] used fractionated microneedle radiofrequency to treat 20 patients with primary axillary hyperhidrosis in two sessions at 4-week intervals. HDSS was used to evaluate clinical improvement. Sweat quantitation was indirectly measured using transepidermal water loss (TEWL). Mean HDSS scores were 3.5, 1.5, 1.8 and 2.3 at baseline, 4 weeks after the first treatment, 4 weeks after the second treatment, and 8 weeks after the second treatment, respectively. This was significant to a level of $p < 0.05$ after repeated-measures ANOVA. Longer term follow-up was not provided. The authors observed a statistically significant decrease in TEWL 1 month after the first treatment, but a gradual increase after the second session and in the follow-up period. They hypothesized that TEWL may have increased due to environmental factors and due to the damage to the epidermal barrier inflicted by the treatment device itself, despite the overall improvement in HDSS. Authors also compared histologic samples obtained at baseline with samples obtained immediately after the first session, 1 month after the first session, and 1 month after the second session. The authors reported that specimens obtained immediately after the first treatment session demonstrated atrophy and necrosis of glands at high magnification. 1 month after the first session, they reported a decrease in density and size of apocrine and eccrine glands compared to baseline.

Fatemi Naeini et al.[32] used fractionated microneedle radiofrequency to treat 25 patients with axillary hyperhidrosis in a single-blind sham randomized controlled study. Each patient had three sessions of treatment at 3-week intervals in one axilla, while the other axilla served as control. After pretreatment with topical anesthesia, the target area was treated with three passes at depths of 2–3 mm. Photographic assessment using starch iodine testing and HDSS measurements were used to assess response. A 10 point visual analog scale in which subjects rated sweating from "no sweating" to "worst possible sweating" was also used. The primary overall efficacy measure was the percentage of subjects with 2 point HDSS reduction. Assessments were made at baseline and posttreatment at 3, 6, and 9 weeks as well as at 3 months. The HDSS index showed a significant decrease after the second treatment for the treated side compared with the control. Visual analog scale sweating intensity score also decreased for the treatment side at 21 weeks relative to that of control. Histopathological examination 30 days after the last treatment demonstrated atrophy of some sweat glands and decrease in number of sweat glands, but quantitative information was not provided. Longer term follow up at 1 year[33] demonstrated significant difference in HDSS score in the treatment versus control side (mean 2.50 vs. mean 3.38, $p < 0.001$). The authors reported that 10 patients had no relapse after 1 year (41.6%), while 11 patients relapsed, and 3 patients did not respond. One patient did not complete the long-term follow-up.

Schick et al.,[34] treated 30 adult patient with pronounced axillary hyperhidrosis using a microneedle fractional RF system with a 5 × 5 array of noninsulated needle electrodes. Following delivery of subcutaneous local anesthesia, axillae were treated at a penetration depth of 3 mm for two consecutive passes followed by a single pass at 2 mm depth. Three treatments were performed at 6-week intervals. Measurements of efficacy included the HDSS score, DLQI, and quantitative gravimetry. Average HDSS score declined from 3.5 before the start of treatment to 2.1 at 6 months following the third treatment ($p < 0.05$). DLQI score improved from an average baseline level of 16 to a final level of 7 ($p < 0.05$). Gravimetric measurement of sweat quantity demonstrated reduction from 221 mg/min at baseline to a final level of 33 mg/min ($p < 0.05$).

CONCLUSION

Primary focal hyperhidrosis remains a challenging condition for millions of people. A variety of treatment avenues are available, including pharmacologic and device-based approaches. Axillary hyperhidrosis is the most frequently studied subtype, but options are available for palmoplantar or other focal hyperhidrosis (often off-label). While many treatments have shown efficacy in clinical trials of varying size, there remain some barriers to their use. Patient compliance (especially for modalities that require frequent use), cost of materials and training, and insurance coverage (especially for expensive options such as onabotulinum toxin and a number of device-based approaches) can be significant though not insurmountable challenges. It is important that patients be reassured that treatment options are available and that a single individual may need to try several before finding the optimal approach for him or her. Realistic expectations of treatment should also be emphasized.

REFERENCES

1. Miller JL. Diseases of the Eccrine and Apocrine Sweat Glands. In: Bolognia JL, Jorizzo JJ, Schaffer JV, Callen JP (Eds). Dermatology, 3rd edition. New York: Elsevier; 2012.
2. Hornberger J, Grimes K, Naumann M, Glaser DA, Lowe NJ, Naver H, et al. Recognition, diagnosis, and treatment of primary focal hyperhidrosis. J Am Acad Dermatol. 2004;51(2):274-86.
3. Strutton DR, Kowalski JW, Glaser DA, Stang PE. US prevalence of hyperhidrosis and impact on individuals with axillary hyperhidrosis: results from a national survey. J Am Acad Dermatol. 2004;51(2):241-8.
4. Doolittle J, Walker P, Mills T, Thurston J. Hyperhidrosis: an update on prevalence and severity in the United States. Arch Dermatol Res. 2016;308(10):743-9.
5. Rachakonda TD, Schupp CW, Armstrong AW. Psoriasis prevalence among adults in the United States. J Am Acad Dermatol. 2014;70(3):512-6.
6. Augustin M, Radtke MA, Herberger K, Kornek T, Heigel H, Schaefer I. Prevalence and disease burden of hyperhidrosis in the adult population. Dermatology. 2013;227(1):10-3.
7. Liu Y, Bahar R, Kalia S, Huang RY, Phillips A, Su M, et al. Hyperhidrosis Prevalence and Demographical Characteristics in Dermatology Outpatients in Shanghai and Vancouver. PLoS One. 2016;11(4):e0153719.
8. Fujimoto T, Kawahara K, Yokozeki H. Epidemiological study and considerations of primary focal hyperhidrosis in Japan: from questionnaire analysis. J Dermatol. 2013;40(11):886-90.
9. Holzle E, Braun-Falco O. Structural changes in axillary eccrine glands following long-term treatment with aluminium chloride hexahydrate solution. Br J Dermatol. 1984;110(4):399-403.
10. Pariser DM, Ballard A. Topical therapies in hyperhidrosis care. Dermatol Clin. 2014;32(4): 485-90.
11. Doft MA, Hardy KL, Ascherman JA. Treatment of hyperhidrosis with botulinum toxin. Aesthet Surg J. 2012;32(2):238-44.
12. Baumann L, Frankel S, Welsh E, Halem M. Cryoanalgesia with dichlorotetrafluoroethane lessens the pain of botulinum toxin injections for the treatment of palmar hyperhidrosis. Dermatol Surg. 2003;29(10):1057-60.
13. Lowe NJ, Glaser DA, Eadie N, Daggett S, Kowalski JW, Lai PY, et al. Botulinum toxin type A in the treatment of primary axillary hyperhidrosis: a 52-week multicenter double-blind, randomized, placebo-controlled study of efficacy and safety. J Am Acad Dermatol. 2007;56(4):604-11.
14. Naumann M, Lowe NJ. Botulinum toxin type A in treatment of bilateral primary axillary hyperhidrosis: randomised, parallel group, double blind, placebo controlled trial. BMJ. 2001;323(7313):596-9.
15. Glaser DA. Oral medications. Dermatol Clin. 2014;32(4): 527-32.
16. Dolianitis C, Scarff CE, Kelly J, Sinclair R. Iontophoresis with glycopyrrolate for the treatment of palmoplantar hyperhidrosis. Australas J Dermatol. 2004;45:208-12.
17. Davarian S, Kalantari KK, Rezasolani A, Rahimi A. Effect and persistency of botulinum toxin iontophoresis in the treatment of palmar hyperhidrosis. Australas J Dermatol. 2008;49: 75-9.
18. Pariser DM, Ballard A. Iontophoresis for palmar and plantar hyperhidrosis. Dermatol Clin. 2014;32(4):491-4.
19. Kreyden OP. Iontophoresis for palmoplantar hyperhidrosis. J Cosmet Dermatol. 2004;3(4): 211-4.
20. Stolman LP. Treatment of excess sweating of the palms by iontophoresis. Arch Dermatol. 1987;123(7):893-6.
21. Kim DH, Kim TH, Lee SH, Lee AY. Treatment of palmar hyperhidrosis with tap water iontophoresis: a randomized, sham-controlled, single-blind, and parallel-designed clinical trial. Ann Dermatol. 2017;29(6):728-34.
22. Karakoc Y, Aydemir EH, Kalkan MT, Unal G. Safe control of palmoplantar hyperhidrosis with direct electrical current. Int J Dermatol. 2002;41(9): 602-5.
23. Johnson JE, O'Shaughnessy KF, Kim S. Microwave thermolysis of sweat glands. Lasers Surg Med. 2012;44(1):20-5.
24. Glaser DA, Coleman WP 3rd, Fan LK, Kilmer SL, Nossa R, Smith SR, et al. A randomized, blinded clinical evaluation of a novel microwave device for treating axillary hyperhidrosis: the dermatologic reduction in underarm perspiration study. Dermatol Surg. 2012;38(2): 185-91.
25. Nestor MS, Park H. Safety and Efficacy of Micro-focused Ultrasound Plus Visualization for the Treatment of Axillary Hyperhidrosis. J Clin Aesthet Dermatol. 2014;7(4): 14-21.
26. Leclère FM, Moreno-Moraga J, Alcolea JM, Vogt PM, Royo J, Cornejo P, et al. Efficacy and safety of laser therapy on axillary hyperhidrosis after one year follow-up: a randomized blinded controlled trial. Lasers Surg Med. 2015;47(2):173-9.
27. Goldman A, Wollina U. Subdermal Nd-YAG laser for axillary hyperhidrosis. Dermatol Surg. 2008;34(6):756-62.

28. Bechara FG, Georgas D, Sand M, Stücker M, Othlinghaus N, Altmeyer P, et al. Effects of a long-pulsed 800-nm diode laser on axillary hyperhidrosis: a randomized controlled half-side comparison study. Dermatol Surg. 2012;38(5):736-40.
29. Aydin F, Pancar GS, Senturk N, Bek Y, Yuksel EP, Canturk T, et al. Axillary hair removal with 1064-nm Nd:YAG laser increases sweat production. Clin Exp Dermatol. 2010;35(6):588-92.
30. Letada PR, Landers JT, Uebelhoer NS, Shumaker PR. Treatment of focal axillary hyperhidrosis using a long-pulsed Nd:YAG 1064 nm laser at hair reduction settings. J Drugs Dermatol. 2012;11(1):59-63.
31. Kim M, Shin JY, Lee J, Kim JY, Oh SH. Efficacy of fractional microneedle radiofrequency device in the treatment of primary axillary hyperhidrosis: a pilot study. Dermatology. 2013;227(3):243-9.
32. Fatemi Naeini F, Abtahi-Naeini B, Pourazizi M, Nilforoushzadeh MA, Mirmohammadkhani M. Fractionated microneedle radiofrequency for treatment of primary axillary hyperhidrosis: a sham control study. Australas J Dermatol. 2015;56(4):279-84.
33. Abtahi-Naeini B, Naeini FF, Saffaei A, Behfar S, Pourazizi M, Mirmohammadkhani M, et al. Treatment of primary axillary hyperhidrosis by fractional microneedle radiofrequency: is it still effective after long-term follow-up? Indian J Dermatol. 2016;61(2):234.
34. Schick CH, Grallath T, Schick KS, Hashmonai M. Radiofrequency Thermotherapy for Treating Axillary Hyperhidrosis. Dermatol Surg. 2016;42(5):624-30.

26

CHAPTER

Laser Treatment of Onychomycosis

Christine Chen, Meera Kohli, Shivani Sharma, Kachiu C Lee

INTRODUCTION

Onychomycosis, a fungal infection of the nail bed, occurs in 2–13% of the population.[1] Dermatophyte infections, the most common pathogen being *Trichophyton rubrum*, cause 99% of onychomycosis cases.[2] Non-dermatophyte molds such as *Fusarium* species. and *Aspergillus* species. or yeasts such as *Candida* species. can also cause onychomycosis.[3]

DIAGNOSTIC TOOLS

Physicians can diagnose onychomycosis in three ways: (1) Clinical observation, (2) Pathology, and (3) Culture of the causative pathogen. Nail clippings are used for fungal cultures as well.[4] Clinical signs associated with onychomycosis include visible residual changes in 10% of the nail plate, orange-brown or white-yellow streaks or patches in or beneath the nail, lateral onycholysis with debris, or hyperkeratosis on the lateral nail fold edge[5] (**Figs. 1** and **2**). Onychomycosis can also be characterized by thickening and yellowing of the nails. Oftentimes, subungual debris may be present (**Fig. 3**). Superficial onychomycosis can present with white discoloration on the surface of the nail plate (**Fig. 4**). The white superficial fungus can sometimes be scraped off fully (**Fig. 5**) or partially (**Figs. 6A** and **B**).

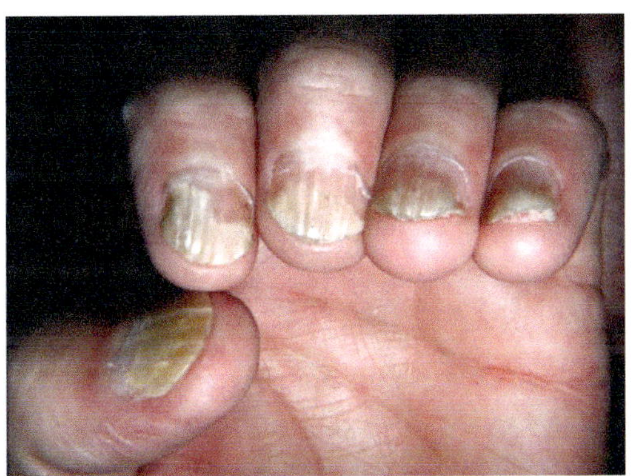

FIG. 1: Yellowing and hyperkeratosis of all 5 nails characteristic of onychomycosis.

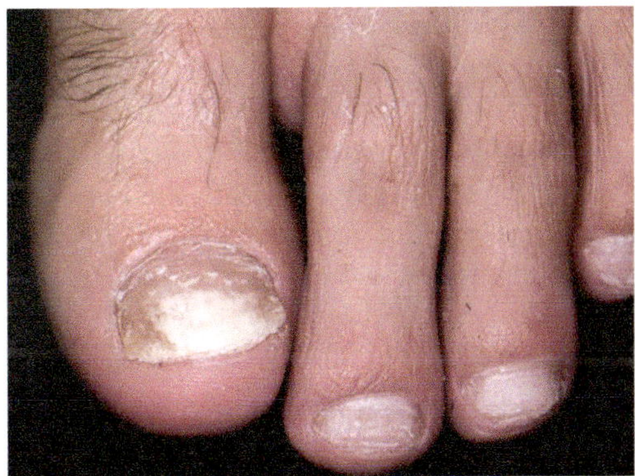

FIG. 2: Large toenail with onychomycosis characterized by white discoloration.

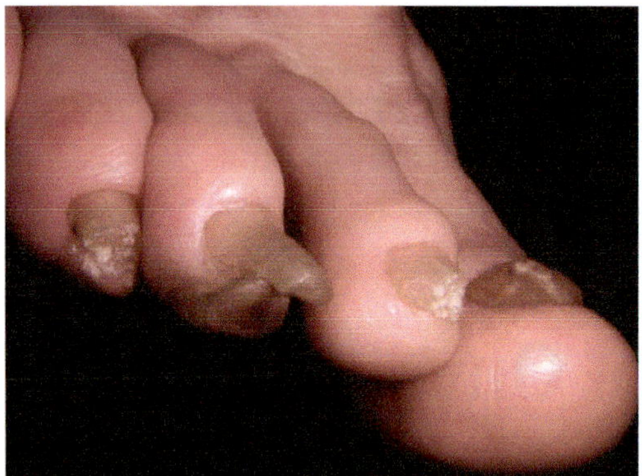

FIG. 3: Thickening of nail plate with evidence of subungual debris.

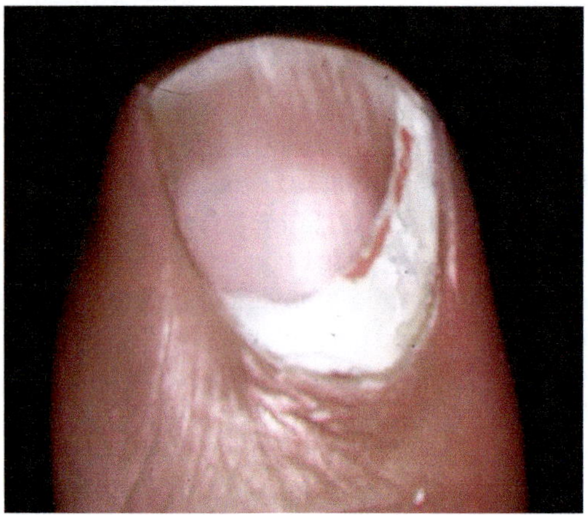

FIG. 4: Superficial onychomycosis characterized by white discoloration on top of the nail plate.

Microscopic tests are evaluated through taking nail clippings and staining with potassium hydroxide visualization.[4] More commonly, nail clippings are taken from the diseased nail. These clippings are treated with the Periodic acid-Schiff stain for improved visualization of the pathogen within the nail.

PRETREATMENT CONSIDERATIONS

Pretreatment considerations include efficacy of previous oral or topical treatment and the extent of involvement. Physicians must also evaluate the thickness of the nails to relate the

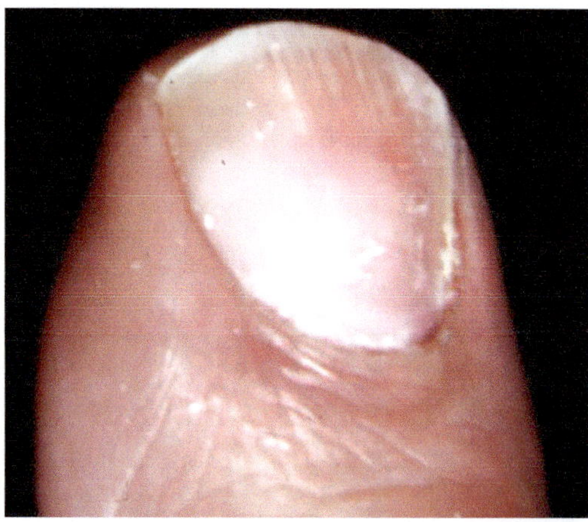

FIG. 5: Superficial white discoloration can be scraped off fully.

depth of the nail with the depth the laser can penetrate. Other pretreatment considerations include determining whether the patient has realistic expectations regarding the degree of improvement, the number of treatments needed, and the likelihood of recurrence. Understanding the patient's medical history and types of previous treatments used for onychomycosis is essential.

DEFINITION OF A CURE

The United States Food and Drug Administration (FDA) has provided three definitions for a cure of onychomycosis: a visual evaluation of a clear nail, a mycological cure, and a complete cure.[6] First, an improvement in nail clarity occurs with ≥6 mm of clear nail growth, 60 mm^2 outward nail growth after 6 months, or complete clearance of the nail if the involvement of onychomycosis is ≤6 mm.[6]

MANAGEMENT

Clinicians often find onychomycosis difficult to treat. The current treatment methods, including topical antifungals, oral antifungals, and surgical removal all have limitations with limited efficacy. Topical antifungals cannot penetrate the nail to reach the affected

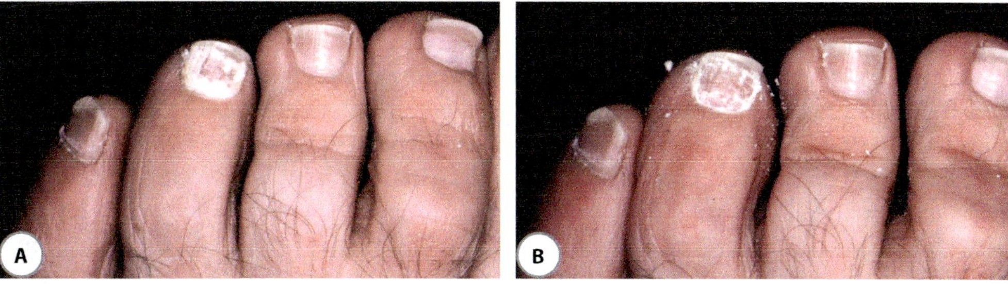

FIGS. 6A AND B: (A) Superficial white onychomycosis of left 4th toenail; (B) After scraping.

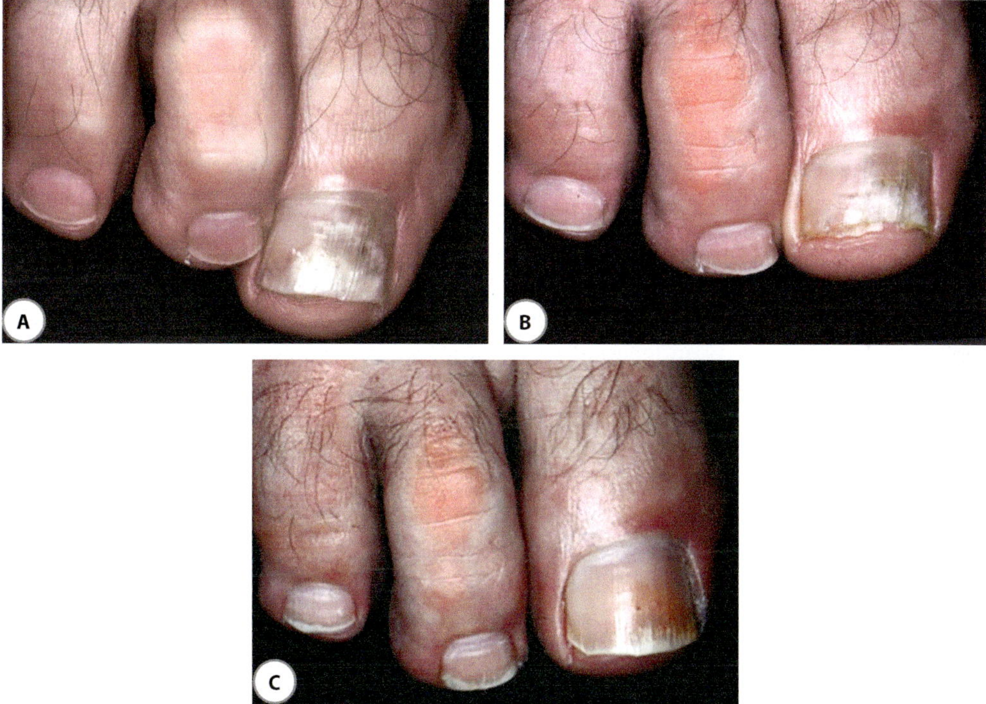

FIGS. 7A TO C: (A) Baseline onychomycosis of the right large toe; (B) 6 weeks after starting oral terbinafine 250 mg daily; (C) 12 weeks after starting oral terbinafine 250 mg daily.

area, making them a less effective treatment option.[7] Additionally, topical treatments often require daily application over a span of 48 weeks, reducing patient compliance rates. Oral antifungals, such as terbinafine, serve as the current "gold standard" treatment (**Figs. 7A** to **C**). Two medications, itraconazole and terbinafine have cure rates of 50–80%.[8] However, oral treatment can interact with other medications and may cause serious side effects such as liver toxicity.[9] Therefore, vulnerable populations such as children, the elderly, and individuals with comorbidities cannot take oral antifungals. Additionally, oral medications have high relapse rates ranging from 3 to 20% for terbinafine and 21 to 27%

for itraconazole in follow-up durations of up to 3 years.[10] The final option, surgical removal of the nail, can expose the nail to further infection and is highly invasive. Nail removal is also cosmetically undesirable for many patients due to the high risk of permanent scarring or permanent loss of nail.

Given the limitations in onychomycosis treatment options, researchers and physicians are evaluating lasers as alternatives or adjuvant treatments. Currently, the FDA has approved lasers for esthetic purposes, with a goal of achieving complete nail clarity.[6] More research on lasers needs to be done to evaluate their efficacy in onychomycosis treatment. The purpose of this chapter is to evaluate the current literature on laser treatment for onychomycosis.

MECHANISM OF ACTION

The mechanisms of action behind different lasers' modalities are poorly understood. One explanation for the effectiveness of lasers is photothermolysis. Temperatures of 55°C have been found to have a fungicidal effect; however, heating of dermal tissue up to 40°C leads to necrosis.[11] Therefore, lasers must be pulsed to allow for heat dissipation during treatment or lasers must deliver treatment at lower energy levels to prevent harming surrounding dermal tissue.

Bhatta et al. evaluated several potential mechanisms for laser treatment of onychomycosis.[12] Their systematic review reported that nonspecific tissue heating via the long-pulsed (LP) 1,064 nm neodymium-doped yttrium aluminum garnet (Nd:YAG) laser led to vasodilation under the nail bed, increasing the immunological response.[12] Therefore, the photothermolytic effect was not solely responsible for the effectiveness of laser treatment on onychomycosis. A lingering immunologic response may also play a role in eliminating fungal pathogens from the nail plate. Bhatta et al. also described the mechanism of action of the CO_2 laser as having a photothermal effect, where the fungal tissue is heated, causing water to convert to steam and increase the pressure within the fungus cell. This action leads to ablation of the fungal cells.[12]

Other studies proposed that the high peaks of energy transmitted through lasers led to mechanical damage of the fungi, leading to onychomycosis clearance.[12] Another theory argued that the Q-switched Nd:YAG laser attacks the xanthomegnin and melanin pigments within the cell wall of *Trichophyton rubrum,* the main dermatophyte responsible for onychomycosis, therefore inhibiting its growth.[12] Laser energy may also become absorbed by the water within the fungal cells, causing increased heating, and killing components of the cell that are needed for further growth.[13]

Laser treatment may also activate the mitochondrial apoptotic pathway, leading to fungi cell death.[12] Additionally, the activation of the mitochondrial apoptotic pathway may release reactive oxygen species (ROS) which would continue to induce apoptosis in surrounding fungal cells.[12] Researchers also argue that lasers irradiate the nail matrix, allowing for accelerated nail growth and increased nail clearance. In addition to theories concerning the mechanisms of action behind the Nd:YAG laser, other studies theorized potential mechanisms used by the CO_2 laser and the diode laser.

Fractional CO_2 lasers can create small pores in the nail bed, allowing for improved drug delivery. This means that if topical antifungals are applied in combination with the fractional CO_2 laser, the topical treatment may be able to effectively interact with the area of interest under the nail. Some researchers also attribute the effectiveness of the near-infrared diode to thermal effects or decreasing the mitochondrial membrane potential and

TABLE 1: US Food and Drug Administration (FDA) definition of a cure.[6]

Cure types	Mycological cure	Complete cure	Linear increase in nail clarity
Definition	Negative culture and Negative microscopy	Negative culture and Negative microscopy and Completely clear nail	>6 mm of nail growth after 6 months; or 60 mm^2 of nail growth with outward growth of infected area after 6 months; or Complete nail clearance if affected area is <6 mm

TABLE 2: US Food and Drug Administration (FDA) approved Lasers for treatment of onychomycosis.[35]

Lasers	Pulse Length	Laser Type	Wavelength (nm)
Dualis SP™ (Fotona)	35 ms	Long pulse Nd:YAG	1,064
PinPointe™ FootLaser (Nuvolase)	100–3,000 µs	Short pulse Nd:YAG	1,064
GenesisPlus™ (Cutera)	300 µs	Short pulse Nd:YAG	1,064
VARIA™ (CoolTouch)	600 µs	Short pulse Nd:YAG	1,064
LightPod® Neo™ (Aerolase)	650 µs	Short pulse Nd:YAG	1,064
JOULE ClearSense™ (Sciton)	0.3–200 ms	Short pulse Nd:YAG	1,064
CoolTouch CT3 Plus™ (CoolTouch)	450 µs	Short pulse Nd:YAG	1,320
Mira® 900 (Coherent Laser Group)	200 fs	Mode-locked Ti:Sapphire	800
Noveon® (Nomir Medical Technologies)	–	Diode	870, 930 (dual wavelength)
V-Raser® (ConBio/Cynosure)	–	Diode	980
(Nd:YAG: neodymium-doped yttrium aluminum garnet)			

causing an increased production of ROS for fungal cell apoptosis.[14]

TYPES OF LASERS AND FDA APPROVED LASERS

Several lasers that have been approved by the FDA are being evaluated as potential treatments for onychomycosis. The most common FDA-approved lasers are within (Nd:YAG category of lasers.[14] Currently, the FDA approved lasers for the treatment of onychomycosis are presented in **Table 2**.

TREATMENT EFFICACY

CO_2 Fractional Laser Analysis

Based on limited available research, CO_2 fractionated lasers appear to be generally effective via laser assisted drug delivery. In this approach, CO_2 fractionated lasers are first used over the nail plate to create small channels within the keratin. These channels theoretically allow for enhanced drug penetration into the nail plate. **Figures 8A** and **B** shows the combination of CO_2 fractionated laser for laser-assisted drug delivery of efinaconazole 10% solution.

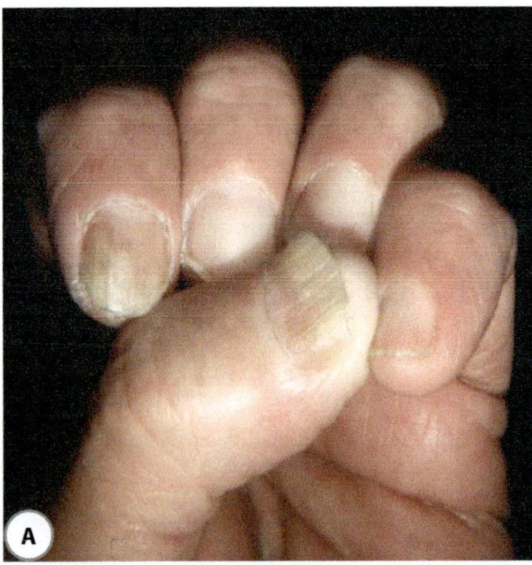

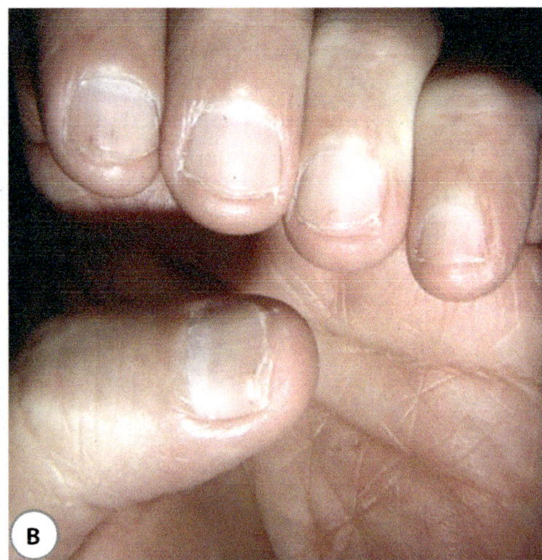

FIGS. 8A AND B: (A) Baseline and (B) 16 weeks after CO_2 fractionated laser for laser-assisted drug delivery of daily application of efinaconazole 10% solution. Treatments were performed monthly.

A prior randomized controlled study showed higher clearance rates with laser-assisted drug delivery of luliconazole 1% compared to the placebo. Clinical efficacy rates were 69.6% ($p = 0.004$) and mycological cure rates were 57.4% ($p = 0.006$) at 6 months.[12] However, there were high relapse rates after discontinuation of CO_2 laser treatment.

Factors that predict efficacy of this treatment method include thickness of the nail and type of onychomycosis infection. Thicker nails, such as nail plates >2.2 mm were much less likely to achieve clinical or mycological cure compared to thinning nails.[15] This is possibly related to the depth of the channels created with the CO_2 laser, as some CO_2 fractionated devices may be unable to penetrate through a depth ≥2.2 mm. Cases infected with *Candida albicans* often did not respond as well to topical agents, such as terbinafine, due to lack of sensitivity to this medication.

870 nm and 930 nm Near-infrared Diode Laser

These wavelengths have only been investigated in two studies, one of which was funded by the laser company with employees of the company as coauthors.[16] The other study was an *in vitro* study evaluating the use of an 870 and 930 nm laser on *T. rubrum* and *Candida* cultures. Both wavelengths caused decreased colony growth at 19 and 20 hours, respectively.[13] However, clinical studies are needed to confirm these findings.

1,320 nm Nd:YAG Laser versus Cryogenic Cooling

One notable study by Ortiz et al. evaluated the efficacy of 4 treatments of 1,320 nm Nd:YAG laser (*CT3 Plus CoolBreeze*) in treating toenails.[17] The treatment group received 4 sessions over 2 months, while the control group received a sham treatment with cryogenic cooling. 3 months after the last treatment, 50% of the patients had negative mycological results. However, the patients were not evaluated long term and relapse rates were not determined.[13]

1,064 nm ND:YAG Lasers

The 1,064 nm lasers are the most popular devices for laser treatment of onychomycosis, likely due to this wavelength's ability to penetrate the deepest among commercially available lasers. As such, these devices have the most clinical trials and evidence investigating their efficacy. Most of the remaining chapters will discuss the efficacy and evidence behind use of 1,064 nm lasers for treatment of onychomycosis.[18,19] Long-pulsed lasers are defined as those in the millisecond range, whereas Q-switched lasers are defined as those in the nanosecond range.

Q-switch 1,064 nm Nd:YAG Laser

The Q-switch (QS) laser delivers high pulses of energy over a nanosecond pulse range, theoretically killing pathogens before fungal hyphae can recover. **Table 3** presents a summary of several studies evaluating the efficacy of QS lasers for treatment of onychomycosis.

Overall, QS 1,064 nm devices appear to have efficacy in vitro and in clinical settings, with higher number of treatments showing improved efficacy.

TABLE 3: Use of Q-switch (QS) lasers for treatment of onychomycosis.

Author	Study Type	*n*	Follow-up	Treatment	Results	Side effects
Garcia et al.[36]	Prospective	120	9 months	QS 1,064 nm, 1 session	100% clinical cure; no data on mycological cure	N/A
Gupta et al.[30]	Retrospective	23	31 weeks on average	QS 1,064 nm, 4 sessions: Group A (3 patients) - 2 weeks in between Group B (13 patients) - 4 weeks in between Group C (7 patients) - Variable intervals	9% clinical cure 50% improvement in 46% of patients as a measure of nail involvement -no data on mycological cure	N/A
Hees et. al.[37]	Randomized control trial	15	3 and 6 days	Group A: QS 1064 nm Group B: QS 532 nm Group C: long-pulsed Nd:YAG 1,064 nm (all groups treated once) Group D: Control Sham	0% improvement in vitro across all groups at both follow-ups	N/A
Kalokasidis et al.[38]	Prospective	131	3 months	QS 1,064 nm, 2 sessions, 1 month interval	95% clinical and mycological cure	None
Rivers et al.[39]	Retrospective	199	4 weeks	QS 1,094 nm, at least 2 sessions, 4 weeks in-between	Statistically significant improvement of 52.8% nail involvement to 50% nail involvement	Mild discomfort during treatment
Wiznia et al.[15]	Retrospective (Literature Review)	NA	NA	Group B:QS Nd:YAG	Group B:little evaluation given no controlled or randomized trials of the QS laser but author suggests potential	N/A

(Nd:YAG: neodymium-doped yttrium aluminum garnet; QS; Q switch)

Long Pulsed 1,064 nm Nd:YAG Laser

Table 4 presents a selection of studies evaluating the use of long-pulsed (LP) 1,064 nm Nd:YAG lasers for treatment of onychomycosis. The lack of uniformity in study design makes it difficult to directly compare results or to conduct a meta-analysis. Some studies combined LP 1,064 nm lasers with oral and/or topical terbinafine, while others evaluated the efficacy of LP 1,064 nm alone.

In randomized trials comparing monotherapy (1,064 nm laser alone, oral antifungal

TABLE 4: Use of long-pulsed lasers for treatment of onychomycosis.

Author	Study type	*n*	Follow-up	Treatment	Results	Side effects
El-Tatawy et al.[21]	Randomized control trial	40	6 months	2 groups: • LP 1,064nm (Group A), 4 sessions • Topical terbinafine (Group B), twice daily	All Group A patients had significant improvement and 80% had mycological cure. All Group B patients still had positive culture results and 50% had moderate improvement	Mild-to-moderate pain
Hochman et al.[40]	Prospective	8	4–6 months	LP 1,064 nm, 2 or 3 sessions	7 out of 8 patients had negative culture results	Temporary darkening under the nail plate occurred in 2 patients
Karsai et al.[41]	Randomized controlled trial	20	12 months	2 groups: • Treatment group: 1,064nm, 4 sessions • Control group: Sham tx	Mycological remission was not achieved in either groups; condition worsened for both groups	Mean score of 5 for pain on a scale of 1–10
Kim et al.[27]	Randomized controlled trial	56	24 weeks	3 groups: • LP 1,064 nm (L), 3 or 4 sessions • 10 mg/mL of topical naftifine HCL spray (T), daily • Combined (L + T)	Approximately 70% of both the L and L + T groups had a clinical response; 15.2% of L and 22.5% of L+T were cured. Both groups had significantly greater clinical and cure rates than the T group	None

Cont'd...

Cont'd...

Author	Study type	*n*	Follow-up	Treatment	Results	Side effects
Li et al.[22]	Self-controlled trial	19	24 weeks	2 groups: • Group A (mild to moderate involvement); 4 sessions of LP 1,064 nm with oral itraconazole 200 mg twice daily or med only (control) • Group B (severe involvement); 4 sessions of LP 1,064 nm with oral itraconazole 200 mg twice daily or med only (control)	Efficacy between Group A patients given pure medication and combination therapy revealed no significant differences. Patients in Group B given pure medication had half the percent of improvement of the combination therapy	None
Li et al.[42]	Randomized controlled trial	37	24 weeks	2 groups: • Group 1 (fingernails), LP 1,064 nm, once weekly • Group 2 (toenails), LP 1,064 nm, once weekly	On week 24, response rate was 52% for Group 1 and 71% for Group 2, which revealed a statistically significant difference	None
Lu et al.[43]	Comparative design study	31	6 months	2 groups: • Group 1, LP 1,064 nm, 4 sessions • Group 2, topical 5% amorolfine nail lacquer twice a week	41.3% of Group 1 had negative mycological examinations compared with 60.6% of Group 2, a statistically significant difference	Some with darkening under or over the nail plate
Moon et al.[44]	Prospective?	13	1 month	LP 1,064 nm, 5 sessions with 4 week intervals	Of 43 nails, 9.3% had complete cure, 18.6% had excellent outcomes, and 72% had good outcomes	None
Okan et al.[45]	Prospective	15	4 weeks	LP 1,064 nm, 4 sessions	60% had mycological cure; 47% had complete clinical cure	None

Cont'd...

Cont'd...

Author	Study type	*n*	Follow-up	Treatment	Results	Side effects
Piccolo et al.[46]	Prospective	20	2 months	LP 1,064 nm, 4 sessions	70% had excellent results; severe cases had the best results	Mild pain and burning during laser treatments
Wanitphakedeedecha et al.[47]	Prospective	35	6 months	LP 1,064 nm, 4 sessions	40.7% had mycological clearance after the first series of tx; 59.3% underwent second tx. Overall cure rate was 51.9%	Mild erythema and swelling after procedure
Xu et al.[20]	Randomized controlled trial	53	24 weeks	3 groups: • Oral terbinafine (T), 250 mg daily • LP 1,064 nm (L), weekly • Combined (L + T)	Mycological clearance rates and clinical clearance rates increased in all groups, but were significantly higher in the L+T group than the L and T groups	No adverse effects in the L or L+T group; one patient in T group had temporary increase of alanine and aspartate aminotransferases
(L: laser; LP: long-pulsed; T: topical; tx: treatment)						

medication alone, topical antifungal alone) with combination therapy (1,064 nm laser plus oral or topical antifungal), combination treatments were usually superior to monotherapy. Combination therapy consistently showed higher mycological and clinical cure rates compared to monotherapy.[20-22]

SYSTEMIC REVIEWS

Two systematic reviews evaluated many different types of lasers to determine the efficacy of lasers overall compared with other treatment options. Francuzik et al. evaluated 22 studies. Among the studies, 47% concluded that lasers in general were effective.[23]

Additionally, 60% of the studies found that use of lasers led to a complete mycological cure in at least 50% of patients in each clinical trial. However, Gupta et al., evaluated 21 random control trials[24] and found that while in general lasers do demonstrate evidence of clinical improvement and clear nail growth, they are not as effective when compared to the efficacy rates of topical and oral therapies.

OTHER LASER MODALITIES

Other laser or light-based modalities have been used to treat onychomycosis. **Table 5** summarizes the efficacy of a dual-diode laser with wavelengths 635 nm and 405 nm, a 1,064 nm diode laser, a 1,319 nm laser, a Broad Band Light, and a 2,940 nm erbium-yttrium-aluminum-garnet (Er:YAG) laser. All of these lasers have shown varying efficacy, with the

TABLE 5: Other laser modalities for the treatment of onychomycosis.

Author	Study type	*n*	Follow-up	Treatment	Results	Side effects
Nestor et al.[48]	Retrospective	50	6 months	635 nm and 405 nm dual-diode laser, 4 sessions	67% of nails had ≥3 mm of clear nail growth; 89% of nails showed increase in achieving clear nail	None
Renner et al.[31]	Prospective	23	3.2 months	1,064 nm diode laser, 2–3 sessions	Approximately 41% of the patients showed clinical improvement; 25% of patients showed improvement in onychomycosis severity index	None
Waibel et al.[25]	Prospective	21	6 months	1,064 nm laser, 1,319 nm laser, or Broadband light (BBL), 4 sessions	100% of patients treated with 1,064 nm laser and BBL had negative cultures; 1 patient treated with 1,319 nm laser had positive culture	None
Zhang et al.[28]	Self-controlled trial	9	24 weeks	2 groups: • 2,940 nm Er:YAG, 6 sessions and 5% amorolfine lacquer twice weekly (Group 1) • 5% amorolfine lacquer twice weekly (Group 2)	75% of group 1 and 20% of group 2 had negative mycological examination; 60% of group 1 and 20% of group 2 had complete clinical cure with mycological cure	Mild bleeding in 2 cases following laser treatment

(Er:YAG: erbium-yttrium-aluminum-garnet)

1,064 nm and 1,319 nm lasers appearing to be the most effective.[25] These other modalities have *little-to-no* side effects associated with their treatment of onychomycosis.

COMBINATION THERAPY

Based on the results of the studies evaluated, it appeared as if combination treatments, laser treatment combined with topical treatments or oral treatments, proved more effective than monotherapies. **Table 6** highlights combination therapies referenced above. The improvement achieved through combination treatments varied among the studies reviewed here. Studies that included controls[26-28] cited a significant difference in nail clearance and clinical improvement in the combination group versus the monotherapies. For example, Zhang et al.[28] compared Er:YAG 2,940 nm and 5% amorolfine lacquer treatment with amorolfine lacquer only. At the 24% week follow-up, 60% of nails in the combination group achieved complete mycological cure compared to 20% in the amorolfine only group.

However, many of the studies[29-32] did not include controls, making it difficult to compare the relative efficacy of combination treatment with monotherapies. Of these, the most convincing data in favor of combination treatment was produced by Bhatta et al.[32] 75 patients were treated with CO_2 fractional

TABLE 6: Combination therapies.

Study	Study type	*n*	Combination treatment	Results
Bhatta et al.[32]	Clinical trial	75	Fractional carbon-dioxide laser + 1% topical terbinafine	After 3 months, around 92–94% of patients were culturally and microscopically negative. This decreased to 80–84% after 6 months due to recurrence of onychomycosis
Zhou et al.[26]	Non-blind, random-ized, positive-controlled trial	60	Fractional carbon-dioxide laser + luliconazole 1% cream	Clinical efficacy rate and mycological clearance rate of the combination group were 69.6% and 57.4%, respectively. The results of the combination group were significantly higher than the laser treatment only group
Kim et al.[27]	Random-ized com-parative study	56 (8 received combi-nation treat-ment)	1,064 nm Nd:YAG laser + 10 mg/mL naftifine HCL spray	Around 72% of patients in the combination group had clinical responses. Around 23% were cured after 24 weeks. The results of the combination group were significantly greater than the topical treatment monotherapy group
Lim et al.[29]	Clinical trial	24	Fractional carbon-dioxide laser + amorolfine cream	92% of patients had some improvement and 50% had a negative microscopic result
Renner et al.[31]	Prospective clinical trial	24	Diode Laser + topical ciclopiroxolamine, amorolfine, or clotrimazole (*n* = 15) or oral terbinafine (3)	All nails showed an improvement from 14 to 56%

Cont'd...

Cont'd...

Study	Study type	*n*	Combination treatment	Results
Gupta et al.[30]	Retro-spective chart review	23	Nd:YAG 1064-nm laser + debridement + 1% topical terbinafine	A temporary improvement was found in 78% of patients' nails. 46% of patients had nails cleared to 50% of baseline. Better outcomes were found after four or more treatments
Li et al.[22]	Self-controlled study	19	Long pulsed 1,064-nm Nd:YAG laser + oral itraconazole	Those in the combination treatment group with mild/medium onychomycosis severity improved 100%, 95.2%, and 90.5% on the 8th, 16th, and 24th week after follow-up, respectively. The differences between the combination and monotherapy medication groups were not significant. For those in the combination treatment group with high severity onychomycosis had 95.2%, 90.5%, and 100% of improvement during the 8th, 16th, and 24th weeks after treatment, respectively. The combination therapy group had statistically significant improved results compared to the oral medication monotherapy group
Zhang et al.[28]	Self-controlled study	9	Er:YAG laser + 5% amorolfine lacquer	At week 24, 90% nails in the combination group had a clinical response. The mean OSI (onychomycosis severity index) score showed a significant decrease (5.24) and the average maximum linear clear nail growth was 3.1 mm

(Er:YAG: erbium-yttrium-aluminum-garnet)

laser (3 sessions, 4 week intervals) and prescribed 1% topical terbinafine (daily). The results cited 92–94% mycological clearance at the 3-month follow-up.

Interestingly, Li et al.[22] cited a higher efficacy of treatment in nails with severe onychomycosis compared to mild/moderate cases. Patients were divided into two groups based on disease severity. Within these two groups, half were treated with the Nd:YAG 1,064 nm laser (4 sessions, 1 week intervals) and oral itraconazole (1 ×/day for 1 week) and half were treated with oral itraconazole only. The group with higher disease severity at onset achieved 30–40% higher improvements compared with the oral itraconazole group. The moderate severity group still achieved a higher efficacy than the oral itraconazole group, although the difference was not statistically significant.

Overall, the studies reviewed in **Table 3** demonstrate a potential for greater improvement through combination therapies as compared to monotherapies. However, there is still more research to be done to evaluate the best conditions and circumstances for using combination therapy.

RANDOMIZED CONTROL TRIALS

While many studies have been published on laser therapy for onychomycosis, few randomized control trials have been conducted to prove the efficacy of laser therapy. **Table 7** shows all the randomized control trials discussed earlier. These studies are a valuable tool for evaluating the variable efficacy of oral or topical medication, laser, and combination treatments. Three studies[20,26,27] compared the efficacy of all combination therapy versus monotherapy and all found that the combination produced a greater improvement than monotherapy, both laser only and medication only, as measured by mycological cure.

Similarly, two studies which evaluated laser therapy allowed for a substantiated demonstration of the efficacy of laser therapy. El-Tatawy et al.[21] compared laser only with

TABLE 7: Randomized control trials.

Study	Type of laser	*n*	Objective	Results
Zhou et al.[26*]	Fractionated Carbon Dioxide	60	Compare the efficacy of combination therapy of carbon dioxide (CO_2) laser with luliconazole 1% cream versus fractional CO_2 laser alone	After 6 months: • The combination therapy group had a significantly higher clinical efficacy rate and mycological clearance rate compared to the laser treatment group • The clinical efficacy rate was 69.6% for the combination group • The mycological clearance rate was 57.4% for the combination group
Kim et al.[27]	Short pulsed 1,064 nm Nd:YAG	56	Compare the efficacy of 1,064 nm Nd:YAG laser with topical treatments and combination therapy	At 24 weeks: • 76% of the group receiving laser treatment had clinical responses • 71.8% of the group receiving combination therapy had clinical responses • 15.2% of the laser group was cured • 22.5% of the combination group was cured • Both laser and combination groups had significantly greater results than the group that received only topical treatment
Xu et al.[20]	Long pulsed 1,064 nm Nd:YAG	53	Compare the efficacy of combination therapy with a long-pulsed 1,064-nm Nd:YAG laser and oral terbinafine with laser treatment alone and with topical treatment alone	At weeks 8, 12,16, and 24: • The mycological clearance rate and the clinical clearance rate was significantly higher in the group that received combination therapy compared to the groups that received monotherapies

Cont'd...

Cont'd...

Study	Type of laser	*n*	Objective	Results
El-Tatawy et al.[21]	Long Pulsed 1,064 nm Nd:YAG	40	Compare the efficacy of long pulsed 1,064 nm Nd-YAG laser with the terbinafine treatment	After 6 months: • Every patient in the group treated (with 4 sessions) of long pulsed 1,064 nm Nd-YAG laser showed improvement, while only 50% of patients in the group treated with terbinafine (applied twice daily for 6 months) had mild to moderate improvement • 80% of the patients who received laser treatment had mycological cure while the patients who received topical treatment still had positive cultures
Lands-man et al.[33]	870 nm and 930 nm Near-Infrared Diode	34	To test the efficacy of The Noveon, a 870 and 930 nm near-infrared diode laser, developed to treat onychomy-cosis	After 180 days: • 85% of the eligible treated toenails showed improvements • 65% showed clear nail growth up to at least 3 mm • 26% showed at least 4 mm of clear nail growth. • The 16 toes with more severe involvement had a 63% clear nail growth of at least 3 mm • 30% had negative cultures and Periodic acid–Schiff
Holl-mig et al.[34*]	1,064 nm Nd:YAG	27	Compare the ef-ficacy of 1,064-nm neodymium:yttrium-aluminum-garnet laser with no treatment	At 3 months: • 33% of patients treated with laser had negative cultures • 20% of the control group had negative cultures At 12 months: • No difference was found between both groups for nail plate clearance
Ortiz et al.[17]	1,320 nm Nd:YAG	10	Determine effi-cacy of 1,320-nm neodymium:yttrium aluminum garnet (Nd:YAG) laser in improving the appear-ance of onychomy-cosis	At 3 months: • 50% of the group that received laser treatment had negative mycologic cultures • 70% of the control group had negative mycologic cultures

*Non-blinded randomized control studies.

topical terbinafine only and produced promising data in favor of laser treatment. Patients were divided in two groups of 20. Group A was treated with Nd:YAG 1,064 nm (4 sessions, 1 week intervals), and Group B received topical terbinafine (2 ×/day for

6 months). At the 6 months follow-up, 100% of patients in Group A improved clinically while only 50% of patients in Group B showed any improvement. Similarly, Landsman et al.[33] evaluated the 870 nm and 930 nm Nd:Yag, however without a control group, and 85% of samples showed improvement (measured by clear nail growth) at the 180-day follow-up.

Importantly, two of the studies reviewed here[17,34] showed no statistically significant improvement in the laser therapy group versus the control sham group. Hollmig et al.[34] found no significant improvement (measured as nail plate clearance) in the Nd:YAG 1,064 nm (2 treatments, 2 weeks apart) laser treatment group compared with the sham control group. Similarly, Ortiz et al.[17] not only found no statistically significant difference in improvement between the laser group (1,320 nm Nd:Yag) versus the sham control, but also reported that 70% of control group cultures were negative compared to 50% of the laser group.

Through controlled methods, regarding frequency of treatment and treatment intervals, these studies allow for a more substantiated evaluation of laser therapy for onychomycosis. Overall, the majority of these studies demonstrated a markedly higher efficacy of laser therapy and combination therapy as compared to oral or topical medication in treating onychomycosis.

CONCLUSION

There is still much to understand about the use of lasers for treatment of onychomycosis. Photothermolysis is one explanation for the effectiveness of using lasers. Certain temperatures can have a fungicidal effect, but lasers must be pulsed or delivered at low energy levels to prevent tissue necrosis of the underlying nail bed.[11] Bhatta et al. evaluated other potential mechanisms for laser treatment of onychomycosis, and suggested that nonspecific tissue heating may increase immunological response and therefore eliminate fungal pathogens.[12] Still, some studies proposed that laser energy cause mechanical damage of the fungi and inhibit growth, while others argued that laser treatment may activate the mitochondrial apoptotic pathway, resulting in fungal cell death.[12,13] In addition, some researchers believe that lasers can create small pores in the nail bed, allowing for improved drug delivery and thus improved efficacy in the treatment of onychomycosis.[14]

While there are many laser treatment studies examining the effectiveness in treating onychomycosis, few are randomized controlled trials. Many studies highlight the long-pulsed 1,064 nm laser, suggesting that the particular wavelength may have the best depth of penetration of nails. Additionally, the results of these trials favor combination treatment versus monotherapy. Of the studies reviewed here, laser + topical was the most commonly studied combination therapy although both the lasers and topicals used varied. Both fractional carbon-dioxide laser and the 1,064 nm Nd:YAG laser were used in three combination studies each and topical terbinafine was the only medication used in two studies.

However, while many studies demonstrate promising improvement in onychomycosis through laser treatment, the degree of improvement varies greatly. For example, Kim et al.[27] evaluated laser and topical treatment (1,064 nm Nd:YAG and 10 mg/mL naftifine HCl spray) versus topical only and 22.5% of the combination group were mycologically cured. Meanwhile, Zhou et al.[26] evaluated laser and topical combination treatment (fractional CO_2 laser and luliconazole 1% cream) versus laser only and achieved a 57.4% mycological cure rate in the combination group. Additionally, relapse of onychomycosis was not uncommon

TABLE 8: Complications.

Study	Type of laser	*n*	Side effects
Carney et al.[19]	Submillisecond 1,064 nm Nd:YAG laser	10	One patient had treatment-related onycholysis
Helou et al.[49]	Short-pulsed 1,064 nm Nd:YAG	30	Of the 30 patients, 4 had pain within 48 hours and 3 had a burning sensation in the treated area. Twenty seven did not report any side effects
Helou et al.[50]	0.65 ms pulsed Nd-YAG 1,064 nm laser	1	Patients who had ring block anesthesia on toe before laser treatment had extreme pain, edema, oozing, and erythema following treatment
Karsai et al.[41]	Short-pulsed 1,064 nm Nd:YAG	20	Patients described the pain to be a mean of 5 from a scale of 1–10
Moutran et al.[51]	Short-pulsed 1,064 nm Nd-YAG	1	Diabetic patient with neuropathy had necrotic lesions and needed to have two big toes amputated after treatment
Wanitphakdeedecha et al.[47]	Long-pulsed 1,064 nm nd:YAG	35	Side effects were limited to mild erythema and swelling after the laser procedure

(Nd:YAG: neodymium-doped yttrium aluminum garnet)

among study patients. For these reasons, it is important to manage patient expectations in regards to degree of improvement and number of treatment sessions required as this impacts overall patient satisfaction.

Finally, side effects of laser treatments typically involved only moderate pain except in the few cases outlined in **Table 8.** Therefore, given the necessary precautions, these treatments are safe for patient use and demonstrate a meaningful opportunity to improve onychomycosis.

REFERENCES

1. Ghannoum MA, Hajjeh RA, Scher R, Konnikov N, Gupta AK, Summerbell R, et al. A large-scale North American study of fungal isolates from nails: the frequency of onychomycosis, fungal distribution, and antifungal susceptibility patterns. J Am Acad Dermatol. 2000;43(4):641-8.
2. Evans EG. Causative pathogens in onychomycosis and the possibility of treatment resistance: a review. J Am Acad Dermatol. 1998;38(5 Pt 3):S32-36.
3. Welsh O, Vera-Cabrera L, Welsh E. Onychomycosis. Clin Dermatol. 2010;28(2):151-9.
4. Clinicalkey. Onychomycosis. [online] Available from: https://www.clinicalkey.com/#!/content/21-s2.0-1014880. [Last Accessed March, 2021].
5. Scher RK, Tavakkol A, Sigurgeirsson B, Hay RJ, Joseph WS, Tosti A, et al. Onychomycosis: diagnosis and definition of cure. J Am Acad Dermatol. 2007;56(6):939-44.
6. Food and Drug Administration. (2016). Medical Devices and Clinical Trial Design for the Treatment or Improvement in the Appearance of Fungally-Infected Nails. [online] Available from https://www.fda.gov/regulatory-information/search-fda-guidance-documents/medical-devices-and-clinical-trial-design-treatment-or-improvement-appearance-fungally-infected. [Last Accessed March, 2021].
7. Bhatta AK, Huang X, Keyal U, Zhao JJ. Laser treatment for onychomycosis: a review. Mycoses. 2014;57(12):734-40.
8. Evans EG, Sigurgeirsson B. Double blind, randomised study of continuous terbinafine compared with intermittent itraconazole in treatment of toenail onychomycosis. The LION Study Group. BMJ. 1999;318(7190):1031-5.
9. UpToDate. (2017). Onychomycosis: Management (Goldstein A, Bhattia N). [online] Available from: https://www.uptodate.com/contents/onychomycosis-management?source=search_result&search=Terbinafine&selectedTitle=6~40. [Last Accessed March, 2021].

10. Tosti A, Piraccini BM, Stinchi C, Colombo MD. Relapses of onychomycosis after successful treatment with systemic antifungals: a three-year follow-up. Dermatology. 1998;197(2):162-6.
11. Hira K, Yamada H, Takahashi Y, Ogawa H. Successful treatment of chromomycosis using carbon dioxide laser associated with topical heat applications. J Eur Acad Dermatol Venereol. 2002;16(3):273-5.
12. Bhatta AK, Keyal U, Wang X, Gellén E. A review of the mechanism of action of lasers and photodynamic therapy for onychomycosis. Lasers Med Sci. 2017;32(2):469-74.
13. Ortiz AE, Avram MM, Wanner MA. A review of lasers and light for the treatment of onychomycosis. Lasers Surg Med. 2014;46(2):117-24.
14. Nenoff P, Grunewald S, Paasch U. Laser therapy of onychomycosis. J Dtsch Dermatol Ges. 2014;12(1):33-8.
15. Wiznia LE, Quatrano NA, Mu EW, Rieder EA. A Clinical Review of Laser and Light Therapy for Nail Psoriasis and Onychomycosis. Dermatol Surg. 2017;43(2):161-72.
16. Bristow IR. The effectiveness of lasers in the treatment of onychomycosis: a systematic review. J Foot Ankle Res. 2014;7:34.
17. Ortiz AE, Truong S, Serowka K, Kelly KM. A 1,320-nm Nd: YAG laser for improving the appearance of onychomycosis. Dermatol Surg. 2014;40(12):1356-60.
18. Kimura U, Takeuchi K, Kinoshita A, Takamori K, Hiruma M, Suga Y. Treating onychomycoses of the toenail: clinical efficacy of the sub-millisecond 1064 nm Nd:YAG laser using a 5 mm spot diameter. J Drugs Dermatol. 2012;11(4):496-504.
19. Carney C, Cantrell W, Warner J, Elewski B. Treatment of onychomycosis using a submillisecond 1064-nm neodymium:yttrium-aluminum-garnet laser. J Am Acad Dermatol. 2013;69(4):578-82.
20. Xu Y, Miao X, Zhou B, Luo D. Combined oral terbinafine and long-pulsed 1064-nm Nd: YAG laser treatment is more effective for onychomycosis than either treatment alone. Dermatol Surg. 2014;40(11):1201-7.
21. El-Tatawy RA, Abd El-Naby NM, El-Hawary EE, Talaat RA. A comparative clinical and mycological study of Nd-YAG laser versus topical terbinafine in the treatment of onychomycosis. J Dermatology Treat. 2015;26(5):461-4.
22. Li Y, Xu J, Zhao JY, Zhuo FL. Self-controlled Study of Onychomycosis Treated with Long-pulsed Nd:YAG 1064-nm Laser Combined with Itraconazole. Chin Med J (Engl). 2016;129(16):1929-34.
23. Francuzik W, Fritz K, Salavastru C. Laser therapies for onychomycosis - critical evaluation of methods and effectiveness. J Eur Acad Dermatol Venereol. 2016;30(6):936-42.
24. Gupta AK, Versteeg SG. A critical review of improvement rates for laser therapy used to treat toenail onychomycosis. J Eur Acad Dermatol Venereol. 2017;31(7):1111-8.
25. Waibel J, Wulkan AJ, Rudnick A. Prospective efficacy and safety evaluation of laser treatments with real-time temperature feedback for fungal onychomycosis. J Drugs Dermatol. 2013;12(11):1237-42.
26. Zhou BR, Lu Y, Permatasari F, Huang H, Li J, Liu J, et al. The efficacy of fractional carbon dioxide (CO_2) laser combined with luliconazole 1% cream for the treatment of onychomycosis: a randomized, controlled trial. Medicine (Baltimore). 2016;95(44):e5141.
27. Kim TI, Shin MK, Jeong KH, Suh DH, Lee SJ, Oh IH, et al. A randomised comparative study of 1064 nm Neodymium-doped yttrium aluminium garnet (Nd:YAG) laser and topical antifungal treatment of onychomycosis. Mycoses. 2016;59(12):803-10.
28. Zhang J, Zhang Y, Qin J, Lu S, Cai W, Li J, et al. Combination therapy for onychomycosis using a fractional 2940-nm Er:YAG laser and 5 % amorolfine lacquer. Lasers Med Sci. 2016;31(7):1391-6.
29. Lim EH, Kim HR, Park YO, Lee Y, Seo YJ, Kim CD, et al. Toenail onychomycosis treated with a fractional carbon-dioxide laser and topical antifungal cream. J Am Acad Dermatol. 2014;70(5):918-23.
30. Gupta AK, Paquet M. A retrospective chart review of the clinical efficacy of Nd:YAG 1064-nm laser for toenail onychomycosis. J Dermatolog Treat. 2015;26(4):376-8.
31. Renner R, Grusser K, Sticherling M. 1064-nm diode laser therapy of onychomycosis: results of a prospective open treatment of 82 toenails. Dermatology. 2015;230(2):128-34.
32. Bhatta AK, Keyal U, Huang X, Zhao JJ. Fractional carbon-dioxide (CO2) laser-assisted topical therapy for the treatment of onychomycosis. J Am Acad Dermatol. 2016;74(5):916-23.
33. Landsman AS, Robbins AH, Angelini PF, Wu CC, Cook J, Oster M, et al. Treatment of mild, moderate, and severe onychomycosis using 870- and 930-nm light exposure. J Am Podiatr Med Assoc. 2010;100(3):166-77.
34. Hollmig ST, Rahman Z, Henderson MT, Rotatori RM, Gladstone H, Tang JY. Lack of efficacy with 1064-nm neodymium:yttrium-aluminum-garnet laser for the treatment of onychomycosis: a randomized, controlled trial. J Am Acad Dermatol. 2014;70(5):911-7.
35. Gupta A, Simpson F. Device-Based Therapies for Onychomycosis Treatment. 2012;17(9):4-9..
36. Galvan Garcia HR. Onychomycosis: 1064-nm Nd:YAG q-switch laser treatment. J Cosmet Dermatol. 2014;13(3):232-5.

37. Hees H, Raulin C, Baumler W. Laser treatment of onychomycosis: an in vitro pilot study. J Dtsch Dermatol Ges. 2012;10(12):913-8.
38. Kalokasidis K, Onder M, Trakatelli MG, Richert B, Fritz K. The Effect of Q-Switched Nd:YAG 1064 nm/532 nm Laser in the Treatment of Onychomycosis In Vivo. Dermatol Res Pract. 2013;2013:379725.
39. Rivers JK, Vestvik BJ, Berkowitz J. Real-World Efficacy of 1064-nm Nd:YAG Laser for the Treatment of Onychomycosis. J Cutan Med Surg. 2017;21(2):108-13.
40. Hochman LG. Laser treatment of onychomycosis using a novel 0.65-millisecond pulsed Nd:YAG 1064-nm laser. J Cosmet Laser Ther. 2011;13(1): 2-5.
41. Karsai S, Jäger M, Oesterhelt A, Weiss C, Schneider SW, Jünger M, et al. Treating onychomycosis with the short-pulsed 1064-nm-Nd:YAG laser: results of a prospective randomized controlled trial. J Eur Acad Dermatol Venereol. 2017;31(1):175-80.
42. Li Y, Yu S, Xu J, Zhang R, Zhao J. Comparison of the efficacy of long-pulsed Nd:YAG laser intervention for treatment of onychomycosis of toenails or fingernails. J Drugs Dermato. 2014;13(10):1258-63.
43. Lu S, Zhang J, Liang Y, Li X, Cai W, Xi L. The Efficacy and Prognostic Factors for Long Pulse Neodymium: Yttrium-Aluminum-Garnet Laser Treatment on Onychomycosis: a Pilot Study. Ann Dermatol. 2016;28(3):406-8.
44. Moon SH, Hur H, Oh YJ, Choi KH, Kim JE, Ko JY. Treatment of onychomycosis with a 1064-nm long-pulsed Nd:YAG laser. J Cosmet Laser Ther. 2014;16(4):165-70.
45. Okan G, Tarikci N, Gokdemir G. The Effect of Long-Pulsed Nd:YAG Laser for the Treatment of Onychomycosis. J Am Podiatr Med Assoc. 2017;107(1):54-9.
46. Piccolo D, Kostaki D, Del Duca E, Cannarozzo G, Sannino M, Nisticò S. Long-Pulsed 1064-nm Nd:YAG Laser for the Treatment of Onychomycosis. Photomed Laser Surg. 2017;35(4):213-6.
47. Wanitphakdeedecha R, Thanomkitti K, Bunyaratavej S, Manuskiatti W.. Efficacy and safety of 1064-nm Nd:YAG laser in treatment of onychomycosis. J Dermatolog Treat. 2016;27(1):75-9.
48. Nestor M, Andriessen A, Berman B, Katz BE, Gilbert D, Goldberg DJ, et al. Photobiomodulation with non-thermal lasers: Mechanisms of action and therapeutic uses in dermatology and aesthetic medicine. J Cosmet Laser Ther. 2017:1-9.
49. Helou J, Maatouk I, Hajjar MA, Moutran R. Evaluation of Nd:YAG laser device efficacy on onychomycosis: a case series of 30 patients. Mycoses. 2016;59(1):7-11.
50. Helou J, Korkomaz J, Haber R, Habre M, Tomb R. Laser treatment of onychomycosis: beware of ring block anesthesia! Lasers Med Sci. 2015;30(9):2399-400.
51. Moutran R, Maatouk I, Helou J. Diabetic neuropathy and Nd-YAG (1064 nm) laser for onychomycosis: be careful. J Eur Acad Dermatol Venereol. 2015;29(6):1239-40.

27

CHAPTER

Laser Treatment of Actinic Keratosis and Nonmelanoma Skin Cancer

Oge C Onwudiwe, Zeina Tannous

INTRODUCTION

Millions of Americans are diagnosed annually with nonmelanoma skin cancer (NMSC) or its premalignant precursor, actinic keratosis (AK). Chronic UV exposure is the main risk factor for development. A variety of treatment options exists that range from topical immunotherapy to Mohs micrographic surgery. Lasers have also been used in the treatment of NMSC, although many laser treatment protocols have been published but no gold standard exists. Traditional ablative lasers, ablative and nonablative fractional lasers as well as vascular-selective lasers have been studied. Herein, the use of lasers in the treatment of AK and NMSC will be reviewed as well as the associated risks, benefits, and complications.

ACTINIC KERATOSIS AND NONMELANOMA SKIN CANCER

Actinic Keratosis

Actinic keratosis (AK) is a relatively common cutaneous condition consisting of cytologically atypical epidermal keratinocytes. They are most commonly seen in lighter skin phototypes, but can be seen in all races. AK is considered a premalignant condition as it can progress to nonmelanoma skin cancer (NMSC). These lesions predominantly arise in cosmetically sensitive sun-exposed areas such as the face and scalp. Other common areas of involvement include the ears, neck, hands, and forearms. It has been reported that the risk of malignant degeneration is approximately 10–20% per lesion over a 10-year period.[1]

Traditional Treatment of Actinic Keratosis

Various treatment options are geared toward preventing progression of AK to NMSC. These options can be patient-performed topical applications or office-based procedures. Some topical applications include 5-fluorouracil (5-FU), imiquimod, diclofenac, and tretinoin. Procedural interventions include cryotherapy, curettage, dermabrasion, chemical peels, laser and photodynamic therapy (PDT). Combination methods such as laser resurfacing with PDT and fractionated laser therapy with drug delivery have also been reported.

Laser Treatment of Actinic Keratosis

In light of the fact that AK has the propensity to develop into NMSC, it is not only crucial to treat this condition, but utilize therapies that are efficacious as well as yield acceptable to great cosmetic outcomes. For example, cryotherapy with liquid nitrogen is most commonly used due to ease of use and efficacy; however, it bears a high risk of permanent hypopigmentation. For this purpose, laser intervention as both a treatment and preventative strategy has been investigated. Results with a 1,550 nm fractionated erbium-doped fiber laser at 32–40% surface area coverage per treatment and 5 treatment sessions at 2–4-week intervals showed a 73% clinical clearance rate at 1 month. Clinical clearance dropped to 55% at 6 months, after 4 treatments, signifying recurrence. Histological findings showed that the vast majority of the lesions persisted at month 1 and month 6, concluding that the lesions were never successfully removed entirely.[5] A subsequent study using a fractionated 1,927-nm nonablative thulium laser where subjects underwent 4 treatments at 2–6-week intervals with densities ranging from 40 to 70% showed a decrease in lesion count of 91% at month 1 and 86% at 6 months.[6]

Fully ablative laser resurfacing has also been investigated in the treatment of AK. It has been shown to be an effective option in the reduction of AK and thus, may be useful in preventing the development of nonmelanoma skin cancers. Data from a retrospective analysis of 24 subjects with facial AKs (lesion count 30 or greater) treated with full face CO_2 and/or erbium-doped yttrium aluminum garnet laser (Er:YAG) laser resurfacing showed 87% of the subjects remained lesion free for at least 1 year. At 2 years, fourteen of the 24 patients (58.3%) showed no new lesions.[7] Other studies using fully ablative lasers have shown varying degrees of success as well.[8-10] Limitations with this approach include scarring, infection, downtime, pain and delayed-onset permanent hypopigmentation have restricted its use. As a result, fractionated ablative laser therapy for the treatment of actinic keratosis has been assessed.[11] To enhance these efforts, laser assisted drug delivery has gained traction. It has been shown that fractional laser-assisted topical delivery leads to enhanced, accelerated and deeper penetration of topical agents,[12] which would theoretically lead to higher clearance rates. Other combination treatments such as fractional ablative CO_2 laser-mediated photodynamic therapy have also been described in the literature.[13,14]

Nonmelanoma Skin Cancer

Nonmelanoma skin cancers is the most common type of cancer and includes basal cell carcinoma (BCC) and squamous cell carcinoma (SCC). Data suggest that 1 in 5 persons in the US will develop a NMSC in their lifetime[2] and approximately 5–5.5 million basal and squamous cell skin cancers are diagnosed each year.[3] Reports show average treatment cost to be approximately $8 billion dollars per annum.[4] Although death from these cancers is uncommon, it is estimated that about 2,000 people in the US die each year from NMSC, especially from SCC in high risk locations and in immunocompromised individuals such as renal transplant patients.[3] Data suggests that there are more skin cancers in the US than all other cancers combined and its incidence is rising. Chronic UV light exposure is the major risk factor for development of NMSC. Ionizing radiations, infection with human papillomavirus, immunosuppression, among others, are additional risk factors. In individuals with fairer skin, it has been estimated that up to three-fourths of NMSCs are BCCs and up to one-quarter are SCCs. With mounting incidence, these neoplasms will continue to be a burden on the healthcare system. Of note, NMSC incidence in lightly pigmented versus darkly pigmented is 230 per 100,000 versus 3.4 per 100,000, respectively.[1]

Traditional Treatment of Nonmelanoma Skin Cancer

Bearing in mind the subtype of cancer, location and depth of penetration, various treatment options are considered standard: Topical immunotherapy such as 5-FU, imiquimod, curettage and electrodessication, surgical excision, Mohs micrographic surgery and radiation therapy. Limitations with the aforementioned modalities include risks of structural deformity, functional impairment, recurrence of the tumor, scarring, among other adverse events.

Laser Treatment of Nonmelanoma Skin Cancer

Studies have shown varying degrees of success with the use of lasers in the treatment of NMSCs. The focus herein, however, will be on the use of vascular specific lasers in the treatment of basal and squamous cell carcinomas (**Table 1**).

Skin cancers, such as BCCs and SCCs possess vasculature, which is crucial for tumor growth. Tumor induced angiogenesis is exhibited by the secretion of proangiogenic factors such as vascular endothelial growth factor A and the downregulation of endogenous angiogenesis inhibitors such as thrombospondin 1 and thrombospondin 2.[15] Directly targeting cutaneous tumor vasculature using the theory of selective photothermolysis[16] with pulsed vascular specific lasers has been investigated (**Fig. 1**). By targeting the microvasculature, which is typically greater in diameter than the vasculature of normal skin,[17] it has been shown that tumor regression can occur (**Figs. 2A** to **C**).

Allison et al. performed a preliminary study with a 585 nm PDL. Parameters utilized were an energy density of 6.0 J/cm^2 with a 5 mm diameter spot and pulse duration of 450 µs. Results showed clearance in one of seven superficial BCCs in a single treatment.[18] Campolmi et al. studied twenty patients (eight males and 12 females) with superficial basal cell carcinoma.[19] Five treatments with a 595 nm pulsed-dye laser (PDL) every 20 days with the following parameters: 7.5 J/cm^2, 7 mm spot size and pulse duration of 1.5 ms or 6.5 J/cm^2, 10 mm spot size and pulse duration of 0.5 ms. Follow-up was 12–24 months after the fifth treatment. A complete response was obtained in 16 out of 20 patients. Three recurrences and one failed response were reported.[19] More recently, Shah et al. examined the use of the 595 nm PDL in the treatment of BCC. Variants studied included superficial, nodular, micronodular, and keratinizing. The treatment parameters in this particular study were 15 J/cm^2, 3-millisecond pulse duration, 7-mm spot size with single passes that had 10% overlap. The tumors were treated four times every 2 weeks and were subsequently excised. Results showed clearance of 11/12 of BCCs less than 1.5 cm in size but only 2/8 lesions greater than 1.5 cm were effectively cleared. No evidence of clinical scarring or fibrosis on histology was seen.[20] In a follow-up study conducted by Konnikov et al. fourteen patients with 20 biopsy-proven BCCs were treated with four consecutive PDL treatments at 3–4 week intervals. The lesions were located on the trunk and extremities and ranged in size from 8 to 35 mm in diameter. A 4 mm margin of clinically normal skin was also treated. The following parameters were used: pulse energy of 15.00 J/cm^2, pulse duration of 3 milliseconds, and a 7 mm spot size. A complete clinical response was reported in 19 of 20 treated BCCs, irrespective of size and histologic subtype. Of the 19 BCCs, only one recurrence was noted at 17 months follow-up. In summary, 90% (18/20 tumors) of the treated BCCs in this study showed no clinical or histologic evidence of BCC greater than 12 months after PDL treatment.[21]

It has been suggested that pulse stacking may increase the depth of injury. Tran et al.

TABLE 1: NMSC treatment with vascular lasers: Summary of the literature.

Author	Laser type	Parameters	Type of NMSC treated	Number of treatments	Clearance rate
Alison et al.	585 nm PDL	6 J/cm^2, 5 mm spot size, 450 µspulse duration	sBCC	1	1 out of 7
Campolmi et al.	595 nm PDL	7.5 J/cm^2, 7 mm spot size, 1.5 ms pulse duration or 6.5 J/cm^2, 10 mm spot size, 0.5 ms pulse duration	sBCC	5	16 out of 20
Shah et al.	595 nm PDL	15 J/cm^2, 7 mm spot size, 3 ms pulse duration	BCC-multiple subtypes	4	13 out of 20
Konnikov et al.	595 nm PDL	15 J/cm^2, 7 mm spot size, 3 ms pulse duration	BCC-multiple subtypes	4	18 out of 20
Tran et al.	595 nm PDL	• *Group 1*: 15 J/cm^2, 7 mm spot size, 3 ms pulse duration (2 passes) • *Group 2*: 7.5 J/cm^2, 10 mm spot size, 3 ms pulse duration (double pulse)	BCC SCC IS	1	• Group 1: 2 out of 8 • Group 2: 5 out of 7
Jalian et al.	585 nm PDL and 1,064 nm ND:YAG	• 585 nm PDL-8 J/cm^2, 7 mm spot size, 2 ms pulse • 1,064 nm ND:YAG—40 J/cm^2, 15 ms pulse	BCC-multiple subtypes	4	7 out of 12
Ibrahimi et al.	755 nm Alexandrite	100 J/cm^2, 8 mm spot size, 3 ms pulse duration	BCC-multiple subtypes	1	15 out of 18
El-Tonsy et al.	1,064 nm Nd:YAG-continuous wave	10 W, 8 mm spot size	BCC-multiple subtypes	2 to 4	36 out of 37
Ortiz et al.	1,064 nm Nd:YAG-long pulse	• Group 1: 80 J/cm^2, 5 mm spot size, 10 ms pulse duration • Group 2: 120 J/cm^2, 5 mm spot size, 10 ms pulse duration	BCC-multiple subtypes	1	• Group 1:12 out of 13 • Group 2:10 out of 10

(BCC: basal cell carcinoma; Nd:YAG: neodymium-doped yttrium aluminum garnet; NMSC: nonmelanoma skin cancer; PDL: pulsed dye laser; SCC IS: squamous cell carcinoma in situ)

had subjects undergo a single PDL treatment using 2 passes in one treatment arm and double stacked pulses in another. Twenty patients with 23 biopsy-proven BCCs and SCCIS measuring 4–30 mm in size and located on the trunk and extremities were recruited. Parameters were as follows: Group 1 received the 595 nm PDL at pulse energy of 15 J/ cm^2, 3-millisecond pulse duration, a 7-mm spot size with 10% overlap of pulses and two passes and no dynamic cooling. Group 2 received the 595 nm PDL at 7.5 J/cm^2, 3-millisecond

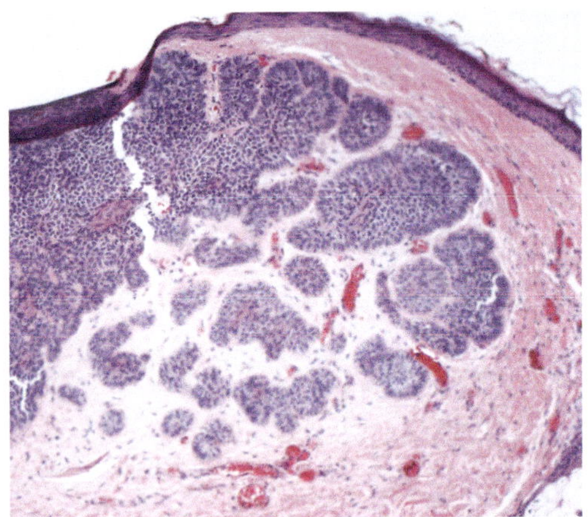

FIG. 1: Histology of nodular basal cell carcinoma immediately following pulsed-dye laser (PDL) treatment, showing selective coagulation of the feeding blood vessels surrounding and infiltrating between the tumor nests.

pulse duration, a 10-mm spot size with 10% overlap of pulses and double stacked pulses with no dynamic cooling. Results showed two out of eight lesions with no residual tumor, representing a clearance rate of 25% for Group 1—similar to the clearance rate of 28% seen in the control group that received no laser treatment. In comparison, group 2 had a clearance rate of 71% (five out of seven lesions). Of note, both treatments arms led to some degree of scarring.[22]

Based on these initial investigations, further studies sought to investigate the use of the neodymium-doped yttrium aluminum garnet (Nd:YAG) laser as solo therapy or in combination with PDL as well as the use of other vascular specific lasers such as the 755 nm alexandrite. It was hypothesized that the use of a combination PDL and Nd:YAG would selectively target the superficial and deep vasculature of the tumor, respectively. In addition, PDL converts hemoglobin to deoxyhemoglobin which is a prime target for the Nd:YAG. The use of these two lasers successively was theorized to potentially improve clearance rates.

Jalian et al. performed a study where ten subjects with 13 biopsy-proven BCCs received four combined PDL and Nd:YAG treatments at 2–4 week intervals. Seven of twelve tumors (58%) showed a complete response. When size was taken into account, 75% of all tumors less than 1 cm in diameter showed complete response. Notably, the authors found that all subjects with incomplete responses were on various forms of anticoagulation, which may impede intravascular coagulation after laser irradiation.[23] Ibrahimi et al. sought to use the 755 nm alexandrite laser hypothesizing that its deeper penetrating wavelength would reach some of the deeper-seated vessels not reached by PDL leading to higher clearance rates. This particular study in a patient with basal cell nevus syndrome (BCNS) treated a total of 18 clinically apparent BCCs. The parameters were two passes at an energy of 100 J/cm^2, pulse length of 3 milliseconds, no dynamic cooling mode and 8 mm spot size. It is important to reference that patients with BCNS typically have more aggressive forms of BCC, which may pose a challenge in terms of clearance with lasers. Due to the total number of tumors, biopsies were not performed prior to laser treatment and hence the histologic subtype(s) were not identified. At 2- and 7-month clinical follow-up visits, fifteen of eighteen of laser treated lesions showed a complete clinical response.[24]

The solo use of 1,064 nm Nd:YAG due to its deeper penetration and affinity for arterial vasculature has also been explored. One study, using a continuous-wave 1,064 nm Nd:YAG laser for the treatment of BCC reported a 97.3% clearance rate in 36 subjects after 2–4 treatments. The delivery of continuous rather than pulsed light primarily causes thermal damage due to bulk heating. This can lead to burns and subsequent scarring. In this study, 11% of patients developed a depressed scar.[25] In contrast, selective photothermolysis causes destruction to a preferential target thereby

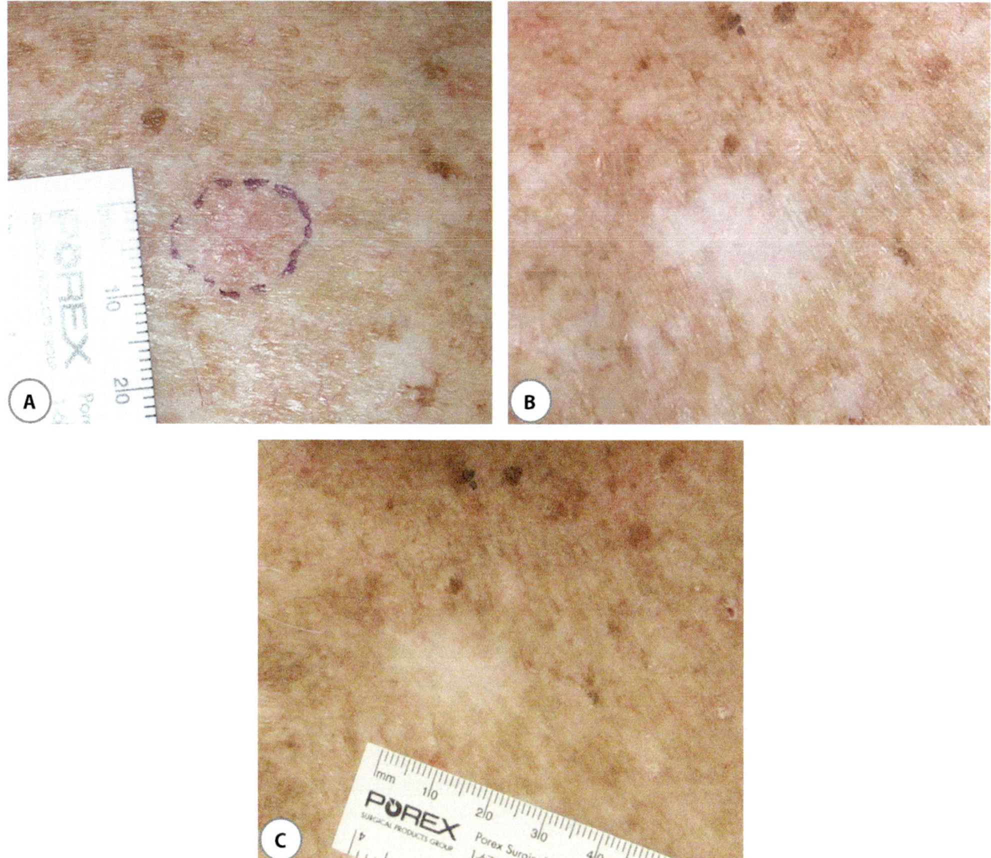

FIGS. 2A TO C: Basal cell carcinoma (BCC) on the chest before pulsed-dye laser (PDL) treatment (A). Six months (B) and 1 year (C) follow-up pictures after 4 PDL treatments showing complete disappearance of the BCC with no recurrence.

sparing local surrounding tissue. Ortiz et al. conducted a clinical study to assess efficacy of long-pulsed 1,064 nm Nd:YAG laser using high fluence in the treatment of BCCs on the trunk and extremities. Parameters consisted of a 5 mm spot size, fluence of 80 or 120 J/cm^2, a pulse duration of 10 milliseconds and no epidermal cooling. Three passes were performed on the visible tumor and a 4 mm margin of adjacent skin in addition to three stacked pulses to the center of the tumor. BCC tumors had a 92% (12 of 13 BCC tumors) histologic clearance rate after one treatment with the long-pulsed 1,064 nm Nd:YAG laser. The clearance rate increased to 100% (10 of 10 BCC tumors) after the fluence was increased from 80 to 120 J/cm^2.[26]

The use of water as a chromophore with ablative lasers in the treatment of NMSCs has been reported. Clinical studies to date have shown relative success. The literature suggests more research has been conducted with the traditional ablative CO_2 laser when compared to Erbium YAG. Combination treatments such as traditional ablative CO_2 and PDT have also been reported. These lasers work by ablating tissue through the vaporization of tissue water. Optimal outcomes occur when the target is vaporized with minimal nonspecific collateral damage to the surrounding tissue. Er:YAG lasers have a higher affinity for water and thus, less penetration depth per pass when compared to CO_2 lasers, which may influence clearance rates. Humphreys et al. set out to determine whether a pulsed CO_2 laser could effectively ablate superficial multifocal basal cell carcinoma and squamous cell carcinoma in situ (SCCIS). Seventeen BCCs and thirteen SCCs were treated with 2–3 passes of a pulsed CO_2 laser (500 mJ, 2–4 W). A 3 mm rim of surrounding skin was also treated. The treated areas were subsequently excised and histologically analyzed. The authors reported an average tumor thickness of SCC in situ that extended significantly deeper than that of superficial BCC (0.57 vs. 0.34 mm; $p = 0.01$). Results showed complete clearance for 9 of 9 patients with sBCC treated with 3 passes. Residual deep margin involvement was seen in 5 of 8 patients with sBCC treated with 2 passes ($p = 0.005$). Incomplete clearance with SCC IS was reported in both arms: 3 of 7 patients treated with 3 passes and in 2 of 6 patients treated with 2 passes. The SCCs incompletely treated were significantly thicker than those with complete clearance (0.65 vs. 0.41 mm; $p = 0.01$). Positive lateral margins were seen in 1 BCC and 3 SCC specimens.[27] Horlock et al. treated fifty-one BCCs (21 superficial, 28 nodular and 2 infiltrative types), ranging from 4 to 35 mm, with a carbon dioxide laser. They concluded that BCCs of the superficial type could be dependably cleared but these findings were not so for nBCC. They did, however, note complete ablation in a subset of nodular BCCs less than 10 mm suggesting size may influence response rates.[28]

Other studies have shown good treatment outcomes with the use of fully ablative CO_2 lasers in the treatment of BCC.[29-31] The use of erbium lasers in the treatment of BCCs has not been widely studied when compared to carbon dioxide lasers. Šmucler and Vic set out to determine effectiveness of reducing tumor mass with Er:YAG laser ablation. Three methods for the treatment of recurring nodular basal cell carcinomas were employed: PDT with topical application of ALA methyl ester, solitary Er:YAG laser ablation, and Er:YAG laser ablation followed by PDT with topical application of ALA methyl ester. The combination therapy was the most effective treatment with clearance rates of 98.97% versus 94.85% (PDT only) and 91.75% (Er:YAG laser only) Owing to the simplicity of treatment, 67% of patients preferred solitary Er:YAG laser treatment over the PDT method (20%) and the combined treatment (13%).[32] Ablative fractional laser treatments have also been shown to enhance outcomes when combined with PDT in the treatment of BCCs.[33-35] A major limiting factor in treating NMSC with PDT is the depth of penetration of the photosensitizer (5-aminolevulinic acid). Lippert et al. conducted a study where 56 nBCCs received fractionated carbon dioxide laser prior to ALA-PDT and another 56 nBCCs received curettage prior to PDT. Fifty-two of 56 nBCCs in the fractional laser treatment group were successfully treated, compared with only 45 of 56 in the control group.[33] In comparison, Haak et al. conducted a study with 32 facial nodular BCCs of a diameter >15 mm were randomized into two groups: (1) Fractional ablative CO_2 with PDT (AFXL-PDT) or PDT alone. Of note, all tumors were debulked prior. Histology 12 months posttreatment showed similar tumor clearance after AFXL-PDT (63%, 10 of 16) and PDT (56%, 9 of 16) and thus no superior method was elucidated in this study.[34]

There is limited data in the literature with respect to laser use in cutaneous SCCs when compared to BCCs. Data is even more scarce with respect to the use of vascular specific lasers in the treatment of cutaneous SCC.

Pulsed-dye laser has been used to target tumor vasculature in treating glottal dysplasia[36] and SCCIS using 585 nm PDL. In one study, the 585 nm PDL was used in conjunction with 5-aminolevulanic acid on cutaneous SCC in situ at an energy level of 10 J/cm^2 and a 7 mm spot size with a 5 mm treatment margin. Thirteen patients with a total of 17 lesions were treated. Of the 17 lesions treated, 14 (82%) exhibited a complete clinical response at 1 year.[37] In the Tran et al. study, previously referenced above, patients with 23 biopsy-proven BCCs and SCCIS were utilized. The lesions measured 0.4–3 cm in size and were located on the trunk and extremities. The lesions were randomly placed into three study arms: a control group (no treatment), first treatment group (S1), and second treatment group (S2). In the control group, 2/7 lesions showed complete clearance. The S1 treatment arm had 2/8 lesions with complete clearance–a clearance rate of 25%. The S2 treatment group had a clearance rate of 71% (5/7). The results here may suggest that a deeper penetrating spot size and pulse stacking may increase clearance rates of NMSC with PDL.[22]

Some success with ablative lasers in the treatment of SCCs-in-situ has been documented. Martinez-Gonzalez et al. recruited 44 patients with 48 biopsy proven SCCIS. The lesions were treated with one or more passes of super-pulsed CO_2 laser at 2 W/cm^2. Of note, the number of passes needed was determined clinically during the treatment. Postprocedure assessment was performed at weeks 2 and 4, and then every 6 months (range 8–52 months). Clearance after one treatment was seen in 86.3% of cases, of these, 7.9% developed recurrence of the lesion. Clearance after more than one treatment was seen in an additional 11.3% of the cases. The authors noted a total response rate of 97.6%.[38] Fader and Lowe sought to optimize clearance rates in laser treated SCCIS present in hair-bearing areas. They found complete clearance in 3/3 patients with the concomitant use of high-energy pulsed CO_2 followed by high-energy diode. Preprocedure histopathologic evaluation showed full-thickness epidermal atypia with focal follicular extension. Postprocedure analysis revealed epidermal ablation with follicular necrosis. No evidence of recurrence was seen at 4 months and all patients had good cosmetic results.[39] Other small case series have also exhibited good efficacy with traditional ablative CO_2 lasers in the treatment of SCC *in situ*.[40-43]

Data is even more scarcer with the use of ablative fractional devices to treat SCCs. In one study, ten patients with Bowen's disease were enrolled to evaluate the efficacy of PDT with ablative carbon dioxide fractional laser. Five of the ten (50%) lesions showed a complete response (CR) after three PDT sessions. After four treatment sessions, the response rate increased to 90%. All lesions except one penile shaft lesion achieved a complete response.[44] Ko et al. evaluated twenty-one patients with a total of 58 Bowen's disease (BD) lesions in an effort to directly compare the efficacy of MAL-PDT with and without fractional ablative Er:YAG. The subjects received either one session of AFXL Er:YAG-PDT or two sessions of MAL-PDT 1 week apart. At 3 months, AFXL Er:YAG-PDT was more effective (93.8%) than MAL-PDT (73.1%), and the recurrence rate was significantly lower for AFXL Er:YAG -PDT (6.7%) than MAL-PDT (31.6%) at 12 months. Of note, no appreciable difference was noted with respect to cosmesis or safety (**Boxes 1** to **5**).[45]

Nguyen et al. with a follow-up study by Hsu et al. showed successful treatment with ablative fractional laser (AFXL)-assisted delivery of topical fluorouracil in the treatment of superficial basal cell carcinoma (sBCC) and SCCIS. Overall treatment success at a mean follow up of 15 months was 79–92% (11/12) for SCC IS and 67% (8/12) for sBCC.[46,47]

BOX 1: Pretreatment Considerations.

- Histologic subtype of NMSC
- Location: On or off the face
- Skin phototype
- Current Tan or Sunburn
- Medications: Anticoagulants (ASA, warfarin), isotretinoin
- Past medical history: HSV, MRSA, comorbidities
- Pain control
- Need for antiviral prophylaxis

(ASA: acetylsalicylic acid; HSV: herpes simplex virus; MRSA: methicillin-resistant *Staphylococcus aureus*)

BOX 2: Key consultation questions.

- Accutane use
- Use of anticoagulants
- HSV history
- History of previous actinic keratosis, other skin cancers or recurrent NMSC
- History of chronic UV exposure and sunburns
- History of keloids or hypertrophic scars

(HSV: herpes simplex virus; NMSC: nonmelanoma skin cancer; UV; ultraviolet rays)

BOX 3: Diagnostic tools.

- Preprocedure biopsy for clinical and histopathological typing
- Standardized photography
- Dermoscopy
- Imaging: Confocal laser scanning microscopy

BOX 4: Tips for efficacy.

- If medically possible, place a perioperative hold on aspirin and anticoagulants
- When applicable, apply the theory of selective photothermolysis to target specific structures such as hemoglobin in blood vessels and avoid complications from bulk heating such as ulceration and scarring

BOX 5: Treatment complications.

- Infection
- Dyschromia
- Scarring
- Ulceration
- Bruising
- Erythema
- Swelling

CONCLUSION

Nonmelanoma skin cancers are the most common cause of cancer worldwide and incidence continues to rise. Laser treatments for NMSCs have shown varying success. Studies investigating the use of visible and infrared light lasers for the treatment of NMSCs have shown mixed results. This in part may be secondary to varying approaches including tumor type, tumor size, tumor location, wavelength, spot size, fluence, pulse duration, pulse stacking, use of cooling, and the use of anticoagulation by the subjects. Various methods to test clearance (clinical assessment, biopsy, and excision) were also employed and thus, no standardized methodology for comparison was identified. Controversy exists as to whether superficial BCCs respond better to laser secondary to its superficial nature or its lack of response due to the lack of robust vasculature when compared to the nodular variant. With respect to SCCs, they possess a thicker stratum corneum and are more dysplastic and typically extend deeper into the dermis than BCCs[1] and thus, these histological differences may render laser treatments less effective when treating the former.

With the increasing incidence of actinic keratosis and nonmelanoma skin cancers, it is prudent to develop other treatment options for those whose cancers are not amenable to current therapies due to factors such as location, size, comorbidities, sheer number of lesions in conditions such as BCNS or eruptive keratoacanthomas or those who elect alternatives due to scar risks. Arguably, the use of lasers in the treatment of NMSCs and its precursor has shown promise. Based on the theory of selective photothermolysis, lasers can be used to selectively target the tumor's vascular supply without collateral destruction of normal surrounding tissue. Ablative lasers have been documented as well, but likely carry a higher risk of scarring, dyschromia and atrophy secondary to its mechanism of action. Current literature suggests ablative fractional laser (AFL) and AFL-assisted combination chemotherapy may represent promising treatment modalities for non-melanoma skin cancer.[48-52]

Factors such as size and type of the tumor, laser wavelength, energy, and pulse duration, location, and the presence of anticoagulation can all impact the outcomes. Adverse events such as bleeding, infection, dyschromia and scarring have been reported. Bearing in mind the aforementioned studies were pilot studies with varying parameters, further research is needed to determine which vascular specific and/or ablative laser(s) are optimal alternatives to conventional therapy to help standardize treatment parameters for optimal outcomes. Dissimilarities in treatment protocols referenced above preclude the determination of a standard method.

In authors' opinion, the most promising lasers for treatment of basal cell carcinomas are vascular specific lasers, specifically pulsed dye laser, utilizing the theory of selective photothermolysis. However, increasing the fluences of these vascular lasers will produce bulk heating and loss of vascular selectivity, with resulting scar formation, as seen with ablative lasers. Although the PDL is limited in depth of penetration, it has proven to be very effective in treating all types of BCC. PDL induces coagulation of the superficial vessels resulting in a cascade of coagulation that reaches the deeper connecting vessels associated with the tumor, with selective destruction of the tumor lobules and with no surrounding histologic fibrosis or clinical scarring.

REFERENCES

1. Rigel DS, Cockerell CJ, Carucci J, Wharton J. Actinic Keratosis, Basal Cell Carcinoma, Squamous Cell Carcinoma. In: Bolognia J, Jorizzo J, Rapini R (Eds). Dermatology, 2nd edition. St. Louis: Mosby Elsevier; 2008. pp. 1641-59.
2. Rigel DS, Friedman RJ, Kopf AW. Lifetime risk for development of skin cancer in the US population: current estimate is now 1 in 5. J Am Acad Dermatol. 1996;35(6):1012-3.
3. American Cancer Society. Key Statistics for Basal and Squamous Cell Skin Cancers. [online] Available from https://www.cancer.org/cancer/basal-and-squamous-cell-skin-cancer/about/key-statistics.html. Accessed June 2017.
4. Guy GP Jr, Machlin SR, Ekwueme DU, Yabroff KR. Prevalence and costs of skin cancer treatment in the U.S., 2002-2006 and 2007-2011. Am J Prev Med. 2015;48(2):183-7.
5. Katz TM, Goldberg LH, Marquez D, Kimyai-Asadi A, Polder KD, Landau JM, et al. Nonablative fractional photothermolysis for facial actinic keratoses: 6-month follow-up with histologic evaluation. J Am Acad Dermatol. 2011;65(2):349-56.
6. Weiss ET, Brauer JA, Anolik R, Reddy KK, Karen JK, Hale EK, et al. 1927-nm fractional resurfacing of facial actinic keratoses: a promising new therapeutic option. J Am Acad Dermatol. 2013;68(1):98-102.
7. Iyer S, Friedli A, Bowes L, Kricorian G, Fitzpatrick RE. Full face laser resurfacing: therapy and prophylaxis for actinic keratoses and non-melanoma skin cancer. Lasers Surg Med. 2004; 34:114-9.
8. Hantash BM, Stewart DB, Cooper ZA, Rehmus WE, Koch RJ, Swetter SM. Facial resurfacing for nonmelanoma skin cancer prophylaxis. Arch Dermatol. 2006;142:976-82.
9. Jiang SB, Levine VJ, Nehal KS, Baldassano M, Kamino H, Ashinoff RA. Er:Yag laser for the treatment of actinic keratoses. Dermatol Surg. 2000;26:437-40.
10. Ostertag JU, Quaedvlieg PJ, Neumann MH, Krekels GA. Recurrence rates and long-term follow-up after laser resurfacing as a treatment for widespread actinic keratoses on the face and scalp. Dermatol Surg. 2006;32:261-7.

11. Gan SD, Hsu SH, Chuang G, Konnikov N, Liang CA. Ablative fractional laser therapy for the treatment of actinic keratosis: A split-face study. J Am Acad Dermatol. 2016;74(2):387-9.
12. Wenande E, Olesen UH, Nielsen MM, Janfelt C, Hansen SH, Anderson RR, et al. Fractional laser-assisted topical delivery leads to enhanced, accelerated and deeper cutaneous 5-fluorouracil uptake. Expert Opin Drug Deliv. 2017;14(3): 307-17.
13. Togsverd-Bo K, Haak CS, Thaysen-Petersen D, Wulf HC, Anderson RR, Hædersdal M. Intensified photodynamic therapy of actinic keratoses with fractional CO_2 laser: a randomized clinical trial. Br J Dermatol. 2012;166(6):1262-9.
14. Kessels JP, Nelemans PJ, Mosterd K, Kelleners-Smeets NW, Krekels GA, Ostertag JU. Laser-mediated Photodynamic Therapy: an Alternative Treatment for Actinic Keratosis? Acta Derm Venereol. 2016;96(3): 351-4.
15. Velasco P, Lange-Asschenfeldt B. Dermatological aspects of angiogenesis. Br J Dermatol 2002; 147(5):841-52.
16. AndersonRR, ParrishJA. Selective photothermolysis: precise microsurgery by selective absorption of pulsed radiation. Science. 1983; 220(4596):524-7.
17. Bedlow AJ, Stanton AW, Cliff S, Mortimer PS. Basal cell carcinoma—an in-vivo model of human tumour microcirculation. Exp Dermatol. 1999;8(3):222-6.
18. Allison KP, Kiernan MN, Waters RA, Clement RM. Pulsed dye laser treatment of superficial basal cell carcinoma: Realistic or not? Lasers Med Sci. 2003;18(2): 125-6.
19. Campolmi P, Mavilia L, Bonan P, Cannarozzo G, Lotti TM. 595 nm pulsed dye laser for the treatment of superficial basal cell carcinoma. Lasers Med Sci. 2005;20(3-4): 147-8.
20. Shah SM, Konnikov N, Duncan LM, Tannous ZS. The effect of 595 nm pulsed dye laser on superficial and nodular basal cell carcinomas. Lasers Surg Med. 2009;41(6):417-22.
21. Konnikov N, Avram M, Jarell A, Tannous Z. Pulsed dye laser as a novel non-surgical treatment for basal cell carcinomas: response and follow up 12–21 months after treatment. Lasers Surg Med. 2011;43(2):72-8.
22. Tran HT, Lee RA, Oganesyan G, Jiang SB. Single treatment of non-melanoma skin cancers using a pulsed-dye laser with stacked pulses. Lasers Surg Med. 2012;44(6):459-67.
23. Jalian HR, Avram MM, Stankiewicz KJ, Shofner JD, Tannous Z. Combined 585nm pulsed-dye and 1,064nm Nd:YAG lasers for the treatment of basal cell carcinoma. Lasers Surg Med. 2014;46(1):1-7.
24. Ibrahimi OA, Sakamoto FH, Tannous Z, Anderson RR. 755 nm alexandrite laser for the reduction of tumor burden in basal cell Nevus syndrome. Lasers Surg Med. 2011;43(2): 68-71.
25. El-Tonsy MH, El-Domyati MM, El-Sawy AE, El-Din WH, Anbar T, Raouf D. Continuous-wave HA, Nd:Yag laser hyperthermia: a successful modality in treatment of basal cell carcinoma. Dermatol Online J. 2004;10(2):3.
26. Ortiz AE, Anderson RR, Avram MM. 1064nm long-pulsed Nd:YAG laser treatment of basal cell carcinoma. Lasers Surg Med. 2015;47(2):106-10.
27. Humphreys TR, Malhotra R, Scharf MJ, Marcus SM, Starkus L, Calegari K. Treatment of superficial basal cell carcinoma and squamous cell carcinoma in situ with a high-energy pulsed carbon dioxide laser. Arch Dermatol. 1998;134(10):1247-52.
28. Horlock N, Grobbelaar AO, Gault DT. Can the carbon dioxide laser completely ablate basal cell carcinomas? A histological study. Br J Plast Surg. 2000;53(4):286-93.
29. Campolmi P, Brazzini B, Urso C, Ghersetich I, Mavilia L, Hercogova J, et al. Superpulsed CO_2 laser treatment of basal cell carcinoma with intraoperatory histopathologic and cytologic examination. Dermatol Surg. 2002; 28:909-11.
30. Ebrahimi A, Rezaei M, Kavoussi R, Eidizadeh M, Madani SH, Kavoussi H. Superpulsed CO_2 laser with intraoperative pathologic assessment for treatment of periorbital basal cell carcinoma involving eyelash line. Dermatol Res Pract. 2014;2014:931657.
31. Kavoussi H, Ebrahimi A, Mansour R. Treatment and cosmetic outcome of superpulsed CO_2 laser for basal cell carcinoma. Acta Dermatovenerol Alp Pannonica Adriat. 2013;22:57-61.
32. Smucler R, Vlk M. Combination of Er. Yag laser and photodynamic therapy in the treatment of nodular basal cell carcinoma. Lasers Surg Med. 2008;40:153-8.
33. Lippert J, Smucler R, Vlk M. Fractional laser pretreatment increases the fluorescence and clinical effectiveness of ALA-PDT for the treatment of nBCC. Dermatol Surg. 2013;39(8):1202-8.
34. Haak CS, Togsverd-Bo K, Thaysen-Petersen D, Wulf HC, Paasch U, Anderson RR, et al. Fractional laser-mediated photodynamic therapy of high-risk basal cell carcinomas--a randomized clinical trial. Br J Dermatol. 2015;172(1):215-22.
35. Roozeboom MH, Aardoom MA, Nelemans PJ, Thissen MR, Kelleners-Smeets NW, Kuijpers DI, et alK. Fractionated 5-aminolevulinic acid photodynamic therapy after partial debulking versus surgical excision for nodular basal cell carcinoma: a randomized controlled trial with at least 5-year follow-up. J Am Acad Dermatol. 2013;69(2):280-7.

36. Zeitels SM, Franco RA Jr, Dailey SH, Burns JA, Hillman RE, Anderson RR. Office-based treatment of glottal dysplasia and papillomatosis with the 585-nm pulsed dye laser and local anesthesia. Ann Otol Rhinol Laryngol. 2004;113(4):265-76.
37. Britton JE, Goulden V, Stables G, Stringer M, Sheehan-Dare R. Investigation of the use of the pulsed dye laser in the treatment of Bowen's disease using 5-aminolaevulinic acid phototherapy. Br J Dermatol. 2005;153(4):780-4.
38. Martinez-Gonzalez MC, Pozo JD, Paradela S, Fernández-Jorge B, Fernández-Torres R, Fonseca E. Bowen's disease treated by carbon dioxide laser. A series of 44 patients. J Dermatolog Treat. 2008;19(5):293-9.
39. Fader DJ, Lowe L. Concomitant use of a high-energy pulsed CO_2 laser and a long-pulsed (810 nm) diode laser for squamous cell carcinoma in situ. Dermatol Surg. 2002;28:97-9.
40. Dave R, Monk B, Mahaffey P. Treatment of Bowen's disease with carbon dioxide laser. Lasers Surg Med. 2003;32:335.
41. Gordon KB, Robinson J. Carbon dioxide laser vaporization for Bowen's disease of the finger. Arch Dermatol. 1994;130:1250-2.
42. Gordon KB, Garden JM, Robinson JK. Bowen's disease of the distal digit. Outcome of treatment with carbon dioxide laser vaporization. Dermatol Surg. 1996;22:723-8.
43. Tantikun N. Treatment of Bowen's disease of the digit with carbon dioxide laser. J Am Acad Dermatol. 2000;43:1080-3.
44. Kim SK, Park J, Song HS, Kim Y, Kim YC. Photodynamic Therapy with Ablative Carbon Dioxide Fractional Laser for Treating Bowen Disease. Ann Dermatol. 2013;25(3):335-9.
45. Ko DY, Kim KH, Song KH. A randomized trial comparing methyl aminolaevulinate photodynamic therapy with and without Er:YAG ablative fractional laser treatment in Asian patients with lower extremity Bowen disease: results from a 12-month follow-up. Br J Dermatol. 2014;170:165-72.
46. Nguyen BT, Gan SD, Konnikov N, Liang CA. Treatment of Superficial Basal Cell Carcinoma and Squamous Cell Carcinoma in Situ on the Trunk and Extremities With Ablative Fractional Laser-Assisted Delivery of Topical Fluorouracil. J Am Acad Dermatol. 2015;72(3):558-60.
47. Hsu SH, Gan SD, Nguyen BT, Konnikov N, Liang CA. Ablative Fractional Laser-Assisted Topical Fluorouracil for the Treatment of Superficial Basal Cell Carcinoma and Squamous Cell Carcinoma In Situ: A Follow-Up Study. Dermatol Surg. 2016;42(9):1050-3.
48. Wenande E, Olesen UH, Boesen MR, Persson DP, Lerche CM, Stürup S, et al. Laser-assisted delivery enhances topical uptake of the anticancer agent cisplatin. Drug Deliv. 2018;25(1):1877-85.
49. Wenande E, Tam J, Bhayana B, Schlosser SK, Ishak E, Farinelli WA, et al. Laser-assisted delivery of synergistic combination chemotherapy in in vivo skin. J Control Release. 2018;275:242-53.
50. Olesen UH, Clergeaud G, Lerche CM, Andresen TL, Haedersdal M. Topical delivery of vismodegib using ablative fractional laser and micro-emulsion formulation in vitro. Lasers Surg Med. 2019;51(1):79-87.
51. Togsverd-Bo K, Paasch U, Haak CS, Haedersdal M. Lesion dimensions following ablative fractional laser treatment in non-melanoma skin cancer and premalignant lesions. Lasers Med Sci. 2012;27(3):675-9.
52. Olesen UH, Clergeaud G, Hendel KK, Yeung K, Lerche CM, Andresen TL, et al. Enhanced and Sustained Cutaneous Delivery of Vismodegib by Ablative Fractional Laser and Microemulsion Formulation. J Invest Dermatol. 2020:140(10):2051-9.

28

CHAPTER

Photodynamic Therapy for Actinic Keratosis and Nonmelanoma Skin Cancer

Samantha L Schneider, David M Ozog

INTRODUCTION

Actinic Keratoses and Nonmelanoma Skin Cancer

Actinic keratosis (AK) and nonmelanoma skin cancer (NMSC) [specifically squamous cell carcinoma (SCC)] exist on a disease spectrum. AKs represent dysplastic keratinocytes in the epidermis related to chronic sun damage.[1] AKs are extremely common in the United States and have been estimated at ~40 million cases[2] in 2004 with an annual treatment cost of upward of 1 billion US dollars.[1] Similarly, AKs have been estimated as a diagnosis in >10% of dermatology visits.[1,2] They are thought to exist on a spectrum with SCC such that AKs have the potential to progress to SCC at a rate of 0.06% annually in elderly patients,[1] but ranges have been widely reported varying from <0.025% to 16% per year.[3] Actinic cheilitis is a related clinical entity that represents premalignant keratinocytes on the cutaneous lips that has the potential to progress to SCC.[4]

In the United States, NMSC represents the fifth most costly cancer to treat for medicare patients.[5] Nonmelanoma skin cancer consists primarily of basal cell carcinoma (BCC) and SCC. BCC is the most common type of skin cancer, particularly in Caucasian patients, and the incidence is continuing to grow.[6] This type of NMSC arises from the basal layer of the epidermis. It can have several different histologic subtypes including superficial, nodular/micronodular, and morpheaform (which is also known as sclerosing or infiltrative).[4] There are various risk factors for the development of BCC including ionizing radiation, chronic sun exposure, genetic variance/mutation, family history, and skin type (particularly type I). SCC is the second most common type of skin cancer and frequently arises on sun exposed areas and represents dysplastic epidermal keratinocytes.[7] Bowen's disease or SCC in situ (SCCIS) represents full-thickness epidermal atypia without dermal invasion,[4] whereas invasive SCC demonstrates disease in the dermis. SCC can arise de novo or can exist on a spectrum with AKs and Bowen's disease.[7]

Photodynamic Therapy

Photodynamic therapy (PDT) is a Food and Drug Administration (FDA)-approved treatment for nonhyperkeratotic AKs on the face and scalp.[4,8] PDT utilizes three components: A photosensitizer, light, and oxygen[4,9] to generate reactive oxygen species (ROS) within cells for selective destruction of premalignant or malignant cells.[4] The photosensitizer can be either endogenous or exogenous and topical or systemic.[4] The most common photosensitizer utilized for PDT is 5-aminolevulinic acid (5-ALA) or one of derivatives, mainly methyl aminolevulinate (MAL).[4] 5-ALA works as a photosensitizer through the creation of porphyrin intermediates, specifically protoporphyrin IX (PpIX) (**Fig. 1**). The rate limiting step of the heme biosynthesis pathway is the synthesis of ALA via ALA synthase; however, topical ALA application bypasses this enzyme leading to an excess of PpIX.[4] When exposed to a light source within its visible active light spectrum (peak at 400–410 nm and smaller peak at 635 nm) (**Fig. 2**), PpIX leads to the generation of ROS and ultimately cell death.[4,8] Neoplastic cells generate higher concentrations of PpIX due to their increased metabolic activity, which creates a selective destruction of these cells via the ROS.[3,4,8] As a derivative of 5-ALA, MAL gets demethylated in vivo to ALA via intracellular enzymes. The methyl group is the main advantage of MAL as it makes the molecule more lipophilic thereby enhancing penetration and ultimately leading to higher intracellular concentrations with a shorter incubation period.[4,10]

As aforementioned, PpIX has a strong absorption peak in the Soret band (405–415 nm) and additional smaller absorption peak bands from 500 to 635 nm.[4] Knowing the absorption spectrum of PpIX has allowed clinicians to determine the appropriate light sources to efficiently excite PpIX

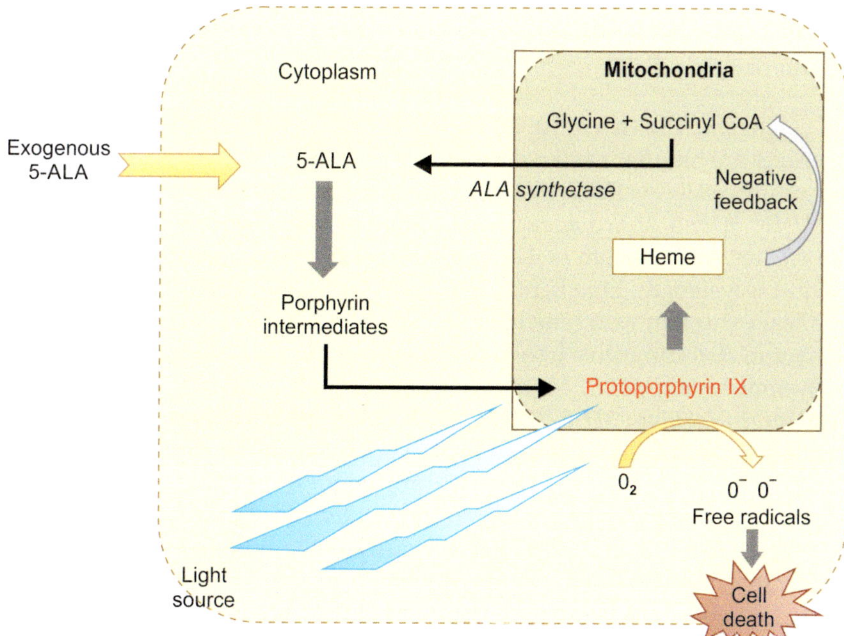

FIG. 1: Mechanism of action: 5-aminolevulinic acid (5-ALA) is a component of the heme biosynthetic pathway. It is the direct result of the rate limiting step involving the enzyme ALA synthetase. Applying exogenous 5-ALA bypasses the rate limiting step in the heme pathway leading to an access of this substrate in the cytoplasm of the cell. The excess 5-ALA leads to the creation of porphyrin intermediates including protoporphyrin IX (PpIX). The excess PpIX is the active target of photodynamic therapy ultimately leading to the creation of free oxygen radicals and cell death.

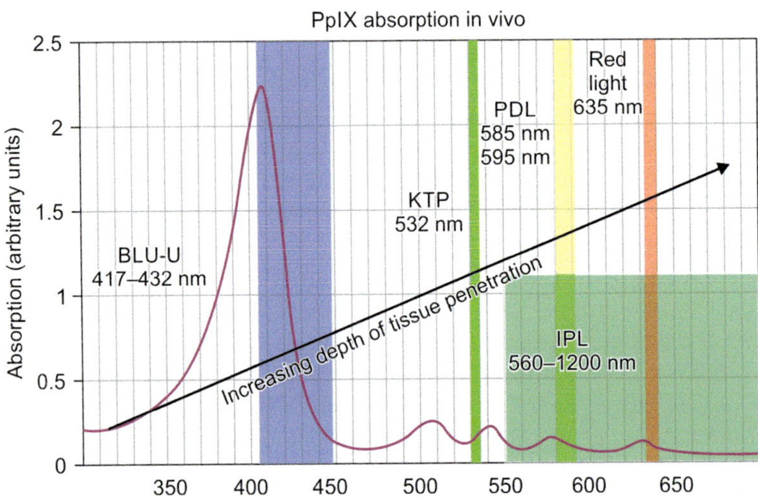

FIG. 2: PpIX absorption in vivo: PpIX is the photoactive substrate utilized in photodynamic therapy. It has activity within the visible active light spectrum. The first main peak of PpIX is at 400–410 nm and it has a smaller peak of activity at 635 nm. BLU-U targets the first main peak with activity from 417–432 nm whereas red light targets the second peak at 635 nm. As the wavelengths lengthen, the depth of tissue penetration increases thus red light penetrates deeper into the dermis than blue light photodynamic therapy.

and induce cell death. The two most widely used light sources are blue light and red light. A common commercially available blue light source, BLU-U© (Dusa Pharmaceuticals) (**Figs. 3A** to **C**), has a wavelength of 405 nm. Given the short wavelength, blue light has a more superficial treatment with penetration depths of ~2 mm. On the other hand, red light photodynamic therapy such as with the Aktilite© (Galderma) (**Figs. 3D** to **F**) has a longer wavelength at 635 nm allowing for deeper penetration (>2 mm) making it a more useful treatment for thicker lesions; however, red light PDT is not as efficient at exciting the PpIX molecules.[4] For a discussion of other commercially available light sources, please see **Table 1**.

When considering the light source, fluence (J/cm^2) and irradiance (mW/cm^2) are key concepts to keep in mind. Fluence needed will depend on the light source and will impact the time to photobleach. Photobleaching is defined as the loss of fluorescence of the photosensitizing agent after exposure to the light source. The effective photobleaching dose for a light source at 405 nm is 10 J/cm^2; whereas, a light source at 635 nm would require a 10-fold increase (100 J/cm^2) for a similar effect. This example demonstrates the importance of fluence because if the fluence for blue and red light were identical, blue light would take a lot less time than a treatment with red light.[4] Irradiance is similarly important to consider and should be kept within the range of 150-200 mW/cm^2 to avoid consuming too much oxygen too quickly thereby increasing the risk for tissue hypoxia.[4,11,12]

An additional light source under investigation is daylight. Daylight PDT was first described in the literature in 2008. The action spectrum of visible light is 380-780 nm which includes the absorption peaks of PpIX.[3,10]

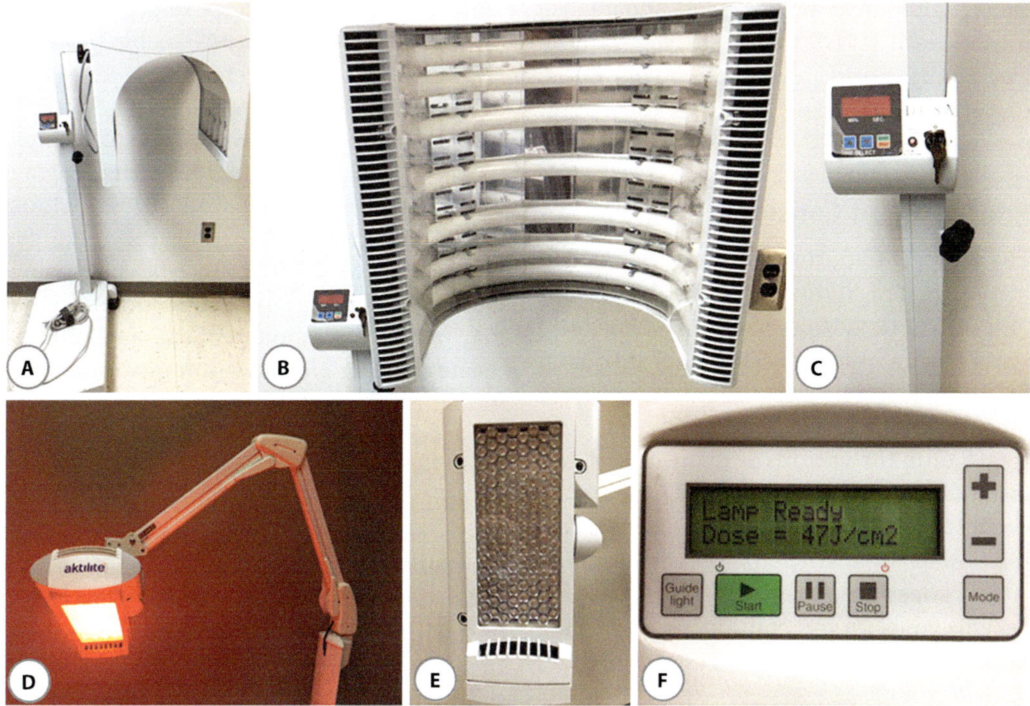

FIGS. 3A TO F: Panel A-C demonstrates images of the most frequently used commercial blue light device named the BLU-U©. Panels D-F illustrate the most common red light device used for photodynamic therapy named the Aktilite©.

Courtesy: David M Ozog, MD.

TABLE 1: Commercially available light sources. This table lists the most common commercially available PDT light sources.

	Company	Red light	Blue light	Comments
BLU-U©	Dusa Pharmaceuticals		X	Indicated for Aks with ALA
				Indicated for acne without photosensitizer
Aktilite CL 128©	Galderma	X		Cooling fan incorporated into device
				7–10 min to deliver
				37 J/cm^2 for MAL PDT
Clear light	CureLight		X	Indicated for acne
Omnilux blue	Omnilux		X	Indicated for acne
Omnnilux red	Omnilux	X		Indicated for NMSC and severe acne
				Can be used in combination with Omnilux Blue for mild-to-moderate acne or cystic acne

(ALA: aminolevulinic acid; MAL: methyl aminolevulinate; NMSC: nonmelanoma skin cancer; PDT: photodynamic therapy)

Other light sources include lasers and intense pulsed light (IPL), which utilize specific wavelengths and ranges of wavelengths, respectively, to target the PpIX absorption peaks (**Table 2**).[4,13-15]

Pretreatment Considerations

The only FDA-approved indication for PDT in the United States is for the treatment of nonhyperkeratotic AKs on the face and scalp with a blue light source;[4,8] however, PDT is used for a variety of other therapies off-label and we have performed over 6,000 treatments for various indications at our institution. PDT can be used for AKs, actinic cheilitis, superficial NMSC, photoaging, acne, rosacea, sebaceous hyperplasia, verrucae, and "field cancerization".[4,10,15-19] In this chapter, we will focus on the common uses of PDT for AKs, actinic cheilitis, NMSC, and "field cancerization."

When considering the use of PDT for the aforementioned conditions, it is important to consider the location of the target and surface area involved. For example, PDT for AKs is highly effective, particularly on the head and neck. It has similar or improved efficacy compared to other FDA-approved treatments with better cosmesis.[1,4]

Furthermore, PDT is useful when a large surface area needs to be treated. "Field cancerization" refers to an area with diffuse photodamage with multiple actinic keratosis admixed with SCCIS and likely high p53 mutations throughout. It is challenging to treat with nonfield modalities such as liquid nitrogen or other physical methods. Additionally, Mohs surgery can be challenging when SCC arises since superficial atypia may be present in much of the surrounding tissue making clear pathological margins difficult. PDT can be a valuable adjunct in these areas of high photodamage (such as the scalp, face, or upper extremities) to reduce keratinocyte atypia and potentially prevent future AKs or NMSC. The goal of therapy is to reduce any visible photodamage, AKs, and treat subclinical lesions as well.[10] For cases of superficial NMSC, patients can be initially treated with field therapy either as a definitive treatment or to clear the background area prior to surgery (**Figs. 4A** and **B**). Multiple treatment options can be considered depending on the clinical scenario including repeat treatment with PDT, surgical excision, electrodessication and curettage (ED&C), Mohs or biopsy for invasive disease.[4] Additionally, although SCCIS is uncommon in children, PDT has been successfully used as a treatment modality in

TABLE 2: Laser light sources for PDT: In addition to commercially available light sources, clinicians can utilize lasers to target the PpIX absorption peaks. This table highlights some of the more common lasers utilized for PDT as well as their wavelengths.

Laser	Wavelength (nm)
Tunable argon dye laser	450–530
Copper vapor laser-pumped dye laser	510–574
Long-pulse pulsed dye laser	585–595
Nd:YAG KTP dye laser	532
Gold vapor laser	629
Solid-state diode laser	630

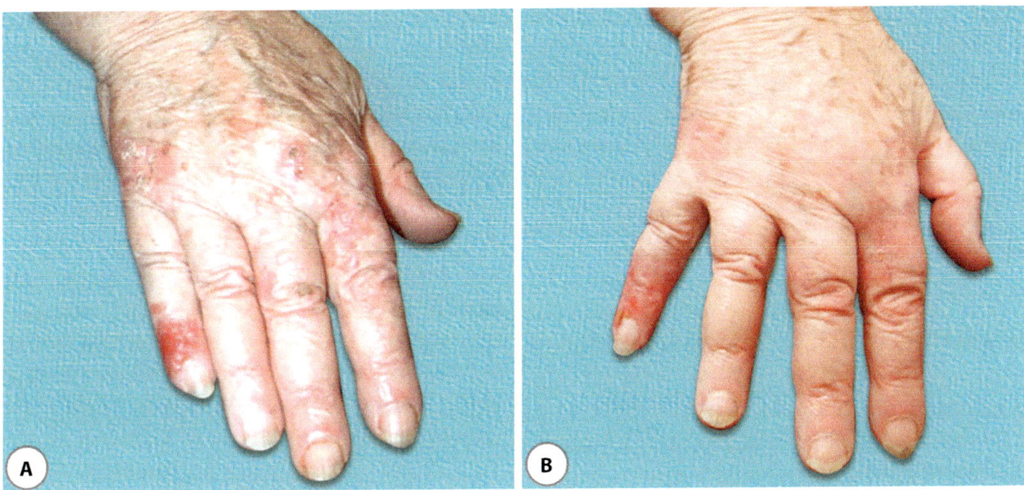

FIGS. 4A AND B: (A) Right hand with multiple Bowen disease; and (B) after two session of PDT using 20% aminolevulinic acid and blue light combined with pulse-dyed laser. Of note, the residual lesion on the fifth digit was treated with Mohs surgery.
Courtesy: David M Ozog, MD.

this patient population.[9,20] Similarly, PDT has been studied in children with BCCs and found to be safe and efficacious.[21-23]

There are multiple advantages of PDT as compared to surgical interventions including covering a large surface area, which allows for treatment of subclinical lesions. There is little to no risk of scarring even with treating such a large area. Patients have faster recovery and improved cosmesis compared to surgical excision and cryotherapy. Overall, patients prefer PDT over 5-fluorouracil (5-FU) or imiquimod.[4,24] An additional potential benefit that is still being explored involves BCC antibody protection with PDT treatment. Researchers have found that after treatment with PDT, patients develop antibodies to proteins in the sonic hedgehog signaling pathway, which is important in the genesis of BCC tumors. It has been hypothesized that these antibodies may improve the efficacy of treatment and may even decrease recurrence rates.[4,25]

Key Consultation Questions

There are important concepts to consider when determining whether to utilize PDT. The contraindications for PDT include the following: History of photosensitizing disorder, porphyrias, or documented allergy to ALA or MAL, planned sun exposure within the next 48 hours, isotretinoin use in the last 6 months, and pregnancy.[4,9] We do not recommend herpes simplex virus (HSV) prophylaxis prior to treatment. There is likely different immune pathway activation with PDT versus ablative laser injury to tissue. At our institution, we have not had a case of herpetic outbreak attributed to PDT in over 6,000 treatments. Additionally, any hyperkeratotic skin conditions (such as seborrheic dermatitis) should be optimized prior to treatment as the hyperkeratosis can absorb the ALA making the treatment less effective. Lastly, it is important to keep in mind that PDT is not an effective treatment for invasive SCC. Biopsies must be performed on clinically suspicious lesions. Characteristics of SCC that should preclude treatment with PDT include an SCC > 2 cm, lesions with multiple histologic subtypes present, and lesions with any dermoscopic characteristics of invasive SCC.[4]

MANAGEMENT

Treatment Options

In the United States, conventional PDT is performed with ALA while MAL is widely available worldwide. ALA is available as a 20% solution called Levulan Kerastick© that is packaged as two sealed glass ampules within a cardboard tube. One ampule contains 354 mg of δ-ALA hydrochloride powder and the other contains 1.5 mL of solvent that mix together upon breaking the glass immediately before use. Additionally, ALA has been recently approved by the FDA as a 10% gel preparation called Ameluz© (**Figs. 5A** and **B**). MAL is available in Europe and comes as a 16.8% cream.[4,8]

When performing PDT, there are several steps to perform which will increase efficacy (**Box 1**). First, patients should be cleansed to ensure uniform penetration of the photosensitizing agent. This is commonly performed with acetone but hibiclens, soaps, alpha-hydroxy/salicyclic acid cleansers, or towelettes are alternatives.[3,4] After cleansing, the stratum corneum is typically irritated to increase penetration of the photosensitizing agent most commonly via gauze abrasion, which consists of a 4×4 gauze pad rubbed on the skin. Other methods include oscillating brushes, microdermabrasion,[26] microneedling,[27] or fractional nonablative or ablative laser.[4,28-31] Next, the photosensitizing agent (either ALA or MAL) is applied with cotton-tipped applicators or a gloved hand. Two coats ensures even application. If the extremities are being treated, occlusion with plastic wrap or a warm blanket can help increase penetration and ultimately efficacy.[32,33] Ideally, the medication is then left to incubate with the patient in a dark room. Times dependent upon the clinical indication for treatment with times ranging from 1 to 4 hours if blue or red light devices are used (**Table 3**). If daylight PDT is employed, patients may begin exposure shortly after application. AKs on the face should incubate for 1–2 hours, the scalp for 2 hours, and the extremities for 3 hours prior to blue or red light treatment.[4]

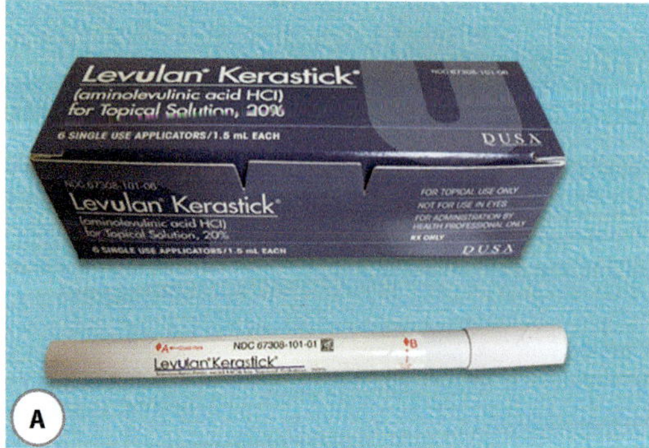

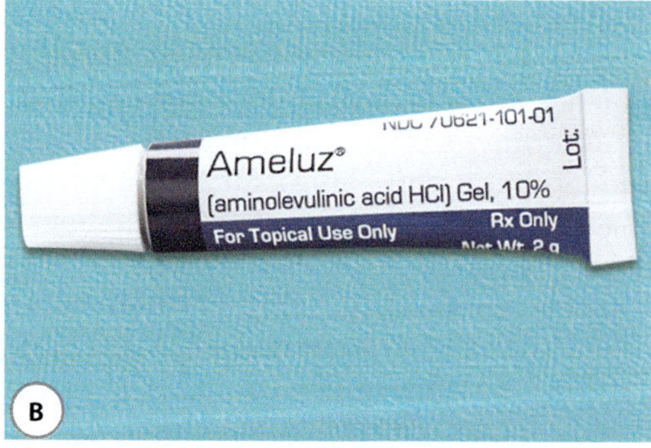

FIGS. 5A and B: Available preparations of aminolevulinic acid (ALA) in the United States. Panel A illustrates the classic preparation of the Levulan Kerastick© and panel B represents a new FDA-approved preparation of ALA gel called Ameluz©.

BOX 1: Protocol for photodynamic therapy (PDT): This Box outlines a general protocol that clinicians can use for performing PDT.

Protocol for photodynamic therapy:

- Wash the treatment area. Options include: Acetone, hibiclens, alcohol, soaps, alpha-hydroxy/salicyclic acid cleansers, or towelettes
- Irritate the stratum corneum (optional). Options include gauze abrasion, oscillating brushes, microdermabrasion, microneedling, or fractional nonablative or ablative laser
- Apply (ALA or MAL) in an even layer using a gloved hand or cotton tipped applicators. Two layers allow for even application
- Incubate for up to 4 h-preferably in a dark room for treatment with red (best) or blue light. Daylight PDT requires minimal to no incubation period
- Wash with soap and water to remove residual photosensitizing agent
- Apply the activating light source or send patient outside with physical block sunscreen (daylight PDT)
- Discuss aftercare including avoidance of direct sunlight for 48 h, if using red/blue light activation
- Re-evaluate patients at 3 months for possible repeat treatment

TABLE 3: Photodynamic therapy treatment protocols: This table highlights the different topical photosensitizers utilized and the recommended incubation period for different clinical indications of photodynamic therapy. It also discusses the various light sources and dosing regimens by clinical indication.

Indication	Topical photosensitizer	Incubation period	Light source	Dosing	Additional information
Actinic keratosis	ALA	1–4 h	Blue light	10 J/cm^2	Requires 1–2 sessions
		1–4 h	Red light	75–150 J/cm^2	
		10–30 min	Daylight	1–3 h	Requires physical blockade sunscreen
	MAL	1–3 h	Red light	37–75 J/cm^2	
Bowen's disease	ALA	4 h	Red light	≥100 J/cm^2	Requires 2–3 sessions
	MAL	3 h	Red light	75–100 J/cm^2	
Superficial BCC	ALA	3–6 h	Red light	≥60 J/cm^2	Requires 2–3 sessions
	MAL	3 h	Red light	37–75 J/cm^2	

At the completion of the incubation time, wash the target area with soap and water which may remove excess photosensitizer. Then, the patient proceeds with treatment with the light source. The light source can be either blue or red light, but for many practitioners, red light has become the device of choice due to higher tissue penetration leading to improved efficacy. Eye protection is paramount for everyone present in the room to protect the retina and avoid cataracts from blue light exposure. It is important to discuss the after-treatment effects with the patients for realistic expectations (**Box 2**). Patients may develop erythema and edema related to the treatment. They should remain indoors from dawn until dusk for 36 hours after treatment as well as six feet from any window to avoid any additional activation by visible light. It is also recommended that patients cover the treated areas with opaque clothing as even a physical sunblock may not protect their skin from the visible light (unless it is applied in a thick opaque coating).[4] Patients should be reevaluated at 3 months and offered a repeat treatment if necessary.[3]

Daylight PDT has multiple advantages over conventional PDT including minimal incubation time, no additional equipment, and minimal clinical time required. Because patients are receiving their light source outside via natural sunlight, challenges include determining standard exposure times and treatment in inclement weather.[3,4] The most common procedure in Europe is MAL-PDT in combination with sunlight as visible light contains both blue and red light.

The protocol is as follows: The patient applies the ALA/MAL to the face and/or scalp using 1–2 g without occlusion for 10–30 minutes. After the incubation period, patients apply chemical sunscreen (to protect against UV light at 100–380 nm without physically blocking the sunlight) and proceed outside for 2 hours of

BOX 2: Patient home care instructions: This is a sample of patient home care instructions that practitioners can utilize to provide patients with a handout of information.

Patient home care instructions

On the day of treatment:

- Avoid direct sunlight for 36 h. This includes light from windows as well
- Wash your face twice daily with a gentle cleanser
- Apply a gentle noncomedogenic facial moisturizer frequently (up to four times daily)
- Swelling is a common side effect of the procedure and is most common around the eyes. It is also more obvious in the morning
- Your face may be red for the first 1–2 days
- For pain:
  - You can take pain medications such as ibuprofen per packaging instructions
  - You can apply ice packs to the treated areas for 5–10 min every 2–3 h. The cooling sensation helps minimize pain and reduces swelling

Over the next week:

- Wash your face twice daily with a gentle cleanser
- Apply a gentle noncomedogenic facial moisturizer twice daily (to help alleviate the dry and tight feeling on your face)
- Your face may remain red throughout this next week
- Once the crusted lesions have healed, you may apply make-up to cover any residual redness
- Apply physical blocking sunscreen with either zinc oxide or titanium dioxide to protect your skin from the sun. Use a minimum of sun protective factor (SPF) 30

Please contact the office with any questions or concerns.

Note: The authors give permission for these recommendations to be used for patient handouts.

sunlight exposure to achieve the activating dose of light.[3,4,10] This is obviously not an exact science but patients can be counseled that the "tingling" feeling during daylight exposure will continue until all of the ALA/MAL is photobleached (used up). Importantly, sunny weather is not necessary for treatment but avoid treatment on rainy days. Given seasonal variance in sunlight, certain countries can perform daylight PDT throughout the year (i.e., Australia, Latin America, and Southern Europe); however, other countries should perform daylight PDT from March/April through September/October.[10] After the 2 hours of sunlight exposures, patients may wash off any residual photosensitizer. Daylight PDT is thought to limit the build-up of PpIX before (given the short incubation period) and during the treatment (via the longer exposure to lower energy visible light) all of which leads to decreased pain during treatment.[3,4]

Treatment Efficacy

PDT for the treatment of AKs is highly effective. The initial FDA studies demonstrated clearance rates of 85–90% after 1–2 treatments with good cosmesis.[8] As in other modalities, studies were performed primarily on facial lesions which have the highest overall response rate. A multicenter double-blind study of AKs treated with MAL-PDT found clearance rates of 67% after the first treatment and 90% after retreatment.[34] Furthermore, a Cochrane report found that ALA-PDT or MAL-PDT with blue or red light had similar efficacy in treating AKs but ALA-PDT with prolonged incubation times (4 h) had better cosmesis likely due to the significant peeling associated with longer incubation (and additional pain). The study also demonstrated that 4-hour incubation ALA-PDT was more efficacious than cryotherapy but 1 hour incubation was not significantly different from treatment with 5-FU. Lastly, the Cochrane review found that MAL-PDT had similar efficacy regardless of the light source used.[4,35] Additional studies have compared MAL-PDT (3-h incubation with broad-spectrum red light) for the treatment of AKs with cryotherapy (two freeze thaw cycles) and they found no significant difference in the treatment between groups but improved cosmesis with MAL-PDT.[36] The bottom line is that longer incubation improves efficacy but the cost is increased discomfort during treatment and brisk inflammatory response afterward. Most practices have moved to 1 hour or less incubation (at the cost of additional treatments) for that reason.

To improve efficacy, one can use multiple sequential light sources (i.e., intense pulsed light, pulse dye laser, blue light, and red light). Studies have shown improved efficacy compared to blue light treatment alone without an increase in adverse effects. The proposed mechanism is that the different light sources are activating the PpIX along different peaks of its absorption spectrum leading to improved efficacy.[4,15] However, this is impractical and time consuming for most offices.

Multiple studies have shown increased efficacy of PDT with pretreatment of lesions with ablative fractional laser. Ko et al. treated 236 facial AKs with MAL-PDT with half of the treatment group receiving pretreatment with 2,940 nm ablative fractional Erbium:yttrium-aluminum-garnet (Er:YAG) laser. The pre-treatment group demonstrated better treatment results at 1 year (86.9% vs. 61.2%) with a lower recurrence rate (9.7% vs. 26.6%).[4,37] A similar study of facial and scalp AKs treated with MAL-PDT (3 h-incubation) versus pretreatment with Er:YAG ablative fractional laser also had improved cure rates compared to traditional MAL-PDT (91.7% vs. 65.6%) at 1 year.[4,38] Another group combined fractional Er:YAG with daylight PDT in the treatment of AKs on the scalp, chest, and extremities in transplant patients. Pre-treatment with the

Er:YAG ablative fractional laser had the highest cure rate at 74% in 3 months.[4,39] This is a major clinical improvement and the evidence is strong. Equipment and cost/time is a limiting factor for most practices. It will be interesting to determine if needling with myriad inexpensive devices on the market will yield similar results.

It is important to note that AKs on the trunk are more challenging to treat with PDT and thus have decreased efficacy with standard treatment protocols. To improve efficacy, clinicians can increase the incubation time, curette the lesions prior to treatment, apply the photosensitizer under occlusion, pretreat with fractional ablation, utilize sequential laser and light sources, warm the skin during treatment, and/or pretreat with topical agents.[4]

Like the extremities, actinic cheilitis is not treated as effectively with conventional PDT (29–47% cure rate); however, laser-assisted PDT has a clearance rate of up to 85%.[4] Studies of ALA and MAL PDT with incubation times ranging from 2 to 4 hours using red light demonstrated a complete response in 62% of patients but histologic clearance was only 47%.[4,40] This is a much lower efficacy than standard treatment with surgical excision (96–99% cure) but it has much lower morbidity and pain as well. Choi et al. pretreated patients with actinic cheilitis with Er:YAG followed by MAL-PDT (one or two sessions 1 week apart). They found that pre-treatment with the ablative fractional laser was much more effective than even two sessions of MAL-PDT (85 vs. 29%) with lower recurrence rate at 1 year (8% vs. 50%).[4,28] Another group treated 19 patients with 595 nm pulsed dye laser with 1–3 treatments at 1 month intervals. They found a complete response rate of 68% after 1.8 treatments.[4,41] This combination of fractional laser and PDT is the first addition to the clinical armamentarium for actinic cheilitis in many years.

Bowen's disease (or SCCIS) is thought to have increased efficacy when treated with PDT compared to cryotherapy or 5-FU with an overall clearance rate of 80–82%.[4,42,43] Ko et al. also examined pretreatment of SCCIS lesions with fractional Er:YAG laser on the extremities followed by MAL-PDT and found that pretreatment with ablative fractional laser was significantly more effective than two treatments of MAL-PDT (93.8% vs. 73.1%) with a lower recurrence rate at 1 year (6.7% vs. 31.6%).[4,29] Other pretreatment lasers can be utilized including pulsed-dye laser with good efficacy and cosmesis (**Figs. 6A** to **D**).

Organ transplant patients represent a unique population that is at high risk of developing NMSC, particularly SCC. Cyclic PDT is a treatment regimen that involves repeating therapy every 4–8 weeks over a course of a year or more, which could culminate in 12–24 treatments total over that time period. It has been studied in solid organ transplant patients at 1–2 month intervals and has been shown to decrease the incidence of new lesions by 79% at 1 year and 95% at 2 years.[44] The European guidelines for topical PDT also found that a single treatment of MAL-PDT has the potential to delay the incidence of new NMSC in organ transplant patients by 9.8 months (compared to 6.7 months in controls).[4,45] It has been suggested that cyclic PDT in this patient population may be an effective method of reducing AKs and NMSC in this high risk patient population. This is an outstanding option for these patients and regular treatments should be considered for patients at high risk of SCC.

PDT is highly effective in the treatment of superficial BCCs (sBCC) with efficacy approaching that of simple excision.[4,21,46] Fernandez-Guarino et al. completed a 6-year longitudinal study of BCC lesions treated with MAL-PDT (2 sessions, and 2 weeks apart with red light) and they found a 95% cure rate

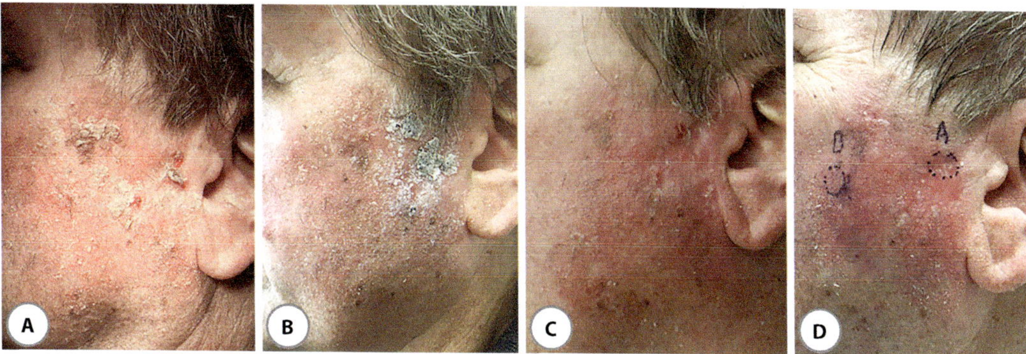

FIGS. 6A TO D: PDT for superficial NMSC: This patient presented with diffuse photodamage and multiple lesions of Bowen's disease on the left cheek extending to the preauricular area. Panel A demonstrates his initial presentation. He was treated with laser assisted red light PDT with the fractional CO_2 laser and his post-treatment is demonstrated in panel B. He was then treated with curettage and postcurettage is evident in panel C. He then received laser assisted ALA daylight PDT (with fractional CO_2 laser) with end results in Panel D when he presented for Mohs micrographic surgery to treat two residual lesions that were found to be superficial SCC (lesion A) and Bowen's disease (lesion B).

for sBCC, 49% for nodular BCC, and 46% for morpheaform BCC. Additionally, they found that certain anatomical areas (such as the cheeks and scalp) had higher response rates than others (such as the chin, lips, forehead, and temples). This study demonstrated that the histologic subtype of the BCC tumor is the most important factor in predicting the response.[4,47] Shkorollahi et al. examined combined therapy with fractional CO_2 laser and MAL-PDT in patients with BCCs on the head and neck of various histologic subtypes. They found a total recurrence free rate of 97.1% and that 88.1% of lesions required a single treatment. Their overall recurrence rate was 2.82% with 2/7 morpheaform lesions recurring.[4,30] Another group examined the efficacy of fractional CO_2 followed by PDT versus conventional PDT for high-risk nodular BCC, which was defined as morpheaform or infiltrative tumors, thick tumors (>7 mm), tumor diameter >15 mm on face, scalp and extremities and >20 mm on trunk, and tumors on central face. Patients were initially treated with tumor debulking, then proceeded with their treatment arm. The clinical cure rate was at 3 months was 100% for the CO_2 group versus 88% for conventional PDT and the recurrence rate at 1 year was 19% with CO_2 versus 44% with conventional CO_2 (however the histologic recurrence was 63% vs. 56%).[4,21] Clearly laser (or needling) assisted delivery of the photosensitizer yields consistently improved efficacy across all cutaneous malignancies. However, only results for superficial lesions have acceptable cure rates.

COMPLICATIONS

There are advantages to PDT making it a good treatment option for many patients; however, there are also a few disadvantages to consider including a large in-office time commitment, the potential need for multiple treatment sessions (versus one for standard therapies such as ED&C and surgical excision), and pain. The main adverse events associated with PDT include pain, phototoxicity, infection, and dyspigmentation. These are significantly less with incubation times under 1 hour and almost nonexistent for daylight PDT. There are other site specific complications such as erythema, burning, and swelling when treating actinic cheilitis.[4,28]

Pain is the most concerning adverse event. It is thought to occur due to an interaction between the inflammation caused by cell necrosis and myelinated A delta or unmyelinated C fibers. Most patients describe the pain as a burning sensation with a peak in discomfort within the first few minutes of treatment. The main factors that contribute to pain include the incubation time type of photosensitizer, location of lesions, type of lesion treated, type of light source utilized, rate of energy delivered, and number of sessions.[4] MAL-PDT is less painful than ALA-PDT. There are two main hypotheses for this difference in pain perception. The first is that MAL is more specifically absorbed by the atypical keratinocytes making it less painful due to less normal keratinocyte destruction. The second is that ALA is thought to be transported into nerve endings whereas MAL is not.[4,48] Lesions located in areas with higher density of nerve endings (such as the head and hands) as well as lesions with larger surface areas (>130 mm^2) tend to be more uncomfortable. Interestingly, AKs tend to be more painful to treat than Bowen's or BCC.[4] It is unclear whether this is solely related to larger areas of treatment for diffuse actinic keratosis versus focal SCCIS or sBCC.

Strategies to ameliorate the pain with PDT treatments include cool air, injectable anesthetics, interruption of treatment reducing irradiance, a protocol for in-office painless PDT, and daylight PDT (**Table 4**). Cool air helps with the discomfort during PDT by stimulating the A delta fiber, which inhibits pain transmission.[4] Strangeland and Kroon examined the effect of cool air on pain perception in PDT and found a statistically significant difference in overall pain scores at 3 and 9 minutes with the addition of air cooling devices in the treatment of AKs.[4,49] However, Tyrell et al. found that patients who utilized air cooled devices had significantly less photobleaching and reduced clinical clearance at 3 months.[4,50] Although uncommonly required, injectable anesthetics can be utilized to reduce pain either through nerve blocks or

TABLE 4: Methods to minimize pain during photodynamic therapy. Multiple methods exist to attempt to ameliorate pain during treatment. The most effective with the least impact on treatment efficacy is interruption of treatment with or without cold spray.

Method	Advantage	Limitations
Cool air	Minimizes pain	Reduces clinical efficacy
Interruption of treatment (breaks +/- cold spray)	• Minimizes pain • Cold spray does not decrease efficacy	Longer treatment session
Increase distance to device	Minimizes pain	• Reduces clinical efficacy • Longer treatment session due to decreased irradiance
Topical anesthetics	Not effective	
Injectable anesthetics	Minimal pain reduction	Not practical
Daylight photodynamic therapy	Minimizes pain	Weather limitations

local infiltration. It is important to avoid using a vasoconstrictor with the anesthesia to ensure adequate flow of oxygen to the treatment area. Paoli et al. performed unilateral facial nerve blocks for patients treated with PDT for AKs and found a significant reduction in pain scores in a side to side comparison (1.3 compared to 7.5).[4,51] Additionally, another group compared nerve blocks to cold air and found that nerve blocks are more effective at reducing pain; however, they require more time and are more costly.[4,52] Topical anesthetics have been studied in reducing pain in PDT including topical eutectic mixture of local anesthetics, lidocaine, tetracaine, and capsaicin, and these do not significantly ameliorate discomfort and are thus not recommended.[4,48] Furthermore, topical anesthetics can increase the penetration of MAL/ALA, which should be kept in mind to prevent overaggressive treatment. Interruption of treatment (at 3 min intervals) has been shown to help with pain reduction while maintaining efficacy. Some providers also utilize cold spray during the episodes of interruption.[4,53] Lastly, an in-office painless PDT protocol has been developed that works by limiting the buildup of PpIX before and during PDT. The protocol is as follows: 15-minutes incubation with ALA followed by 1 hour of blue light PDT. This protocol does need a larger study to definitively establish the protocol.[4]

Phototoxicity is very common with PDT with erythema and edema being the most common manifestations. These side effects peak 1–2 hours after irradiation and generally resolve within 1–2 weeks but can rarely persist for months.[4,54] Infection is a very rare complication; however, it is recommended to culture patients that have received PDT that present with increased pain and burning, which could mean a higher intensity of pain or pain that subsides after the procedure and then recurs during the postprocedure recovery. Additionally, these patients should be started on prophylaxis antibiotics to cover *Staphylococcus aureus.*[4,55] As aforementioned, HSV reactivation is rare and thus prophylaxis is not routinely recommended.[4] Dyspigmentation is another complication that can occur after treatment with PDT. It is more common when ALA is used as a photosensitizer and there is a higher incidence in phototypes IV–VI. Patients can develop hyper- or hypopigmentation and both generally resolve with time.[4,8] The potential for erythema and edema should be thoroughly discussed with patients. Fortunately, this reaction usually leads to significant improvement in lesions and cosmesis.

CONCLUSION

In the United States, PDT is only FDA-approved for nonhyperkeratotic AKs on the face and scalp; however, it is being studied for sBCC. Commonly PDT is used off-label for many indications including AKs, actinic cheilitis, field cancerization, and NMSC. Advantages of PDT include the ability to treat a large surface area with little risk of scarring and improved patient satisfaction. The main disadvantages include time commitment (by both the patient and the office staff) as well as equipment and the cost. The main side effect is pain which can be managed through in-office pain reduction strategies. In summary, PDT is a highly efficacious and well-tolerated treatment for AKs and NMSC.

REFERENCES

1. Siegel JA, Korgavkar K, Weinstock MA. Current perspective on actinic keratosis: a review. Br J Dermatol. 2017;177(2):350-8.
2. Bickers DR, Lim HW, Margolis D, Weinstock MA, Goodman C, Faulkner E, et al. The burden of skin diseases: 2004 a joint project of the American Academy of Dermatology Association and the Society for Investigative Dermatology. J Am Acad Dermatol. 2006;55(3):490-500.

3. See JA, Shumack S, Murrell DF, Rubel DM, Fernández-Peñas P, Salmon R, et al. Consensus recommendations on the use of daylight photodynamic therapy with methyl aminolevulinate cream for actinic keratoses in Australia. Australas J Dermatol. 2016;57(3):167-74.
4. Ozog DM, Rkein AM, Fabi SG, Gold MH, Goldman MP, Lowe NJ, et al. Photodynamic Therapy: A Clinical Consensus Guide. Dermatol Surg. 2016;42(7):804-27.
5. Chren MM, Sahay AP, Bertenthal DS, Sen S, Landefeld CS. Quality-of-life outcomes of treatments for cutaneous basal cell carcinoma and squamous cell carcinoma. J Invest Dermatol. 2007;127(6):1351-7.
6. Blixt E, Nelsen D, Stratman E. Recurrence rates of aggressive histologic types of basal cell carcinoma after treatment with electrodesiccation and curettage alone. Dermatol Surg. 2013;39(5):719-25.
7. Lansbury L, Bath-Hextall F, Perkins W, Stanton W, Leonardi-Bee J. Interventions for non-metastatic squamous cell carcinoma of the skin: systematic review and pooled analysis of observational studies. BMJ. 2013;347:f6153.
8. Babilas P, Schreml S, Landthaler M, Szeimies RM. Photodynamic therapy in dermatology: state-of-the-art. Photodermatol Photoimmunol Photomed. 2010;26(3):118-32.
9. Kumar N, Warren CB. Photodynamic therapy for dermatologic conditions in the pediatric population: a literature review. Photodermatol Photoimmunol Photomed. 2017;33(3):125-34.
10. Philipp-Dormston WG, Sanclemente G, Torezan L, Tretti Clementoni M, Le Pillouer-Prost A, Cartier H, et al. Daylight photodynamic therapy with MAL cream for large-scale photodamaged skin based on the concept of 'actinic field damage': recommendations of an international expert group. J Eur Acad Dermatol Venereol. 2016;30(1):8-15.
11. Calzavara-Pinton PG, Venturini M, Sala R. Photodynamic therapy: update 2006. Part 1: Photochemistry and photobiology. J Eur Acad Dermatol Venereol. 2007;21(3):293-302.
12. Peng Q, Warloe T, Berg K, Moan J, Kongshaug M, Giercksky KE, et al. 5-Aminolevulinic acid-based photodynamic therapy. Clinical research and future challenges. Cancer. 1997;79(12):2282-308.
13. Kalka K, Merk H, Mukhtar H. Photodynamic therapy in dermatology. J Am Acad Dermatol. 2000;42(3):389-413.
14. Clark C, Bryden A, Dawe R, Moseley H, Ferguson J, Ibbotson SH. Topical 5-aminolaevulinic acid photodynamic therapy for cutaneous lesions: outcome and comparison of light sources. Photodermatol Photoimmunol Photomed. 2003;19(3):134-41.
15. Friedmann DP, Goldman MP, Fabi SG, Guiha I. The effect of multiple sequential light sources to activate aminolevulinic Acid in the treatment of actinic keratoses: a retrospective study. J Clin Aesthet Dermatol. 2014;7(9):20-5.
16. Friedmann DP, Goldman MP, Fabi SG, Guiha I. A Retrospective Study of Multiple Sequential Light and Laser Sources to Activate Aminolevulinic Acid in the Treatment of Acne Vulgaris. Skinmed. 2017;15(2): 105-11.
17. Friedmann DP, Goldman MP, Fabi SG, Guiha I. Multiple sequential light and laser sources to activate aminolevulinic acid for rosacea. J Cosmet Dermatol. 2016;15(4):407-12.
18. Friedmann DP, Goldman MP, Fabi SG, Guiha I. Multiple sequential light and laser sources to activate aminolevulinic acid in the treatment of photodamage: A retrospective study. J Cosmet Dermatol. 2016;15(4): 407-12.
19. Rivard J, Ozog D. Henry Ford Hospital dermatology experience with Levulan Kerastick and blue light photodynamic therapy. J Drugs Dermatol. 2006;5(6): 556-61.
20. Hyun DJ, Seo SR, Kim DH, Yoon MS, Lee HJ. Periungual Bowen's Disease in a 12-Year-Old Boy Treated with Photodynamic Therapy. Pediatr Dermatol. 2016;33(2):e82-3.
21. Oseroff AR, Shieh S, Frawley NP, Cheney R, Blumenson LE, Pivnick EK, et al. Treatment of diffuse basal cell carcinomas and basaloid follicular hamartomas in nevoid basal cell carcinoma syndrome by wide-area 5-aminolevulinic acid photodynamic therapy. Arch Dermatol. 2005;141(1):60-7.
22. Girard C, Debu A, Bessis D, Blatiere V, Dereure O, Guillot B. Treatment of Gorlin syndrome (nevoid basal cell carcinoma syndrome) with methylaminolevulinate photodynamic therapy in seven patients, including two children: interest of tumescent anesthesia for pain control in children. J Eur Acad Dermatol Venereol. 2013;27(2):e171-5.
23. Loncaster J, Swindell R, Slevin F, Sheridan L, Allan D, Allan E. Efficacy of photodynamic therapy as a treatment for Gorlin syndrome-related basal cell carcinomas. Clin Oncol (R Coll Radiol). 2009;21(6):502-8.
24. Tierney EP, Eide MJ, Jacobsen G, Ozog D. Photodynamic therapy for actinic keratoses: survey of patient perceptions of treatment satisfaction and outcomes. J Cosmet Laser Ther. 2008;10(2):81-6.
25. Kabingu E, Oseroff AR, Wilding GE, Gollnick SO. Enhanced systemic immune reactivity to a Basal cell carcinoma associated antigen following photodynamic therapy. Clin Cancer Res. 2009;15(13):4460-6.

26. Kalisiak MS, Rao J. Photodynamic therapy for actinic keratoses. Dermatol Clin. 2007;25(1):15-23.
27. Mikolajewska P, Donnelly RF, Garland MJ, Morrow DI, Singh TR, Iani V, et al. Microneedle pre-treatment of human skin improves 5-aminolevulininc acid (ALA)- and 5-aminolevulinic acid methyl ester (MAL)-induced PpIX production for topical photodynamic therapy without increase in pain or erythema. Pharm Res. 2010;27(10):2213-20.
28. Choi SH, Kim KH, Song KH. Efficacy of ablative fractional laser-assisted photodynamic therapy for the treatment of actinic cheilitis: 12-month follow-up results of a prospective, randomized, comparative trial. Br J Dermatol. 2015;173(1):184-91.
29. Ko DY, Kim KH, Song KH. A randomized trial comparing methyl aminolaevulinate photodynamic therapy with and without Er:YAG ablative fractional laser treatment in Asian patients with lower extremity Bowen disease: results from a 12-month follow-up. Br J Dermatol. 2014;170(1): 165-72.
30. Shokrollahi K, Javed M, Aeuyung K, Ghattaura A, Whitaker IS, O'Leary B, et al. Combined carbon dioxide laser with photodynamic therapy for nodular and superficial basal cell carcinoma. Ann Plast Surg. 2014;73(5):552-8.
31. Haak CS, Togsverd-Bo K, Thaysen-Petersen D, Wulf HC, Paasch U, Anderson RR, et al. Fractional laser-mediated photodynamic therapy of high-risk basal cell carcinomas--a randomized clinical trial. Br J Dermatol. 2015;172(1):215-22.
32. Willey A, Anderson RR, Sakamoto FH. Temperature-Modulated Photodynamic Therapy for the Treatment of Actinic Keratosis on the Extremities: A One-Year Follow-up Study. Dermatol Surg. 2015;41(11):1290-5.
33. Willey A, Anderson RR, Sakamoto FH. Temperature-modulated photodynamic therapy for the treatment of actinic keratosis on the extremities: a pilot study. Dermatol Surg. 2014;40(10):1094-102.
34. Pariser DM, Lowe NJ, Stewart DM, Jarratt MT, Lucky AW, Pariser RJ, et al. Photodynamic therapy with topical methyl aminolevulinate for actinic keratosis: results of a prospective randomized multicenter trial. J Am Acad Dermatol. 2003;48(2):227-32.
35. Gupta AK, Paquet M, Villanueva E, Brintnell W. Interventions for actinic keratoses. Cochrane Database Syst Rev. 2012;12(12):CD004415.
36. Morton C, Campbell S, Gupta G, Keohane S, Lear J, Zaki I, et al. Intraindividual, right-left comparison of topical methyl aminolaevulinate-photodynamic therapy and cryotherapy in subjects with actinic keratoses: a multicentre, randomized controlled study. Br J Dermatol. 2006;155(5):1029-36.
37. Ko DY, Jeon SY, Kim KH, Song KH. Fractional erbium: YAG laser-assisted photodynamic therapy for facial actinic keratoses: a randomized, comparative, prospective study. J Eur Acad Dermatol Venereol. 2014;28(11):1529-39.
38. Choi SH, Kim KH, Song KH. Efficacy of ablative fractional laser-assisted photodynamic therapy with short-incubation time for the treatment of facial and scalp actinic keratosis: 12-month follow-up results of a randomized, prospective, comparative trial. J Eur Acad Dermatol Venereol. 2015;29(8):1598-605.
39. Togsverd-Bo K, Lei U, Erlendsson AM, Taudorf EH, Philipsen PA, Wulf HC, et al. Combination of ablative fractional laser and daylight-mediated photodynamic therapy for actinic keratosis in organ transplant recipients - a randomized controlled trial. Br J Dermatol. 2015;172(2):467-74.
40. Yazdani Abyaneh MA, Falto-Aizpurua L, Griffith RD, Nouri K. Photodynamic therapy for actinic cheilitis: a systematic review. Dermatol Surg. 2015;41(2):189-98.
41. Alexiades-Armenakas MR, Geronemus RG. Laser-mediated photodynamic therapy of actinic cheilitis. J Drugs Dermatol. 2004;3(5):548-51.
42. Morton C, Horn M, Leman J, Tack B, Bedane C, Tjioe M, et al. Comparison of topical methyl aminolevulinate photodynamic therapy with cryotherapy or Fluorouracil for treatment of squamous cell carcinoma in situ: Results of a multicenter randomized trial. Arch Dermatol. 2006;142(6):729-35.
43. Salim A, Leman JA, McColl JH, Chapman R, Morton CA. Randomized comparison of photodynamic therapy with topical 5-fluorouracil in Bowen's disease. Br J Dermatol. 2003;148(3):539-43.
44. Willey A, Mehta S, Lee PK. Reduction in the incidence of squamous cell carcinoma in solid organ transplant recipients treated with cyclic photodynamic therapy. Dermatol Surg. 2010;36(5):652-8.
45. Morton CA, Szeimies RM, Sidoroff A, Braathen LR. European guidelines for topical photodynamic therapy part 2: emerging indications--field cancerization, photorejuvenation and inflammatory/infective dermatoses. J Eur Acad Dermatol Venereol. 2013;27(6):672-9.
46. Szeimies RM, Ibbotson S, Murrell DF, Rubel D, Frambach Y, de Berker D, et al. A clinical study comparing methyl aminolevulinate photodynamic therapy and surgery in small superficial basal cell carcinoma (8-20 mm), with a 12-month follow-up. J Eur Acad Dermatol Venereol. 2008;22(11):1302-11.
47. Fernandez-Guarino M, Harto A, Perez-Garcia B, Royuela A, Jaen P. Six years of experience in photodynamic therapy for Basal cell carcinoma: results and fluorescence diagnosis from 191 lesions. J Skin Cancer. 2014;2014:849248.

48. Tierney E, Mahmoud BH, Srivastava D, Ozog D, Kouba DJ. Treatment of surgical scars with nonablative fractional laser versus pulsed dye laser: a randomized controlled trial. Dermatol Surg. 2009;35(8):1172-80.
49. Stangeland KZ, Kroon S. Cold air analgesia as pain reduction during photodynamic therapy of actinic keratoses. J Eur Acad Dermatol Venereol. 2012;26(7):849-54.
50. Tyrrell J, Campbell SM, Curnow A. The effect of air cooling pain relief on protoporphyrin IX photobleaching and clinical efficacy during dermatological photodynamic therapy. J Photochem Photobiol B. 2011;103(1):1-7.
51. Paoli J, Halldin C, Ericson MB, Wennberg AM. Nerve blocks provide effective pain relief during topical photodynamic therapy for extensive facial actinic keratoses. Clin Exp Dermatol. 2008;33(5):559-64.
52. Serra-Guillen C, Hueso L, Nagore E, Vila M, Llombart B, Requena Caballero C, et al. Comparative study between cold air analgesia and supraorbital and supratrochlear nerve block for the management of pain during photodynamic therapy for actinic keratoses of the frontotemporal zone. Br J Dermatol. 2009;161(2):353-6.
53. Wiegell SR, Haedersdal M, Wulf HC. Cold water and pauses in illumination reduces pain during photodynamic therapy: a randomized clinical study. Acta Derm Venereol. 2009;89(2):145-9.
54. Lehmann P. Side effects of topical photodynamic therapy. Hautarzt. 2007;58(7):597-603.
55. Wolfe CM, Hatfield K, Cognetta AB Jr. Cellulitis as a postprocedural complication of topical 5-aminolevulinic acid photodynamic therapy in the treatment of actinic keratosis. J Drugs Dermatol. 2007;6(5):544-8.

INDEX

Page numbers followed by b refer to box, *f* refer to figure, and *t* refer to table.

C

D

L

M

N

O

P

T

U

V

W

Y

Z

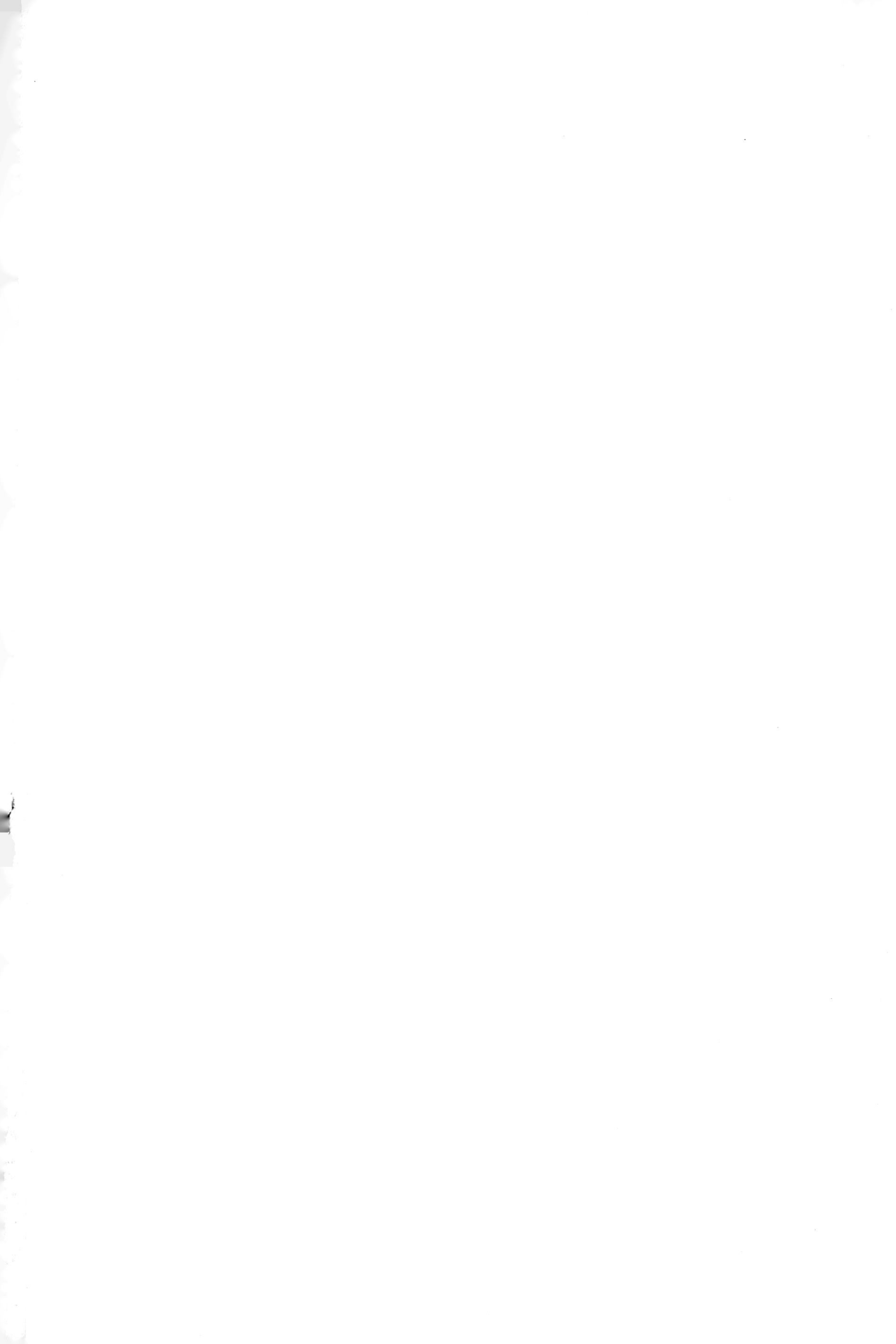

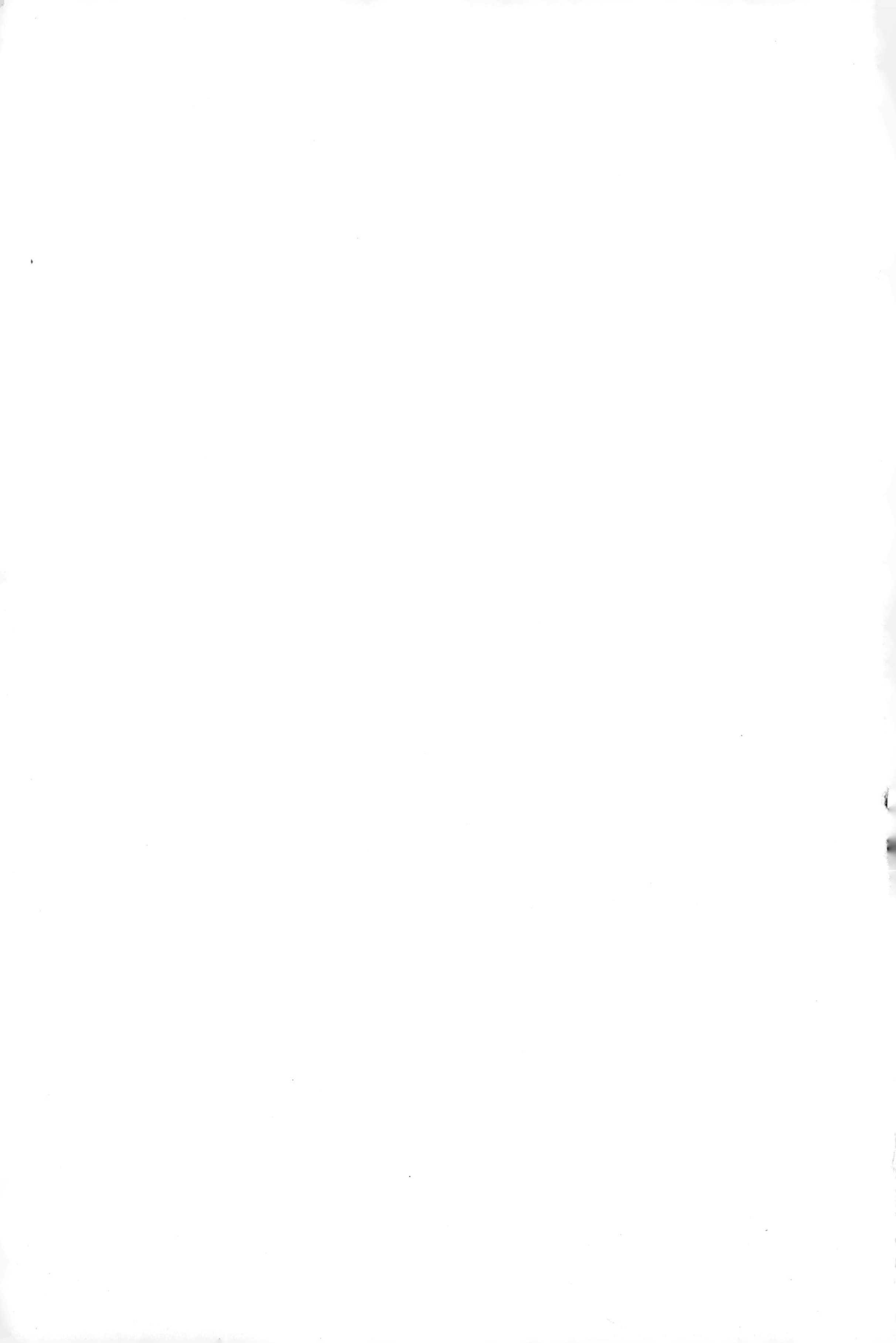